Review of

AIIMS/PGI/JIPMER PATTERN

MAY 2017

Review of
AIIMS/PGI/JIPMER PATTERN
MAY 2017

Editors

Bahram Gor
Jyotsana Priya

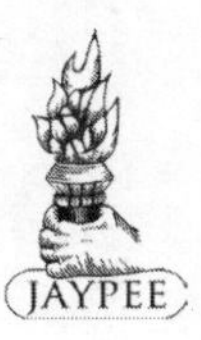

The Health Sciences Publisher
New Delhi | London | Panama

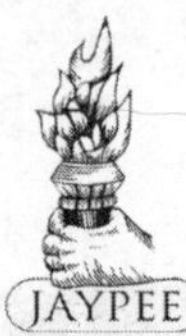

Jaypee Brothers Medical Publishers (P) Ltd.

Headquarters
Jaypee Brothers Medical Publishers (P) Ltd.
4838/24, Ansari Road, Daryaganj
New Delhi 110 002, India
Phone: +91-11-43574357
Fax: +91-11-43574314
E-mail: jaypee@jaypeebrothers.com

Disclaimer

If the question in JIPMER Pattern Based was actually asked in JIPMER May 2017, then it is merely a coincidence.

Overseas Offices

J.P. Medical Ltd.
83, Victoria Street, London
SW1H 0HW (UK)
Phone: +44-20 3170 8910
Fax: +44(0)20 3008 6180
E-mail: info@jpmedpub.com

Jaypee-Highlights Medical Publishers Inc.
City of Knowledge, Bld. 235, 2nd Floor, Clayton
Panama City, Panama
Phone: +1 507-301-0496
Fax: +1 507-301-0499
E-mail: cservice@jphmedical.com

Jaypee Brothers Medical Publishers (P) Ltd.
17/1-B, Babar Road, Block-B, Shaymali
Mohammadpur, Dhaka-1207
Bangladesh
Mobile: +08801912003485
E-mail: jaypeedhaka@gmail.com

Jaypee Brothers Medical Publishers (P) Ltd.
Bhotahity, Kathmandu, Nepal
Phone: +977-9741283608
E-mail: kathmandu@jaypeebrothers.com

Website: www.jaypeebrothers.com
Website: www.jaypeedigital.com

Inquiries for bulk sales may be solicited at: jaypee@jaypeebrothers.com

Review of AIIMS/PGI/JIPMER PATTERN

First Edition: **2018**

ISBN: 978-93-5270-317-3

Printed at Sanat Printers

Dedication

Dedicated to my honorable mentor A. S. Niazi

—Bahram Gor

Dedicated to all the readers

—Jyotsana Priya

Editorial Board

Microbiology

Author: Bahram Gor

Co-author: Rashmi M Sangolikar MD (Microbiology)
Vijayanagar Institute of Medical Sciences
Bellary, Karnataka, India

Forensic Medicine and Toxicology

Author: Bahram Gor

Co-author: Krishna Kumar Singh MD (Forensic Medicine and Toxicology)
All India Institute of Medical Sciences
New Delhi, India

Orthopedics

Author: Bahram Gor

Co-author: Naveen Kumar A MS (Orthopedics)
Vijayanagar Institute of Medical Sciences
Bellary, Karnataka, India

Ophthalmology

Author: Jyotsana Priya

Co-author: Shivani Sinha MD (Ophthalmology) MBBS
King George's Medical University
Lucknow, Uttar Pradesh, India

ENT

Author: Jyotsana Priya

Co-author: Vishakha Gupta MS (ENT) MBBS
King George's Medical University
Lucknow, Uttar Pradesh, India

Preventive and Social Medicine

Author: Bahram Gor

Co-author: Abhishek Pathania MD (PSM)
All India Institute of Medical Sciences,
New Delhi, India

Medicine

Author: Bahram Gor

Surgery

Author: Jyotsana Priya

Pediatrics

Author: Jyotsana Priya

Co-author: Muhammad Awais SR (Pediatrics)
All India Institute of Medical Sciences,
New Delhi, India

Obstetrics and Gynecology

Author: Jyotsana Priya

Co-author: Sayeda Sarah MS (Obstetrics and Gynecology)
Mahadevappa Rampure Medical College
Gulbarga, Karnataka, India

Dermatology

Author: Jyotsana Priya

Anesthesia

Author: Bahram Gor

Co-author: Abhijit MD (Anesthesia)
Maulana Azad Medical College
New Delhi, India

Radiology

Author: Jyotsana Priya

Co-author: Anjuna R MD (Radiodiagnosis)
Vardhaman Mahavir Medical College
New Delhi, India

Psychiatry

Author: Bahram Gor

Co-author: Pawan Vilas Khot MD (Psychiatry)
Assistant Professor and Head
Department of Psychiatry
RCSM GMC and CPR Hospital
Kolhapur, Maharashtra, India

Preface

Dear Reader,

The idea of writing such a book developed during our postgraduate entrance preparation days, as the difficulty we faced was due to the non-availability of books for the upcoming PGI or JIPMER examination. It is very well known that one should be perfect in recently asked topics, as the topic itself may repeat or sometimes even the exact question. Here, we present you with a book that contains solved papers of AIIMS, PGI, JIPMER Pattern examinations. Also you all know, NEET has changed its pattern to 'single day single session' examination, this book will be a valuable aid for NEET preparation also.

The questions are original to the best of our knowledge, and providing explanation was extremely time-consuming task. All efforts have been made to provide correct answers and explanations to each question. The questions have been rearranged in subject-wise manner for ease of understanding. All individual subjects have been reviewed by experts in the concerned specialty. There were few questions that were incomplete, but to make sure readers do not miss out that topic we have added such questions in last of concerned subject, to have a glance. If you do not find completeness of the topic in the explanation, you may go through the reference for clarifying your doubts.

Finally, all the best for your upcoming examinations, hope you do the best. Hope we did best to shorten the time between you and your dream PG seat. If you feel this book has helped you in your preparation, then that itself will be rewarding for us. This is our first book, if you notice any mistake or any suggestions for future work or any compliments or complains; feel free to contact at 'drbahramghor@gmail.com'.

Regards

Bahram Gor

Jyotsana Priya

Contents

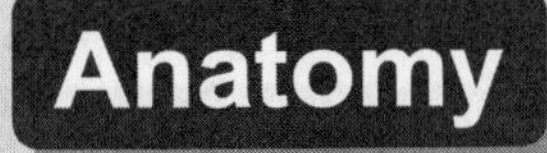

Author: Bahram Gor, Co-author: Rajesh Kumar

AIIMS MAY 2017

1. A 5-year-child presented with absence of thymus, hypoparathyroidism and tetany. Which of the following marked area is defective in this case?

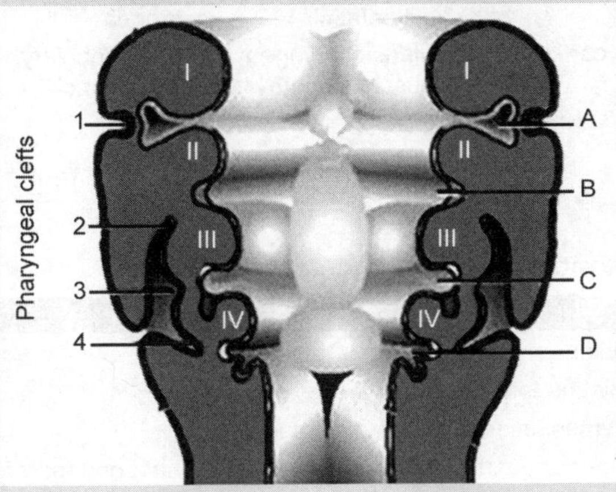

a. A
b. B
c. C
d. D

Ans. c. C *Ref: Gray's Anatomy 41st/ed p607; Langman's Medical Embryology 13th/ed p279 to 292*

EXPLANATION

In the figure
I, II, III, IV, VI: Pharyngeal arches
1, 2, 3, 4: Pharyngeal clefts
A, B, C and D: Pharyngeal pouches

Derivatives of pharyngeal arches:

Pharyngeal arches	Cartilage derived	Muscles derived	Nerves	Artery
1. Mandibular (quadrate or meckel)	Incus, malleus, anterior ligament of malleus, spine of sphenoid, sphenomandibular ligament, genial tubercle of mandible	Tensor tympani, Muscle of mastication, Mylohyoid, anterior belly of digastric, Tensor veli palatini	Mandibular division of trigeminal	First aortic arch artery

Contd...

Contd...

Pharyngeal arches	Cartilage derived	Muscles derived	Nerves	Artery
2. Hyoid (Re-ichert)	Stapes, styloid process of temporal bone, stylohyoid ligament, Lesser horn and upper part of body of hyoid bone	Stapedius, Stylohyoid, Facial muscles, also buccinator, Platysma, posterior belly of digastric	Facial	Stapedial artery
3. Third	Greater horn and lower part of body of hyoid bone	Stylopharyngeus	Glossopharyngeal	Common carotid artery, 1st part of internal carotid
4. Fourth	Thyroid cartilage, corniculate cartilage and cuneiform cartilage	Pharyngeal and extrinsic laryngeal muscles, levator veli palatini	Vagus (superior laryngeal branch)/ Pharyngeal branch	Subclavian artery or part of arch of aorta
5. Sixth	Arytenoid cartilage	Intrinsic laryngeal muscle, cricothyroid	Recurrent laryngeal branch of vagus	Ductus arteriosus (Between pulmonary trunk and dorsal aorta of left) Right side disappear

Pharyngeal pouches derivatives:

Pharyngeal pouch	Derivatives
1st	Middle ear cavity, auditory tube
2nd	Palatine tonsil, tonsillar fossa
3rd	Thymus, inferior parathyroid gland
4th	Superior parathyroid gland, ultimobranchial body (parafollicular C cells of thyroid gland)

Derivatives of pharyngeal clefts:

Pharyngeal cleft	Derivatives
1st	External auditory meatus and eardrum
2nd, 3rd and 4th	Cervical sinus—finally disappear

2. Nucleus pulposus originate from which of the following marked area?

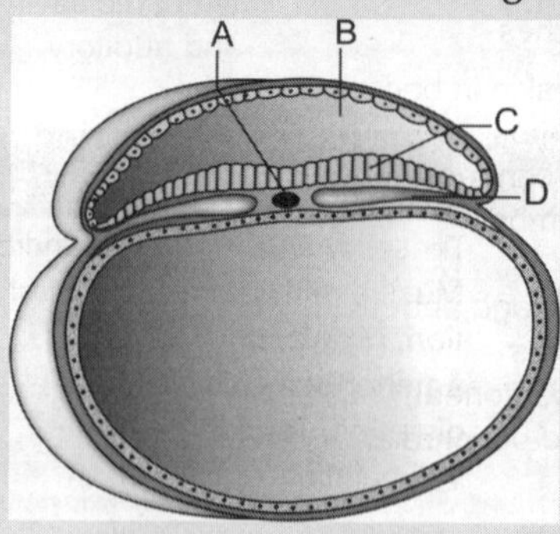

a. A b. B
c. C d. D

Ans. a. A *Ref: Langman's Medical Embryology 13th/ed p152-153,79*

Explanation

In the given figure
A. Notochord
B. Amniotic cavity
C. Ectoderm
D. Mesoderm

- **Vertebrae and vertebral column development:**
  - Vertebrae—develops from sclerotome portion of somite-derived from paraxial mesoderm.
  - Resegmentation occurs in sclerotome
  - Each vertebrae formed by caudal half on one somite and cranial half of neighbor.
  - Mesenchymal cell contribute to intervertebral disc.
  - Notochord forms nucleus pulposus ***(Answer)***.
  - Nucleus pulposus is surrounded by annulus fibrosus forming intervertebral disc
  - Two primary curvatures—thoracic and sacral curvatures
  - Two secondary curvature—cervical when child holds up head, lumbar when child walks.
- **Development of various tissues is as follows:**

Ectoderm	Mesoderm	Endoderm	Neural crest cells
• Central nervous system • Peripheral nervous system • Sensory epithelium of ear, nose and eye • Epidermis including hair and nails • Subcutaneous glands • Mammary glands • Pituitary gland • Enamel of teeth	• **Paraxial:** Somites: • Mesenchyme of head • Axial skeleton Sclerotome: • Vertebrae • Ribs Dermomyotome: • Dermis for skin of back, muscles of back, intercostal muscles and limb muscles • **Intermediate mesoderm-** Urogenital structures • **Lateral plate mesoderm**. Parietal layer: • Dermis of skin in body wall and limbs • Bone and connective tissue of limbs • Sternum • Costal cartilage and limb muscles • Lining of peritoneal, pleural and pericardial cavities	• Epithelial lining of GIT. • Intraembryonic portion of allantois and vitelline duct • Epithelial lining of respiratory tract • Parenchyma of thyroid, parathyroid, liver and pancreas • Reticular stroma of Tonsils and thymus • Epithelial lining of urinary bladder and urethra • Epithelial lining of tympanic cavity and auditory tube.	• Connective tissue and bones of face and skull • Cranial nerve ganglia • C cells of thyroid gland • Conotruncal septum of heart • Odontoblast • Dermis in face and neck • Dorsal root ganglia • Sympathetic chain and preaortic ganglia • Parasympathetic ganglia of GIT • Adrenal medulla • Schwann cells • Glial cells • Meninges • Melanocytes • Smooth muscle cells to blood vessels of face and forebrain

Contd...

Contd...

Ectoderm	Mesoderm	Endoderm	Neural crest cells
	Visceral layer: 1. Wall of gut tube 2. Serous membrane around each organ 3. **Blood cells and blood vessels**		

Number of somites with age of embryo:

Age (day)	Somites in pairs
20	1–4
21	4–7
22	7–10
23	10–13
24	13–17
25	17–20
26	20–23
27	23–26
28	26–29
30	34–35

- **Somites:**
  - Appears 1st at 20th day in occipital region
  - At end of 5th week, 42–44 pairs are present
  - Occipital-4, Cervical-8, Thoracic-12, Lumbar-5, Sacral-5, Coccygeal-8–10 pairs
  - 1st occipital and last 5–7 coccygeal disappear.
  - Somites form axial skeleton.
- **Skull:**
  - Membranous neurocranium: From neural crest cells and paraxial mesoderm-membranous ossification
  - Chondrocranium: Skull base-from neural crest cells and paraxial mesoderm-endochondral ossification
- **Face:**
  - Viscerocranium: From 1st two pharyngeal arches.

3. The area marked in the following picture of cut section of lymphatic follicle:

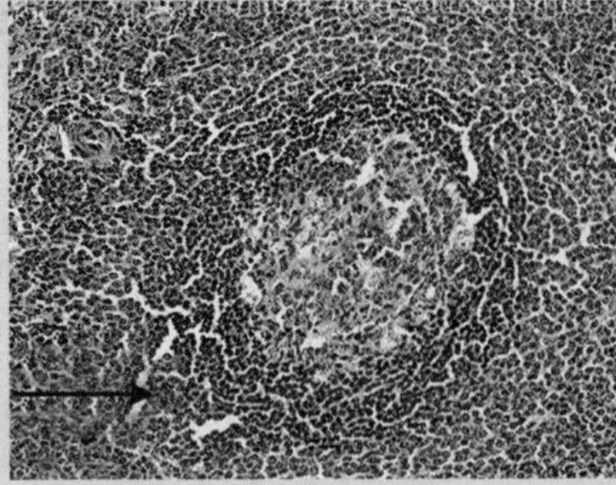

a. Germinal Center
b. Mantle zone
c. Paracortical area
d. Marginal zone

Ans. d. Marginal zone *Ref: Gray's Anatomy 41st/ed p74-75; Histology: A Text and Atlas by Ross 7th ed p458-462*

Explanation

- Figure shows cut section of lymphoid follicle with 4 layers.
- Center to periphery → Germinal center (lightly stained) → Mantle zone (heterochromatic or deeply stained) → Marginal zone (between mantle and paracortex) and → paracortex or deep cortex (between cortical follicle and medulla).

Germinal center: Lightly stained central area.

- Allows maturation of B-cell response and increases affinity between antigen and antibody.
- **A-Dark zone:** B-cells (centroblasts) undergo rapid proliferation.
- **B-Light zone:** B-cells (centrocytes) interact with FDC forming immune complex.
- Macrophage phagocytose apoptotic lymphocytes.

Mantle zone: Darkly stained area (heterochromatic) because of small lymphocytes.

- Quiescent B-cells with condensed heterochromatic nuclei and little cytoplasm.
- Few helper T-cells, FDCs and macrophages are present.

Marginal zone: Surrounding cells come to periphery having similar cells as primary follicle

Deep cortex or Paracortex: Lies between cortical follicles and medulla having T-cells.

- Consists of CD4 and CD8 T-cells, dendritic cells and Langerhan's cells.

Medulla: Innermost part having less densely packed lymphocytes.

- Irregular branching medullary cords with reticulin network.
- Macrophages like plasma cells, granulocytes are more numerous than cortex.

4. Which cell is inhibited by the cell given in the slide?

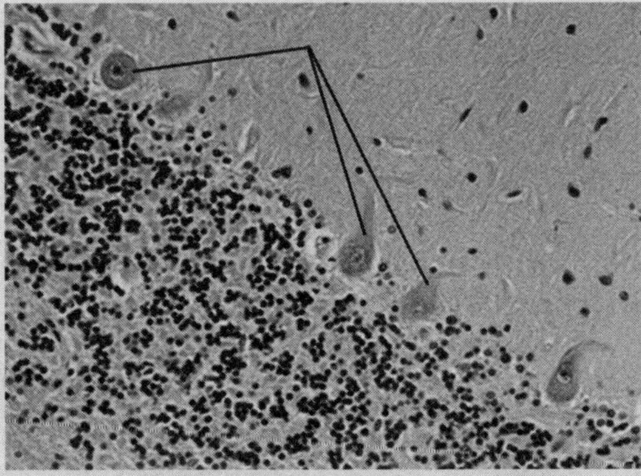

a. Vestibular nuclei
b. Deep nuclei of cerebellum
c. Anterior horn of spinal
d. Basal ganglia

Ans. b. Deep nuclei of cerebellum *Ref: Barr's The Human Nervous System: An Anatomical Viewpoint 10th/ed p159-173*

Explanation

Figure given here is of cytoarchitecture of cerebellar cortex (Cut section of cerebellar folia): Cell shown here is Purkinje cell—gives inhibitory connection to central nuclei of cerebellum.

Cerebellum:

- Maintain equilibrium and coordinate muscle contraction without conscious awareness.
- May have role in conscious awareness.
- Consists of Cortex (Gray matter plus central body of white matter), 4 pairs of nuclei in white matter and three cerebellar peduncles.
- Three lobes: Flocculonodular lobe, anterior lobe and posterior lobe.
- Flocculonodular lobe is most caudal in unrolled cerebellum.
- **3 fissures:** Primary fissure-separates anterior and posterior lobe; Horizontal fissure-present in posterior lobe; Dorsolateral (posterolateral) fissure—separates flocculonodular lobe and 1st fissure to appear.
- Tonsils present inferiorly is close to medulla and herniation may cause compression of vital Centers.

Morphological division of cerebellum:

- **Archicerebellum:** Oldest-flocculonodular lobe and lingula.
- **Paleocerebellum:** Anterior lobe, pyramid and uvula.
- **Neocerebellum:** Newest-posterior lobe except pyramid and uvula.

Functional division of cerebellum:

- **Vestibulocerebellum:** Flocculonodular lobe
- **Spinocerebellum:** Vermis and paravermal zone.
- **Pontocerebellum:** Large lateral part and superior vermis in posterior lobe.

Layers of cerebellar cortex—Three layers:

- **Outer molecular layer:** Synaptic zone containing dendrites of purkinje cells and interneuron (basket cells).
- **Purkinje cell layer:** Large principal cells of cerebellar cortex.
- **Granule cell layer:** Contains interneurons (Granule cells, golgi cells) with axons extend into molecular layer.

Central nuclei of cerebellum: Four pairs of nuclei deep in white matter.

- Lateral to medial—DEGF-Dentate, emboliform, globose and fastigial.
- Dentate nucleus has irregular shape of crumpled purse with hilus facing medially.
- Input to central nucleus from outside the cerebellum is excitatory and input from purkinje cells is inhibitory using GABA.

Afferent

- **Climbing fiber:** From inferior olivary complex to proximal part of purkinje cell dendrites. Each purkinje cell is contacted by single climbing fiber.
- **Mossy fiber:** From other sources synapses with granule cell layer neurons forming **glomerulus** (having astrocyte processes preventing diffusion of neurotransmitter to adjacent synapses.

Cerebellar peduncles

Peduncle	Afferent	Efferent
Superior cerebellar peduncle	• Ventral spinocerebellar tract • Tectocerebellar fibers • From locus Coeruleus (noradrenergic) • Trigeminothalamic fiber	• Cerebellothalamic fibers • Cerebellorubral fibers
Middle cerebellar peduncle	Pontocerebellar fibers	None

Contd...

Contd...

Peduncle	Afferent	Efferent
Inferior cerebellar peduncle	• Olivocerebellar fibers • Dorsal spinocerebellar tract • Cuneocerebellar fibers • Vestibulocerebellar fibers • Arcuate nucleus • Trigeminal sensory nucleus • Precerebellar reticular nucleus	Cerebellovestibular fibers

5. Which of the following marked structure can be palpated in the infraclavicular fossa?

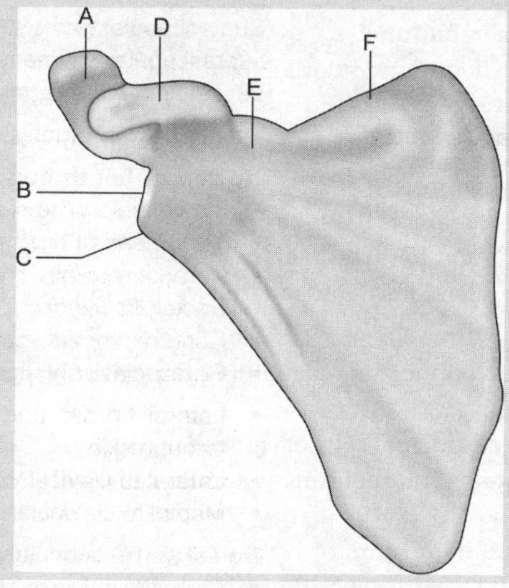

a. A
b. B
c. C
d. D

Ans. d. D *Ref: Gray's Anatomy 41st/ed p786,801-803*

EXPLANATION

In the given figure
A. Acromial process
B. Glenoid fossa
C. Infraglenoid tubercle for long head of triceps
D. Coracoid process
E. Suprascapular notch
F. Superior border of scapula

Scapular parts and attachments:

Parts	Attachment
Costal surface (Subscapular fossa)	Subscapularis
Costal surface (Medial border)	Serratus anterior
Infraglenoid tubercle	Long head of triceps
Supraglenoid tubercle	Long head of biceps
Glenoid fossa	Glenoid labrum

Contd...

Contd...

Dorsal surface	
Supraspinous fossa	Supraspinatus
Infraspinous fossa	Infraspinatus
Lateral border (upper ⅔ rd)	Teres minor
Lateral border (lower ⅓ rd)	Teres major
Medial border (superior angle to root of spine)	Levator scapulae
Medial border (opposite spine)	Rhomboid minor
Medial border (Below spine to inferior angle)	Rhomboid major
Suprascapular notch	Suprascapular nerve and vessels, separated by suprascapular ligament Vessel above the ligament
Superior border near suprascapular notch	Inferior belly of omohyoid
Coracoid process	**Tip can be felt through the skin** • 2.5 cm below the clavicle • Short head of biceps • Coracobrachialis • Pectoralis minor • Coracoacromial ligament • Coracoclavicular ligament
Acromial process	• Lateral border and upper surface can be felt through skin • Lateral to clavicular facet—Deltoid • Medial to clavicular facet—Trapezius
Spine of scapula	Dorsal part is subcutaneous can be felt • Opposite spine of T3 vertebra • Upper lip—Trapezius • Lower lip—Deltoid
Scapular angle (inferior angle of scapula)	Over 7th rib or 7th intercostal space, Spine of T7

6. In the following image of Transversus abdominis, which label denotes conjoint tendon?

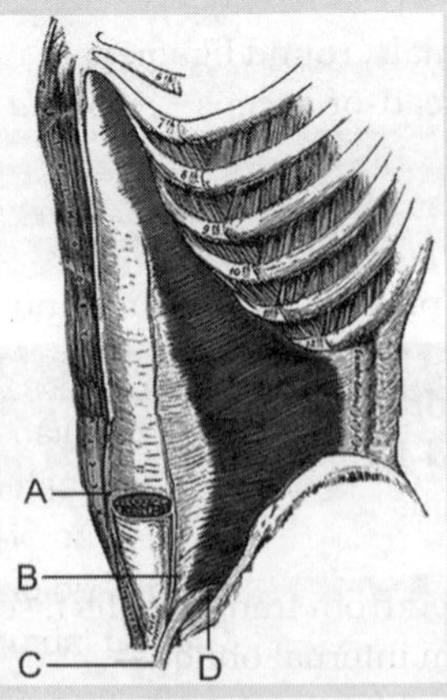

a. A b. B
c. C d. D

Ans. b. B *Ref: Gray's Anatomy 41st/ed p1071, Fig. 61.2, 1074-1078,1272,1278*

EXPLANATION

In the figure:

A. Linea alba
B. Conjoint tendon
C. Spermatic cord
D. Inguinal ligament

- **Conjoint tendon:** Formed from lower fibers of internal oblique and lower part of aponeurosis of transversus abdominis.
  - Attached to pubic crest and extends along pectineal line.
  - Strengthen medial portion of posterior wall of inguinal canal.
- **Linea alba:** Lies between two recti from xiphoid to pubic crest and symphysis.
  - Formed by interlacing fibers of internal oblique, external oblique and transversus abdominis.
  - Relatively bloodless area so named alba (pale).
- **Rectus sheath:** Aponeurosis of anterior abdominal muscles covering recti muscles.

Above the arcuate line	
Anterior rectus sheath	Aponeurosis of both leaf of external oblique aponeurosis and anterior leaf of internal oblique aponeurosis
Posterior rectus sheath	Aponeurosis of anterior leaf of internal oblique and both leaf of transversus abdominis
Below the arcuate line	
Anterior rectus sheath	Aponeurosis of all three muscles.
Posteriorly	Only fascia transversalis. No aponeurosis.

- **Arcuate line:** Junction between upper 2/3 rd and 1/3 rd of rectus abdominis.
  - Corresponds with upper 1/3rd part between umbilicus and pubic symphysis.
- **Inguinal ligament:** Thick lower border of aponeurosis of external oblique.
  - Extends from anterior superior iliac spine to pubic tubercle (not symphysis).
- **Inguinal canal:** Oblique tunnel between the muscle layer of anterior abdominal wall from deep to superficial inguinal ring.
  - Transmits spermatic cord in male, round ligament of uterus in female and ilioinguinal nerve in both sexes.
- **Contents of spermatic cord:**
  1. Ductus deferens/vas deferens
  2. Artery, vein and lymphatics to vas deferens
  3. Artery, veins (pampiniform plexus), lymphatics and nerve supplying testis
  4. Ilioinguinal nerve
  5. Genital branch of genitofemoral nerve
  6. Cremasteric artery, veins and lymphatics
  7. Remains of processus vaginalis

Note:

- Internal spermatic fascia is derived from transversalis fascia.
- Cremasteric fascia is derived from internal oblique.
- External spermatic fascia is derived from external oblique aponeurosis.

- Testicular artery is branch of abdominal aorta.
- Artery to vas deferens is branch of superior vesical artery, branch from internal iliac.
- Cremasteric artery is branch of inferior epigastric artery.
- **Superficial inguinal ring:** Hiatus in aponeurosis of external oblique aponeurosis, just above and lateral to pubic crest.
- **Deep inguinal ring:** Opening in transversalis fascia midway between anterior superior iliac spine and pubic symphysis, 1 cm above the inguinal ligament.
- Hesselbach triangle:
  - **Inferiorly:** Medial third of inguinal ligament
  - **Medialy:** Lower lateral border of rectus abdominis
  - **Laterally:** Inferior epigastric vessels
  - This is divided by medial and lateral part by obliterated umbilical artery.
  - Medial and lateral direct hernia occurs through this triangle.
- **Lacunar ligament**: Triangular band of fibrous tissue lying posterior to medial end of inguinal ligament.
  - Formed by fibers from inguinal ligament and fascia lata from thigh.

7. Which of the following forms the superior boundary of epiploic foramen?

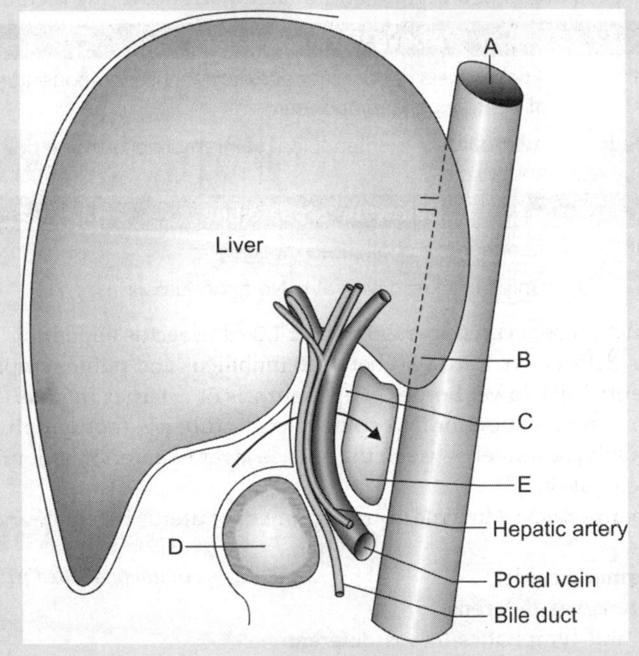

a. A
b. B
c. C
d. D

Ans. b. B *Ref: Gray's Anatomy 41st/ed p1059-1061*

Explanation

In the figure

A. Inferior vena cava
B. Caudate process of liver

C. Right free margin of lesser omentum
D. 1st part of duodenum
E. Epiploic foramen

Epiploic foramen: (Foramen of Winslow, Aditus or opening of lesser sac)

- ❑ Vertical slit like opening through which lesser sac communicates with greater sac
- ❑ Present behind the right free margin of lesser omentum—at T12 vertebra level
- ❑ Boundaries
  - **Anteriorly:** Right free margin of lesser omentum containing portal vein, proper hepatic artery and bile duct.
  - **Posteriorly:** Inferior vena cava.
  - **Superiorly:** Caudate process of liver.
  - **Inferiorly:** First part of duodenum.

Note: Free border of lesser omentum contains—Portal vein (p for posteriorly), Bile duct (anteriorly to right) and Hepatic artery proper (anteriorly to left).

8. Which of the following marked structure is Pelvic Diaphragm?

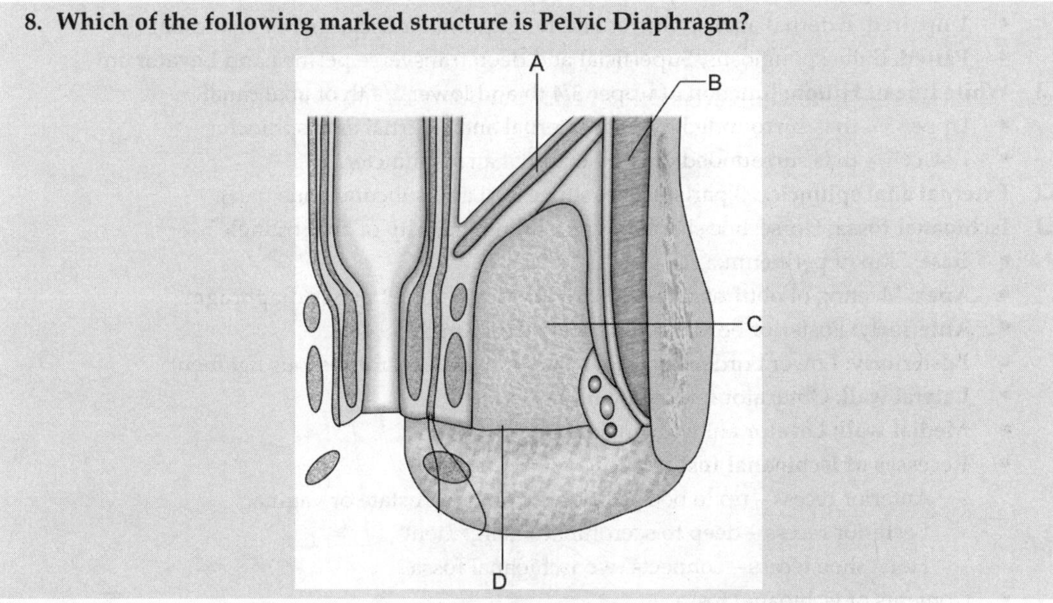

a. A
b. B
c. C
d. D

Ans. a. A *Ref: Gray's Anatomy 41st/ed p1154, 1224, 1231, 1233*

EXPLANATION

The given figure is coronal section through ischioanal fossa

A. Pelvic diaphragm (Levator ani muscle with superior and inferior fascia)
B. Obturator internus muscle
C. Ischioanal space filled with fat
D. Perianal fascia

- ❑ Also seen are internal anal sphincter, three parts of external anal sphincter, pudendal canal with pudendal nerve and internal pudendal vessels, lunate fascia covering ischioanal space from above can be seen.

- **Pelvic diaphragm:** Combination of two fascial layer and intervening levator ani muscle.
  - Superficial fascia is thicker than inferior fascia.
  - Inferior fascia covers the medial wall of ischioanal space and laterally continuous with obturator fascia. Superficial fascia medially blends with visceral pelvic fascia and contribute to endopelvic fascia.
  - **Levator ani**: 3 parts:
    - Pubococcygeus (puboperinealis, puboprostaticus, pubovaginalis, puboanalis, puborectalis)
    - Iliococcygeus
    - Puborectalis
    - Ischiococcygeus (coccygeus) is a separate muscle in posterosuperior portion of levator.
  - **Nerve supply:** Nerve to levator ani (S2-S4), pubococcygeus also by pudendal nerve.
  - **Actions:** Anorectal and urinary continence, support pelvic viscera, increasing intra-abdominal pressure, prevent prolapse.
- **Perineal Body-10 muscles-**2 unpaired and 4 paired
  - **Unpaired:** External anal sphincter and longitudinal muscle coat of anal canal
  - **Paired:** Bulbospongiosus, Superficial and deep transverse perinea and Levator ani
- **White line of Hilton:** Junction of upper 3/4 th and lower 1/4 th of anal canal
  - Upper 3/4 th is surrounded by both internal and external anal sphincter
  - Lower 1/4 th is surrounded only by external anal sphincter.
- **External anal sphincter:** 3 parts (Deep, superficial and subcutaneous part).
- **Ischioanal fossa:** Horseshoe shaped region filling majority of anal triangle.
  - **Base:** Skin of perineum.
  - **Apex:** Meeting of obturator fascia with inferior fascia of pelvic diaphragm
  - **Anteriorly:** Posterior border of perineal membrane
  - **Posteriorly:** Lower border of gluteus maximus and sacrotuberous ligament
  - **Lateral wall:** Obturator internus with fascia
  - **Medial wall:** Levator ani with anal fascia
  - **Recesses of Ischioanal fossa:**
    - Anterior recess—up to body of pubis close to prostate or vagina.
    - Posterior recess—deep to sacrotuberous ligament
    - Horseshoe recess—connects two ischioanal fossa
  - Contents of Ischioanal fossa:
  - Ischioanal pad of fat
  - Inferior rectal nerve and vessels
  - Pudendal canal with contents
  - Posterior scrotal or posterior labial nerve and vessels
  - Perineal branch of S4
  - Perforating cutaneous branch of S2, S3
- **Pudendal canal:** Fascial canal in lateral wall of ischioanal fossa
  - **Laterally:** Obturator fascia
  - **Medially:** Perianal fascia
  - **Above:** Lunate fascia
  - **Below:** Falciform process of sacrotuberous ligament
  - **Contents:** Pudendal nerve and internal pudendal vessels.

9. Mandibular branch of trigeminal nerve passes through which of the following marked structure?

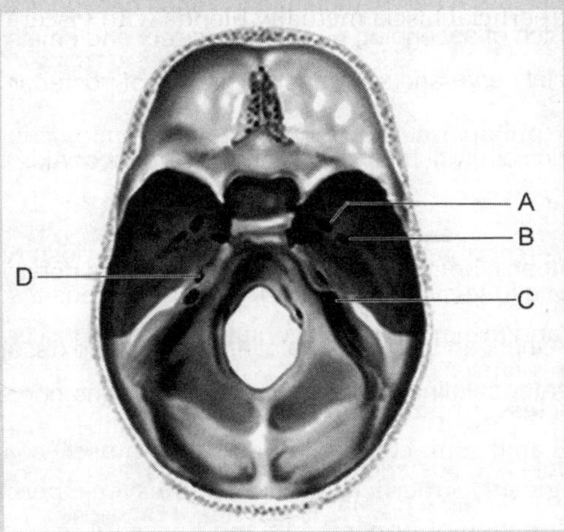

a. A
b. B
c. C
d. D

Ans. a. A *Ref: Gray's Anatomy 41st/ed p429-432*

EXPLANATION

Given figure is of floor of cranial cavity showing cranial fossae and foramina.

A. **Foramen ovale:** Male-mandibular nerve, accessory meningeal artery, lesser petrosal nerve and emissary vein connecting cavernous sinus with pterygoid venous plexus.

B. **Foramen spinosum:** Middle meningeal vessels and meningeal branch of mandibular nerve (nervous spinosus).

C. **Jugular foramen:** Three parts by intrajugular process
   1. **Anterior part:** Inferior petrosal sinus and meningeal branch of ascending pharyngeal
   2. **Middle part:** IX, X and XIth cranial nerves
   3. **Posterior part:** Sigmoid sinus and meningeal branch of occipital artery

D. **Internal acoustic meatus:** VII and VIIIth nerve, nervus intermedius and labyrinthine vessels.

Other foramina:

Foramen or canal	Structures passing through
1. Carotid canal	Internal carotid artery, venous and sympathetic plexus around artery
2. Foramen lacerum	Generally filled with cartilage—no structure passes through it. Sometimes, Nerve of pterygoid canal (vidian nerve) passes
3. Petrotympanic fissure	Chorda tympani nerve, anterior ligament of malleus and anterior tympanic branch of maxillary artery
4. Foramen magnum	1. **Anterior part:** Apical ligament of dens, vertical band of cruciate ligament, membrana tectoria 2. **Posterior part:** Lower part of medulla, meninges 3. **Through subarachnoid space:** Spinal accessory nerve, anterior and posterior spinal artery, Vertebral arteries and sympathetic plexus around artery

Contd...

Contd...

Foramen or canal	Structures passing through
5. Hypoglossal canal	Hypoglossal nerve, meningeal branch of hypoglossal nerve, meningeal branch of ascending pharyngeal artery and emissary vein
6. Stylomastoid foramen	Facial nerve and stylomastoid branch of posterior auricular artery
7. Mastoid canaliculus (Arnold's canal)	Auricular branch of vagus (Arnold's nerve or Alderman's nerve)
8. Tympanic canaliculus	Tympanic branch of IXth nerve (Jacobson's nerve)
9. Incisive foramen	Terminal part of greater palatine vessels and nasopalatine nerve
10. Greater palatine foramen	Greater palatine vessel and anterior palatine nerve
11. Lesser palatine foramen	Middle and posterior palatine nerves
12. Palatovaginal cnal	Pharyngeal branch of pterygopalatine ganglia and pharyngeal branch of maxillary artery
13. Vomerovaginal canal	Generally closed, sometimes pharyngeal branch of pterygopalatine ganglia
14. Foramen of vesalius (emissary sphenoidal F)	Emissary vein connecting cavernous sinus with pterygoid plexus of veins
15. Foramen cecum	Generally closed, occasionally veins from nasal mucosa to superior sagittal sinus. Failure of closure causes Nasal dermoid and nasoethmoidal encephalocoele
16. Foramen rotundum	Maxillary nerve
17. Dorello's canal	Interdural space near petrous apex, petroclival venous confluence, filled with blood from sinuses
18. Facial hiatus	Greater petrosal nerve

10. Third part of vertebral artery is related to which of the marked structure in the given picture?

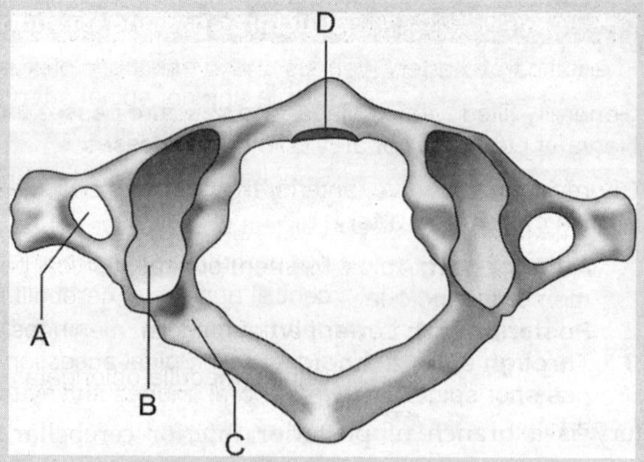

a. A
b. B
c. C
d. D

Ans. c. C *Ref: Gray's Anatomy 41st/ed p720-724,283,458*

Explanation

Given figure is of Atlas (C1) vertebra

A. Foramen transversarium
B. Superior articular Facet—for occipital condyle articulation
C. Groove for 3rd part of vertebral artery on posterior arch
D. Facet for odontoid process (Dens) of Axis (C2) articulation on anterior arch

Recognizing typical cervical vertebrae:

- Foramen transversarium in transverse process
- Spinous process is bifid
- Triangular vertebral canal for cervical enlargement of spinal cord
- **Atlas (C1):** No centrum or body, two lateral masses connected by smaller anterior and larger posterior arch, anterior arch having a tubercle and posterior arch have groove laterally for 3rd part of Vertebral artery. Facet for odontoid process on anterior arch.
- **Axis (C2):** Odontoid process and large bifid spine.
  - **Note:** Attachment on Dens and body of axis from above downward:
    - Apical ligament: Alar ligament-lower vertical band of cruciate ligament-membrana tectoria-posterior longitudinal ligament.
    - Attachment on occipital bone of same structures are just opposite from above downward
- **C6 vertebra:** Anterior tubercle of transverse process is longest, termed carotid tubercle of chassaignac. Carotid artery can be pressed and palpated against it.
- C7 vertebra (vertebra prominens)—long spinous process.
  Costal element of transverse process of C7 may get elongated to form cervical rib.
  Vertebral Artery: Arises from superoposterior aspect of 1st part of subclavian artery.
- **1st part (V1):** Does not passes through foramen of C7. Transverse process of C7 lies posterior to 1st part of vertebral artery.
- **2nd part (V2):** Foramen transversarium of C6 to C1.
- **3rd part (V3):** Groove on upper surface of posterior arch of Atlas (C1).
- **4th part (V4):** Passes through foramen magnum—pierces dura and arachnoid mater, incline anterior to medulla oblongata and unites with other side vertebral artery forming Basilar Artery at junction of Pons and Medulla.

Branches of vertebral artery:

Spinal branches	Single anterior spinal artery and 2 posterior spinal arteries
Muscular branches	Supply muscles of suboccipital region
Posterior inferior cerebellar artery	Largest branch of vertebral artery. Supplies posterior part of cerebellar hemisphere, inferior vermis, central nucleus of cerebellum and choroid plexus of IVth ventricle.
Medullary branches	Supply medulla oblongata

Note: Posterior spinal artery is a branch of posterior inferior cerebellar artery but may arise directly from vertebral artery.

11. In this cross section of head, the action of structure marked on the Mandible is:

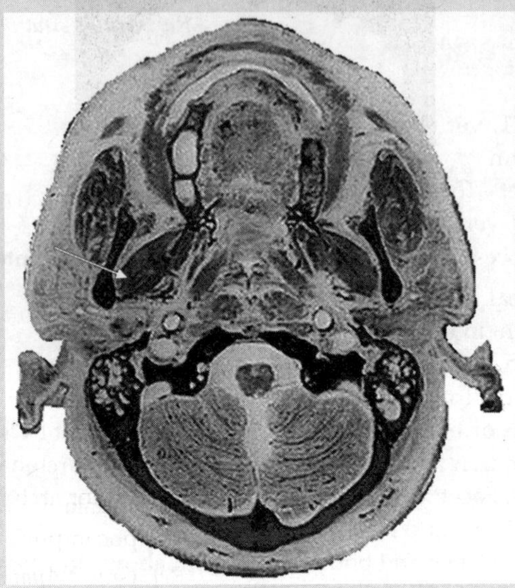

a. Protraction
b. Retraction
c. Elevation
d. Depression

Ans. a. Protraction *Ref: Gray's Anatomy 41st/ed p546-548*

Explanation

Muscle shown here is lateral pterygoid. Major function is opening of Jaw mainly by protraction. Only muscle of mastication that opens mouth.

Muscles of mastication

Muscle	Attachment on mandible	Action	Innervation
Masseter	Lateral surface of mandibular ramus	Elevates mandible (closure) Small side to side movement, protraction and retraction	Anterior trunk of mandibular nerve
Temporalis	Medial surface, apex, anterior and posterior border of coronoid process	Elevates mandible (closure) Main retractor	Anterior trunk of mandibular nerve
Lateral pterygoid	Pterygoid fovea (depression on front of neck)	Mandibular opening by protrusion, grinding food between teeth of same side	Anterior trunk of mandibular nerve
Medial pterygoid	Posteroinferior part of medial surface of ramus and angle	Elevating mandible (closure), help in protrusion by lateral pterygoid and chewing	Nerve to medial pterygoid from main trunk of mandibular nerve

12. The arrow marked structure in the given picture connects which of the following structure?

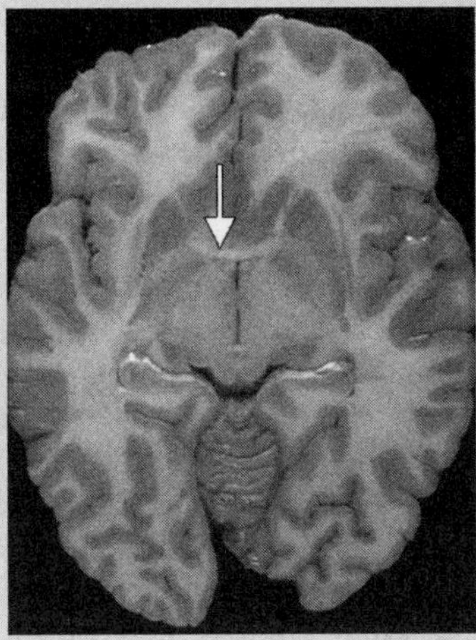

a. Mamillary body
b. Amygdala
c. Habenular nuclei
d. Hippocampus

Ans. b. Amygdala

Ref: Gray's Anatomy 41st/ed p359,362,388-395, Barr's The Human Nervous System: An Anatomical Viewpoint 10th/ed p269-281

EXPLANATION

The figure is of transverse section of brain showing anterior commissure by arrow.
Also seen are frontal lobe, temporal lobe, occipital cortex, insular cortex, putamen globus pallidus, fornix and septum pellucidum can be seen here.

- **Anterior commissure:** Compact bundle of 3.5 million myelinated axons.
  - Runs within basal forebrain and goes laterally to temporal lobe.
  - **2 components:**
    - Anterior or olfactory component—**connects olfactory bulb, olfactory tubercle, anterior perforated substance, Amygdala.**
    - Posterolateral or hemispheric part—anterior region of middle and inferior temporal gyrus, parahippocampal gyrus up to occipital lobe.
- **Diagonal band of Broca:** White matter within the anterior perforated substance efferent fibers from amygdala passes through it.
- **White matter in cerebral hemisphere:** 3 categories of myelinated axons.

Association Fibers	Links different cortical areas in same hemisphere	Fornix, Cingulum, superior longitudinal fasciculus, inferior longitudinal fasciculus, Uncinate fasciculus, middle longitudinal fasciculus
Commissural Fibers	Links corresponding cortical areas in two hemisphere	Corpus callosum, Anterior commissure, Hippocampal commissure, Posterior Commissure, Habenular commissure.
Projection Fibers	Connects cerebral cortex with diencephalon, Corpus striatum brainstem and spinal cord	Internal capsule

- **Amygdala**: Present between anterior end of temporal horn of lateral ventricle and lentiform nucleus. It is a part of limbic system. 2 division:
  - Dorsomedial division—contains corticomedial group of nuclei. Part of lateral olfactory area, afferent comes from olfactory bulb.
  - Ventrolateral division—contains basolateral and central group of nucleus, no direct connection with olfactory bulb, connected with corticomedial group and entorhinal area
  - **Connections:**
    - Afferent: Temporal and prefrontal cortex, cholinergic and catecholaminergic nuclei
    - Efferent: Nucleus accumbens, mediodorsal thalamic nuclei, hypothalamus and septal area
  - Functions: Behavioral and emotional function, fear, anger, irritability.
- **Limbic system:** Consists of limbic lobe (parahippocampal and cingulate gyri), septal area, hippocampal formation (subiculum, hippocampus and dentate gyrus), amygdaloid body.
- *Option d:* **Hippocampus (Cornu ammonis)**-C-shaped-3 areas (CA1, CA2 and CA3)
  - **3 layers:** Molecular layer, pyramidal cell layer and polymorphic layer
  - **Dentate gyrus:** 3 layers-Molecular layer, granule cell layer and polymorphic layer
  - Afferents
    - Fibers from entorhinal area of parahippocampal gyrus
    - Cholinergic fibers from septal area and basal forebrain nuclei
    - Dopaminergic fibers from ventral tegmental area
    - Noradrenergic fibers from locus coeruleus
    - Serotonergic fibers from raphe nucleus
  - Efferents
    - Papez circuit (subiculum, fornix, mamillary body, anterior thalamic nuclei, cingulate and Parahippocampal gyrus)
    - Fibers to septal area, hypothalamus and substantia innominata
    - Mamillo-thalamic fasciculus (Bundle of Vicq d'Azyr)
    - Association fibers to cortex of frontal and temporal lobe
  - Function of Hippocampus
    - Retention of information in short-term memory and its transfer into long-term declarative memory by repetition and practice.
- **Epithalamus:** Consists of anterior and posterior paraventricular nuclei, medial and lateral habenular nuclei, stria medullaris thalami, posterior commissure and pineal body.
- *Option c:* **Habenular nuclei**
  - At dorsomedial aspect of the thalamus deep to ependyma of 3rd ventricle.
  - **Medial H nuclei:** Deep staining-cholinergic neurons
  - **Lateral H nuclei:** Pale staining
  - **Functions:** Involved in sleep mechanism, role in regulation of visceral and neuroendocrine function.
  - **Afferent:** Via stria medullaris thalami from prepiriform cortex, nucleus basalis of Meynert and hypothalamus. Mostly end in lateral nucleus.
  - Efferent: Interpeduncular nucleus of midbrain, substantia nigra, ventral tegmental area, hypothalamus and basal forebrain.
- *Option a:* **Mamillary body:** Nucleus in posterior region of hypothalamus present medially.
  - Most of the fibers of fornix end here.
  - Mamillothalamic tract goes to anterior nucleus of thalamus.
  - Concerned with memory.

13. Disease caused by the structure marked in the picture below is:

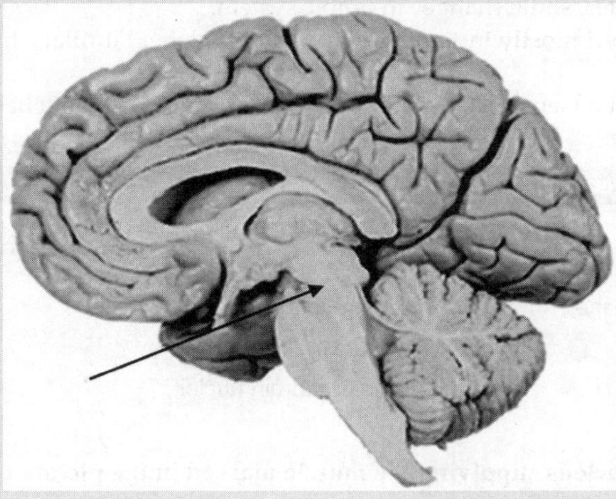

a. Huntington's chorea
b. Alzheimer's disease
c. Dementia
d. Paralysis agitans

Ans. d. Paralysis agitans

Ref: Barr's The Human Nervous System: An Anatomical Viewpoint 10th/ed p107-108,211,212,242

EXPLANATION

Structure shown here is Substantia Nigra—can be recognized at the level of midbrain by black color caused by dopaminergic neurons of pars compacta; cells containing granules of melanin pigment.

Paralysis agitans (Parkinson's Disease): Mainly caused by degeneration of melanin containing cells in pars compacta of substantia nigra.

- **Substantia nigra:** Large nucleus situated between tegmentum and basis pedunculi throughout the midbrain. Extends into subthalamic region of diencephalon.
  - **2 parts:** Pars compacta and Pars reticulate.
  - **Pars compacta:** Contains cytoplasmic inclusion granules of melanin pigment (Neuromelanin), giving its characteristic black color. Neuromelanin is by-product of Dopamine, neurotransmitter used by these cells. Connected with corpus striatum through nigrostriatal fibers, forming functional system of basal ganglia.
  - **Pars reticulata:** Near basis pedunculi, lacks melanin. Detached part of globus pallidus. Connected to thalamus and sends fibers to superior colliculus, pathway for basal ganglis in eye movement.
- **Parkinson's disease:** Disturbances in motor function showing triad of muscular rigidity, slow tremor and bradykinesia. Bradykinesia includes mask like face, difficulty in initiating movement and loss of associated involuntary movement. Shuffling Gait
  - **Causes:** Degeneration in melanin containing cells in pars compacta.
    - Idiopathic, poisons (manganese compound, MPTP and heroin), drugs.
  - **Treatment:** Antiparkinson drugs, thalamotomy and pallidotomy.
- ***Option a:*** **Huntington's chorea:** Autosomal dominant disorder with onset of clinical sign in middle age showing choreiform movements (brisk, jerky and purposeless movements).
  - Atrophy of corpus striatum mainly caudate nucleus.

- ❑ ***Option b:* Alzheimer's disease**
  - Degeneration of magnocellular basal forebrain nuclei. Large cholinergic neurons at base of brain degenerates, some changes in limbic system.
  - Shrinkage of gyri mostly in temporal and parietal lobe. Fibrillary tangles and Plaques are present.
- ❑ ***Option c:* Dementia:** Generalized deterioration of memory and intellect. Can occur in many disorder, see below:

Disorder with dementia	Area involved
Acquired sociopathy	Ventral and medial part of prefrontal cortex
Anosognosia	Right ventral prefrontal cortex
General paralysis of insane	Bilateral prefrontal cortex
Pick's disease	Unknown etiology
Alzheimer's disease	Basal forebrain nuclei

14. Location of the nucleus supplying the muscle marked in the picture is:

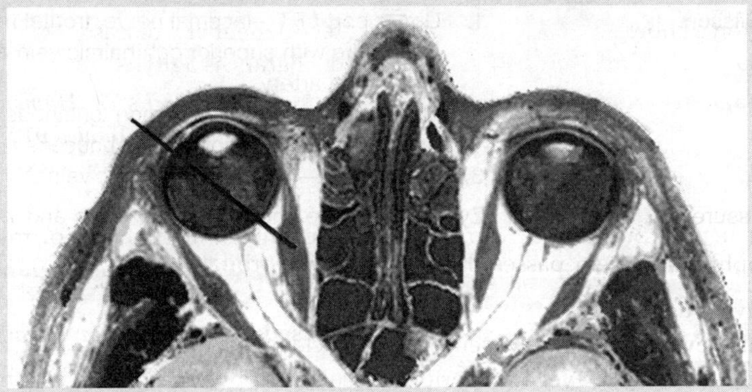

a. Superior colliculus
b. Inferior colliculus
c. Facial colliculus
d. Inferior salivatory nucleus

Ans. a. Superior colliculus

Ref: Gray's Anatomy 41st/ed p666-672; Barr's The Human Nervous System: An Anatomical Viewpoint 10th/ed p96-106;

EXPLANATION

Structure shown here is medial rectus-supplied by occulomotor nerve-nucleus of III nerve present in periaqueductal gray matter of midbrain, ventral to aqueduct at the level of the superior colliculus.

- ❑ **Extraocular muscles:** 7 in number
  - Levator palpebrae superioris, four recti (Superior, inferior, medial and lateral) and two obliques (superior and inferior).
  - Nerve supply-SO4LR6 rest by III nerve.
    - Superior oblique by IVth nerve, Lateral rectus by VIth nerve.
    - Superior rectus by superior division of IIIrd nerve.
    - IR, MR and IO by inferior division of IIIrd nerve.
    - Levator palpebrae superioris by superior division of IIIrd and by sympathetic fibers from plexus around internal carotid artery.

❑ **Actions:**

Muscles	Actions
LPS	Elevates the upper eyelid. Antagonist to this is palpebral part of orbicularis oculi
SR	Elevation, Adduction and medial rotation
IR	Depression, Adduction and Medial rotation
MR	Adduction
LR	Abduction
SO	Rotates visual axis downward with Abduction and Intortion
IO	Rotates visual axis upward with Abduction and Extortion
SR + IO	Upward movement alone
IR + SO	Downward movement alone

Canal/Fissure	Structures passing through
Optic canal	Optic nerve with its meninges and ophthalmic artery
Superior orbital fissure	1. Upper part-LFT—lacrimal nerve, frontal nerve and trochlear nerve with superior ophthalmic vein and recurrent meningeal artery 2. Middle part within the common tendinous ring-NOA—nasociliary, occulomotor and Abducens nerve 3. Inferior part—Inferior ophthalmic vein
Inferior orbital fissure	Zygomatic nerve and Infraorbital nerve and vessels

Note: Inferior ophthalmic vein passes through superior orbital fissure.

❑ **Cranial nerve Nuclei**

- **Midbrain level:** III, IV and mesencephalic nucleus of Vth nerve.
  - **IIIrd nerve N:** At level of superior colliculus-supplying 5 extraocular muscles.
  - Edinger-Westphal nucleus: at same level-supplying ciliary and sphincter pupillae.
  - **Trochlear N:** At level of inferior colliculus-supply SO.
  - Mesencephalic nucleus of Vth at level of superior colliculus.
- **Pons level:** V, VI, VII and VIII nerve nuclei
  - Vth N
  - *Pontine trigeminal nucleus* (chief or principal): Caudal half of pons-discriminative touch
  - *Motor nucleus:* Medial to chief N. supply muscles of mastications.
  - *Mesencephalic nucleus:* Column extending up to midbrain—proprioception from mastication. **Note:** Only true unipolar cell is mesencephalic nucleus.
  - *VIth nerve N:* Beneath the facial colliculus formed by internal genu of VIIth N fibers-LR supply
  - *VIIth nerve N:* At ventrolateral part of tegmentum—forms internal genu looping around abducens nerve nuclei forming facial colliculus.
  - *VIIIth nerve N:* Superior vestibular N. present in Pons. Axons of ventral cochlear nuclei ends in superior olivary nucleus.
- Medulla: VIII, IX, X, XI and XII Nerve Nuclei
  - *VIIIth nerve N*-Inferior, medial and lateral vestibular N. present in Medulla.
  - IXth, Xth and XIth nerve N Shares common nuclei

- *Nucleus ambiguus*: Dorsal to inferior olivary nucleus—supplies muscles of soft palate, pharynx, larynx and upper esophagus. Also to cardiac ganglia.
- *Dorsal nucleus of Vagus*: Largest parasympathetic nucleus of brainstem. Regulates activities of smooth muscles and glandular elements of thoracic and abdominal viscera.
- *Solitary nucleus* (Nucleus of Tractus solitarius): For visceral reflex and taste—IX, X and VII (Taste).

PGI MAY 2017

1. Prophase of meiosis-1, true is/are:

a. Sister chromatids replicate
b. Sister chromatid separate
c. Result in haploid
d. Chromosome separate
e. Cell will be diploid

Ans. e. Cell will be diploid *Ref: Gray's Anatomy 41st/ed p18-21*

EXPLANATION

Meiosis I-4 Stages

1. Prophase I	5 substages–leptotene, zygotene, pachytene, diplotene and diakinesis. • 3 Special features. 1. Pairing or synapsis of homologous chromosomes of paternal and maternal origin to form Bivalent. 2. Organization of nucleoli by autosomal bivalents. 3. Non-ribosomal RNA synthesis by autosomal bivalents. • Female prophage I starts during fetal gonadogenesis and arrested at diplotene stage from 5th month in utero and remains at this stage till puberty. • Male meiosis starts at puberty.
a. Leptotene	• Homologous chromosomes replicated in S-phase locate one another within the nucleus ***(Option a)***. • Process of genetic recombination initiated. • Chromosomes begin to condense. • Attaches via telomere to nuclear envelope.
b. Zygotene	• Pairing or synapsis occurs here. • Bouquet stage: Chromosomes resemble bouquet of flowers because telomeres clusters to one side of nucleus. • Bivalents are linked by Tripartite ribbon (synaptonemal complex): Having 2 lateral dense elements and central less dense element. • Pseudoautosomal region: Synaptic region in male sex chromosome. • Sex vesicles: XY bivalents adopts special condensed structure. • **Chiasmata:** Site for genetic exchange turning in special structure.
c. Pachy-tene	• Genetic recombination between non-sister chromatids is completed. • Crossing over occurs here. • Crossing over points appear as recombination nodules in center of synaptonemal complex. **Note:** Genetic recombination starts at leptotene stage.

Contd...

Contd...

d. Diplotene	• Disjunction: Synaptonemal complex disassembles and homologous chromosomes shortened, separated except where crossing over occurs. ***(Option b and d)***-not complete separation. • At least 1 and up to 5 chiasma have been found.
e. Diakinesis	• Prometaphase of first meiotic division. • Still bivalents becoming shortened and thicker. ***(Option c and e)*** • Gradually attach to spindle and become aligned at metaphase plate. • In eggs spindle form without centromeres only involving microtubules and other motor molecules.
2. Metaphase I	• Homologous pairs occupy equatorial plane of spindle. • Homologous chromosomes are pulled towards opposite spindle poles but held paired at spindle midzone by chiasmata. • Non-disjunction can occur here leading to aneuploidy: Major cause of fetal loss during 1st trimester. • Most common viable aneuploidy is Down's syndrome (Trisomy 21) showing increase with increasing maternal age.
3. Anaphase I	• Begins with release of cohesion between sister chromatids. • Sister centromeres and chromatids does not separate.
4. Telophase I	• Separation of homologous chromosomes occurs with asymmetric cytoplasmic division. • Forming one egg and a polar body in female.

Meiosis II: Nearly similar to mitosis but separated chromatids are different because of previous genetic recombination.

2. Prostaglandin structure:

a. One double bond
b. One ring
c. 20°C structure
d. Consists of 5 membered ring
e. Structural unit is referred as prostanoic acid

Ans. b. One ring; c. 20°C structure; d. Consists of 5 membered ring and e. Structural unit is referred as prostanoic acid *Ref: Prostaglandin: A useful strategy for new drug development; (sethy et. al, 2012); Prostaglandins-basic Chemistry and Action (Zreik et al, 2008); Harper 28th/ed p409-414*

Explanation

Prostaglandins: A type of eicosanoid.

- 20-carbon fatty acids derived enzymatically from the essential fatty acids by cyclization and oxidation (**Option c**)
- Consist of an oxygenated cyclopentane/pentene ring with a heptenoic or heptanoic acid side and a octanoyl side chain on adjacent carbon atoms of the ring (**Option b and d**)
- Basic structural unit is prostanoic acid (**Option e**)
- Classified as PGA, PGB, PGC, PGD, PGE, PGF, PGG and PGH based on cyclopentane or pentene sidechain.

- Subclassified on basis of degree of unsaturation (e.g. PGE1, PGF1, PGF2 etc.), number indicates number of double bonds (**Option a**).

Eicosanoid	Biochemical and physiologic action
PGD2	Weak inhibitor of platelet aggregation
PGE1	Bronchial vasodilation Inhibitor of lipolysis Inhibitor of platelet aggregation Contraction of GI smooth muscle
PGE2	Hyperalgesic response Renal and bronchial vasodilation Inhibitor of platelet aggregation Uterine muscle relaxation Cytoprotection: Protects GI epithelial cells from acid degradation Reduces gastric acid secretion Elevates thermoregulatory set-point in anterior hypothalamus (fever) Promotes inflammation
PGF2	Uterine muscle contraction Bronchoconstrictor
PGI2	Potent inhibitor of platelet aggregation Bronchodilator Uterine relaxant Sensitize/amplify nerve pain response
TXA2	Potent inducer of platelet aggregation Potent vasoconstrictor (bronchioles, renal) Decreases cAMP levels in platelets Stimulates the release of ADP and 5-HT from platelets
LTB4	Increases leukocyte chemotaxis and aggregation
LTC/D4	Slow-reacting substance of anaphylaxis Bronchoconstriction in humans
5-or 12-PETE	Aggregates human leukocytes Promotes leukocyte chemotaxis

3. Anterior interosseous nerve supplies:

a. Flexor carpi ulnaris
b. Pronator teres
c. Brachioradialis
d. Flexor digitorum superficialis
e. Flexor pollicis longus

Ans. e. Flexor pollicis longus *Ref: Gray's Anatomy 41st/ed p848-862*

Explanation

Anterior interosseous nerve: Branch of median nerve between two heads of pronator teres.

- Descends anterior to interosseous membrane.
- Supply flexor pollicis longus, lateral part of flexor digitorum profundus (for index and middle fingers) and pronator quadratus.
- Articular branches to distal radioulnar, radiocarpal and carpal joints.

Forearm muscles:

Muscles	Action	Innervation
Superficial flexor compartment		
Pronator teres ***(option b)***	Pronation, weak flexor	Median nerve (C6-C7)
Flexor carpi radialis	Wrist flexor	Median nerve (C6-C7)
Flexor digitorum superficialis ***(option d)***	Flexor of wrist, metacarpophalangeal and proximal interphalangeal joints	Median nerve (C8-T1)
Palmaris longus	Anchor for skin and fascia of hand, weak wrist flexor	Median nerve (C8-T1)
Flexor carpi ulnaris ***(option a)***	Powerful flexor and also adductor (ulnar deviator) of wrist	Ulnar nerve (C7, C8, T1)
Deep flexor compartment		
Flexor digitorum profundus	Flexes distal interphalangeal joint	Medial part (little and ring finger) by ulnar nerve Lateral part (middle and index finger) by anterior interosseous branch.
Flexor pollicis longus ***(option e)***	Flexion of thumb phalanges and carpometacarpal joint	Anterior interosseous branch (C7-C8)
Pronator Quadratus	Pronation	Anterior interosseous branch
Superficial extensor compartment		
Brachioradialis ***(option c)***	Powerful flexor of elbow	Radial nerve (C5-C6)
Extensor carpi radialis longus	Extensor and abductor of wrist	Radial nerve (C6-C7)
Extensor carpi radialis brevis	Dorsiflexor of wrist Fist making with flexors	Posterior interosseous nerve branch of radial
Extensor digitorum	Extension of wrist, metacarpophalangeal, proximal and distal interphalangeal joint	Posterior interosseous nerve (C7-C8)
Extensor digiti minimi	Extends any joint of little finger	Posterior interosseous nerve (C7-C8)
Extensor carpi ulnaris	Help in power grip with clenched fist	Posterior interosseous nerve (C7-C8)
Anconeus	Extensor of elbow	Radial nerve (C6, C7, C8)
Deep extensor compartment		
Abductor pollicis longus	Radial abductor of thumb	Posterior interosseous nerve
Extensor pollicis longus	Extend a distal phalanx of thumb	Posterior interosseous nerve
Extensor pollicis brevis	Extends proximal phalanx and metacarpal of thumb	Posterior interosseous nerve

Contd...

Contd...

Muscles	Action	Innervation
Extensor indicis	Extends index finger	Posterior interosseous nerve
Supinator	Supination together with biceps brachii	Posterior interosseous nerve

Innervation of intrinsic muscles of hand

Nerve	Muscles
Median nerve	• Flexor pollicis brevis (superficial head) • Abductor pollicis brevis • Opponens pollicis (Also by deep branch of ulnar) • 1st and 2nd lumbricals
Ulnar nerve	• Adductor pollicis • Abductor digiti minimi • Flexor digiti minimi brevis • Opponens digiti minimi • All interossei • Third and 4th lumbricals • Palmaris brevis (by superficial branch) • Opponens pollicis (also by median)

4. Abduction:

a. Serratus anterior and trapezius causes it
b. Supraspinatus main abductor
c. Acromial fibers of deltoid is strong abductor
d. Axillary nerve injury has no effect on abduction
e. Rotator cuff stabilizes shoulder during abduction

Ans. a. Serratus anterior and trapezius causes it; b. Supraspinatus main abductor; c. Acromial fibers of deltoid is strong abductor and e. Rotator cuff stabilizes shoulder during abduction

Ref: Gray's Anatomy 41st/ed p815-826, 830-834

EXPLANATION

Shoulder girdle and shoulder joint musculature:

Muscle	Attachment	Innervation	Action
Trapezius	Origin-medial third of superior nuchal line, external occipital protuberance, ligamentum nuchae, C7-C12 spinous process Insertion—posterior border of lateral 1/3rd of clavicle and medial acromial margin	Motor Spinal accessory nerve Proprioceptive C3-C4	Upper fibers with levator scapulae—elevates as in shrugging Middle fibers with rhomboids—retracts **Lower fibers with serratus—protract and rotate scapula medially, also in overhead abduction *(option a)*** Steadies scapula

Contd...

Contd...

Muscle	Attachment	Innervation	Action
Pectoralis major	Origin—anterior surface of sternal half of clavicle (clavicular head) Half of anterior surface of sternum up to 6th or 7th costal cartilage (sternal head) 1st to 7th costal cartilage (costal head)	Medial and lateral pectoral nerve	Adduction and medial rotation Active in deep inspiration
	Aponeurosis of external oblique (rectus head) Insertion—lateral lip of intertubercular sulcus		
Pectoralis minor	Origin—outer margin of 3rd to 5th rib (2nd to 4th also) Insertion—medial border and upper surface of coracoid process of scapula	Medial and lateral pectoral nerve	Assists serratus in protraction Active in forced inspiration
Subclavius	Origin—1st rib and costal cartilage Insertion—groove on under surface of middle third of clavicle	Nerve to subclavius (C5, C6)	Resists accelerated elevation and rotation of clavicle Stabilizes sternoclavicular joint
Levator scapulae	Origin—transverse process of C1-C4 Insertion—medial border of scapula between superior angle and spine	C3-C4 cervical spinal nerves C5 via dorsal scapular nerve	Elevates superior angle of scapula Lateral rotation of scapula
Rhomboid minor	Origin—spine of C7-T1 and ligamentum nuchae Insertion—medial border of scapula at spine of scapula	Dorsal scapular nerve (C4, C5)	Retraction of shoulders
Rhomboid major	Origin—2nd to 5th thoracic spines Insertion—Medial border of scapula between spine and inferior angle	Dorsal scapular nerve (C4, C5)	Retraction of shoulders
Serratus anterior	Origin—outer surface and superior border of upper 8–10 ribs Upper fibers—1-2 ribs Middle fibers—3-6 ribs Lower fibers—interdigitate with upper 5 slips of external oblique Insertion- 1st digitation—superior angle of scapula 2nd–4th—costal surface along whole medial border Lower 4 or 5 digitation-costal surface of inferior angle	Long thoracic nerve (C5, C6 and C7) Paralysis causes winging of scapula	Protracts scapula Pushing and punching movement Overhead abduction

Contd...

Contd...

Muscle	Attachment	Innervation	Action
Deltoid	Origin—anterior border and superior surface of lateral third of clavicle Lateral margin and superior surface of acromion Lower edge of crest of scapular spine Insertion–deltoid tubercle of lateral aspect of midshaft of humerus	Axillary nerve (C5, C6)	Anterior fibers—rotating arm forward and medially Posterior fibers—drawing arm backward (external rotation) **Acromial part—multi pinnate** **strong abductor up to inferior joint capsule *(option c)***
Coracobra-chialis	Origin—apex of coracoid process Insertion—medial border of humeral shaft between medial head of triceps and brachialis	Musculocutane-ous nerve (C5, C6 and C7)	Antagonist to deltoid Flexes arm forward and medially
Latissimus dorsi	Origin—spine of lower six thoracic vertebrae • Posterior layer of thoracolumbar fascia • Posterior part (outer lip) of iliac crest • Slips from 3–4 lower ribs interdigitating with external oblique • May attach to inferior angle of scapula • Insertion—floor of intertubercular sulcus	Thoracodorsal nerve (C6, C7 and C8)	Adduction, extension and medial rotation Violent expiratory effort like coughing, sneezing
Rotator cuff/ musculotendi-nous apparatus	Supraspinatus Infraspinatus Teres minor Subscapularis Teres major—also included now in rotator cuff functionally (Ref Gray's 823)		Stabilizes humeral head on glenoid **Stabilizes shoulder joint during all movement *(Option e)***
Supraspinatus	Origin: Medial 2/3 rd of supraspinatus fossa Insertion—highest facet on greater tubercle of humerus	Suprascapular nerve (C5, C6)	Initiation and also throughout range of abduction.
Infraspinatus	**Origin:** Infraspinous fossa **Insertion:** Middle facet on greater tubercle of humerus	Suprascapular nerve (C5, C6)	Lateral rotator of humerus
Teres minor	**Origin:** Upper 2/3 rd of lateral border on dorsal aspect of scapula **Insertion:** Lowest facet on greater tubercle of humerus	Axillary nerve (C5, C6)	Lateral rotator and weak adductor of humerus

Contd...

Contd...

Muscle	Attachment	Innervation	Action
Subscapularis	**Origin:** Subscapular fossa **Insertion:** Lesser tubercle of humerus	Upper and lower subscapular nerve (C5, C6)	Medial rotator of humerus
Teres major	**Origin:** Dorsal surface on inferior scapular angle **Insertion:** Medial lip of intertubercular sulcus	Lower subscapular nerve (C5, C6)	Draws humerus backward and rotates medially

Note: In complete axillary nerve lesions (Irreversible deltoid palsy)—supraspinatus along with other cuff muscles can initiate, regulate, achieve and maintain full abduction of arm but endurance is limited ***Option (d).***

5. Which structure is most anterior at tibial plateau?

a. Anterior horn of lateral meniscus
b. Anterior cruciate ligament
c. Posterior cruciate ligament
d. Anterior horn of medial meniscus
e. Posterior horn of medial meniscus

Ans. d. Anterior horn of medial meniscus *Ref: Gray's Anatomy 41st/ed p1387-1388*

EXPLANATION

Structures of Tibial Plateau (means superior surface of tibial condyle): Anterior to posterior

- Medical College of Lucknow
  - Anterior horn of medial meniscus
  - Anterior cruciate ligament
  - Anterior horn of lateral meniscus
  - Posterior horn of lateral meniscus
  - Posterior horn of medial meniscus
  - Posterior cruciate ligament

Menisci: Fibrocartilaginous laminae

- Act to widen, deepen and prepare tibial articulating surface to receive femoral condyle
- Spread load, provide stability, cushion, proprioception
- Lateral meniscus covers larger area than medial meniscus
- Popliteus Hiatus: Lateral meniscus has no peripheral bony attachment in region of popliteus.

6. Regarding fibrous skeleton on heart, true statement/s is/are:

a. Formed of collagen with fibroareolar extensions
b. Related to AV valves and aortic and pulmonary valves
c. Provides support for cardiac valves
d. Strongest at junction of aortic, mitral and tricuspid valve
e. Ensures electrophysiological discontinuity between atria and ventricle
f. Tendon of todaro is part of it

Ans. a. Formed of collagen with fibroareolar extensions; d. Strongest at junction of aortic, mitral and tricuspid valve and e. Ensures electrophysiological discontinuity between atria and ventricle

Ref: Gray's Anatomy 41st/ed p1012-1013

Explanation

Fibrous skeleton of Heart:

- ❑ Complex framework of dense collagen with membranous, tendinous and fibroareolar extensions. *(Option a)*
- ❑ Intimately related to AV valves and aortic orifice ***(Option b-not pulmonary).***
  - Leaflets of pulmonary valve are supported on free standing sleeve of right ventricular infundibulum and can be removed from heart without disturbing fibrous skeleton.
- ❑ Fibrous skeleton does not provide support for valve (Old concept was that it supports-***Option c***).
  - Mitral and tricuspid valve are supported by overall structure of AV junction.
  - Arterial valves are supported by valvular sinuses.
- ❑ Strongest at junction of aortic, mitral and tricuspid valve called central fibrous body ***(Option d).***
- ❑ **Fibrous skeleton comprises of:**
  - **Fila coronaria:** Two pairs of collagenous prongs extending from central fibrous body.
    - Stronger on the left extending partially around mitral and tricuspid orifice.
  - **Subaortic curtain:** Two leaflets of aortic valve are in fibrous continuity with aortic leaflet of mitral valve.
  - **Fibrous trigone:** Right and left ends of curtain—strongest parts of skeleton.
    - Right trigone with membranous septum constitute central fibrous body—penetrated by atrioventricular bundle of His.
  - Membranous septum is divided by tricuspid valve into atrioventricular and interventricular components.
  - **Anulus:** Aortic root is central within fibrous skeleton termed as anulus.
  - **Subaortic spans**: Three triangular areas that separates aortic bulbous sinuses that houses valvular leaflets.
    1. First span: Between non-coronary and left coronary sinuses.
    2. Second span: Between non-coronary and right coronary sinuses.
    3. Third span: Between two coronary aortic sinuses.
  - **Conus/conal ligament** (tendon of infundibulum): Found at the level of sinotubular junction at site of fusion of distal outflow cushion.
  - **Longitudinal raphe:** At site of proximal fusion in muscular subpulmonary infundibulum.
  - Atrioventricular valves are supported by discrete circular fibrous rings in reality D-shaped structure attached to fibrous skeleton.
- ❑ **Functions**:
  1. Electrophysiological discontinuity between atrial and ventricular myocardial masses except at sites of penetration of conduction tissue ***(Option e).***
  2. Provides direct attachment for myocardium and fibrous tissue in heart.
  3. Support matrix for 3D meshwork of cardiomyocytes.
- ❑ **Note:** Tendon of todaro is not part of fibrous skeleton (***Option f***).

7. Taste sensation of tongue:

a. Glossopharyngeal
b. Chorda tympani
c. Facial
d. Lingual nerve
e. Vagus

Ans. a. Glossopharyngeal; b. Chorda tympani; c. Facial and e. Vagus

Ref: Gray's Anatomy 41st/ed p511-517

Explanation

	Anterior 2/3rd	Posterior 1/3rd	Posterior most part
Taste sensation	Chorda tympani (branch of facial N) ***(option b and c)***	Glossopharyngeal N ***(option a)***	Internal laryngeal N (Branch of vagus N) ***(option e)***
General sensation	Lingual N (branch of mandibular N V_3) ***(option d)***	Glossopharyngeal N	Internal laryngeal N (Branch of vagus N)
Motor supply	All intrinsic and extrinsic muscles are supplied by hypoglossal N, except palatoglossus which is supplied by cranial root of accessory N		

Innervation of tongue for taste sensation:

1. **Chorda tympani:** A branch of VIIth nerve, travels via lingual nerve and supplies anterior part of tongue excluding circumvallate papillae.
   Note: *Lingual nerve gives only sensory innervation*—no taste sensation.
2. **Facial nerve:** Also innervates inferior part of soft palate for taste sensation.
3. **Glossopharyngeal nerve:** Taste sensation in circumvallate papillae, post sulcal part of Tongue, palatoglossal arch and oropharynx.
4. **Vagus Nerve:** Extreme pharyngeal part of tongue and epiglottis via internal laryngeal branch.
   Tongue: Highly muscular organ of deglutition, taste and speech.

- ❑ Divided in two parts by Sulcus Terminalis (V shaped) with median depression—Foramen Cecum upper end of embryonic thyroid diverticulum (thyroglossal duct).

1. **Oral (presulcal) part:** Anterior 2/3 rd. papilla present here.
2. **Pharyngeal (post sulcal part):** Posterior 1/3 rd. devoid of papillae.

Muscles of tongue:

1. **Intrinsic:** Superior and inferior longitudinal, transverse and vertical.
2. **Extrinsic:** 4 pairs of muscles.
   a. **Genioglossus:** Protrude its apex from mouth, also diverses tongue to opposite side.
   b. **Hyoglossus:** Depresses tongue.
   c. **Styloglossus:** Up and backward movement.
   d. **Palatoglossus:** Elevates root of tongue.
   Chondroglossus-also present nearly similar to hyoglossus but has separate fibers.

Note: All muscles of tongue supplied by Hypoglossal nerve except Palatoglossus. Palatoglossus is supplied by pharyngeal plexus (formed by IX, X and superior cervical sympathetic ganglia).

- ❑ **Arterial supply:** by Lingual artery-branch from anterior surface of external carotid artery.
  3 branches: dorsal lingual, sublingual and deep lingual artery.
- ❑ **Venous drainage:** by Lingual veins
  Joins facial and anterior division of retromandibular vein to form common facial vein. Finally drains into internal jugular vein.
- ❑ **Lymphatic drainage:** Lingual tonsils present in mucosa of pharyngeal part of dorsal surface of tongue. Three lymphatic vessels.
  - Anterior part drain in-marginal and central vessels
  - Posterior part drain in-dorsal lymph vessels
  - Central part drain in-bilaterally-important to dissect both side in malignancy.
  - Finally all drain in submental, submandibular, jugulo-omohyoid and jugulo-digastric nodes
- ❑ Sensory innervation of tongue (for general sensation):
  - Anterior 2/3rd: Lingual nerve branch of mandibular division of trigeminal nerve.
  - Posterior 1/3rd: Glossopharyngeal nerve.
  - Near valleculae: Internal laryngeal branch of vagus.
  - Taste: Salt (NaCl), Sour (acidic), Sweet (sugar), Bitter (quinine) and Umami (delicious taste).

8. Inferior ophthalmic vein true is/are:

a. Passes through the inferior orbital fissure
b. Communicates with pterygoid venous plexus
c. Drains into cavernous sinus
d. Passes through superior orbital fissure
e. Begins near orbital floor and lateral wall

Ans. b. Communicates with pterygoid venous plexus; c. Drains into cavernous sinus and d. Passes through superior orbital fissure *Ref: Gray's Anatomy 41st/ed p676-677*

EXPLANATION

- Venous drainage of orbit and eyeball
  - **Orbit:** Drained by superior and inferior ophthalmic veins and infraorbital vein.
  - **Eyeball:** Veins of eyeball drain into Vortex veins, Retinal veins drain into Central retinal vein.
- **Superior ophthalmic vein:** Formed by tributaries connecting anteriorly with facial and supraorbital veins, two superior vortex veins and central vein of retina.
  - Traverses in superior orbital fissure above the common ring of recti
  - Ends in cavernous sinus.
- **Inferior ophthalmic vein:** Begins near anterior region of orbital floor and medial wall.
  - Passes through superior orbital fissure below common tendinous ring.
  - May join superior ophthalmic vein or may drain directly in cavernous sinus
  - Communicates with pterygoid venous plexus by small branch which goes through inferior orbital fissure.
  - Receives tributaries from inferior rectus, inferior oblique, nasolacrimal duct, eyelids and two inferior vortex veins.
- **Infraorbital vein:** Runs with infraorbital nerve and artery in floor of orbit.
  - Joins pterygoid venous plexus by passing through inferior orbital fissure.
  - Communicates with inferior ophthalmic vein or facial vein
- **Ophthalmic artery:** Branch of internal carotid artery.
  - Runs in optic canal inferolateral to optic nerve.
  - **Branches:** Central retinal artery, Muscular branches, Ciliary artery, Lacrimal artery, Supraorbital artery, Posterior ethmoidal artery, Anterior ethmoidal artery, Meningeal branch, Medial palpebral artery, Supratrochlear artery, Dorsal nasal artery.

Note: Recurrent meningeal artery and infraorbital branch of maxillary artery also supply orbit.

9. Thyroid anatomy true is/are:

a. Enseathed by pretracheal layer of deep cervical fascia
b. Attached to cricoid cartilage by Berry ligament
c. Isthmus lies at level of second and third tracheal cartilage
d. Musculus levator glandulae thyroideae connects hyoid to pyramidal lobe
e. Most frequent location of ectopic thyroid is base of tongue
f. Superior thyroid artery is related to recurrent laryngeal nerve
g. Thyroidea ima artery is branch of subclavian artery

Ans. a. Enseathed by pretracheal layer of deep cervical fascia; b. Attached to cricoid cartilage by Berry ligament; c. Isthmus lies at level of second and third tracheal cartilage; d. Musculus levator glandulae thyroideae connects hyoid to pyramidal lobe and e. Most frequent location of ectopic thyroid is base of tongue *Ref: Gray's Anatomy 41st/ed p470-471*

EXPLANATION

Thyroid gland: Located anteriorly in lower neck level with C5-T1 vertebrae

- Ensheathed by pretracheal layer of deep cervical fascia.
- Right and left lobe connected by isthmus, opposite 2nd and 3rd tracheal cartilages.
- Heavier in females and enlarges during menstruation and pregnancy.
- **Berry ligament:** Posteromedial aspect of lobe connected to cricoid cartilage by lateral thyroid ligament termed Berry ligament.
- **Pyramidal lobe:** Present in 40% of cases—ascends from either isthmus or left lobe to hyoid bone. Connected by hyoid through levator glandulae thyroideae.
- **Ectopic thyroid:** Most frequent at base of tongue near foramen cecum; anywhere along thyroglossal duct or neck.
- **Relations:**
  - External laryngeal nerve related to superior thyroid artery.
  - Recurrent laryngeal nerve related to inferior thyroid artery.
- **RIA SEN:**
  - Recurrent laryngeal nerve related to inferior thyroid artery—tie it away from gland.
  - Superior thyroid artery is related to external laryngeal nerve—tie it near to gland.

Blood supply

- **Superior thyroid artery:** Branch of external carotid artery.
- **Inferior thyroid artery:** Branch of thyrocervical trunk—branch from 1st part of subclavian.
- **Thyroidea ima artery:** Branch from brachiocephalic trunk or aortic arch.
- **Venous drainage:** Superior, middle and inferior thyroid veins—draining in internal jugular vein

Lymphatics: Prelaryngeal, pretracheal, paratracheal and deep cervical nodes.

Nerve supply: Superior, middle and inferior cervical sympathetic ganglia.

Histology: Thyroid follicle is structural and functional unit.

- Lined by simple cuboidal or low columnar epithelium.
- Central colloid contains iodothyroglobulin—inactive form of T3 and T4.
- Can regulate metabolic activity of body for 3 months.
- 2 types of cells:
- **Follicular (principal cells):** Produces T3 and T4. Basophilic staining.
- **Parafollicular (C-cells):** Produces calcitonin—pale staining.

Embryology: Appears as epithelial proliferation in floor of pharynx between tuberculum impar and copula, later indicated by foramen cecum.

- Descends as bilobed diverticulum.
- Remains connected to tongue by thyroglossal duct, which later disappears.
- Final position reached by 7 week, begins functioning after 3 month.
- Parafollicular (C-cells) derived from ultimobranchial body.

10. Parotid true is/are:

a. 2nd largest salivary gland
b. Divided by facial nerve
c. Deep lobe contains majority of lymph nodes.
d. Opens in vestibule of mouth opposite 2nd upper molar tooth.
e. Innervated by lesser petrosal branch of Glossopharyngeal nerve.

Ans. b. Divided by facial nerve; d. Opens in vestibule of mouth opposite 2nd upper molar tooth and e. Innervated by lesser petrosal branch of Glossopharyngeal nerve.

Ref: Gray's Anatomy 41st/ed p504-505

Explanation

Parotid gland:

- Largest of salivary gland. Completely serous.
- Inverted pyramidal in shape with 4 surfaces—superior (base), superficial, anteromedial and posteromedial; 3 borders—anterior, posterior and medial; and a apex directed downward.
- Superior surface contains facial branches of greater auricular nerve, superficial parotid lymph nodes and posterior belly of platysma.
- Divided into large superficial and small deep part by facial nerve.
- **Relations:** AVN-deep to superficial.
  1. **External carotid artery:** Dividing into maxillary and superficial temporal artery—deepest part of gland on posteromedial surface.
  2. **Retromandibular vein:** Formed by superficial temporal and maxillary vein. Emerges near apex at lower part of gland.
  3. **Facial nerve**: Divides into terminal branches within the gland. Divides it into large superficial and small deep part. Five branches leave at anterior border.
     a. **Temporofacial branch:** Divides into temporal and zygomatic.
     b. **Cervicofacial branch:** Divides into buccal, marginal mandibular and cervical.
- **Parotid capsule:** Derived from investing layer of deep cervical fascia.
  - Pain of acute sialadenitis occurs due to stretching of capsule and stimulation of great auricular nerve.
  - **Lymph nodes:** Mainly lie in superficial part-lesser in deep part. Finally to deep cervical node.
  - **Blood supply:** By external carotid artery. Drain into external jugular vein.
  - **Nerve supply:** Preganglionic fibers comes via lesser petrosal nerve of Glossopharyngeal-synapses in Otic ganglia—postganglionic fibers as secretomotor supply parotid via auriculotemporal nerve.

Frey's syndrome (Gustatory sweating): Aberrant innervation of sweat gland of face by parasympathetic nerve innervating parotid.

- Generally occurs after parotid region surgery or trauma.
- Sweating, warmth and redness of face by gustatory stimulation.
- t/t—subcutaneous infiltration of botulinum toxin.

JIPMER Pattern Based

1. Which of the following is from the sixth branchial arch?

a. Thyrohyoid
b. Stylopharyngeus
c. Cricothyroid
d. Posterior cricoarytenoids

Ans. d. Posterior cricoarytenoids *Ref: Gray's Anatomy 41st/ed p594-595,607*

For explanation refer question number 1 of AIIMS anatomy

2. Sinus draining in anterior border of Sternocleidomastoid is from which branchial arch extending to tonsillar fossa?

a. Third arch
b. Second arch
c. Fourth arch
d. 1st arch

Ans. b. Second arch *Ref: Gray's Anatomy 41st/ed p449; Langman's Medical Embryology 13th/ed p288*

Explanation

- **Branchial fistula:** Persistent connection between 2nd branchial pouch and cervical sinus.
  - Presents as small pit at anterior border of lower 1/3rd of sternocleidomastoid.
  - Extends through carotid bifurcation into distal tonsillar fossa and opens in pharynx.
  - Occurs when 2nd pharyngeal arch fails to grow caudally over 3rd and 4th arch.
- **Internal branchial fistula:** Cervical sinus connected to lumen of pharynx by small canal which usually opens in tonsillar region.
- **Branchial cyst:** Present in early adulthood as fluctuant swelling.
  - At junction of upper and middle 1/3rd of anterior border of sternocleidomastoid.
  - Passes through carotid bifurcation to end at pharyngeal constrictor muscle.
  - IX, XI and XII nerve is intimately associated with it.
  - Treatment—surgical excision.

3. 6th branchial arch forms:

a. In between left common carotid and left subclavian/arch of aorta
b. Ductus arteriosus
c. Right brachiocephalic
d. Arch of aorta

Ans. b. Ductus arteriosus *Ref: Gray's Anatomy 41st/ed p607; Langman's Medical Embryology 13th/ed p279-292*

Refer question 1 of AIIMS anatomy

4. Recognize the structures marked C:

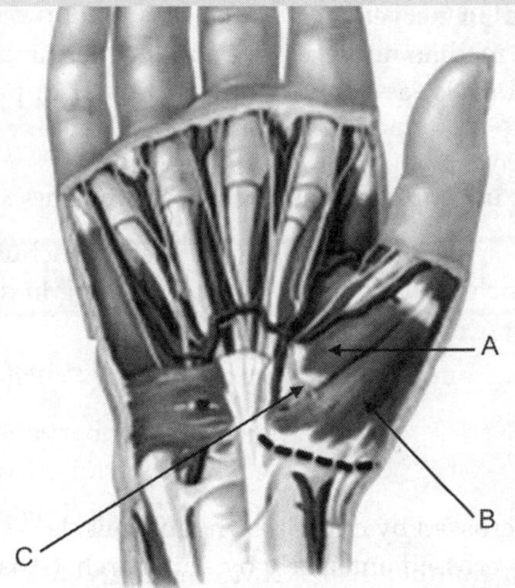

a. Recurrent median nerve
b. Palmar branch of median nerve
c. Deep palmar branch of ulnar nerve
d. Communicating branch of median and ulnar nerve

Ans. a. Recurrent median nerve *Ref: Gray's Anatomy 41st/ed p886, 888, Fig. 50.35*

EXPLANATION

Structures shown here are:

A. Flexor pollicis brevis
B. Abductor pollicis brevis
C. Recurrent branch of median nerve

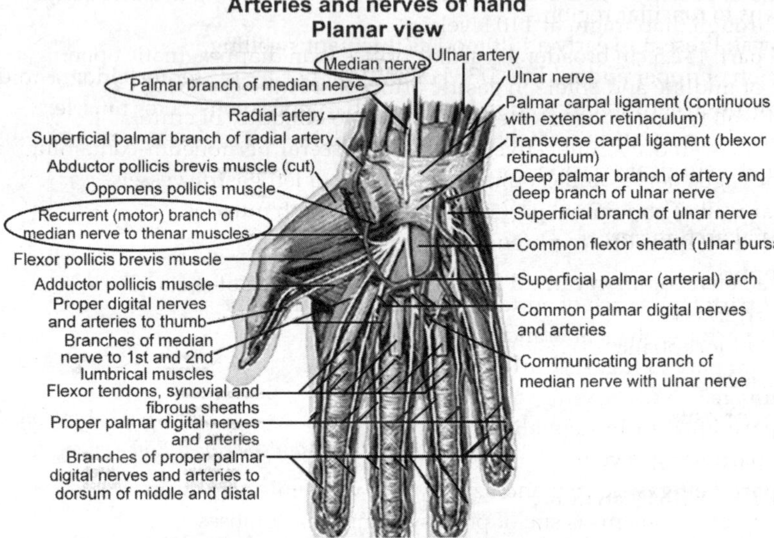

Rest explanation about muscles and nerves in **PGI question no. 3**

Recurrent branch of median nerve:

- ❑ Arises from lateral side of median nerve as 1st palmar or terminal branch.
- ❑ Supplies flexor pollicis brevis, abductor pollicis brevis, opponens pollicis and 1st dorsal interosseous.

5. Foreign body/coin stuck in esophagus at 25 cm from incisors situated at which level?

a. Arch of aorta
b. Left bronchus level
c. Cricopharyngeal sphincter
d. Opening in diaphragm
e. Cricoid

Ans. a. Arch of aorta *Ref: Gray's Anatomy 41st/ed p986-987,1111-1112*

EXPLANATION

Constriction of esophagus:

- ❑ 1st: 15 cms from incisor—crossed by cricopharyngeus muscle.
- ❑ 2nd: 23 cms from incisor—crossed anteriorly by aortic arch. (Answer)
- ❑ 3rd: 28 cms from incisor—due to left principal bronchus.
- ❑ 4th: 40 cms from incisor—esophageal hiatus in diaphragm.

Esophagus: 25 cms long connecting pharynx to stomach

- ❑ **Cervical part** and **Thoracic part:**
  - ▪ Begins at lower border of cricoid cartilage and C6 vertebrae.
  - ▪ Ends in gastric orifice at T11 level.
  - ▪ Recurrent laryngeal nerve ascends on each side in Tracheo-esophageal groove.

- **Azygoesophageal recess:** Long recess of right pleural sac between esophagus anteriorly and azygous vein posteriorly in posterior mediastinum.
- Thoracic duct is posterior and to right of esophagus in lower part and crosses to left at T5 vertebrae level.
- Right vagus nerve remains behind and left in front of esophagus.
- Little left in superior mediastinum between trachea and vertebrae.
- Descends in posterior mediastinum along right of descending thoracic aorta.
- Passes through diaphragm at T10 level.

❑ **Abdominal part**: 1–2.5 cm broader at cardiac orifice than diaphragmatic opening.
- Lies left of midline and enters in gastric orifice at T11 level.
- Anterior wall is longer than posterior wall due to obliquity of crura.
- Surface is covered by connective tissue and visceral peritoneum containing anterior and posterior vagus nerves and esophageal branches of left gastric vessels.
- Muscular wall of abdominal part is entirely of smooth muscles.
- Tethered at margins due to phreno-esophageal ligament.

❑ **Arterial supply:**
- **Cervical part:** Up to arch of aorta by inferior thyroid artery
- **Thoracic part:** Esophageal branch of aorta
- **Abdominal part:** Left gastric artery

❑ **Venous drainage**:
- **Upper part:** Into brachiocephalic vein
- **Middle part:** Azygos vein
- **Lower part:** Left gastric vein and azygos vein via hemiazygos vein.
- Lower end of esophagus is site of portosystemic anastomoses.

❑ **Nerve supply:**
- Parasympathetic: Sensory, motor and secretomotor.
  - **Upper half:** Recurrent laryngeal nerve
  - **Lower half:** Esophageal plexus formed by two vagi.
- Sympathetic-vasomotor
  - **Upper half:** Middle cervical ganglia
  - **Lower half:** Esophageal plexus by upper four thoracic ganglia.

6. Not related to boundary of Koch triangle is/are:

a. Tendon of todaro
b. IVC opening
c. Septal leaflet of tricuspid
d. Coronary sinus ostium

Ans. b. IVC opening *Ref: Gray's Anatomy 41st/ed p1000-1001*

EXPLANATION

Koch triangle: Present internally in Right atrium, contains AV node and its atrial connections. It is bounded by **(Answer below)**

1. Septal leaflet of tricuspid valve
2. Ostium of coronary sinus
3. Collagenous subendocardial Tendon of Todaro

Right atrium: Anterior and right of left atrium

❑ Forms right superior sternocostal surface, convex right pulmonary surface and right side of base.
❑ Superior and inferior vena cava opens into it.
❑ Sulcus terminalis on right side between openings of vena cavae.

- ❑ Internally sulcus terminalis corresponds with Crista terminalis, site of origin of pectinate muscle, arises at right angle.
- ❑ Upper part of sulcus terminalis contains SA node (pacemaker of heart).
- ❑ Right atrioventricular groove contains right coronary artery and small cardiac veins.
- ❑ Tributaries of right atrium: 1. Superior vena cava, 2. Inferior vena cava, 3. Coronary sinus, 4. Anterior cardiac veins, 5. Vena cordis minimae (Thebesian veins), 6. Right marginal veins.
- ❑ Right atrium has 3 important internal regions:

1. **Smooth posterior part/sinus venarum:** Derived from sinus venosus of embryonic heart.
    - Receives vena cavae and coronary sinus and vena cordis minimae.
    - Eustachian valve: Lateral to IVC opening—forming eustachian ridge continuous inferiorly with sinus septum leading to valve of coronary sinus. In embyo guides blood from IVC towards foramen ovale.
    - Coronary sinus: Opens between opening of IVC, fossa ovalis and vestibule of atrioventricular opening. Guarded by Thebesian valve. Joins the tendinous structure Tendon of Todaro, running from commissure to sinus septum, inserting into central fibrous body. Sinus returns most of the blood from heart.
    - Tendon of Todaro: Landmark for triangle of Koch.
    - Crista terminalis: C shaped muscular ridge anterior to orifice of SVC. Corresponds externally to terminal groove (sulcus terminalis). SA node located in superior part of groove. Musculi pectinati extends from crista.
2. **Rough anterior part of Pectinate part:** Derive from primitive atrial chamber.
    - Presents series of musculi pectinati. Teeth of comb appearance.
3. **Septal wall (Interatrial septum):** Derived from septum primum and septum secundum.
    - **Fossa ovalis:** Site of embryonic septum primum. Saucer shaped.
    - **Annulus ovalis** (limbus fossa ovalis): Margin of fossa ovalis—lower free edge of embryonic septum secundum.

7. Structure between right ventricular inlet and outlet:

a. Septomarginal trabeculation
b. Supraventricular crest
c. Chordae tendineae
d. Moderator band

Ans. b. Supraventricular crest *Ref: Gray's Anatomy 41st/ed p1001-1003*

EXPLANATION

Right ventricle: Extends from Tricuspid valve nearly to cardiac apex.

- ❑ RV forms inferior border, 2/3 rd of sternocostal surface and 1/3 rd part of inferior surface.
- ❑ **Wall thickness of RV:** LV = 1:3.
- ❑ Its has 3 components
    - **Inlet component:** Support and surround tricuspid valve-from proximal portion of bulbus cordis.
    - Coarse trabeculated apical component: Develops from proximal portion of bulbus cordis.
    - **Outlet or Infundibulum:** Surrounds attachment of pulmonary valve-from mid-portion of bulbus cordis.
- ❑ Inlet and outlet are separated by muscular ridge called Supraventricular crest/infundibulo-ventricular crest *(Answer)*.
- ❑ Internal features are:
    - Trabeculated appearance is due to irregular muscular ridge and protrusions called Trabeculae carneae.
    - Chordae Tendineae are collagenous cord attached to tricuspid valve.

- Papillary muscles are attached from ventricular wall to chordae tendineae.
- Septomarginal Trabeculations present in septal surface dividing in two limbs to enclose supraventricular crest. Also supports anterior papillary muscles and extends to parietal wall of ventricle termed **Moderator Band.**
- Moderator band prevents over distention of ventricle: Also part of conduction system involving Right atrioventricular bundle.
- Papillary muscles: 3 papillary muscles-Anterior, Posterior and septal.
  - Anterior Papillary muscle is largest. Rest are smaller.

8. Structure related to floor of sphenoidal sinus is:

a. Vidian nerve
b. Maxillary nerve
c. Mandibular nerve
d. Greater petrosal nerve
e. Optic nerve

Ans. a. Vidian nerve. *Ref: Gray's Anatomy 41st/ed p535-537, 567-568, Zoukaa et al, 2007 (Surgical Anatomy of Paranasal Sinus), Sareen et al, 2005 (Study of Sphenoid Sinus Anatomy in Relation to Endoscopic Surgery)*

EXPLANATION

Sphenoid sinus:

- Two large irregular cavity within body of sphenoid, posterior to upper part of nasal cavity
- Opens into sphenoethmoidal recess via aperture on anterior wall of sinus.
- Separated from each other by a septum which is deviated to one side.
- **Relations**:
  1. Superiorly: Optic chiasma and hypophysis cerebri
  2. Laterally: Bulge of internal carotid artery and optic canal
  3. Inferiorly: Nasal cavity
  4. Lateral recess: Sometimes present having canal for maxillary nerve superiorly and canal for **vidian nerve in floor or inferiorly (Answer).**
- Growth starts between 3rd and 4th month of fetal development.
- **Pneumatization** starts at 3 years and finishes in mid teen age. It is of **3 types** on basis of pneumatization:
  1. Chonchal: Area below sella is solid no pneumatization.
  2. Presellar: Pneumatization at the level of frontal plane of sella.
  3. Sellar: Pneumatization extends in body of sphenoid beyond floor of sella reaching clivus. Most common type.
- **Onodi cell**: When posterior ethmoidal sinus extends postero-superior to smaller sphenoid sinus; sphenoid sinus is medial to highly developed spheno-ethmoidal cell termed onodi cells.

9. Content of sinus of morgagni:

a. Levator veli palatini
b. Eustachian tube
c. Ascending palatine artery
d. All

Ans. d. All *Ref: Gray's Anatomy 41st/ed p581-582*

EXPLANATION

Sinus of Morgagni

- Large crescentic gap between upper border of superior constrictor and cranial base.
- Closed by upper strong fibers of pharyngobasilar fascia.
- **Structure passing:** 1. Auditory tube, 2. Levator veli palatini, 3. Ascending palatine artery, 4. Palatine branch of ascending pharyngeal artery.

Gaps between	Structures passing
1. Superior constrictor and skull base (Sinus of Morgagni)	1. Auditory tube (Eustachian tube) 2. Levator veli palatini muscle 3. Ascending palatine artery 4. Palatine branch of ascending pharyngeal artery
2. Superior and middle constrictor	1. Stylopharyngeus muscle 2. Glossopharyngeal nerve
3. Middle and inferior constrictor	1. Internal laryngeal nerve 2. Superior laryngeal vessels *(Pierce thyrohyoid membrane)
4. Below inferior constrictor	1. Recurrent laryngeal nerve 2. Inferior laryngeal vessels

10. Retropharyngeal abscess lies between which two fascia?

a. Between buccopharyngeal and Alar fascia
b. Between buccopharyngeal and pharyngobasilar fascia
c. Between Buccopharyngeal and prevertebral fascia
d. Alar fascia and prevertebral fascia

Ans. a. Between buccopharyngeal and Alar fascia *Ref: Gray's Anatomy 41st/ed p445-447*

Explanation

Cervical fascia and spaces	Facts
Superficial cervical fascia	Zone of loose connective tissue between dermis and deep fascia covers platysma • In lower region, platysma fans out in this.
Deep cervical fascia	Three layers—superficial investing, middle and deep layers
1. Investing layer	• Encircles neck covering trapezius and sternocleidomastoid • Related to parotid gland between mandible and mastoid process. • Forms suprasternal space of burn between its two layers contains areolar tissues, anterior jugular veins, jugular venous arch, sternal head of sternocleidomastoid and lymph node. • Forms supraclavicular space contains external jugular vein, supraclavicular nerves, cutaneous vessels and lymphatics. • Forms stylomandibular ligament • Forms pulley for digastric and omohyoid.
2. Middle layer	Divided into **Muscular layer:** Surrounding infrahyoid strap muscles. **Visceral layers:** Pretracheal and buccopharyngeal fascia.
3. Deep layer	**Dorsal layer:** Prevertebral fascia **Ventral layer:** Alar fascia
a. Pretracheal fascia	• Encloses thyroid gland forming its false capsule. Posterior layer of capsule is thick forming suspensory ligament of thyroid called ligament of berry. • Continues into superior mediastinum fusing with fibrous pericardium.

Contd...

Contd...

Cervical fascia and spaces	Facts
b. Buccopharyngeal fascia	Covers superior constrictor and extends on superficial aspect of buccinator
c. Pharyngobasilar fascia	• Lies deep to pharyngeal muscles. • Thickened between upper border of superior constrictor and base of skull related to foramen of morgagni
d. Carotid sheath	• Condensation of deep cervical fascia around common and internal carotid artery, internal jugular vein, vagus nerve and ansa cervicalis • Thicker around artery than vein • Anteriorly formed by pretracheal fascia • Posteriorly formed by prevertebral fascia
e. Prevertebral fascia	• Lies closest to vertebral bodies covering prevertebral muscles • Blends inferiorly with anterior longitudinal ligament • Cervical and brachial plexus lie behind this • Brachial plexus and subclavian artery passes between scalenus anterior and scalenus medius carrying this fascia as axillary sheath into axilla
f. Alar fascia	• Attached to transverse process of cervical vertebrae • Lies anterior to prevertebral fascia separated by danger space ***(Option d)*** • Lies posterior to pharynx, esophagus and visceral layer separated by retropharyngeal space ***(Option a)*** • Fuses with visceral layer at C7 (C6-T4) level limiting retropharyngeal and danger spaces
Spaces	
1. Visceral space	• Between muscular layer of deep cervical fascia and alar fascia • Divided into anterior visceral (pretracheal) space and posterior visceral (retropharyngeal space)
a. Pretracheal space	• Contains trachea, thyrois and parathyroid glands, larynx, cervical esophagus, recurrent laryngeal nerves and cervical sympathetic trunk • Separated from posterior visceral space by dense tissue surrounding inferior thyroid artery
b. Retropharyngeal space	• Lies between buccopharyngeal fascia and alar fascia ***(Option a)*** • Open and continuous with superior mediastinum • Limited at C7 (C6-T4) level • Contains retropharyngeal lymph nodes, pharyngeal plexus of vessels and nerves and loose areolar tissues
2. Prevertebral space	• Between prevertebral fascia and vertebral column enclosing prevertebral muscles • TB of spine may form Pott's abscess here
3. Danger space	• Between alar and prevertebral fascia • Contains loose areolar tissues • Offers potential route for downward spread of infection from retropharyngeal, parapharyngeal or prevertebral space to posterior mediastinum
4. Carotid space	• Potential space within the carotid sheath • May spread infections from upper neck to lower neck and mediastinum

11. Path of cavernous sinus thrombosis in nose septum infection:

a. Facial vein—maxillary vein—cavernous sinus
b. Posterior vein—sphenopalatine vein—Pterygoid venous plexus—cavernous sinus
c. Anterior vein—facial vein—cavernous sinus
d. Posterior vein—ophthalmic vein—cavernous sinus

Ans. b. Posterior vein—sphenopalatine vein—Pterygoid venous plexus—cavernous sinus

Ref: Gray's Anatomy 41st/ed p564, 438

EXPLANATION

Venous drainage of nasal septum

- Rich submucosal cavernous venous plexus in posterior part of septum and in middle and inferior turbinates.
- **Routes**:
  1. Posterior part of nose (posterior veins): Sphenopalatine vein—pterygoid venous plexus—emissary veins—cavernous sinus ***(option b)***
  2. Anterior part of nose (anterior vein): Facial vein—deep facial vein—pterygoid venous plexus—cavernous sinus ***(option c)***
  3. Anterior part of nose (anterior veins): Ophthalmic vein—cavernous sinus (directly or through) facial vein or pterygoid venous plexus ***(option d)***

Cavernous sinus

- Two large venous plexuses lie on either side of body of sphenoid.
- Extends from superior orbital fissure to petrous apex.
- Floor and medial wall formed by endosteal dura mater; and lateral wall and roof formed by meningeal dura mater.
- Superiorly related to optic tract, optic chiasma, olfactory tract, internal carotid artery and anterior perforated substance.

Structures within lateral wall of sinus Above downward	Structures within medial wall of sinus
• Oculomotor nerve • Trochlear nerve • Ophthalmic nerve • Maxillary nerve • Trigeminal ganglia	• Internal carotid artery • Venous and sympathetic plexus • Abducens nerve

Tributaries	
1. From orbit	Superior ophthalmic vein Branch of inferior ophthalmic vein Central vein of retina
2. From brain	Superficial middle cerebral vein Inferior cerebral veins
3. From meninges	Sphenoparietal sinus Frontal trunk of middle meningeal vein
4. Drainage or Communication	Transverse sinus through superior petrosal sinus. Internal jugular vein through inferior petrosal sinus Pterygoid venous plexus through emissary vein Facial vein through superior ophthalmic vein Intercommunicate by anterior and posterior intercavernous sinus

Note: All communications are valveless, blood can flow in either direction.

- **Thrombosis** of sinus can occur by infection in dangerous area of face.
- **Pulsatile exophthalmos:** During head injury if internal carotid artery communicates with cavernous sinus.
- **Dorello's canal:** A dural tunnel through abducens nerve enters cavernous sinus.

12. Nerve passing between posterior cerebral artery and superior cerebellar artery is:

a. Optic b. Abducens
c. Trigeminal d. Oculomotor

Ans. d. Oculomotor *Ref: Snell Clinical Neuroanatomy 7th/ed, Barr's The Human Nervous System: an Anatomical Viewpoint 10th/ed p117*

Explanation

Oculomotor nerve: Nucleus of III nerve present in periaqueductal gray matter of midbrain, ventral to aqueduct at the level of the superior colliculus.

- Myelinated axons curve through tegmentum and emerges from medial side of cerebral peduncle.
- **Passes in between posterior cerebral artery and superior cerebellar artery *(Answer)*.**
- Traverses subarachnoid space, cavernous sinus and superior orbital fissure.
- Supplies superior, medial and inferior rectus; inferior oblique and levator palpebrae superioris.
- Edinger westphal nucleus: Lies dorsal to oculomotor nucleus, axons goes with IIIrd nerve
- Preganglionic parasympathetic neurons terminate in ciliary ganglia.
- Postganglionic fibers carried by short ciliary nerve and supply Sphincter pupillae and ciliary muscle.

Clinical relevance:

- May be compressed by damage by aneurysm of posterior cerebral or superior cerebellar artery.
- **Third nerve palsy:** Ipsilateral slowness of pupillary light response (1st sign), ptosis, lateral strabismus, dilatation of pupil.
- Edinger Westphal nucleus is involved in light reflex and accommodation reflex.
- **Light reflex:** Afferent from optic nerve, optic tract to olivary pretectal nucleus. Then goes to EW nucleus finally to sphincter pupillae.
- **Consensual light reflex:** Both pupil contracts. Due to each optic tract contains fibers from both retinas and pretectal area projects to contralateral and ipsilateral EW nucleus.
- **Accommodation reflex:** Relayed through superior colliculus to EW nucleus then to muscles.
- **Marcus Gunn pupil:** Paradoxical light reflex in optic neuritis mainly due to multiple sclerosis when one eye is blind.
- **Holmes-Adie pupil:** Both light and accommodation reflex is slow due to damage of some neurons in ciliary ganglia.
- **Argyll-Robertson pupil ARP:** Accommodation reflex present. PRA-pupillary reflex absent. Due to syphilitic disease of CNS.

13. Vein of Labbe, true is:

a. Anastomotic channel for superior cerebral veins
b. Drains in superior sagittal sinus
c. Drains in transverse sinus
d. Superior anastomotic channel for superficial middle cerebral vein

Ans. c. Drains in transverse sinus

Ref: Barr's The Human Nervous System: An Anatomical Viewpoint 10th/ed p382-383

Explanation

Vein of Labbe: Inferior anastomotic vein for superficial middle cerebral vein, drains in transverse sinus.

Venous Drainage of Brain

Veins	Area of drainage	Connections	Opens into
External cerebral veins			
1. Superior cerebral veins	Lateral surface 8–12 in number	—	Superior sagittal sinus
2. Superficial middle cerebral vein	Runs along lateral sulcus	1. Vein of Trolard-superior anastomotic vein-opens in superior sagittal sinus. 2. Vein of Labbe-Inferior anastomotic vein-Drain in transverse sinus ***(Answer)***	Cavernous sinus
3. Deep middle cerebral vein	Depth of lateral sulcus, ventral surface of brain	—	—
4. Anterior cerebral vein	Accompanies anterior cerebral artery	—	—
5. Basal vein	Union of deep middle cerebral vein and anterior cerebral vein	Receives tributaries from optic tract, hypothalamus, temporal lobe and midbrain	Great cerebral vein
Internal cerebral veins (Union of thalamostriate and choroidal vein)			
1. Thalamostriate vein	Medial side of curve of tail of caudate nucleus	Tributaries from corpus striatum, internal capsule, thalamus, fornix and septum pellucidum	—
2. Choroidal vein	Drains choroid plexus of lateral ventricle	Tributaries from hippocampus, fornix and corpus callosum	—
Great cerebral vein of Galen	Union of paired internal cerebral veins	Receives basal veins and tributaries from cerebellum	Straight sinus

14. Geniculate ganglion situated in:

a. Near pyramid
b. Facial canal
c. Stylomastoid foramen
d. Aditus

Ans. b. Facial canal

Ref: Snell Clinical Neuroanatomy 7th/ed p346-348, Barr's The Human Nervous System: An Anatomical Viewpoint 10th/ed p129-134; Gray's Anatomy 41st/ed p632-635.

Explanation

Geniculate ganglion: Ganglion of facial nerve containing cell bodies of all sensory fibers.

Facial nerve components and its course is as follows:

- ❑ Facial nerve has 2 sensory component—one supplies taste bud and other to cutaneous fibers to external ear.
- ❑ Motor axons supply muscles of facial expressions.

- ❑ Preganglionic parasympathetic fibers go to ganglia and supply lacrimal, submandibular and sublingual glands.
- ❑ Sensory and preganglionic parasympathetic axons are located in nervus intermedius, located between motor root and vestibulocochlear nerve.
- ❑ **Two roots of facial nerve enters facial canal and joins at geniculate ganglion *(Answer)***, situated at bend of nerve traversing **facial canal *(Answer)***.
- ❑ Greater petrosal nerve leaves facial nerve at ganglion level.
- ❑ Facial canal and nerve bends distal to ganglion, backward and downward, coming to medial wall of middle ear cavity.
- ❑ Motor branch to stapedius muscle is given out.
- ❑ Turns backward above promontory.
- ❑ Comes to floor posterior wall, giving chorda tympani branch.
- ❑ Descends behind pyramid and emerges through stylomastoid foramen.

Physiology

Author: Ambrish Tiwari, Co-authors: Barun Hanjubam Sharma, Sankalp Jha

AIIMS May 2017

1. Calculate forced expiratory volume in 1 sec/forced vital capacity (FEV1/FVC) ratio from the following spirometry curve?

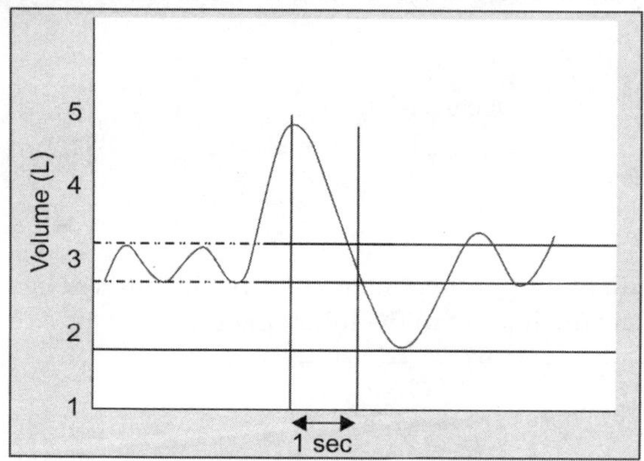

a. 90–99%
b. 80–89%
c. 70–79%
d. 60–69%

Ans. c. 70–79% *Ref: Ganong 24th/ed p629-630; Berne & Levy 6th/ed p443*

Figure given below helps in solving question:

On comparing figure given in question and figure given below

FVC: 5–1 = 4 L

FEV1: 5–2 = 3 L

So FEV1/FVC ratio = 3 L/4 L ~70–79%

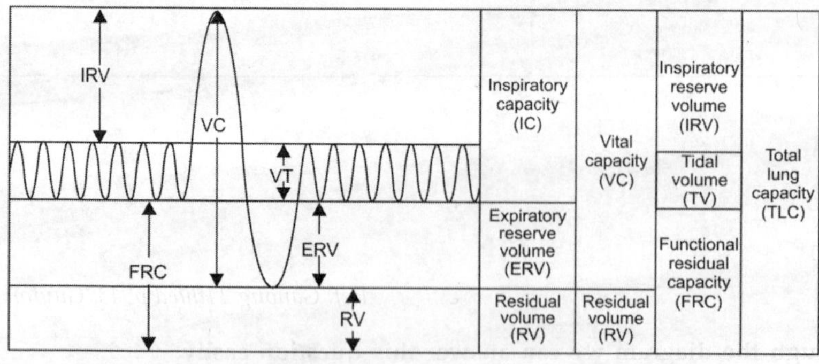

Other important points regarding FEV1 and FVC are:

- FEV1 and the ratio FEV1/FVC help in differentiating between two major patterns of abnormal ventilation — Obstructive and Restrictive (constricted) lung diseases.

Pulmonary function measurement	Obstructive pulmonary disease	Restrictive pulmonary disease
FVC (L)	Decrease	Decrease
FEV1 (L)	Decrease	Decrease
FEV1/FVC	Decrease	Normal
FEF_{25-75} (L/sec)	Decrease	Normal to increased
PEFR (L/sec)	Decrease	Normal
FEF_{50} (L/sec)	Decrease	Normal
FEF_{75} (L/sec)	Decrease	Normal
Slope of FV curve	Decrease	Normal to increased

2. ECG is recorded with phonocardiogram to identify the different heart sounds. Second heart sound will appear at which point in the following diagram?

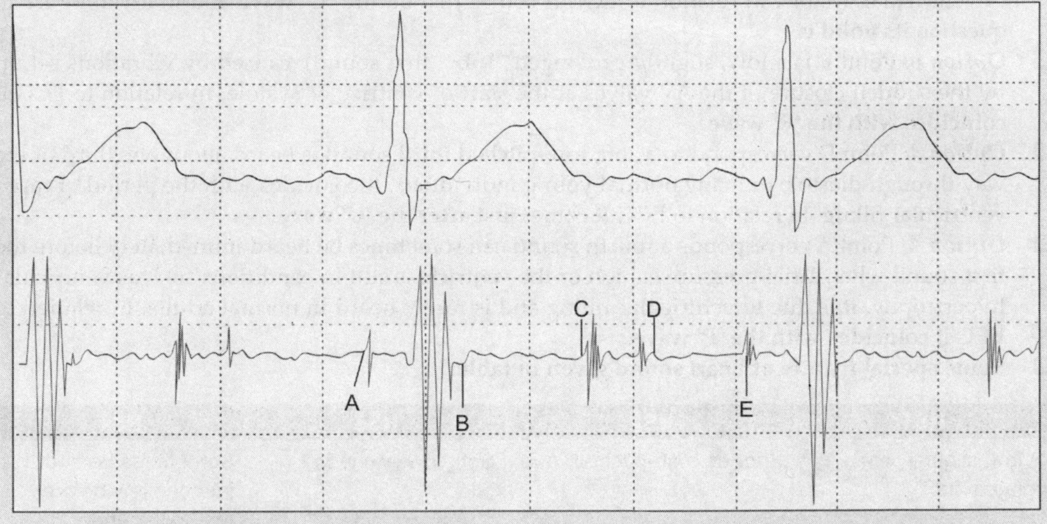

a. Point A
b. Point B
c. Point C
d. Point D

Ans. c. Point C *Ref: Ganong 24th/ed p543; Guyton 13th/ed. p114*

Via going through the diagram we can answer this question easily.

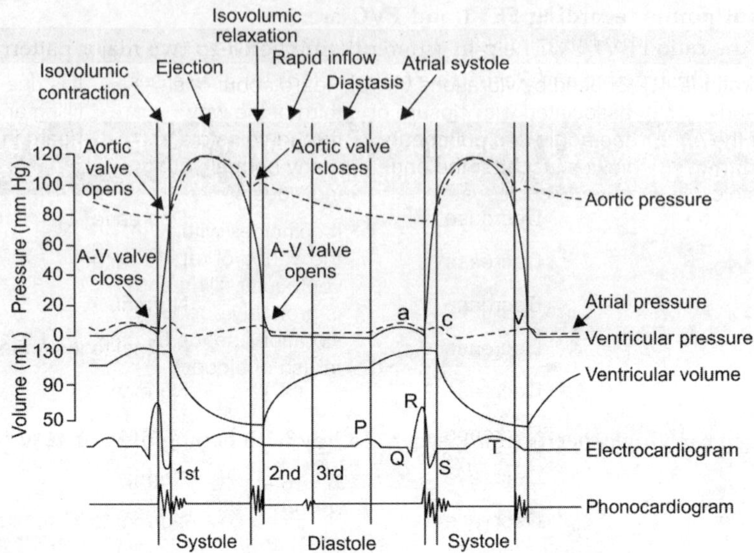

Two sounds are normally heard through a stethoscope during each cardiac cycle.

- *Option c:* is correct because the second is a shorter, high-pitched "dup" (second sound), caused by vibrations associated with closure of the aortic and pulmonary valves just after the end of ventricular systole. In relation to ECG it comes **just before 'U' wave** and in given figure in question its **point c**.
- *Option b:* Point B is a low, slightly prolonged "**lub**" (first sound), caused by vibrations set up by the sudden closure of the AV valves at the start of ventricular systole. In relation to ECG it **coincides with the 'R' wave**.
- *Option d:* Point D correspond to a soft, low-pitched third sound is heard about one third of the way through diastole in many normal young individuals. It coincides with the period of rapid ventricular filling. In relation to ECG it comes just **after the 'U' wave**.
- *Option A:* Point A corresponds a fourth sound can sometimes be heard immediately before the first sound when atrial pressure is high or the ventricle is stiff in conditions such as ventricular hypertrophy. It is due to ventricular filling and is rarely heard in normal adults. In relation to ECG it **coincides with the 'P' wave.**
- **Some special feature of heart sound given in table:**

HS1	HS2	HS3	HS4
A low, slightly prolonged "lub"	Shorter, high-pitched "dup"	Soft, low-pitched	Sometimes be heard immediately before the first sound
A duration of about 0.15 s and a frequency of 25 to 45 Hz	The second sound lasts about 0.12 s, with a frequency of 50 Hz		
	It is loud and sharp when the diastolic pressure in the aorta or pulmonary artery is elevated, diseases		

Contd...

Contd...

HS1	HS2	HS3	HS4
Caused by vibrations set up by the sudden closure of the AV valves at the start of ventricular systole	Caused by vibrations associated with closure of the aortic and pulmonary valves just after the end of ventricular systole	Heard about one third of the way through diastole in many normal young individuals	It is due to ventricular filling and is rarely heard in normal adults
		It coincides with the period of rapid ventricular filling and is probably due to vibrations set up by the inrush of blood	

3. The oxygen carrying capacity of a 18-year-old boy with hemoglobin of 14 g/dL is:

a. 14 b. 16
c. 18 d. 22

Ans. c. 18 *Ref: Textbook of Medical Physiology by RL Bijlani, 4th/ed, p227 and Ganong's Physiology, p642*

Explanation

Carrying capacity (CaO_2) = (SaO_2 × Hb × 1.34) + 0.003 (PaO_2)

- Oxygen content of the artery depends upon oxygen saturation of the blood, Hb concentration and partial pressure of the oxygen
- Saturated hemoglobin has 1.34 mL of O_2
- Hemoglobin concentration in normal blood is about 15 g/dL (14 g/dL in women and 16 g/dL in men).
- 1 dL of blood contains 20.1 mL (1.34 mL × 15) of O_2 bound to hemoglobin when the hemoglobin is 100% saturated.
- The amount of dissolved O_2 is a linear function of the PO_2 (0.003 mL/dL blood/mm Hg PO_2.
- So in given question if Hb is 14g/dL and normal saturation is 97% so
CaO_2 = 0.97 × 14 × 1.34 + 0.003 = 18.2 (Thus the answer)

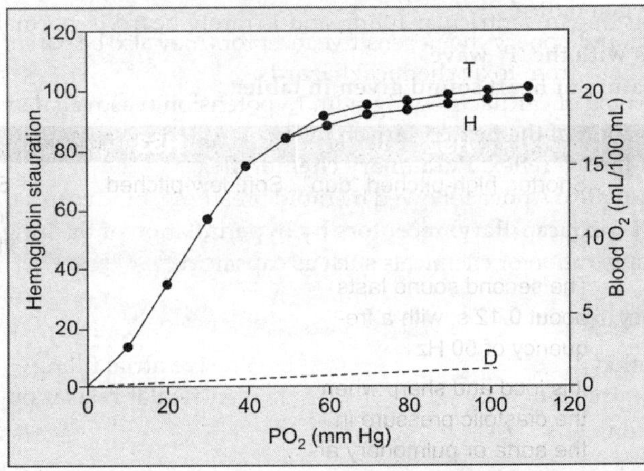

T: Total amount of oxygen carried; H: Oxygen in association with hemoglobin; D: Dissolved oxygen.

In the figure: At the steep portion of the curve between 15 and 40 mm Hg (range of low PO_2), any small increase in PO_2 increases the oxygen carrying capacity of the blood markedly.

Thus at high altitudes, any increase in PO_2 achieved by giving 100% oxygen for breathing is highly beneficial.

4. Bezold-Jarisch reflex is mediated by:

a. Angiotensin b. Histamine
c. Serotonin d. Prostaglandin

Ans. c. Serotonin *Ref: Ganong 25th/ed p592 and 664, Boron p1133*

Bezold-Jarisch Reflex

- ***Option c*** is correct because in experiment on cats rabbit and rodent it is found that stimuli for Bezold-Jarisch reflex are capsaicin, ***serotonin***, phenylbiguanide and veratridine.
- Activation of chemosensitive vagal C fibers in the cardiopulmonary region causes profound bradycardia, hypotension and a brief period of apnea followed by rapid shallow breathing. This response pattern is called the Bezold-Jarisch reflex.
- Vasovagal syncope (VVS) has been attributed to activation of the Bezold-Jarisch reflex.
- ***Option a*** is incorrect because angiotensin is a peptide hormone that cause vasoconstriction and subsequently lead to hypertension.
- ***Option b*** is incorrect because histamine involved in local immune response as well as it also acts as neurotransmitter in uterus and physiological response in gut. It also plays central role in pruritis.
- ***Option d*** is incorrect because prostaglandin has role in constriction or dilation of smooth muscles, platelet aggregation, inducing labor pain, etc.
- ***Other important associated points:***

Receptor	Chemosensitive vagal C fibers in the cardiopulmonary region (e.g. juxtacapillary region of alveoli, ventricles, atria, great veins, and pulmonary artery)
Stimuli	By a variety of substances including capsaicin, serotonin, phenylbiguanide, and veratridine in cats, rabbits, and rodents
Response/effect	Profound bradycardia, hypotension, and a brief period of apnea followed by rapid shallow breathing.

- This reflex may be activated during myocardial ischemia and reperfusion as a result of increased production of oxygen radicals.
- Activation of cardiopulmonary chemosensitive receptors may also be part of a defense mechanism protecting individuals from toxic chemical hazards.
- Finally, the syndrome of cardiac slowing with hypotension **(vasovagal syncope)** has also been attributed to activation of the Bezold-Jarisch reflex.
- Similar to Bezold-Jarisch reflex: **Pulmonary chemoreflex.**
- **Pulmonary chemoreflex:** Apnea followed by rapid breathing, bradycardia, and hypotension due to stimulation of **J (juxtacapillary) receptors by** hyperinflation of the lung or by intravenous or intracardiac administration of chemicals such as capsaicin.

5. In JVP 'a' wave is due to:

a. Atrial contraction b. Passive atrial filling
c. Ventricular contraction d. Ventricular relaxation

Ans. a. Atrial contraction *Ref: Guyton 13th/ed p111*

- ***Option a*** is correct because in **JVP pressure** changes in the atria represented by: a, c, and v waves and the ***a wave*** is caused by ***atrial contraction***

- *Option b* is incorrect because the **c wave** occurs when the **ventricles begin to contract**; it is caused partly by **slight backflow of blood into the atria** at the onset of ventricular contraction but mainly by bulging of the A-V valves backward toward the atria because of increasing pressure in the ventricles.
- *Option c* is incorrect because the **v wave** occurs toward the end of **ventricular contraction**; it results from slow flow of blood into the atria, the A-V valves open, allowing this stored atrial blood to flow rapidly into the ventricles and causing the v wave to disappear.

Answer easily by table and figure given below:

Phases of cardiac cycle:

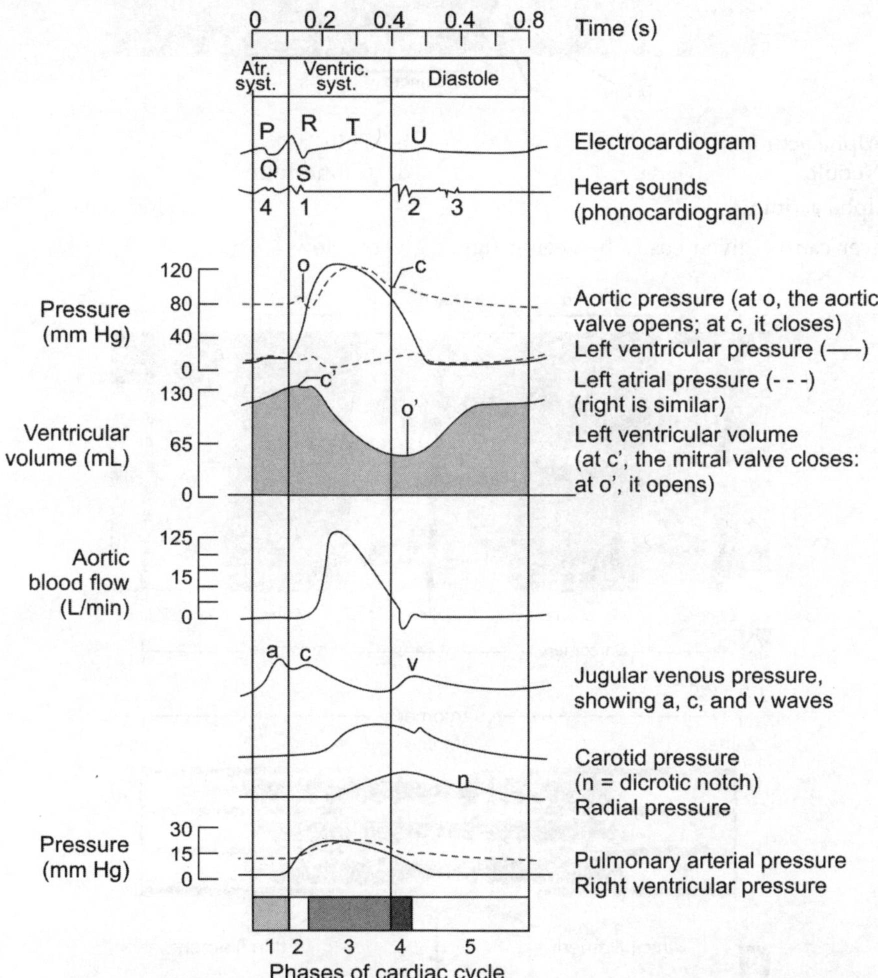

JVP (Jugular Venous Pressure) waves	
a wave	Due to **atrial systole** some blood regurgitates into the great veins when the atria contract.
c wave	It is the transmitted manifestation of the rise in atrial pressure produced by the bulging of the tricuspid valve into the atria during **isovolumetric ventricular contraction**.
v wave	Due to **ventricular contraction**. The jugular pulse waves are superimposed on the respiratory fluctuations in venous pressure.

6. Which of the following is the constituent of the marked area in the electron microscopic picture of muscle?

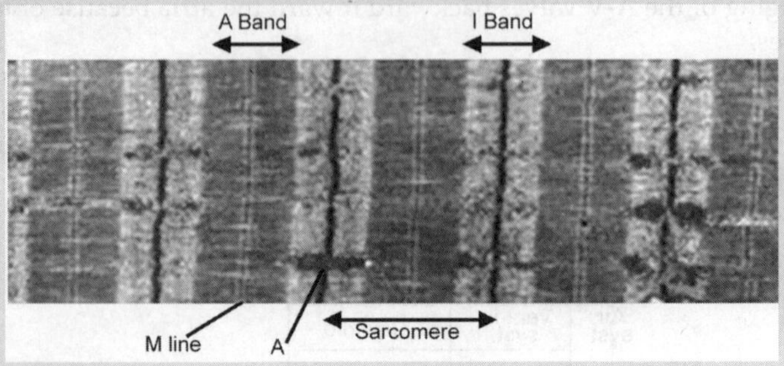

a. Alpha actinin
b. Titin
c. Nebulin
d. Calmodulin

Ans. a. Alpha actinin *Ref: Ganong 25th/ed p101*

Answer can be given easily by seeing figure given below:

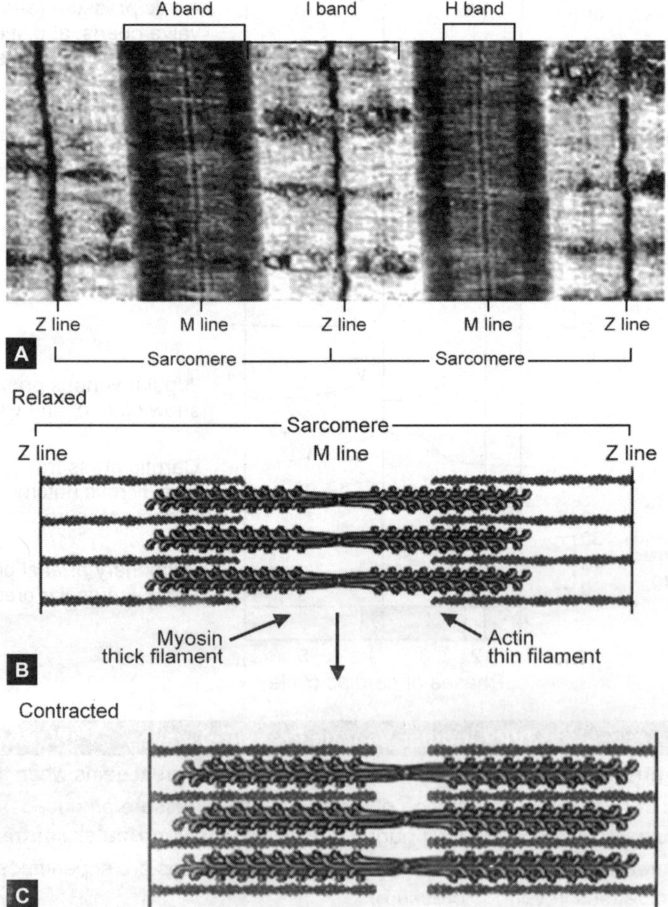

- ❑ Each muscle fiber is a single cell that is multinucleated, long, cylindrical, and surrounded by a cell membrane, the sarcolemma.
- ❑ The contractile mechanism in skeletal muscle largely depends on the proteins myosin-II, actin, tropomyosin, and troponin.
- ❑ The form of myosin found in muscle is myosin-II, with two globular heads and a long tail.
- ❑ The myosin molecules are arranged symmetrically on either side of the center of the sarcomere, and it is this arrangement that creates the light areas in the pseudo-H zone.
- ❑ Each of the three troponin subunits has a unique function.
- ❑ Troponin T binds the troponin components to tropomyosin
- ❑ Troponin I inhibits the interaction of myosin with actin.
- ❑ Troponin C contains the binding sites for the Ca^{2+} that helps initiate contraction.
- ❑ **Actinin** binds actin to the Z lines
- ❑ Titin connects the Z lines to the M lines and provides scaffolding for the sarcomere.
- ❑ Desmin adds structure to the Z lines in part by binding the Z lines to the plasma membrane.

7. Calculate tetanizing frequency of frog gastrocnemius muscle from the graph shown below:

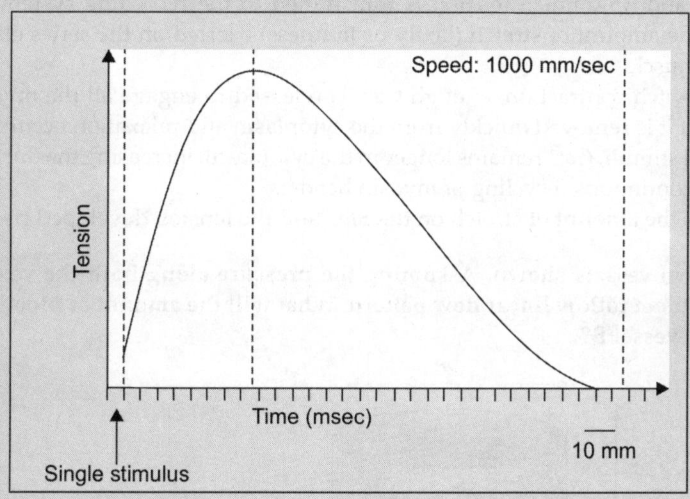

a. 25–30 Hz
b. 30–35 Hz
c. 35–40 Hz
d. 40–50 Hz

Ans. a. 25–30 Hz *Ref: Cl GHAI Experimental Physiology (Amphibian and Mammalian Experiments) 20th/ed p330*

Explanation

In order to produce tetany a muscle must get another stimulus just before it starts relaxing. So if the muscle starts relaxation after T seconds then the frequency of the stimulus must be: one stimulus per T seconds = 1/T sec^{-1} i.e., 1/T Hz

In the figure in question, see the following points:

- ❑ Tetanising frequency is 1/T (where T= time point just before the time of relaxation)
- ❑ Calculate T from the figure in question:
  - ■ Speed is 1000 mm/sec
  - ■ 10 mm = 2 units on the X axis

- Relaxation starts at 8 units, that is at 40 mm
- Convert this 40 mm to seconds, it will be 40/1000 seconds

- Now, tetanising frequency = 1/T = 1000/40 = 25 per sec or 25 Hz, ***thus the answer***

Important terminologies in relation to the above question:

- On applying many successive stimuli, the response of the muscle depends on the frequency of stimulation.
- At low rates of stimulations, the muscle gives jerky or tremulous contractions called subtetanus.
- At high frequencies, the muscle remains in a state of smooth, sustained, and forceful contraction called tetanus.
- The "tetanizing" or "fusion" frequency is that rate of stimulation at which there is complete fusion of individual contractions to produce tetanus.
- In amphibian muscle and in "slow" muscle fibers, the tetanizing frequency is about 30/sec, while in mammalian muscle and in "fast" fibers, it is 60 or more stimuli per second.
- The term tetanus should not be confused with a disease called tetanus (widespread convulsions in the body due to tetanus toxin released by the infecting bacteria).
- How much tension is developed by a muscle depends on the active state of the contractile components; and how much tension is transmitted to the recording system (or to the bone) depends on the amount of stretch (laxity or tautness) exerted on the series elastic components (SEC) of the muscle.
- During one twitch contraction, enough Ca^{2+} is released to engage all the myosin heads to the actin sites, but it is removed quickly from the cytoplasm and relaxation occurs.
- With repeated stimuli, Ca^{2+} remains longer in the cytoplasm, increasing the duration of the active state (due to continuous recycling of myosin heads).
- This increases the amount of stretch on the SEC and the tension developed rises.

8. Below are two vessels shown. Assuming the pressure along both the vessels is the same and both of them follow linear flow pattern. What will the amount of blood flow in vessel A compared to vessel B?

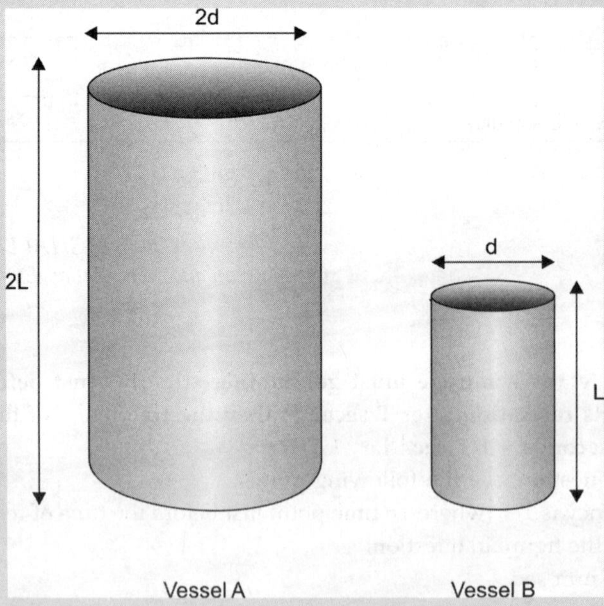

a. 4 times
b. 8 times
c. 16 times
d. 32 times

Ans. b. 8 times *Ref: Ganong 24th/ed p575*

EXPLANATION

- Question asks about blood flow in vessel A compared to vessel B. This can be answered by understanding Poiseuille's law:
- Poiseuille's Law states that the flow of fluid is related to a number of factors:
  - The viscosity (n) of the fluid
  - The pressure gradient across the vessel (P)
  - Length (L) and diameter(r) of the vessel
- The relationship is given by Poiseuille–Hagen formula:

$$F = (P_A - P_B) \times \left(\frac{\pi}{8}\right) \times \left(\frac{1}{\eta}\right) \times \left(\frac{r^4}{L}\right)$$

- Where

  F = Flow
  $P_A - P_B$ = Pressure difference between two ends of the tube
  η = Viscosity
  r = Radius of tube
  L = Length of tube
- Now see the question again,
  - Diameter is doubled, means radius is doubled (consider 2r)
  - Length is doubled (2L)
  - On substituting the values in formula;
    $(2r)^4/(2L)$ = 8 times increase in flow **(Thus the answer is b.)**

9. In a diseased person intrapleural pressure measured –4 mm Hg and –9 mm Hg at the start and end of inspiration having tidal volume 500 mL. Calculate pulmonary compliance in Lit/mm Hg:

a. 0.1 b. 0.2
c. 0.5 d. 0.7

Ans. a. 0.1 *Ref: Respiratory Physiology by John B West, 9th/ed p99*

- The slope of the pressure-volume curve, or the **volume change per unit pressure change**, is known as the *compliance* ***(delta V/ delta P)***
- Tidal volume is change in volume per respiration. So its *delta V = 500 mL*
- So in litre = 0.5 L *and* Delta P given 9–4 = 5 mm Hg
- So compliance = 0.5/5 = **0.1 Lit/mm Hg**
- Compliance of the normal human lung = 200 mL·cm water-1.
- At high expanding pressures lung is stiffer, and its compliance smaller (flatter slope of the curve)
- ***Reduced* compliance**
  - Increase of fibrous tissue in the lung (pulmonary fibrosis)
  - Alveolar edema (prevents the inflation of alveoli)
  - Lung unventilated for a long period
  - If the pulmonary venous pressure is increased and the lung becomes engorged with blood.

- An *increased* compliance
  - Pulmonary emphysema
  - Normal aging lung
  - During an asthma attack

10. A diabetic patient having blood glucose of 200 mg/dL and GFR of 90 mL/min. Transport maximum of glucose = 150 mg/min. What is the amount of glucose excreted in urine?

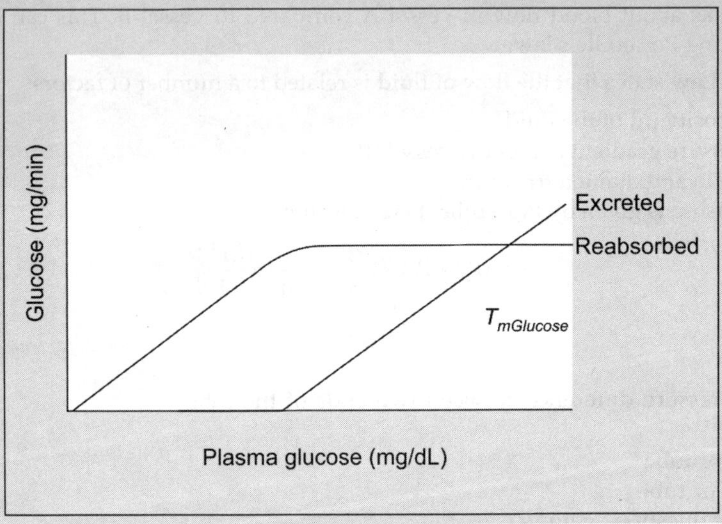

a. 10 mg/min
b. 20 mg/min
c. 30 mg/min
d. 40 mg/min

Ans. c. 30 mg/min *Ref: Guyton, 13th/ed p350*

EXPLANATION

Solution of question:

- Given GFR = 90 mL/min
- Plasma concentration = 200 mg/dL or we can say that 200 mg/100 mL = 2 mg/mL
- So Filtration load = 90 × 2 = 180 mg/min
- But in question they asked excretion rate
- Excretion rate = filtration rate–reabsorption
- And reabsorption is equal to threshold maximum which is given 150 mg/min
- So excretion rate in given question = 180–150 = 30 mg/min
- So correct answer of this question is ***option c***
- Transport maximum is the maximum rate at which glucose can be reabsorbed from the tubules. The threshold for glucose refers to the filtered load of glucose at which glucose first begins to be excreted in the urine
- Transport maximum for substances that are actively reabsorbed
  - There is a limit to the rate at which the solute can be transported, which is often referred to as the transport maximum
  - Limit is due to saturation of the specific transport systems involved when the amount of solute delivered to the tubule (referred to as tubular load) exceeds the capacity of the carrier proteins and specific enzymes involved in the transport process.

  e.g. glucose transport system in the proximal tubule

- Normally, measurable glucose does not appear in the urine because essentially all the filtered glucose is reabsorbed in the proximal tubule.
- However, when the filtered load exceeds the capability of the tubules to reabsorb glucose, urinary excretion of glucose does occur.
- Adult - transport maximum for glucose = 375 mg/min
  - Filtered load of glucose = 125 mg/min

  (GFR × plasma glucose = 125 mL/min × 1 mg/mL).

  With large increases in GFR and/or plasma glucose concentration that increase the filtered load of glucose above 375 mg/min, the excess glucose filtered is not reabsorbed and passes into the urine.

Figure below shows the relation between plasma concentration of glucose, fltered load of glucose, tubular transport maximum for glucose, and rate of glucose loss in the urine.

- Note that when the plasma glucose concentration is 100 mg/100 mL and the filtered load is at its normal level (125 mg/min) there is no loss of glucose in the urine.
- However, when the plasma concentration of glucose rises above about 200 mg/100 mL, increasing the filtered load to about 250 mg/min, a small amount of glucose begins to appear in the urine. This point is termed the threshold for glucose.
- Note that this appearance of glucose in the urine (at the threshold) occurs before the transport maximum is reached.

  One reason for the difference between threshold and transport maximum
  - **Not all nephrons have the same transport maximum** for glucose some of the nephrons therefore begin to excrete glucose before others have reached their transport maximum.
- However, in uncontrolled diabetes mellitus, plasma glucose may rise to high levels, causing the filtered load of glucose to exceed the transport maximum and resulting in urinary glucose excretion.

Substances that are Actively Transported but Do Not Exhibit a Transport Maximum.

- The reason that actively transported solutes often exhibit a transport maximum is that the transport carrier system becomes saturated as the tubular load increases.
- Some substances that are passively reabsorbed do not demonstrate a transport maximum because their rate of transport is determined by:

1. The electrochemical gradient for diffusion of the substance across the membrane
2. The permeability of the membrane for the substance
3. The time that the fluid containing the substance remains within the tubule.

   (Referred to as gradient-time transport because the rate of transport depends on the electrochemical gradient and the time that the substance is in the tubule, which in turn depends on the tubular flow rate).

   e.g. sodium reabsorption in the proximal tubule, where the maximum transport capacity of the basolateral sodium-potassium ATPase pump is usually far greater than the actual rate of net sodium reabsorption since a significant amount of sodium transported out of the cell leaks back into the tubular lumen through junctions of the epithelial cells. Therefore, **sodium transport in the proximal tubules obeys mainly gradient-time transport principles rather than tubular maximum transport characteristics.**

- In the more **distal parts of the nephron**, the epithelial cells have much tighter junctions and transport much smaller amounts of sodium, thus **sodium reabsorption exhibits a transport maximum similar to that for other actively transported substances.**
- Transport maximum can be increased by aldosterone.

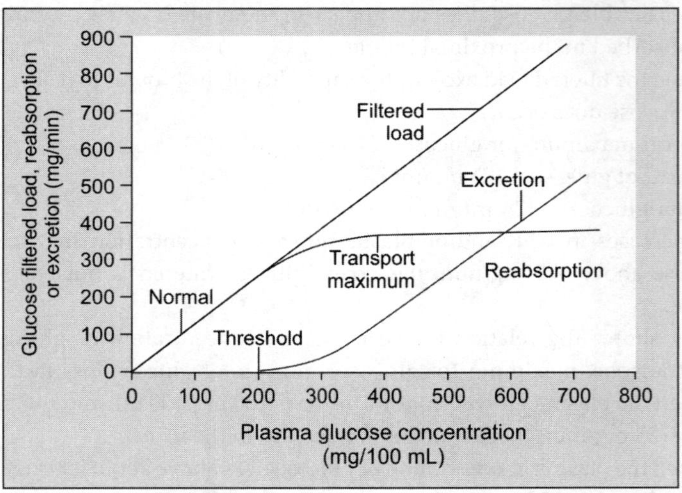

Plasma glucose concentration (mg/100 mL)

PGI MAY 2017

1. Which of the following is/are true regarding Sertoli cells?

a. Are true epithelial cells
b. Spermatids head lie embedded in sertoli cells towards lumen
c. Sertoli cells secrete androgen binding protein
d. Sertoli cells secrete AMH which brings Mullerian involution
e. Inhibin has a negative feedback on gonadotropes
f. Inhibin produced by spermatids
g. Local estrogen production by enzyme CYP19

Ans: a. Are true epithelial cells; c. Sertoli cells secrete androgen binding protein; d. Sertoli cells secrete AMH which brings Mullerian involution; e. Inhibin has a negative feedback on gonadotropes and g. Local estrogen production by enzyme CYP19 *Ref: Ganong, 24th/ed p419*

EXPLANATION

- ❑ ***Option a*** is correct because sertoili cells are true epithelial cells
- ❑ ***Option b*** is incorrect because elongated spermatids lie at the luminal surface with their heads embedded in Sertoli cell cytoplasmic invaginations and the tails extending into the lumen.
- ❑ ***Option c and d*** is Sertoli cells secrete **androgen binding protein (ABP), inhibin, anti-Müllerian hormone (AMH)/MIS.**
- ❑ ***Option d and e*** is correct because inhibin secreted by Sertoli cells in male and granulosa cells in female which has a negative feedback on gonadotropes (FSH regulation).
- ❑ ***Option g*** is correct because even they do not synthesize androgens but they contain **aromatase (CYP19),** the enzyme responsible for local conversion of androgens to estrogens, and they can produce estrogens.

Other important associated points:

- ❑ The regulation of spermatogenesis by FSH and testosterone occurs by the action of these hormones on the Sertoli cells. While the action of testosterone is necessary for spermatogenesis, the action of FSH minimally
- ❑ Reproductive hormones such as FSH and testosterone acts on Sertoli cells and not on germ cells.
- ❑ FSH acts on Sertoli cells by increased levels of cAMP, increased protein synthesis and increased estradiol production.
- ❑ Testosterone receptors are present in Sertoli and peritubular cell.
- ❑ The relationship between the germinal cells and the Sertoli cells is obligatory in testis development as well as in spermatogenesis.
- ❑ Sertoli cells are the somatic cells of the testis essential for testis formation and spermatogenesis.
- ❑ Sertoli cells facilitate the progression of germ cells to spermatozoa via direct contact and by controlling the environment milieu within the seminiferous tubules (in the form of physical support, junctional complexes or barriers, or biochemical stimulation in the form of growth).
- ❑ Serves to promote spermatogenic output by increasing the number of Sertoli cells.
- ❑ Following testis formation Sertoli cells and germ cells undergo rapid proliferation.
- ❑ Puberty involves cessation of mitosis of Sertoli cells formation of tight junctions between adjacent Sertoli cells progression of germ cells through meiosis differentiation into spermatozoa.
- ❑ Persistence of the tight junctional complexes and the two compartment system in the testis is required for spermatogenesis.
- ❑ Sertoli cells make and secrete a number of proteins that form the molecular basis for Sertoli germ cell interactions.
- ❑ The glycoproteins secreted by the Sertoli cells ***transport or bioprotective proteins,*** for example:
  - Metal ion transport proteins such as transferrin and ceruloplasmin
  - Growth factors or paracrine factors
  - Mullerian inhibiting substance (MIS)
  - Inhibin

Figure given below showing arrangements of Sertoli cells and spermatids

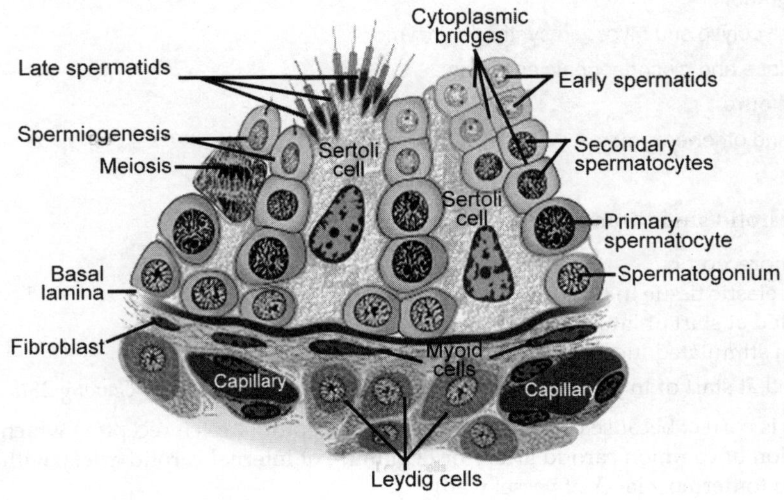

2. Effect of insulin:

a. Import potassium
b. Import calcium
c. Import sodium
d. Export potassium
e. Export sodium

Ans: a. Import potassium and e. Export sodium *Ref: Ganong 24th/ed p434*

- ***Option a and e*** is correct because Insulin activates sodium potassium ATPase which lead to influx of potassium and efflux of sodium ion in cell.
- Other effects are stimulating the uptake of amino acids, facilitating the entry of glucose into adipocytes (glycerol is synthesized from glucose inside cells contributing to its overall anabolic effect)
- Effects of **insulin** on various tissues:
- **Adipose tissue**:
  Increases: Glucose entry, fatty acid synthesis, glycerol phosphate synthesis, triglyceride deposition, activation of lipoprotein lipase, and *K+ uptake.*
  Decreases: Hormone-sensitive lipase
- **Muscle:**
  Increases: Glucose entry, glycogen synthesis, amino acid uptake, protein synthesis in ribosomes, ketone uptake and *K+ uptake.*
  Decreases: Protein catabolism, release of gluconeogenic amino acids.
- **Liver**:
  Increases: Glycogen synthesis, glycolysis. protein synthesis, lipid synthesis.
  Decreases: Ketogenesis and glucose output due to decreased gluconeogenesis.

Time dependent role of Insulin
Fast within second
↑ Transport of glucose, amino acid (AA) and K+ in insulin sensitive cells
Intermediate within minutes
↑ Protein synthesis
↑ Protein degradation
↑ Activity of glycolytic and glycogen synthase enzyme
↓ Phosphorylase and gluconeogenic enzymes
Late within hours
↑ Lipogenic and other enzymes

3. About carotid sinus, true is/are:

a. Chemoreceptor
b. High elastic tissue in tunica media and receptors lie here
c. Located at start of internal carotid artery
d. When stimulated increases sympathetic discharge

Ans. c. Located at start of Internal carotid artery *Ref: Ganong 25th/ed, 2016 p587*

- ***Option c*** is correct because carotid sinus is a baroreceptor (stretch receptor) which is located at termination of common carotid artery or beginning of internal carotid artery within the tunica albuginea (outermost layer of vessel wall)

- ❑ *Option b* is incorrect because it is located within the tunica albuginea (outermost layer of vessel wall) not in tunica media.
- ❑ *Option a* is incorrect because chemoreceptors:
  - **Peripheral arterial chemoreceptors** in the **carotid and aortic bodies:** Primarily activated by a reduction in partial pressure of oxygen **(PaO_2);** also respond to $PaCO_2$ and pH.
  - **Central chemoreceptors** located on the ventrolateral surface of the medulla. Primarily activated by local hypoxia and hypercapnia.

Other associated points associated with receptors:

- ❑ **Baroreceptors:** Sense pressure changes within the vessel and includes:
  - **Carotid sinus** and **aortic arch receptors**: Monitor arterial circulation
  - Cardiopulmonary receptors: Located in low pressure areas: atria, SVC, IVC, pulmonary circulation

Differences between carotid sinus and carotid body given below in tabular form:

	Carotid sinus	Carotid body
Function	Baroreceptor ***(Option a)***	Chemoreceptor
Location	Slight bulge at the termination of common carotid or at the beginning of internal carotid ***(Option c)***	Small structure that lies posterior to the point of bifurcation of common carotid artery
Stimulus	Fall in pressure (pulsatile >> constant pressure)	↓ PaO_2 >> ↓pH or ↑$PaCO_2$
Nerve supply	Glossopharyngeal nerve (branch carotid sinus nerve)	Glossopharyngeal nerve
Response when stimulated	Excess discharge from carotid sinus results in ↓ sympathetic discharge and ↑ vagal discharge	Main effects are on respiration; also cause vasoconstriction

4. Myocardial oxygen demand:

a. Increases with increased contractility
b. Directly proportional to wall tension
c. Proportional to the diameter of the ventricles
d. Major controller of myocardial blood flow

Ans. a. Increases with increased contractility; b. Directly proportional to wall tension; c. Proportional to the diameter of the ventricles and d. Major controller of myocardial blood flow

Ref: Ganong, 24th/ed p550; Physiology of Sport and Exercise, 5th/ed p190

- ❑ ***Option a*** is correct because myocardial oxygen demand (MOD) and myocardial oxygen consumption are not the same but often used interchangeably and depends on the contractile state of myocardium.
- ❑ ***Option b*** is correct because oxygen utilisation get increased when there is high systolic pressure which lead to increase wall tension of vessels. It means oxygen demand is directly proportional to wall tension
- ❑ ***Option c*** is correct because product of diameter of ventricle and its pressure is proportional to muscle tension and muscle tension proportional to oxygen demand so we can say that oxygen demand is proportional to diameter of ventricle.
- ❑ ***Option d*** is correct because MOD depends on need and need can be compensated by increased blood flow.
- ❑ Other associated important points:
  Oxygen consumption by the hearts depends upon:

1. Intramyocardial tension: O_2 requirement increases with increase in tension

2. The contractile state of the myocardium.
3. The heart rate and SBP: Myocardial oxygen uptake and myocardial blood flow are directly related to the product of HR and systolic blood (SBP), called as **rate–pressure product (RPP)**
4. Ventricular work done is the product of stroke volume and mean arterial pressure in the pulmonary artery or the aorta (for the right and left ventricle, respectively).

JIPMER Pattern Based

1. Which is not involved in sound localization?

a. MGB b. LGB
c. Inferior colliculus d. Auditory cortex

Ans: b. LGB *Ref: Boron & Boulpaep 2nd/ed p789*

- ❑ ***Option b*** because to lateral geniculate bodies (LGB) is component of visual pathway.
- ❑ ***Option a, c and d*** is correct because component of auditory pathway which helps in localization of sound.

Other associated points:

- ❑ To localize sound, the brain compares the timing and intensity of input to the ears.
- ❑ Neurons in each of the cochlear nuclei receive information from only the ear on that one side, whereas neurons from the medial superior olivary (MSO) nucleus—and higher CNS centers receive abundant input from both ears.
- ❑ The cochlea does not have any map for sound location. Instead, the CNS localizes low-frequency sounds by calculating an interaural time delay map, using information from both ears together.
- ❑ **The inferior colliculus** receives parallel information on both timing delay and intensity difference; it transforms these two sets of information, combines them, and produces a complete map of sound direction.
- ❑ Figure given below showing central auditory pathway:

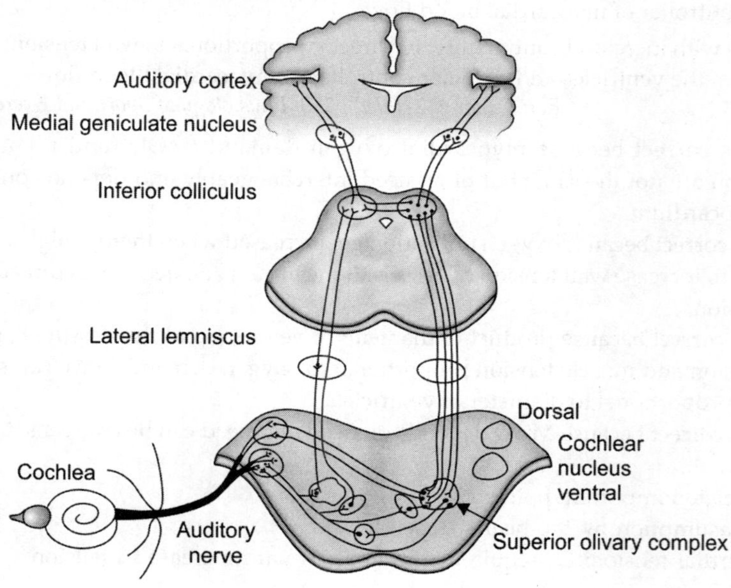

2. What happens when doubling the diffusion capacity of lungs?

a. Increased O_2 uptake from alveolar gas
b. Increased nitrous oxide anaesthesia induction
c. Increased O_2 delivery to tissues
d. Diffusion capacity value becomes 60 mL/min/mm Hg

Ans: d. Diffusion capacity value becomes 60 mL/min/mm Hg *Ref: Ganong 24th/ed p635*

- *Option a b and c* is incorrect because diffusion of O_2 and N_2O are perfusion limited so it does not lead to increase in uptake of O_2 from alveolar gases and delivery to tissue and also not lead to increase induction of anesthesia by N_2O.
- *Option d* is correct by excluding other options.

Other associated points on diffusion capacity:

- Diffusion through lungs occurs through single epithelium thick alveoli and pulmonary capillary each.
- Is reduced in fibrosis especially during exercise and PA-aO_2 gradient is increased, but responds to 100% O_2.
- Like O_2 and CO_2, CO has low solubility in alveolar capillary membrane but has high solubility in blood due to its high affinity for Hb.
- Also, due to high rate of equilibration of O_2 and CO_2 i.e. within 0.25 seconds, the transfer of O_2 and CO_2 is **normally** perfusion limited unlike CO which is diffusion limited.
- In rare conditions like very fit athelete during vigorous exercise and healthy person during exercise at high altitude O_2 uptake becomes diffusion limited, since RBC spends less than 0.25 seconds in capillary bed.

N_2O	O_2	CO
Flow limited	• Intermediate between N_2O and CO • **Perfusion-limited**	**Diffusion-limited**
The amount of N_2O taken up is not limited by diffusion but by the amount of blood flowing through the pulmonary capillaries	O_2 is taken up by hemoglobin, but much less avidly than CO, and it reaches equilibrium with capillary blood in about 0.3s	CO is taken up by hemoglobin in the red blood cells at such a high rate that the partial pressure of CO in the capillaries stays very low and equilibrium is not reached in the 0.75s the blood is in the pulmonary capillaries. Therefore, the transfer of CO is not limited by perfusion at rest, but by diffusion

Graph of diffusion capacity is given below for various gases:

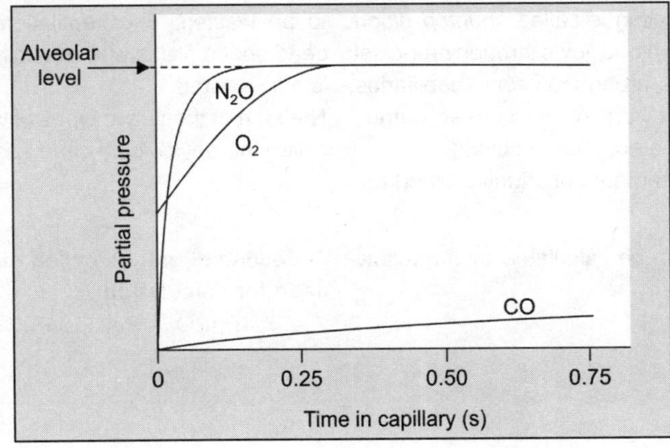

3. Find the amount of pulmonary shunt (Qs/Qt) in a 42-years-old anemic adult male with following findings, if alveolar oxygen concentration is doubled- Hb: h mg/dL, Arterial oxygen content (CaO_2): a mL/100 mL, Mixed venous oxygen content (CvO_2): v mL/100 mL

a. More than double
b. Less than double
c. Equal
d. Qudraple

Ans. b. Less than double *Ref: Respiratory Physiology: The Essentials, J. West, 2005, 7th/ed p169*

EXPLANATION

Option b is correct because

Pulmonary shunt $(Q_s/Q_t) = (CcO_2 - CaO_2)/(CcO_2 - CvO_2)$

$CcO_2 = (1.36 \times Hb) + (0.0031 \times PAO_2)$

Given values in question are:

$Hb = h$ mg/dL

$Ca\ O_2 = a$ mL/100 mL

$CvO_2 = v$ mL/100 mL

So if PAO_2 get doubled then $CcO_2 = 1.36 \times h + (0.0031 \times PAO_2)$

$PAO_2 = CcO2–1.36\ h/0.0031$

New PAO_2 get double then New CcO_2 will be $CcO_2' = 1.36h + (0.0031 \times 2\ [CcO_2–1.36\ h/0.0031])$

Then $CcO_2' = (2\ CcO_2 - 2.72h)$

So New Qs/Qt will be less than double of normal Qs/Qt.

Pulmonary Shunt

- Shunt fraction: Cardiac output fraction which does not equilibrate entirely with alveolar gas.
- Shunting results from the combined effects of anatomical shunt (i.e. no ventilation) and physiological shunt (i.e. V/Q mismatch like low V/Q areas).
- It is used to titrate Oxygen levels, asses breathing capabilities and act as a method of determining the cause of hypoxemia.

Physiologic shunt	Physiologic dead space
V_A/Q is below normal	V_A/Q is greater than normal
There is inadequate ventilation to provide the oxygen needed to fully oxygenate the blood flowing through the alveolar capillaries. Therefore, a certain fraction of the venous blood passing through the pulmonary capillaries does not become oxygenated. This fraction is called *shunted blood.* Also, some additional blood flows through bronchial vessels rather than through alveolar capillaries, normally about 2 per cent of the cardiac output; this, too, is unoxygenated, shunted blood. The total quantitative amount of shunted blood per minute	When ventilation of some of the alveoli is great but alveolar blood flow is low, there is far more available oxygen in the alveoli than can be transported away from the alveoli by the flowing blood. Thus, the ventilation of these alveoli is said to be *wasted.* The ventilation of the anatomical dead space areas of the respiratory passageways is also wasted. The sum of these two types of wasted ventilation is called the *physiologic dead space*
Physiologic shunt can be calculated by the following equation: $\frac{QPS}{QT} = \frac{Ci_{O_2} - Ca_{O_2}}{Ci_{O_2} - Cv_{O_2}}$	**Following equation, called the Bohr equation is used for calculation:** $V_D = V_T\ (PaCO_2 - PeCO_2)/PaCO_2$

Contd...

Contd...

Physiologic shunt	Physiologic dead space
Qps is the physiologic shunt blood flow per minute, Qt is cardiac output per minute, CiO_2 is the concentration of oxygen in the arterial blood if there is an"ideal" ventilation-perfusion ratio, CaO_2 is the measured concentration of oxygen in the arterial blood, and CvO_2 is the measured concentration of oxygen in the mixed venous blood	Where, V_D is the physiologic dead space, V_T is the tidal volume, $PaCO_2$ is the partial pressure of carbon dioxide in the arterial blood, and $PeCO_2$ is is the average partial pressure of carbon dioxide in the entire expired air
The greater the physiologic shunt, the greater the *amount of blood that fails to be oxygenated* as it passes through the lungs.	When the physiologic dead space is great, much of the *work of ventilation* is wasted effort because so much of the ventilating air never reaches the blood.
In the bottom of the lung, there is slightly too little ventilation in relation to blood flow, with, V_A/Q as low as 0.6 times the ideal value. In this area, a small fraction of the blood fails to become normally oxygenated, and this represents a *physiologic shunt.*	At the top of the lung, V_A/Q is as much as 2.5 times as great as the ideal value, which causes a moderate degree of *physiologic dead space* in this area of the lung. During exercise, blood flow to the upper part of the lung increases markedly, so that far less physiologic dead space occurs, and the effectiveness of gas exchange now approaches optimum.

4. Cerebellum input is from:

a. Inferior olive of medulla
b. Superior olive of medulla
c. Superior cerebellar peduncle primarily
d. Inferior cerebellar peduncle rarely

Ans. a. Inferior olive of medulla *Ref: Guyton 11th/ed p700-701*

- ❑ ***Option a*** is correct because all cerebellar nuclei receive special inputs from the inferior olive of the medulla.
- ❑ ***Option b*** is incorrect because superior olive of medulla project fibres to ipsilateral inferior olive nucleus.
- ❑ ***Option c is incorrect because*** superior cerebral peduncle consists mainly of efferent fibers, the **cerebellothalamic tract** that runs from a cerebellar hemisphere to the contralateral thalamus, and the cerebellorubral tract that runs from a cerebellar hemisphere to the red nucleus. It also contains afferent tracts, most prominent of which is the ventral **spinocerebellar tract**. Other afferent tracts are the trigeminothalamic fibers, tectocerebellar fibers, and noradrenergic fibers from the locus coeruleus
- ❑ ***Option d*** is incorrect because inferior cerebellar peduncle carries information leaving cerebellum: from the Purkinje cells to the vestibular nuclei in the dorsal brainstem located at the junction between the pons and medulla oblongata.

Other associated points are:

- ❑ Anatomical locations of the cerebellar nuclei correspond to the cerebellar cortex regions from which they receive input.
- ❑ The medially located fastigial nucleus receives input from the medially located vermis
- ❑ The slightly lateral interposed nuclei receive input from the slightly lateral intermediate zone
- ❑ The most lateral dentate nucleus receives input from the lateral hemispheres.
- ❑ Middle (frontal/parietal cortex to **pontine nuclei** to deep nuclei) and inferior peduncle (frontal/parietal cortex to red nuclei to inferior olive to deep nuclei) brings input from contralateral side

❑ **Figure below showing input and output tracts of cerebellum:**

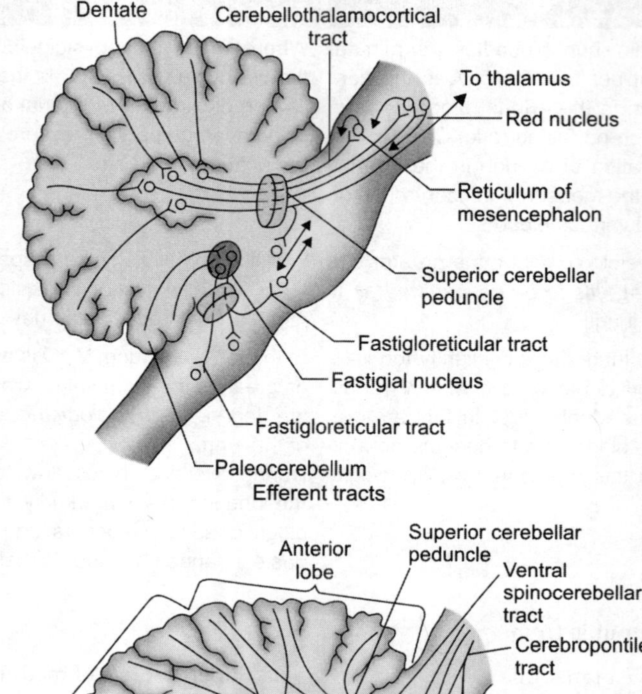

Efferent tracts

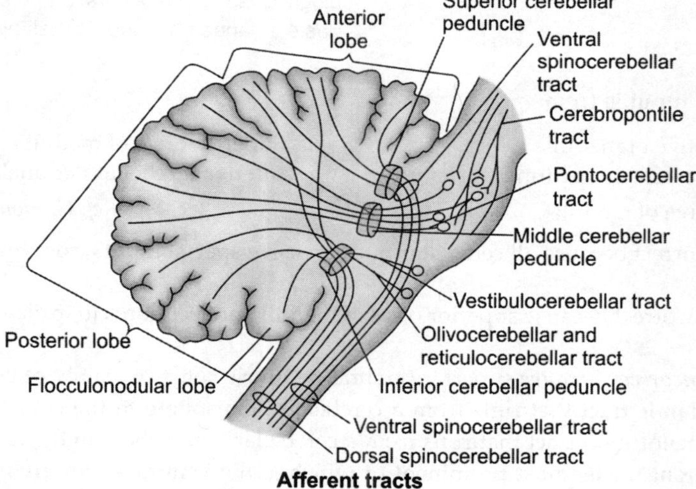

Afferent tracts

5. Glucose uptake in brain is by:

a. GLUT 1 and 3
b. GLUT 2 and 3
c. GLUT 3 and 4
d. GLUT 1 and 4

Ans: a. GLUT 1 and 3 *Ref: Ganong 25th/ed p*

For this question table given below:

Receptor	Location
GLUT 1	***Brain***, kidney, colon, placenta, erythrocytes
GLUT 2	Liver, pancreatic β cell, small intestine, kidney
GLUT 3	***Brain***, kidney, placenta
GLUT 4	Heart and skeletal muscle, adipose tissue

Contd...

Contd...

Receptor	Location
GLUT 5	Small intestine
SGLT 1	Small intestine and kidney

Some other associated points on GLUT:
- Glucose enters cells by facilitated diffusion or, in the intestine and kidneys, by secondary active transport with Na+.
- Seven different GLUTs, named GLUT 1–7, have been characterized (as shown in table).
- They differ from sodium-glucose linked transporters (SGLT-1 and SGLT-2), which are responsible for the secondary active transport of glucose in the intestine and renal tubules.

6. Maximum concentrating ability of kidney in preterm infant:

a. 400 mOsm b. 600 mOsm
c. 800 mOsm d. 500 mOsm

Ans. d. 500 mOsm *Ref: Pol~fiek E, Voeel J, Neugebauerov~, L, ~ebkov~, M, and V~chetov~, E; The osmotic concentrating ability in healthy infants and children, Arch. Dis. Child. 40:291,1965*

- **Option d** is correct because maximum concentrating ability of preterm infant kidney is 500 mOsm.
- Comparison for concentrating ability must be restricted to investigations in which an increased osmotic load or a restriction of fluid intake has been employed or a combination of both.

7. Mast cell degranulation is suggested by rise in .... serum levels.

a. Tryptase b. Major basic protein (MBP)-1
c. RNase3 d. Peroxidase (EPX)

Ans. a. Tryptase *Ref: Allergens and Allergen Immunotherapy, 5th/ed; By Richard F. Lockey, Dennis K. Ledford*

- ***Option a*** is correct because the primary source of tryptase in serum is mast cell. Two forms of tryptase α and β are produced
- ***Option b*** is incorrect because **Major basic protein** is the predominant constituent of the crystalline core of the eosinophil granule. High levels of the proform of this protein are also present in placenta and pregnancy serum, where it exists as a complex with several other proteins including pregnancy-associated plasma protein A **(PAPPA)**, angiotensinogen **(AGT)**, and C3dg
- ***Option c*** is incorrect because RNAse III is mainly present in cell membrane and cytoplasm and its a type of ribonuclease that cleaves rRNA (16s rRNA and 23s rRNA) from transcribed polycistronic RNA operon in prokaryotes.
- ***Option d*** is incorrect because peroxidase is found in mast cell but they are not specific for mast call they are also present in cell membrane and golgi bodies

Other associated points regarding tryptase:
- A pro-tryptase is continuously sectreted in blood but all mast cells as an inactive enzyme along with unprocessed β pro-tryptase and they are elevated in mastocytosis.
- In contrast, mature β-tryptase is released into blood along with prestored histamine following mast cell degranulation that is associated with anaphylaxis.
- The level of mature Beta tryptase is generally reflect the magnitude of mast cell activation.

8. Deglutitive inhibition:

a. Wave of inhibition preceding esophageal peristalsis
b. Inhibition of deglutination
c. Does not involves a higher center d. Can be voluntary

Ans. a. Wave of inhibition preceding esophageal peristalsis

Ref: Ganong: p; & Guyton 11th/ed p781-783

- ❑ ***Option a*** is correct ***and b*** is incorrect because degultitive inhibition is an inhibitory wave induced by swallowing and then a contractile wave appears. A wave of inhibition precedes a swallow-induced peristaltic contraction in the esophageal smooth muscle.
- ❑ ***Option c*** is incorrect because the brain stem controls the inhibition of the esophageal skeletal muscle, the smooth muscles have an intrinsic peripheral control mechanism.
- ❑ ***Option d*** is incorrect because local gradients of inhibitory and excitatory myenteric nerves determines the latency between swallow and contractions.

Deglutition reflex:

Afferent	Center/Nuclei	Efferent
5th, 9th and 10th CN (receptor mainly in tonsillar pillars epithelium, etc.)	NTS, NA–Degulitation center (areas in medulla and lower pons) (inhibit Respiratory center in medulla)	5th, 7th, 9th, 10, 12th CN, few superficial cervical nerves pharyngeal and tongue muscles, etc.

Mastigation reflex:

Afferent	Center/nuclei	Efferent
Via ***5th*** and ***9th*** C.N. (Bolus of food in mouth)	In brainstem (connection with reticular areas in brainstem taste centers, hypothalmus, amygadala and cerebral cortex near sensory area for taste and smell)	Via 5th CN (muscles of mastica-tion) Reflex inhibition of the muscles

9. Increase of blood flow in skeletal muscle during exercise:

a. 3 mL/min/100 g
b. 30 mL/min/100 g
c. 50 mL/min/100 g
d. 100 mL/min/100 g

Ans. d. 100 mL/min/100 g

Ref: Guyton & Hall 13th/ed p203,204,207 and 247

- ❑ **Option d** is correct because during heavy exercise, muscle metabolic activity can increase more than 60-fold and the blood flow as much as 20-fold, increasing to as high as 16,000 mL/min in the body's total muscle vascular bed (or 80 mL/min/100 g of muscle).
- ❑ Resting state, the metabolic activity of the muscles is very low, as is the blood flow—only 4 mL/min/100 g.
- ❑ Extreme exercise can increase the flow by 25-50 times. Peak flows may be as high as 400 mL/min/100 g.
- ❑ During body heating, skin blood flow may increase many fold, to as high as 7 to 8 L/min for the entire body.

	Percent of cardiac output	mL/min	mL/min/100 g of tissue weight
Muscle (inactve muscle state)	15	750	4
Skin cool weather	6	300	3

Contd...

Contd...

	mL/100 g muscle/min
Resting blood flow	3.6
Blood flow during maximal exercise	90

10. Renal artery lumen is reduced by half, what will be the blood flow?

a. Reduce by 1/2
b. Reduce by 1/4
c. Reduce by 1/16
d. Come to normal after autoregulation

Ans: c. Reduce by 1/16 *Ref: Ganong 24th/ed p575*

- **Option c** is correct because the flow of fluids can be described by Poiseuille's Law.
- In which flow of liquid is directly proportional to R^4. So if lumen is reduced to half then blood flow will get reduce by 1/16.
- *Other points related to blood flow...*
- **Poiseuille's Law** states that the flow (Q) of fluid is related to a number of factors:
  - The viscosity (n) of the fluid
  - The pressure gradient across the vessel (P)
  - Length (L) and diameter(r) of the vessel
- **Diameter:** Doubling the diameter of tube increases the flow rate by 16 fold (r^4). The larger the vessels's diameter greater is the blood flow.
- **Viscosity: Flow is inversely proportional to the viscosity of the fluid.**
- Viscosity of blood increases with increasing hematocrit and decreasing temperature
- **Pressure: Increasing pressure further maximizes flow as described by Poiseuille's equation.**
- **The relationship is given by Poiseuille–Hagen formula:**

$$F = (P_A - P_B) \times \left(\frac{\pi}{8}\right) \times \left(\frac{1}{\eta}\right) \times \left(\frac{r^4}{L}\right)$$

Where

F = Flow
$P_A - P_B$ = Pressure difference between two ends of the tube
η = Viscosity
r = Radius of tube
L = Length of tube

- Relationship between arterial blood pressure and blood flow given in graph below:

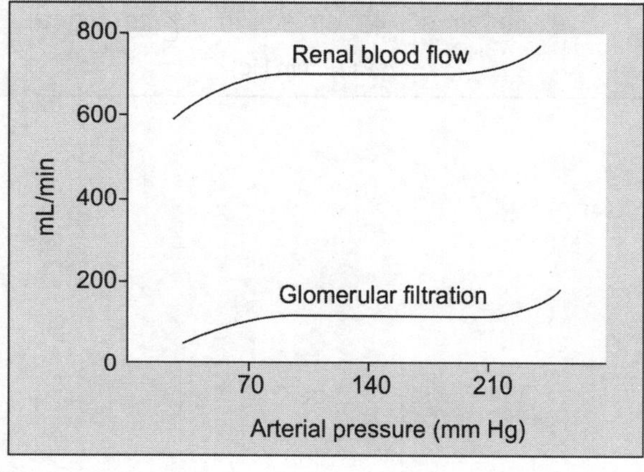

11. If the concentration of inhaled O_2 is doubled in a normal person then the resultant effect will be:

a. O_2 dissolved in plasma increases, but with Hb remains relatively constant
b. O_2 dissolved in plasma increases, but with Hb decreases
c. O_2 dissolved in plasma will remain constant, but with Hb increases
d. O_2 dissolved in plasma will remain constant, but with Hb remains constant

Ans: a. O_2 dissolved in plasma increases, but with Hb remains relatively constant

Ref: Guyton 11th/ed p491,492,507,500; Ganong 24th/ed p642

- ***Option a*** is correct because normally Hb is 97% saturated, so even with increased concentration of inhaled O_2, the % saturation of Hb slightly raises or remains relatively constant. Also the maximum O_2 saturation of Hb can never be more than 100%, which is only 3% above normal.
- There will be increased in amount of dissolved O_2. Normally, only about 3% of the total O_2 is transported in dissolved state, as compared with 97% transported by the Hb.
- According to Henry's law partial pressure = concentration of dissolved gas/solubility and coefficient concentration of dissolved gas = partial pressure × solubility coefficient
- And we know that pressure of gas is directly proportional to the concentration of the gas molecules. So, with increasing concentration of the inhaled O_2, there will be proportionate increase in O_2 dissolved in plasma.
- **Graph of oxyhemoglobin dissociation curve with O_2 concentration given below:**

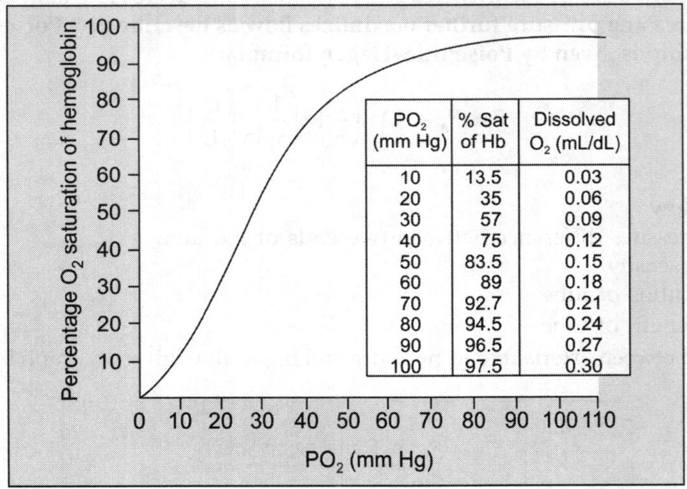

Biochemistry

Author: Bahram Gor, Co-author: Ambrish Tiwari

AIIMS May 2017

1. Maximum thermic energy is seen in:

a. Fat metabolism
b. Carbohydrate metabolism
c. Proteins metabolism
d. Alcohol metabolism

Ans. c. Protein metabolism *Ref: Harper 30th/ed, p148 (Table 14-1)*

Explanation

Thermic energy generated after metabolism of different substrates:

	Energy yielded kJ/g
Carbohydrates	16
Fats	17
Proteins	37
Alcohol	29

2. A girl with habit of eating paint from the wall complaints of acute abdominal pain on and off and tingling sensation of limbs and at times weakness of limbs. She had a history of eating paint from the wall of newly built house. Which of the following enzyme deficiency will be the cause of her condition?

a. ALA synthase
b. ALA dehydratase
c. Heme synthase
d. Coproporphyrinogen oxidase

Ans. b. ALA dehydratase *Ref: Harper 30th/ed, p328 (Table 31-2)*

Explanation

- ALA dehydratase is one of the most important enzyme of heme biosynthesis. In its deficiency patient present with abdominal pain and neuropsychiatric symptoms.
- This enzyme is zinc metalloprotein and sensitive to inhibition by Lead (Pb).
- As given in question that patient had history of wall paint eating which contains lead as constituent.
- In **option a,** ALA synthase have two isoenzymes ALAS 1 and ALAS 2, in which ALAS 2 deficiency present with anemia and ALAS1 is rate limiting enzyme for heme biosynthesis.
- In **option c,** Heme synthase is also known as Ferrochelatase, its inhibition present with photosensitivity. This enzyme takes part in final step of heme synthesis.
- In **option d,** Coproporphyrinogen oxidase converts uroporphyrinogen III into porphyrinogen III and its inhibition present with photosensitivity, abdominal pain and neuropsychiatric symptoms.

Enzyme involved	Type and class	Signs and symptoms
ALA synthase 2	X-linked sideroblastic anemia(erythropoietic)	Anemia
ALA dehydratase	ALA dehydratase deficiency (hepatic)	Abdominal pain and neuropsychiatric symptom
Uroporphyrinogen I synthase	Acute intermittent porphyria (hepatic)	Abdominal pain and neuropsychiatric symptom
Uroporphyrinogen III synthase	Congenital erythropoietic (erythropoietic)	Photosensitivity
Uroporphyrinogen decarboxylase	Porphyria cutanea tarda (hepatic)	Photosensitivity
Coproporphyrinogen oxidase	Hereditary coproporphyria	Photosensitivity, abdominal pain, neuropsychiatric symptoms
Protoporphyrinogen oxidase	Variegate porphyria (hepatic)	Photosensitivity, abdominal pain, neuropsychiatric symptoms
Ferrochelatase	Protoporphyria (erythropoietic)	Photosensitivity

3. A young lady presented with tingling sensation in legs and hands. On examination she had fissure tongue and lesions in angle of mouth. On investigation, she had low RBC glutathione reductase activity. Most likely deficiency is of:

a. Vitamin B1
b. Vitamin B12
c. Vitamin B6
d. Vitamin B2

Ans. d. Vitamin B2 *Ref: Harper 30th/ed, p556*

Explanation

- *Deficiency of Vitamin B2* is characterized by cheilosis, desquamation and inflammation of the tongue, and a seborrheic dermatitis.
- Riboflavin nutritional status is assessed by measurement of the activation of erythrocyte **glutathione reductase** by FAD added in vitro.
- It is a reactive moiety of the coenzymes **flavin mononucleotide (FMN)** and **flavin adenine dinucleotide (FAD)**.
- In **option a**, Vitamin B1 also known as thiamin deficiency lead to three syndromes : Chronic peripheral neuritis, Beriberi and Wernicke encephalopathy with Korsakoff psychosis.
- Thiamin nutritional status can be assessed by activation of **Erythrocyte transketolase**.
- In **option b**, vitamin B12 deficiency can lead to **pernicious anemia** and **spinal cord** degeneration.
- Its source is animal origin so mostly deficient in strict vegetarian and nutritional status assessed by level of **methylmalonic acid in urine**.
- In **option c**, vitamin B6 deficiency can lead to increased sensitivity to steroid hormone action and may be important in the development of **hormone-dependent cancer** of the breast, uterus, and prostate and its excess can lead to sensory neuropathy.
- Its deficiency is rare and can be assessed by assaying **erythrocyte transaminases** activity.

4. Decreased insulin-glucagon ratio is seen in all *except*:

a. Glycogen storage
b. Glycogen breakdown
c. Gluconeogenesis
d. Ketogenesis

Ans. a. Glycogen storage *Ref: Harper 30th/ed, p192 (Table 19-3) and 230*

EXPLANATION

- Insulin and glucagon play a central role in regulating blood glucose.
- Insulin/glucagon ratio is indirect measure of glucose status of blood.
- Insulin enhances long-term uptake of glucose of liver as a result of its action on the enzymes controlling **glycolysis, glycogenesis** and **gluconeogenesis.**
- Glucagon stimulates **glycogenolysis** by activating glycogen phosphorylase, enhances **gluconeogenesis** from amino acids and lactate and also enhances **ketogenesis.**

5. RFLP was used in-order to identify the five different species of staphylococci in a surgical ICU. Which of the following site does the restriction enzyme act?

a. TAGATA/ATCTAT
b. ATGGAC/TACGTG
c. AATATA/TATAAT
d. GATTAC/CATTAG

Ans. d. GATTAC/CATTAG *Ref: Lehninger 6th/ed, p314*

EXPLANATION

- **Restriction endonucleases** (also called restriction enzymes) recognize and cleave DNA at specific sequences (recognition sequences or restriction sites) to generate a set of smaller fragments.
- There are three types of restriction endonucleases, designated I, II, and III.
- Type II restriction endonucleases are used in RFLP.
- The recognition sequences are usually 4 to 6 bp long and palindromic in nature.
- A **palindromic sequence** is a nucleic acid sequence on double-stranded DNA or RNA wherein reading 5′ to 3′ forward on one strand matches the sequence reading 5′ to 3′ on the complementary strand.
- So, in **option d** sequence given are palindromic in nature.

6. Which of the following is true regarding Mitochondrial DNA?

a. It has 3×10^9 base pairs
b. It has less mutations than human DNA
c. 23 pairs inherited from each parents
d. Less than 20% respiratory chain proteins codes from mDNA

Ans. d. Less than 20% respiratory chain proteins codes from mDNA

Ref: Harper 30th/ed, p378 (Table 35-3)

EXPLANATION

- Mitochondrial DNA encodes 13 protein subunits of the respiratory chain (of a total of about 67) which is less than 20%, so option d is correct.
  Seven subunits of NADH dehydrogenase (complex I).
  Cytochrome *b* of complex III.
  Three subunits of cytochrome oxidase (complex IV).

Two subunits of ATP synthase.

- ❑ Mitochondrial DNA is circular, double-stranded, and composed of heavy (H) and light (L) chains or strands.
- ❑ **Option a** is wrong because it contains **16,569 bp**.
- ❑ **Option b** is wrong because there is high mutation rate (5–10 times that of nuclear DNA).
- ❑ **Option c** is wrong because an important feature of human mitochondrial mtDNA is that—because all mitochondria are contributed by the ovum during zygote formation—it is transmitted by maternal non-mendelian inheritance.

Other important points regarding mitochondrial DNA;

- ❑ Encodes large (16S) and small (12S) mt ribosomal RNA.
- ❑ Encodes 22 mt tRNA molecule.
- ❑ Genetic code differs slightly from the standard code.
  UGA (standard stop codon) is read as Trp.
  AGA and AGG (standard codons for Arg) are read as stop codon.
- ❑ Contains very few untranslated sequence.
- ❑ Comparisons of mtDNA sequences provide evidence about evolutionary origins of primates and other species.

7. Thiamin deficiency results in decreased energy production, because TPP interferes with:

a. Alcohol metabolism
b. Transketolase activity
c. Its coenzyme for pyruvate and alpha-ketoglutarate dehydrogenase
d. Energy production from amino acids

Ans. c. Its coenzyme for pyruvate and alpha-ketoglutarate dehydrogenase

Ref: Harper 30th/ed, p555

Explanation

- ❑ **Thiamin** has a central role in energy-yielding metabolism, especially the metabolism of carbohydrates.
- ❑ **Thiamin diphosphate** is the coenzyme for three multienzyme complexes that catalyze oxidative decarboxylation reactions:
  - **Pyruvate dehydrogenase** in carbohydrate metabolism.
  - **α-ketoglutarate dehydrogenase** in the citric acid cycle.
  - **Branched-chain ketoacid dehydrogenase** in the metabolism of leucine isoleucine, and valine.
- ❑ In **option a**, alcohol abuse causes thiamin deficiency it does not have any role in alcohol metabolism.
- ❑ In **option b**, thiamin diphosphate is also the coenzyme for transketolase, in the pentose phosphate pathway. But this pathway is not associated with energy yielding.
- ❑ In **option d**, thiamin is coenzyme for only in metabolism of branched chain ketoacids.
- ❑ Thiamin triphosphate has a role in nerve conduction, it phosphorylates, and activates chloride channel in the nerve membrane.

8. 3 ATPs for each sugar, will be generated if the following substrate is used for anaerobic glycolysis:

a. Fructose
b. Glucose
c. Galactose
d. Glycogen

Ans. d. Glycogen

Ref: Harper 30th/ed, p186 (Fig. 19.1)

EXPLANATION

- Normally when glucose is substrate in anaerobic glycolysis, 4 moles of ATP are generated but 2 moles are get used so net ATP generated is 2 moles.
- In the same way fructose and galactose when substrate for anaerobic glycolysis net 2 moles of ATP generated.
- But if glycogen is substrate then due to glycogenolysis we get glucose-6-phosphate directly, so only 1ATP is used in its anaerobic glycolysis so net gain of 3 ATP occurs.

9. Which of the following is an example of anaplerotic reaction?

a. Pyruvate to oxaloacetate
b. Pyruvate to Acetyl CoA
c. Pyruvate to lactic acid
d. Pyruvate to acetaldehyde

Ans. a. Pyruvate to oxaloacetate *Ref: Harper 30th/ed, p164 (Fig. 16.4)*

EXPLANATION

- **Anaplerotic** reactions are those reactions in which citric acid cycle intermediates get converted into oxaloacetate and then finally to glucose.
- Among all **anaplerotic** reactions the most important is the formation of oxaloacetate by the carboxylation of pyruvate, catalyzed by **pyruvate carboxylase.**
- Reactions given in other option cannot lead to formation of glucose so they are not example of anaplerotic reaction.

10. Phenylbutyrate is used in urea cycle disorders because it:

a. Activates enzymes
b. Maintains renal output
c. Maintains energy level
d. Increases renal excretion of ammonia

Ans. d. Increases renal excretion of ammonia *Ref: Nelson 19th/ed, p449*

EXPLANATION

- Urea cycle disorders are characterized by hyperammonemia, encephalopathy, and respiratory alkalosis.
- Four of the five metabolic diseases, deficiencies of carbamoyl phosphate synthetase I, ornithine carbamoyltransferase, argininosuccinate synthase, and argininosuccinate lyase, result in the accumulation of precursors of urea, principally ammonia and glutamine.
- Ammonia may be toxic to the brain in part because it reacts with α-ketoglutarate to form glutamate result in impairment of TCA cycle due to depletion of α-ketoglutarate.
- An important advance in treatment of hyperammonemia has been the advent of acylation therapy in which exogenously administered organic acids form acyl adducts with endogenous nonessential amino acids.
- These adducts are nontoxic compounds with high renal clearances.
- One mole of phenylbutyrate removes 2 moles of ammonia as glutamine from the body.

11. In uncontrolled diabetes, VLDL and triglycerides are high because of:

a. Increased activity of hepatic lipase
b. Increase in peripheral function of LDL receptors

c. Increased activity of lipoprotein lipase and decreased activity of hormone sensitive lipase
d. Increased activity of hormone sensitive lipase and decreased activity of lipoprotein lipase

Ans. d. Increased activity of hormone sensitive lipase and decreased activity of lipoprotein lipase

Ref: Harper 30th/ed, p164 (Fig. 16.4)

EXPLANATION

- In adipose tissue, **insulin** enhances lipoprotein lipase synthesis in adipocytes and its translocation to the luminal surface of the capillary endothelium.
- Insulin in adipose tissue is to inhibit the activity of **hormone-sensitive lipase,** reducing the release not only of FFA.
- So in uncontrolled diabetes mellitus, due to decreased action of insulin, hormone sensitive lipase get activated and lipoprotein lipase get inhibited.
- Insulin causes increase in LDL receptor so in uncontrolled diabetes it will get decreased.
- **Hormone-sensitive lipase** is distinct from lipoprotein lipase, which catalyzes lipoprotein triacylglycerol hydrolysis before its uptake into extrahepatic tissues.
- In **diabetes mellitus,** where insulin deficiency causes excessive mobilization of FFA and underutilization of chylomicrons and VLDL, leading to **hypertriacylglycerolemia.**

PGI May 2017

1. Which of the following statements is/are correct regarding gluconeogenesis?

a. Hexokinase, phosphofructokinase and pyruvate kinase prevent simple reversal of glycolysis for glucose synthesis in gluconeogenesis
b. Acetyl-CoA as an allosteric activator in gluconeogenesis
c. Glucagon and epinephrine inhibit gluconeogenesis in the liver by increasing the concentration of cAMP
d. Biotin act as coenzyme in carboxylation reactions in gluconeogenesis
e. Superfluity of glucose, lead to increased activity of the enzymes of gluconeogenesis

Ans. a. Hexokinase, phosphofructokinase and pyruvate kinase prevent simple reversal of glycolysis for glucose synthesis in gluconeogenesis; b. Acetyl-CoA as an allosteric activator in gluconeogenesis **and** d. Biotin act as coenzyme in carboxylation reactions in gluconeogenesis *Ref: Harper 30th/ed, p185*

EXPLANATION

- **Option a** is correct because there are three non-equilibrium reactions in glycolysis catalyzed by hexokinase, phosphofructokinase and pyruvate kinase, prevent simple reversal of glycolysis for glucose synthesis in gluconeogenesis.
- **Option b** is correct because gluconeogenesis, pyruvate carboxylase, which catalyzes the synthesis of oxaloacetate from pyruvate, requires acetyl-CoA as an **allosteric activator.**
- **Option c** is incorrect because **glucagon** and **epinephrine,** hormones that are responsive to a decrease in blood glucose, inhibit glycolysis and stimulate gluconeogenesis in the liver by increasing the concentration of cAMP.
- **Option d** is correct because mitochondrial **pyruvate carboxylase** catalyzes the carboxylation of pyruvate to oxaloacetate, an ATP-requiring reaction in which the vitamin biotin is the coenzyme.
- **Option e** is incorrect because the enzymes involved in the utilization of glucose become more active when there is a superfluity of glucose, and under these conditions the enzymes of gluconeogenesis have low activity.

2. DNA gyrase is:

a. Restriction endonuclease
b. Topoisomerase 1
c. Topoisomerase 2
d. RNA polymerase 1
e. RNA polymerase 2

Ans. c. Topoisomerase 2 *Ref: Lehninger 6th/ed, p1019*

EXPLANATION

- DNA gyrase is also known as Topoisomerase 2.
- It is one of the protein required for Initiation of replication in prokaryotes.
- It relieves the topological stress induced **ahead** of the fork by the unwinding reaction.
- Topological stress is due to unwinding **reactions** by helicase.
- In other **option a** restriction endonuclease **is** enzyme which is used for site specific cutting of double stranded DNA.
- In **option d and e** enzyme RNA polymerase 1 and 2 is used during transcription.

3. True about telomerase is/are:

a. Works as reverse transcriptase
b. Elongates the chromosome
c. 3′ to 5′ direction
d. Contains RNA and protein
e. RNA is about 500 nucleotide long

Ans. a. Works as reverse transcriptase; b. Elongates the chromosome and d. Contains RNA and protein *Ref: Lehninger 6th/ed, p1089*

EXPLANATION

- Telomerase **contains both RNA and protein** components.
- DNA replication requires a template and primer, and beyond the end of a linear DNA molecule no template is available for the pairing of an RNA primer.
- So telomerase acts as a cellular reverse transcriptase that provides the active site for RNA-dependent DNA synthesis **(reverse transcriptase).**
- The RNA component is about **150 nucleotide long** and contain 1.5 copies of the appropriate C_yA_x telomere repeat.
- Telomere synthesis requires the 3′ end of a chromosome as primer and proceeds in the usual **5′-3′ direction.**

4. True about HMP pathway:

a. Occurs in cytosol
b. Found in liver, adipose tissue, gonads
c. Does not produce ATP
d. Produce NADP in oxidative phase
e. Irreversible phase generate ribose precursor

Ans. a. Occurs in cytosol; b. Found in liver, adipose tissue, gonads and c. Does not produce ATP *Ref: Harper 30th/ed, p185*

EXPLANATION

- The HMP pathway also known as pentose phosphate pathway is an alternative route for the metabolism of glucose.

- It does not lead to formation of ATP but has two major functions:
  1. The formation of **NADPH** for synthesis of fatty acids and steroids and maintaining reduced glutathione for antioxidant activity.
  2. The synthesis of **ribose** for nucleotide and nucleic acid formation.
- Enzymes of the pentose phosphate pathway are **cytosolic.**
- The sequence of reactions of the pathway may be divided into two phases:
  Irreversible oxidative phase generates NADPH.
  Reversible non-oxidative phase ribose precursors.
- The pentose phosphate pathway is active in liver, adipose tissue, adrenal cortex, thyroid, erythrocytes, testis, and lactating mammary gland.

5. DNA repair defect:

a. Thymidine dimmers
b. Acetylation of base pairs
c. Methylation of base pairs
d. Deletion of base pairs
e. Addition of base pairs

Ans. d. Deletion of base pairs and e. Addition of base pairs *Ref: Lehninger 6th/ed, p1037*

EXPLANATION

- Alterations in DNA repair genes that result in an increased rate of mutation can greatly increase an individual's susceptibility to cancer.
- Defect in the genes encoding the proteins involved in nucleotide excision repair, mismatch repair, recombinational repair, and error-prone translesion DNA synthesis have all been linked to human cancers.
- Nucleotide-excision repair is the sole repair pathway for pyrimidine and thymidine dimers in humans.
- Deletion and addition of base pairs also lead to defect in DNA repair mechanisms **(Answer).**
- Methylation in DNA repair gene lead to defect in repair and development of cancer.
- Histone H4 acetylation participates directly in one or more steps required to repair broken chromatin.

6. UV light causes what kind of defect in the DNA?

a. Pyrimidine dimer defect
b. Strand breaks
c. Bulky adduct
d. Bases mismatch
e. Insertion and deletion

Ans. a. Pyrimidine dimer defect and c. Bulky adduct *Ref: Harper 30th/ed, p390, (Fig. 35-22)*

EXPLANATION

DNA damaging agent	DNA lesion formed	DNA repair pathway
Ionizing radiation, X-rays, antitumor drugs	Double strand breaks, single strand breaks	Non-homologous end joining (NHEJ), Homologous recombination (HR)

Contd...

Contd...

UV-light, chemicals	Bulky adducts, pyrimidine dimers	Nucleotide excision repair (NER)
Oxygen radicals, hydrolysis, alkylating agents	Abasic sites, single strand breaks 8-oxoguanine lesions	Base excision repair (BER)
Replication errors	Bases mismatch, Insertions, deletions	Mismatch repair (MMR)

7. True about genes are:

a. Smallest functional unit of DNA
b. Not capable of independent expression
c. Promoter and enhancer genes are typical example
d. Cistron is single functional unit

Ans. a. Smallest functional unit of DNA; c. Promoter and enhancer genes are typical example and d. Cistron is single functional unit *Ref: Lippincott 4th/ed, p449*

EXPLANATION

- ❑ Gene is a functional unit that is regulated by transcription and encodes a RNA product.
- ❑ Gene locus includes region that are necessary to control its expression called as promoter and enhancer.
- ❑ Capable of independent expression.
- ❑ Cistron is a genetic unit codes structure of the subunit of enzyme and protein.

8. Pyrimidines are:

a. Thymidine
b. Cytidine
c. Adenine
d. Guanidine
e. Uracil

Ans. a. Thymidine; b. Cytidine and e. Uracil *Ref: Harper 30th/ed, p390 (Fig. 35-22)*

EXPLANATION

- ❑ Adenine and guanine are purines and thymine, cytosine and uracil are pyrimidines.

9. True about Proteoglycans is/are:

a. Positively charged
b. Present in extracellular matrix and connective tissue
c. Holds lot of water
d. Formed with binding of glycosaminoglycans to core proteins
e. Sieve nature is due to short polysaccharide chain of GAGs

Ans. b. Present in extracellular matrix and connective tissue; c. Holds lot of water and d. Formed with binding of glycasaminoglycans to core proteins *Ref: Harper 30th/ed, p634*

EXPLANATION

- ❑ **Proteoglycans** are proteins that contain covalently linked **glycosaminoglycans** (GAGs).

- The proteins bound covalently to glycosaminoglycans are called **"core proteins."**
- Proteoglycans vary in tissue distribution, nature of the core protein, attached glycosaminoglycans, and their function.
- Proteoglycans are found in **every tissue** of the body, mainly in the ECM or "ground substance."
- The GAGs present in the proteoglycans are **polyanions** and hence bind polycations and cations such as Na^+ and K^+ due to which attracts water by osmotic pressure into the extracellular matrix and contributes to its turgor.
- Due to its long extended nature of the polysaccharide chains of GAGs and their ability to gel, the proteoglycans can act as **sieves**.

10. Post-translational modifications include:

a. Adding of base pairs at the end
b. Excision of a peptide
c. Hydroxyl groups of AA get phosphorylated
d. Addition of terminal
e. Removal of terminal

Ans. a. Adding of base pairs at the end; d. Addition of terminal and e. Removal of terminal

Ref: Lehninger 6th/ed, p1037

Explanation

- Newly made proteins do not attain their final biologically active conformation until they have been altered by one or more processing reactions called **posttranslational modifications.**
- Amino-terminal and Carboxyl-terminal modifications occurs by deletion of amino acids at both end.
- Amino-terminal end of some proteins play a role in directing the protein to its ultimate destination in the cell. Such **signal sequences** are eventually removed by specific peptidases.
- Hydroxyl groups of certain Ser, Thr, and Tyr residues of some proteins are enzymatically phosphorylated by ATP.
- Extra carboxyl groups may be added to Glu residues of some proteins.
- The carbohydrate side chains of glycoproteins are attached covalently during or after synthesis of the polypeptide.
- Addition of prosthetic groups, proteolytic processing and formation of disulfide cross links are also part of post translational modification.

11. What are uses of hydrogenation of fatty acids?

a. Hydrogenation makes unsaturated into saturated fatty acids
b. In vegetable oils FA are mostly in trans form
c. Hydrogenation converts cis into trans form
d. Trans form leads to higher incidence of CVD
e. Hydrogenation increases shelf life of vegetable oils

Ans. a. Hydrogenation makes unsaturated into saturated fatty acids; c. Hydrogenation converts cis into trans form; d. Trans form leads to higher incidence of CVD and e. Hydrogenation increases shelf life of vegetable oils

Ref: Lehninger 6th/ed, p361

Explanation

- Most natural fats present in vegetable oils, dairy products, and animal fat are complex mixtures of simple and mixed triacylglycerols and contain a variety of fatty acids differing in chain length and degree of saturation.

- Lipid-rich foods when exposed too long to the oxygen in air, they may spoil and become rancid.
- So to improve the shelf life of vegetable oils used in cooking, and to increase their stability at the high temperatures used in deep-frying, commercial vegetable oils are prepared by **partial hydrogenation**.
- Many of the cis double bonds in the fatty acids to single bonds and increases the melting temperature of the oils so that they are more nearly solid at room temperature.
- Also some cis double bonds are converted to trans double bonds which leads to a higher incidence of cardiovascular disease.

12. True about Triacylglycerol:

a. Mono and diacylglycerols are component of tissues
b. Absorption through lymph node and blood vessels
c. Main storage form of FA
d. Hydrolysis by lipase

Ans. a. Mono and diacylglycerols are component of tissues; b. Absorption through lymph node and blood vessels; c. Main storage form of FA and d. Hydrolysis by lipase *Ref: Harper 30th/ed, p255*

EXPLANATION

- The triacylglycerols are esters of the trihydric alcohol, glycerol and fatty acids and they are main storage form of fatty acids.
- Dietary lipids in form of triacylglycerol are transported by chylomicrons in chyle whereas from liver it is transported by VLDL to extrahepatic tissues via blood.
- Mono and diacylglycerols are found in tissues.
- Triacylglycerols must be hydrolyzed by a lipase to their constituent fatty acids and glycerol before further catabolism can proceed.

13. Binding of 2, 3 BPG to hemoglobin leads to:

a. Shift of oxygen dissociation curve to left
b. Shift to oxygen dissociation curve to right
c. Increased affinity to oxygen
d. Decreased affinity to oxygen

Ans. a. Shift of oxygen dissociation curve to left and d. Decreased affinity to oxygen
Ref: Harper 30th/ed, p255

EXPLANATION

- O_2-induces transition of hemoglobin from the low-affinity **T (taut) state** to the high-affinity **R (relaxed) state**.
- The glycolytic pathway in red blood cells also possesses a shunt which isomerizes 1,3-bisphosphoglycerate (1,3,-BPG) to **2,3-bisphosphoglycerate** (2,3-BPG) which binds to and stabilizes hemoglobin in the T-state.
- This lead to decreased affinity of O_2 with Hb due to which O_2 dissociation curve shift to left.
- Catalyzed by the bifunctional enzyme **2,3-bisphosphogylcerate synthase/2-phosphatase**.
- Activity of this enzyme is sensitive to pH so reinforce the impact of the Bohr effect on O_2 binding and delivery by hemoglobin.

JIPMER Pattern Based

1. Enzyme catalyzing substrate level phosphorylation in TCA cycle:

a. Succinyl-CoA synthetase
b. Succinate dehydrogenase
c. α-ketoglutarate dehydrogenase
d. Isocitrate dehydrogenase

Ans. a. Succinyl-CoA synthetase *Ref: Harper 30th/ed, p164*

EXPLANATION

- ❑ Succinyl-CoA is converted to succinate by the enzyme **succinate thiokinase (succinyl-CoA synthetase)** example of substrate level phosphorylation in the citric acid cycle.
- ❑ First dehydrogenation reaction, forming fumarate, is catalyzed by **succinate dehydrogenase,** which is bound to the inner surface of the inner mitochondrial membrane.
- ❑ **Oxidative decarboxylation** in a reaction catalyzed by a multienzyme complex called as **α-ketoglutarate dehydrogenase complex.**
- ❑ **Isocitrate dehydrogenase** have three isoenzymes one, which uses NAD^+, is found only in mitochondria. The other two use $NADP^+$ and are found in mitochondria and the cytosol.

2. Lactate is produced in anaerobic glycolysis for:

a. Use as substrate in glycogenesis
b. Production of ATP and GTP
c. Use in protein synthesis
d. Act as shuttle for reducing equivalents

Ans. d. Act as shuttle for reducing equivalents *Ref: Harper 30th/ed, p172*

EXPLANATION

- ❑ During vigorous exercise, septic shock, and cancer cachexia lactate is produced via anaerobic glycolysis and used in the liver for gluconeogenesis.
- ❑ This lead to increase in metabolic rate to provide the ATP and GTP needed.
- ❑ Some time lactate may be formed in the Cytosol which get enter the mitochondrion to be oxidized to pyruvate for onward metabolism. Acting as shuttle for transfer of reducing equivalents.
- ❑ Liver, kidneys, and heart normally take up lactate and oxidize it.

3. Number of high energy phosphates required in conversion of glucose to 2 moles of pyruvate:

a. 2
b. 5
c. 4
d. 7

Ans. a. 2 *Ref: Harper, 30th/ed, p169 Table 17.1*

EXPLANATION

- ❑ ATP production and utilize during glycolysis.
- ❑ 2 ATP required for reactions of hexokinase and phosphofructokinase by which glucose get converted into 2 moles of pyruvate.

- 2 NADH is produced from one molecule of glucose by reaction catalyzed by Glyceraldehyde-3-phosphate dehydrogenase and then 5 ATP produced by respiratory chain oxidation.
- At Substrate-level phosphorylation 4 moles ATP produced by reaction catalyzed by enzymes phosphoglycerate kinase and pyruvate kinase.
- So net 7 ATP are produced in glycolysis.

4. How many phosphate bonds are used for forming one glucose from lactate?

a. 4 b. 6
c. 12 d. 2

Ans. b. 6 *Ref: Harper 30th/ed, p186 (Fig. 19.1)*

Explanation

- Production of 1 mole of glucose from lactate need 6 phosphate bond.
- 1 ATP needed for conversion of pyruvate to oxaloacetate but for 1 mole of glucose 2 moles of pyruvate is used, so 2 ATP are used for 1 molecule of glucose production.
- In same way 2 ATPs are used in conversion of oxaloacetate to phosphoenolpyruvate and 2 ATPs in conversion of 3-phosphoglycerate to 1,3-bisposphoglycerate.

5. Most common mutation of hypercholesterolemia:

a. LDL receptor mutations
b. Lipoprotein lipase mutation
c. Hepatic lipase deficiency
d. Abnormality in ApoE

Ans. a. LDL receptor mutations *Ref: Harper 30th/ed, p275*

Explanation

- Inherited defects in lipoprotein metabolism lead to the primary condition of either **hypo-** or **hyperlipoproteinemia**.
- **Familial hypercholesterolemia (FH),** causes severe hypercholesterolemia and is also associated with premature atherosclerosis.
- Most common defect is in the gene for the LDL receptor, so that LDL is not cleared from the blood called as Familial hypercholesterolemia (type IIa).
- Types of hyperlipoproteinemias with there features:

Name	Defects	Features
Familial lipoprotein lipase deficiency (Type I)	Deficiency of Lipoprotein lipase or Apo C-II	Increased level of chylomicrons and VLDL. Low levels of LDL and HDL. No increased risk of coronary disease
Familial hypercholesterolemia (Type IIa)	Defective LDL receptors or mutation in ligand region of Apo B-100	Elevated LDL levels and hypercholesterolemia, resulting in atherosclerosis and coronary disease
Familial type III hyperlipoproteinemia (broad beta disease, familial dysbetalipoproteinemia)	Abnormality in Apo E	Increase in chylomicron and VLDL remnants. Causes hypercholesterolemia, xanthomas, and atherosclerosis

Contd...

Contd...

Name	Defects	Features
Familial hypertriglyceridemia (Type IV)	Overproduction of VLDL	Cholesterol levels rise with the VLDL concentration, coronary heart disease, type II diabetes mellitus
Familial hyperalphalipoproteinemia	Increased concentrations of HDL	A rare condition apparently beneficial to health and longevity
Hepatic lipase deficiency	Deficiency of the enzyme	Patients have xanthomas and coronary heart disease
Familial lecithin: Cholesterol acyltransferase (LCAT) deficiency	Absence of LCAT	Cholesteryl esters and lysolecithin are low
Familial lipoprotein(a) excess	Lp(a) consists of 1 mol of LDL attached to 1 mol of apo(a).	Premature coronary heart disease due to atherosclerosis and thrombosis

6. Microsatellite DNA means:

a. 10–15 base pairs
b. Marker for various genome searches
c. Dinucleotide repeats of AG
d. 500,000 to 10,00,000 times in the human genome

Ans. b. Marker for various genome searches *Ref: Harper 30th/ed, p463*

Explanation

- ❑ Microsatellite DNA is a short (2–6 bp), inherited, tandem repeat units of DNA occur about 50,000 to 100,000 times in the human genome.
- ❑ They occur more frequently so they are used as the marker loci for various genome searches replacing RFLPs (which was used earlier). ***(Answer)***.
- ❑ Most commonly are found as dinucleotide repeats of AC (Adenine and Cytosine) on one strand and TG (thymine and guanine) on the opposite strand
- ❑ Most genes are associated with one or more microsatellite markers so the relative position of genes on chromosomes can be assessed.

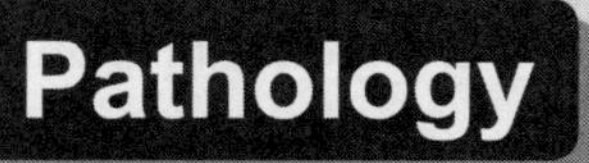

Author: Jyotsana Priya, Co-author: Akanksha Singh

AIIMS May 2017

1. MHC-2 is seen in which cells?

a. Dendritic cells
b. Erythrocyte
c. All nucleated cells
d. Platelets

Ans. a. Dendritic cells *Ref. Robbins and Cotran Pathologic Basis of Diseases 9th/ed p195*

Explanation

Class II MHC molecules are mainly expressed on antigen presenting cells (APCs) that respond to T-cell help

APCs are:

- ❑ Macrophages
- ❑ B lymphocytes
- ❑ Dendritic cells

2. A 29-year-old female with history of polyarthralgia and backache was investigated. She had nucleolar pattern of ANA in immunofluorescence. Which of the following is the best fits in this case?

a. Sclerodactyly, Raynaud's phenomenon, lung fibrosis
b. Raynaud's phenomenon, parotid swelling, dry mouth
c. Glomerulonephritis, malar rash, oral ulcer
d. Genital ulcer, skin nodules, lung fibrosis

Ans. a. Sclerodactyly, Raynaud's phenomenon, lung fibrosis

Ref. Robbins and Cotran Pathologic Basis of Diseases, p125

Explanation

- ❑ Antinuclear antibodies (ANAs) are directed against nuclear antigens and can be grouped into four categories:
  1. Antibodies to DNA
  2. Antibodies to histones
  3. Antibodies to nonhistone proteins bound to RNA
  4. Antibodies to nucleolar antigens.
- ❑ The most widely used method for detecting ANAs is ***indirect immunofluorescence***.
- ❑ The pattern of nuclear fluorescence suggests the type of antibody present in the patient's serum. Four basic patterns are recognized:
  1. **Homogeneous or diffuse nuclear staining:** Usually reflects antibodies to chromatin, histones, and, occasionally, double-stranded DNA.
  2. **Rim or peripheral staining patterns:** Most often indicative of antibodies to double-stranded DNA.

3. **Speckled pattern:** Refers to the presence of uniform or variable-sized speckles. This is one of the most commonly observed patterns of fluorescence and therefore the least specific. It reflects the presence of antibodies to non-DNA nuclear constituents. Examples include Sm antigen, ribonucleoprotein, and SS-A and SS-B reactive antigens.

Nucleolar pattern: Presence of a few discrete spots of fluorescence within the nucleus and represents antibodies to RNA. This pattern is reported most often in patients with systemic sclerosis. Nucleolar ANA → Systemic Sclerosis (Scleroderma)

Some patients with the limited disease also develop a combination of calcinosis, Raynaud's phenomenon, esophageal dysmotility, sclerodactyly, and telangiectasia, called the *CREST syndrome.*

3. **A 40-year-old patient presented with heart burn and increased salivation (sternal tenderness, Dysphagia). UGE scopy was done and biopsy was taken and is as shown below. Likely diagnosis is?**

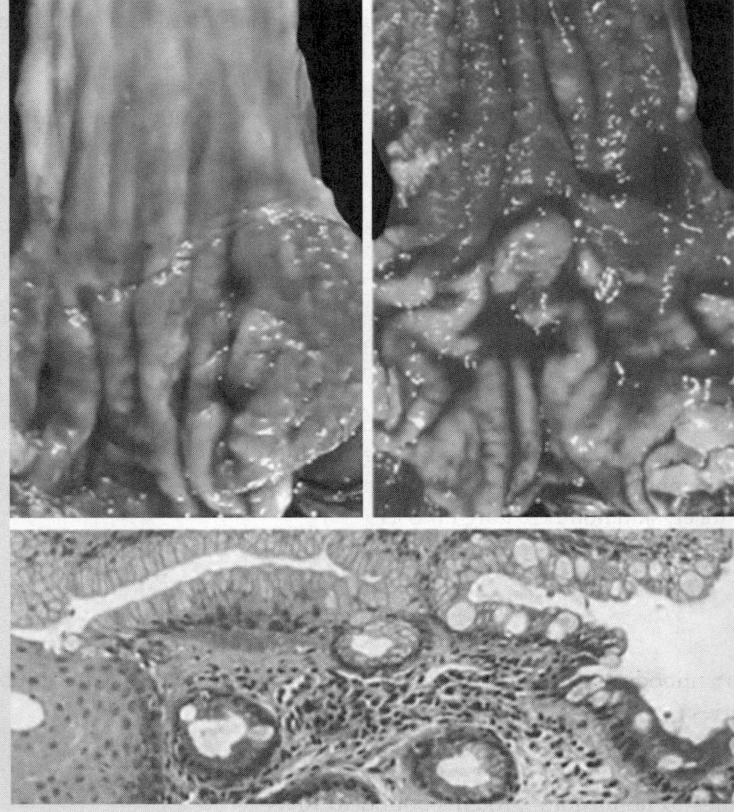

a. Barrett's esophagus
b. Adenocarcinoma
c. Esophagitis
d. Squamous cell carcinoma

Ans. a. Barrett's esophagus *Ref. Robbins and Cotran Pathologic Basis of Diseases 9th/ed p757*

EXPLANATION

Given figure is of Barrett esophagus.

1st image, Normal gastroesophageal junction.

2nd image, Barrett esophagus. Note the small islands of residual pale squamous mucosa within the Barrett mucosa.

3rd image, Histologic appearance of the gastroesophageal junction in Barrett esophagus. Note the transition between esophageal squamous mucosa (left) and Barrett metaplasia, with abundant metaplastic goblet cells (right).

4. Pancreatic cancer has highest association with:

a. Peutz-Jeghers
b. Hereditary pancreatitis
c. FAP
d. FAMMM syndrome

Ans. a. Peutz-Jeghers *Ref. Robbins and Cotran Pathologic Basis of Diseases 9th/ed p894*

EXPLANATION

Inherited predisposition to pancreatic cancer	Disorder gene	Increased Risk of pancreatic cancer (Fold)	Risk of pancreatic cancer by age 70 (%)
Peutz-Jeghers syndrome	*STK11*	130	30–60
Hereditary pancreatitis	*PRSS1, SPINK1*	50–80	25–40
Familial atypical multiple-mole melanoma syndrome	CDKN2A	20–35	10–17
Strong family history (3 or more relatives with pancreatic cancer)	Unknown	14–32	8–16
Hereditary breast and ovarian cancer	Multiple, including *BRCA1, BRCA2, PALP2, BRCA2*	4–10	5
Hereditary non-polyposis colorectal cancer (HNPCC)	Multiple, including *MLH1, MSH2* (2p21)	8–10	4

5. Which of the following is accurate regarding the intracellular iron metabolism in iron deficiency anemia?

a. Transferrin receptor 1 – iron responsive elements (IRE) increases transferrin receptor mRNA concentration and synthesis
b. Transferrin receptor 1 – iron responsive elements (IRE) decreases transferrin receptor mRNA concentration and increases synthesis
c. Apoferritin mRNA – iron response element (IRE) decreases and ferritin synthesis decreases
d. Apoferritin mRNA – iron response element decreases and Ferritin synthesis increases

Ans. a. Transferrin receptor 1 – iron responsive elements (IRE) increases transferrin receptor mRNA concentration and synthesis *Ref. Williams Hematology 8th/ed, Chapter 42*

Explanation

- The regulation of iron metabolism at the cytoplasmic mRNA level by interaction of iron-regulatory protein (IRP-1) and the iron-responsive elements (IREs) to **apoferritin mRNA (Mechanism 1) and transferrin receptor (TfR) mRNA (Mechanism 2).**
- When the cytoplasmic iron concentration is low, IRP-1 binds to the IREs of both mRNAs. ***This represses the translation of apoferritin mRNA***, where the IRE is at the 5′ end of the mRNA, thereby reducing the amount of apoferritin formed.
- It stabilizes ***and increases the translation of TfR mRNA*** where the IRE is at the 3′ end of the mRNA, thereby increasing the amount of TfR formed.
- Conversely, when there is an abundance of iron in the cytoplasm, IRP-1 is displaced from both species of mRNA. This results in derepression of apoferritin synthesis and destabilization and degradation of TfR mRNA.

At low cytosolic mobile iron pool:
IRP levels increase and bind to mRNA-IREs of ferritin and transferrin receptors

IRP IRE
5′ UTR Coding region UTR An 3′
Inactive ferritin mRNA

IRP
IRE
5′ UTR Coding region UTR An 3′
Active transferrin receptor mRNA

At high cytosolic mobile iron pool:
IRP levels decrease causing opposite effects on the mRNAs

IRE
5′ UTR Coding region UTR An 3′
Active ferritin mRNA

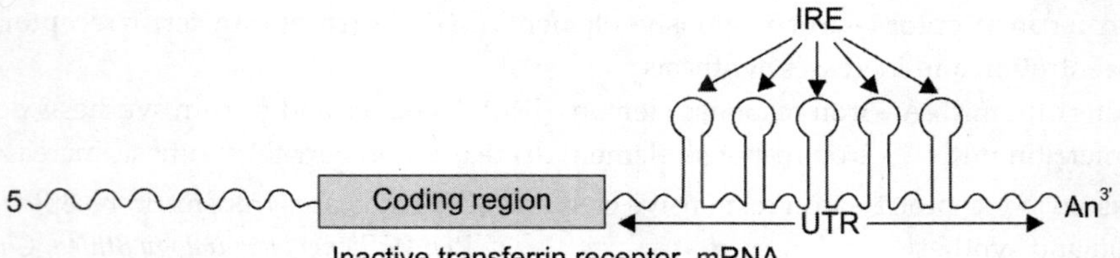

Inactive transferrin receptor mRNA

6. A 50-year-old male diabetic presented with blurring of vision. Urine examination showed proteinuria. Fundus examination showed dot and blot hemorrhages, microaneurysm and cotton wool spots. Histopathology picture of kidney given shows:

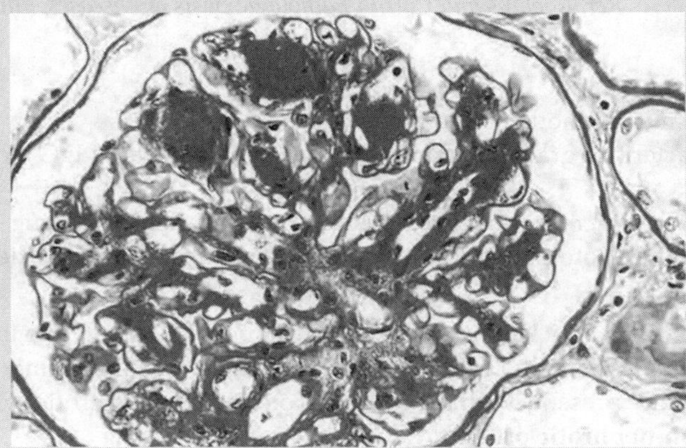

a. Segmental sclerosis
b. Kimmelstiel-Wilson lesions
c. Amyloid
d. Crescents

Ans. b. Kimmelstiel-Wilson lesions *Ref. Robbins and Cotran Pathologic Basis of Diseases, 9th/ed p1110*

Explanation

Above figure shows

- Diffuse and nodular diabetic glomerulosclerosis (PAS stain). Also known as **intercapillary glomerulosclerosis or Kimmelstiel-Wilson disease.**
- The glomerular lesions take the form of ovoid or spherical, often laminated, nodules of matrix situated in the periphery of the glomerulus.
- The nodules are PAS-positive. They lie within the mesangial core of the glomerular lobules and can be surrounded by patent peripheral capillary loops.
- These nodular lesions are frequently accompanied by prominent accumulations of hyaline material in capillary loops ("**fibrin caps**") or adherent to Bowman capsules ("**capsular drops**").

7. A 50-year-old male with frothy urine and periorbital edema proteinuria. The IF and electron microscopic picture of the patient is given below. Diagnosis is:

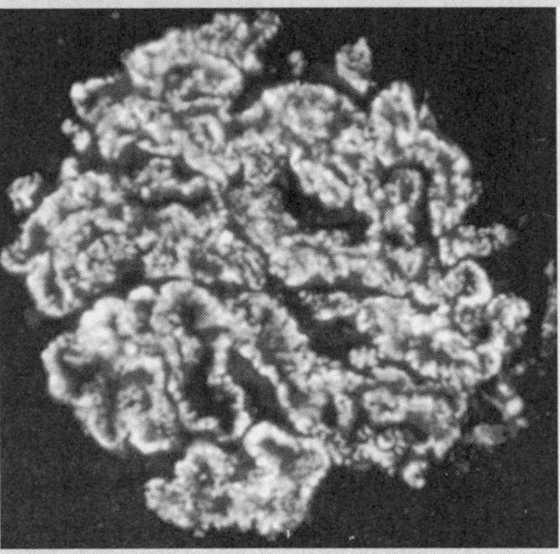

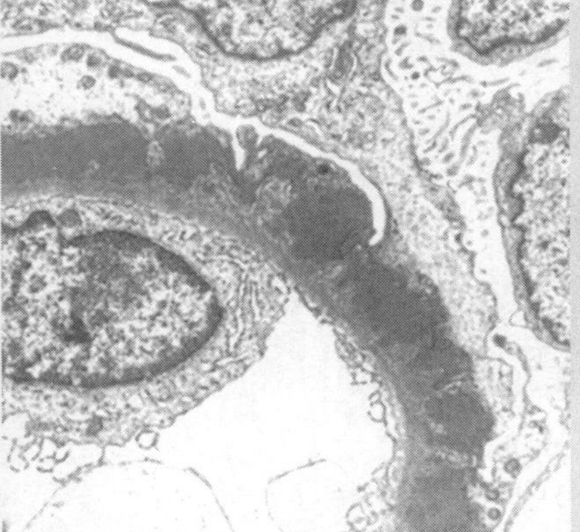

a. FSGS
b. Minimal change disease
c. MPGN
d. Membranous glomerulopathy

Ans. d. Membranous glomerulopathy

Ref. Robbins and Cotran Pathologic Basis of Diseases, 9th/ed p916 Figure 20-12.

EXPLANATION

Given image shows membranous nephropathy.

1st image: Characteristic granular immunofluorescent deposits of IgG along glomerular basement membrane.

2nd image: Electron micrograph showing electron-dense deposits along the epithelial side of the basement membrane. Note the effacement of foot processes overlying deposits.

Membranous nephropathy

- Characterized by diffuse thickening of the glomerular capillary wall due to the accumulation of deposits containing Ig along the subepithelial side of the basement membrane.
- This disorder usually presents with the insidious onset of the nephrotic syndrome or, in 15% of patients, with **non-nephrotic proteinuria.**

8. In order to avoid liver biopsy for diagnosis of fibrosis, new tests were aimed to diagnose liver fibrosis serologically:

a. Alkaline phosphate
b. Transaminase
c. Serum laminin and hyaluronic acid
d. Unconjugated bilirubin and GGT

Ans. b. Transaminase

Ref. Harsh Mohan 6th/ed p595

EXPLANATION

Transaminases

- Transaminase estimations are useful in the early diagnosis of viral hepatitis.
- Very high levels are seen in extensive acute hepatic necrosis such as in severe viral hepatitis and acute cholestasis.
- Alcoholic liver disease and cirrhosis are associated with mild to moderate elevation of transaminases.

9. What is the diagnosis of the below histopathology figure?

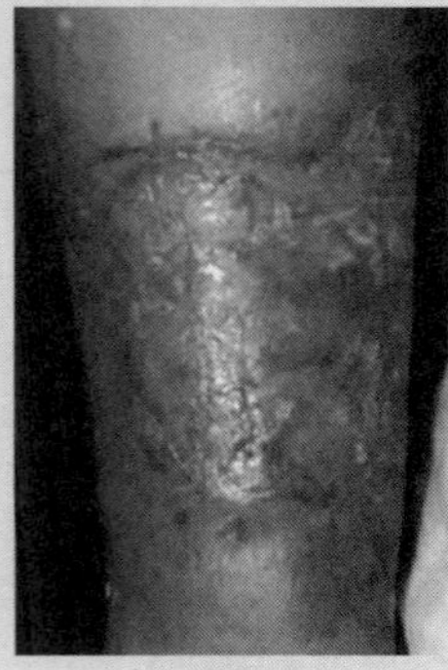
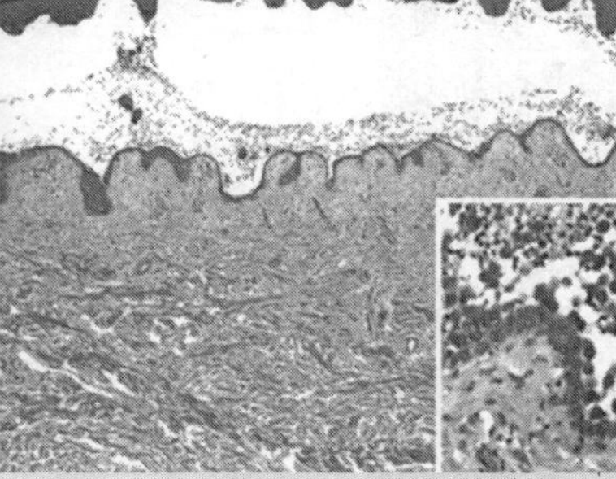
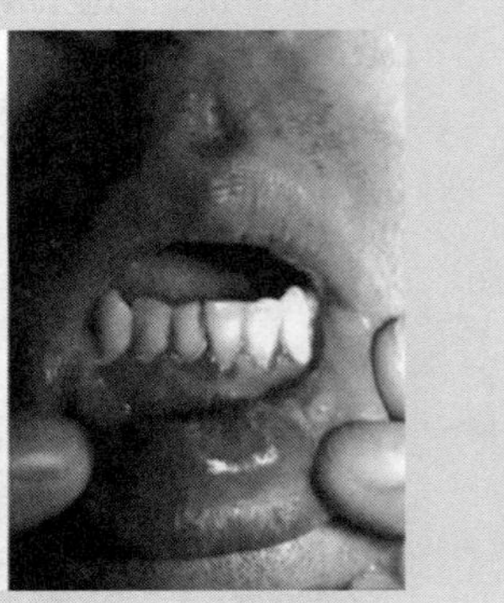

a. Pemphigus
b. Leishmaniasis
c. Mycosis fungoides
d. Psoriasis

Ans. a. Pemphigus

Ref. Robbins Pathology 9th/ed p1169, Figure 25-29

EXPLANATION

Figure above shows pemphigus vulgaris.

1st image: Eroded plaques are formed following the rupture of confluent, thin-roofed bullae, here affecting axillary skin.

2nd image: Suprabasal acantholysis results in an intraepidermal blister in which dyscohesive (acantholytic) epidermal cells are present *(inset).*

3rd image: Ulcerated blisters in the oral mucosa are also common, as seen here on the lip.

Pemphigus

- **A blistering disorder caused by autoantibodies that result in the dissolution of intercellular attachments within the epidermis and mucosal epithelium.**
- The common histologic denominator in all forms of pemphigus is **acantholysis**, the dissolution or lysis of the intercellular bridges that connect squamous epithelial cells.
- Acantholytic cells dissociate from one another, lose their polyhedral shape and become rounded.
- In pemphigus vulgaris and pemphigus vegetans, acantholysis selectively involves the cells immediately above the basal cell layer.

10. Which stain is used in the staining of liver in the following figure?

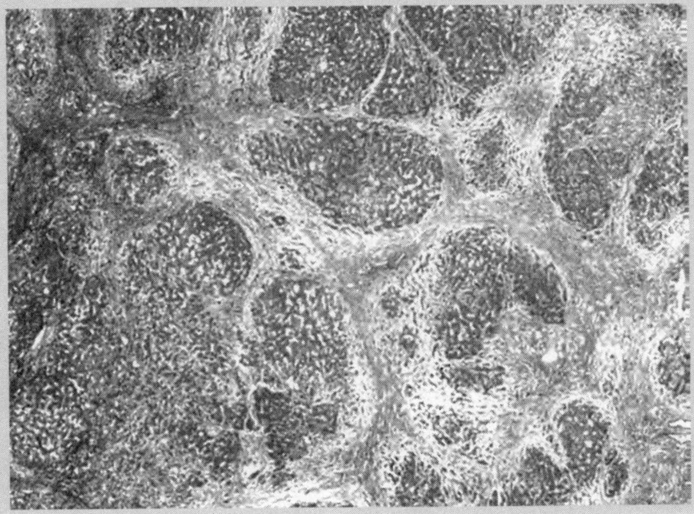

a. Silver stain
b. Masson trichrome
c. Warthin starry silver stain
d. Sweet reticulin silver stain

Ans. b. Masson trichrome

Ref. Robbins and Cotran Pathologic Basis of Diseases, 9th/ed p828, Figure 18-08.

EXPLANATION

Thick bands of collagen separate rounded cirrhotic nodules. (Masson trichrome stain)

11. Which of the following technology is used for gene editing?

a. GeneXpert
b. α PERT
c. CRISPR
d. Big Data

Ans. c. CRISPR

Ref. Genome Editing by Kursad Turksen, p3

Explanation

Clustered regularly interspaced palindromic repeats (CRISPR) are segments of prokaryotic DNA containing short, repetitive base sequences.

- Editing genes can mean removing or replacing an existing gene, switching a gene on or off, or inserting a new gene altogether.
- Whatever the aim, the first step is always to find the stretch of DNA that codes for the gene and grab hold of it is, so a cut can be made.
- CRISPR not only finds the target gene and locks on, it also delivers an enzyme that cuts the DNA with unprecedented accuracy.
- The reason it is able to manage this precision double act is because CRISPR is made of ribonucleic acid (RNA)—a molecule that can be tailor-made to perfectly match a sequence of DNA or to bind to a protein.
- CRISPR RNA does both jobs—one end is custom-made to match the target gene's DNA sequence, and the other end binds to a DNA-cutting enzyme, or nuclease.

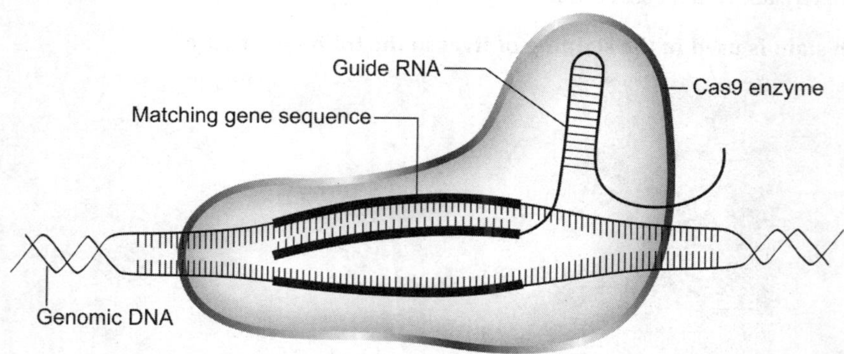

Option A: GeneXpert—used in Nucleic Acid Amplification Tests, e.g. identification of for mycobacterium tuberculosis and rifampicin resistance by polymerase chain reaction—The Xpert MTB/RIF detects DNA.

12. If the phosphorylation of RB gene is blocked what is the effect on cell cycle?

a. Cell cycle gets shorter
b. Affect G1 phase
c. Affect G2 phase
d. It would not affect because normally RB gene is in non-phosphorylated state

Ans. b. Affect G1 phase *Ref. Robbins and Cotran Pathologic Basis of Diseases 9th/ed p292*

Explanation

RB

- **A key negative regulator of the G1/S cell cycle transition.**
- **Directly or indirectly inactivated in most human cancers.**
- It exists in an active hypophosphorylated state in quiescent cells and an inactive hyperphosphorylated state in cells passing through the G1/S cell cycle transition.

The cycling and CDKs promote cell cycle progression, withe the CDK inhibitors stop it. The balance between the two groups of molecules determines whether the cell proliferates or is quiescent

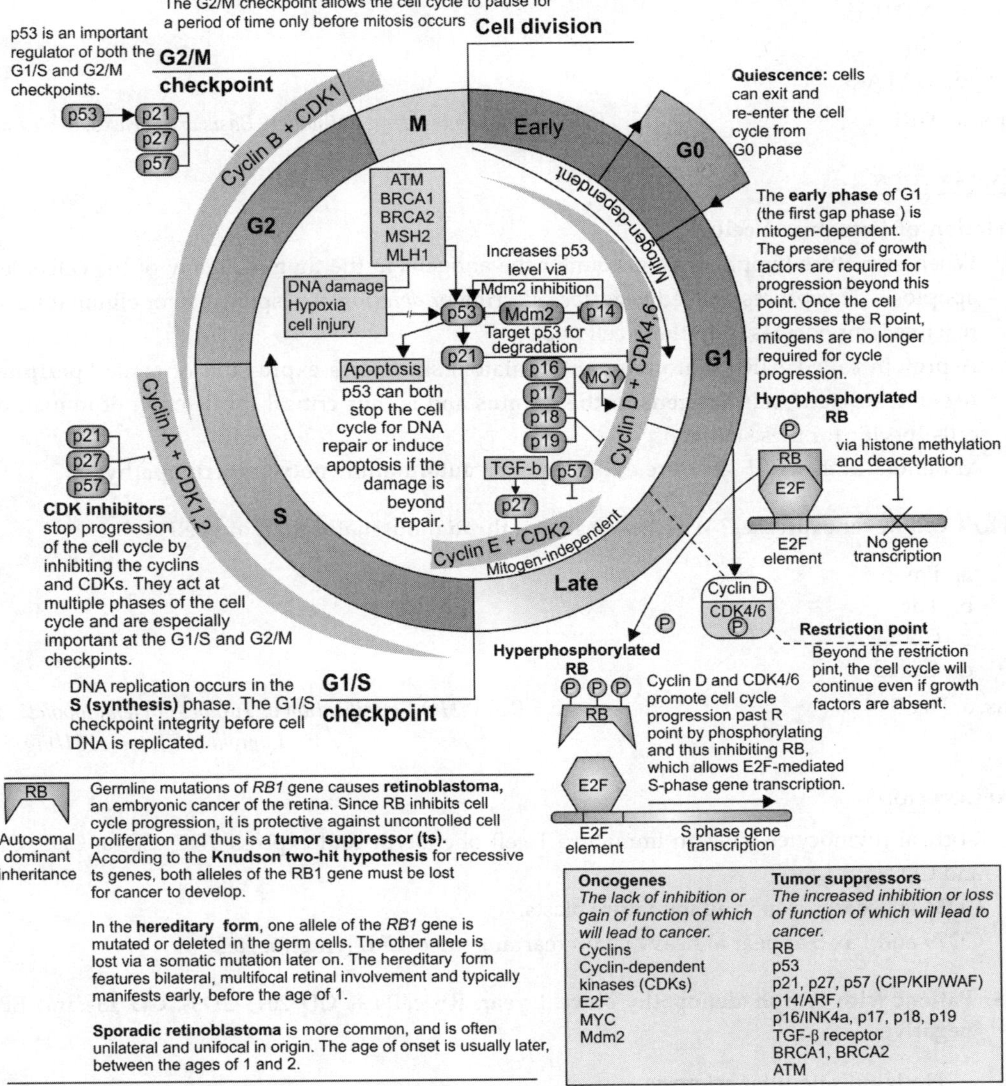

Germline mutations of *RB1* gene causes **retinoblastoma,** an embryonic cancer of the retina. Since RB inhibits cell cycle progression, it is protective against uncontrolled cell proliferation and thus is a **tumor suppressor (ts).** According to the **Knudson two-hit hypothesis** for recessive ts genes, both alleles of the RB1 gene must be lost for cancer to develop.

In the **hereditary form**, one allele of the *RB1* gene is mutated or deleted in the germ cells. The other allele is lost via a somatic mutation later on. The hereditary form features bilateral, multifocal retinal involvement and typically manifests early, before the age of 1.

Sporadic retinoblastoma is more common, and is often unilateral and unifocal in origin. The age of onset is usually later, between the ages of 1 and 2.

Oncogenes	**Tumor suppressors**
The lack of inhibition or gain of function of which will lead to cancer.	*The increased inhibition or loss of function of which will lead to cancer.*
Cyclins	RB
Cyclin-dependent kinases (CDKs)	p53
E2F	p21, p27, p57 (CIP/KIP/WAF)
MYC	p14/ARF,
Mdm2	p16/INK4a, p17, p18, p19
	TGF-β receptor
	BRCA1, BRCA2
	ATM

p53

Autosomal dominant inheritance

Germline mutations of *p53* gene causes **Li-Fraumeni syndrome**, in which multiple cancers develop at a relatively young age (<45). Breast cancer, osteosarcoma, leukemia, lymphoma, and adrenocortical carcinomas are the most common cancers found in Li-Fraumeni syndrome

Similar to retinoblastoma, the **two-hit hypothesis** applies to Li-Fraumeni syndrome as well. One allele of *p53* is lost in the germline and the second allele is lost somatically. The risk of cancer is dominantly inherited.

p53 is called the "guardian of the genome." It is lost in almost every type of cancer because its loss confers a significant survival advantage, leading to rapid, unchecked proliferation and evasion of apoptosis.

13. Which gene is responsible for expression of self-antigen for deletion of immature t cell?

a. AIRE
b. NOTCH- 3
c. Rb
d. GATA-3

Ans. a. AIRE *Ref. Robbins and Cotran Pathologic Basis of Diseases, 9th/ed p213*

Explanation

Deletion of immature t cells

- When immature lymphocytes encounter the antigens in the thymus, many of the cells die by apoptosis. This process, called ***negative selection* or *deletion*,** is responsible for eliminating self-reactive lymphocytes from the T-cell pool.
- A protein called AIRE (autoimmune regulator) stimulates expression of some "**peripheral tissue-restricted" self-antigens in the thymus** and is thus critical for deletion of immature T cells specific for these antigens.
- Mutations in the *AIRE* gene are the cause of **an autoimmune polyendocrinopathy.**

14. T cell never expresses? Which was absent throughout maturation of t cell?

a. Pax-5
b. Tdt
c. CD 34
d. CD 1a

Ans. a. Pax-5 *Ref. WHO Classification of Tumors of Hematopoietic and Lymphoid Tissue/p161/Fig. 8.03*

Explanation

- Cortical thymocytes have an immature T cell phenotype and express TDT, CD1a, CD3, CD5, and CD34.
- CD34 is usually seen in all immature blasts.
- CD79 and Pax-5 appear at heavy chain rearrangement of B lymphocytes.

15. Patient with lymphadenopathy since 1 year. RS cells +, CD 20+, CD3-, CD 15- and EBV negative:

a. Hodgkin's nodular sclerosis
b. Nodular lymphocyte predominant HL
c. HL lymphocyte rich
d. Mixed cellularity

Ans. b. Nodular lymphocyte predominant HL

Ref. Robbins and Cotran Pathologic Basis of Diseases 9ed

Explanation

Subtypes of Hodgkin Lymphoma

Subtype	Morphology and immunophenotype	Typical clinical features
Nodular sclerosis	Frequent lacunar cells and occasional diagnostic RS cells; background infiltrate composed of T lymphocytes, eosinophils, macrophages, and plasma cells; fibrous bands dividing cellular areas into nodules. RS cells CD15+, CD30+; usually EBV−	Most common subtype; usually stage I or II disease; frequent mediastinal involvement; equal occurrence in males and females (F = M), most patients young adults
Mixed cellularity	Frequent mononuclear and diagnostic RS cells; background infiltrate rich in T lymphocytes, eosinophils, macrophages, plasma cells; RS cells CD15+, CD30+; 70% EBV+	More than 50% present as stage III or IV disease; M greater than F; biphasic incidence, peaking in young adults and again in adults older than 55
Lymphocyte rich	Frequent mononuclear and diagnostic RS cells; background infiltrate rich in T lymphocytes; RS cells CD15+, CD30+; 40% EBV−	Uncommon; M greater than F; tends to be seen in older adults
Lymphocyte depletion	Reticular variant: Frequent diagnostic RS cells and variants and a paucity of background reactive cells; RS cells CD15+, CD30+; most EBV+	Uncommon; more common in older males, HIV-infected individuals, and in developing countries; often presents with advanced disease
Lymphocyte predominance	Frequent L&H (popcorn cell) variants in a background of follicular dendritic cells and reactive B cells; RS cells CD20+, CD15−, C30−; EBv−	Uncommon; young males with cervical or axillary lymphadenopathy; mediastinal

16. Variation in gene expression by methylation and acetylation without changing content of the gene:

a. Mutation
b. Inversion
c. Epigenetics
d. Amplification

Ans. c. Epigenetics *Ref. Robbins and Cotran Pathologic Basis of Diseases 9th/ed p613*

Explanation

Epigenetics refers to reversible, heritable changes in gene expression that occur without mutation.

Gene expression is regulated by two types of epigenetic modifications, DNA methylation and posttranslational modifications of histones (e.g. acetylation, methylation, phosphorylation).

Option b: **Inversion** occur when there are two interstitial breaks in a chromosome, and the segment reunites after a complete turnaround.

Option d: Amplification

- Proto-oncogenes may be converted to oncogenes by amplification, with consequent overexpression, of otherwise normal proteins. Such amplification may produce several hundred copies of the proto-oncogene in the tumor cell.

17. Function of acetone free methyl alcohol in staining is:

a. Sterilizes the slide
b. Fixes the cells to the slide
c. Regulates the metabolism of the cells
d. Staining the cell

Ans: b. Fixes the cells to the slide *Ref. Laboratory Hematology Practice p285*

EXPLANATION

- Methyl alcohol acts as fixative in Leishman stain.
- Acetone if present destroys cell membrane.

18. A 26-year-old female with history of breathlessness comes with 5 g/dL hemoglobin and normal WBC count, absolute reticulocyte count was 9. What will be the corrected reticulocyte count?

a. 3
b. 4
c. 4.5
d. 5

Ans. a. 3 *Ref: Clinical hematology by Turgeon. Page 77*

EXPLANATION

Corrected reticulocyte count = Absolute reticulocyte count x Hemoglobin/15
= 9 × 5/15 = 3

19. Red cell distribution width measures:

a. Anisocytosis
b. Polychromasia
c. Poikilocytosis
d. Hypochromasia

Ans: a. Anisocytosis *Ref. Rapid Review of Hematology, 1st/ed p05*

EXPLANATION

- Red cell distribution width is a quantitative measure of anisocytosis.
- RDW is particularly useful in characterizing microcytic anemia, allowing to distinguish between uncomplicated iron deficiency anemia (high RDW, normal to low MCV) and uncomplicated heterozygous thalassemia (normal RDW, low MCV), although other tests are usually required to confirm the diagnosis.
- RDW is also useful in identifying red cell fragmentation, agglutination, or dimorphic cell populations (including patients who have had transfusions, have sideroblastic anemias, or have been recently treated for a nutritional deficiency).
- **Poikilocytosis:** Variation in shape of cells, e.g. Sickle cell, Burr Cell, Schistocytes, Ovalocytes, etc.
- **Polychromasia** (also known as Polychromatophilia) is a disorder where there is an abnormally high number of immature red blood cells found in the bloodstream as a result of being prematurely released from the bone marrow during blood formation. (Poly- refers to many, and -chromasia means color).
- **Hypochromasia:** Hypochromia is characterized by an increase in central pallor. It is said to be present when greater than 1/2 of the cell diameter has central pallor. Hypochromia is caused by a deficiency in the production of hemoglobin, which is usually the result of iron deficiency caused by chronic hemorrhage.

20. Latest marker on mantle cell lymphoma:

a. MYD 88
b. ITRA1
c. SOX 11
d. Annexin 5

Ans. c. SOX 11 *Ref. The 2016 revision of the World Health Organization Classification of Lymphoid Neoplasms, bloodjournal.com*

EXPLANATION

Mantle cell lymphoma (MCL)

- Recognized as an aggressive but incurable small B-cell lymphoma that developed in a linear fashion from naıve B cells.
- Two types of clinically indolent variants are now recognized and reflect, in part, that MCL develops along 2 very different pathways.
- Classical MCL is usually composed of IGHV-unmutated or minimally mutated B cells that usually express SOX11 and typically involves lymph nodes and other extranodal sites.
- Other MCL develop from IGHV-mutated SOX11- B cells.

21. ALK positive cancer:

a. Ewing's sarcoma
b. Synovial sarcoma
c. Fibroma
d. Inflammatory myofibroblastic tumor

Ans. d. Inflammatory myofibroblastic tumor *Ref. Rosai and Ackerman 10th/ed p45*

EXPLANATION

ALK

- Useful for the identification of **anaplastic large cell lymphoma.**
- Expression of the ALK protein also occurs **in inflammatory myofibroblastic tumor** and rare cases of pulmonary adenocarcinoma.

22. Negative acute phase reactant:

a. Ferritin
b. CRP
c. Haptoglobin
d. Albumin

Ans. d. Albumin *Ref. Dacie and Lewis Practical Hematology 11th/ed p101*

EXPLANATION

Inflammatory response to tissue injury includes alteration in serum protein concentration, especially increases in **fibrinogen, haptoglobin, ceruloplasmin, immunoglobulins and CRP, and decrease in albumin.**

Acute Phase Reactant	
Positive acute phase reactant	**Negative acute phase reactant**
CRP (C-Reactive protein) Alpha-1 Antitrypsin Ceruloplasmin Fibrinogen IL- 1, IL -6, TNF-α Haptoglobulin	Albumin and prealbumin Transferrin Retinol binding protein Transthyretin

PGI May 2017

1. Sideroblastic anemia findings include:

a. Coarse basophilic stippling
b. Erythroid hypoplasia in marrow
c. Pappenheimer bodies
d. Dimorphic RBC
e. Increase MCHC

Ans. c. Pappenheimer bodies and d. Dimorphic RBC *Ref: Harsh Mohan,6th/ed p302*

EXPLANATION

Sideroblastic anemias usually show the following hematological features:

- There is generally moderate to severe degree of *anemia.*
- The *blood picture* shows hypochromic anemia which may be microcytic, or there may be some normocytic red cells as well (***dimorphic– Option d***). Iron-containing inclusions (***Pappenheimer bodies***) in the RBCs (***Option c***).
- *Absolute values* (MCV, MCH and **MCHC**) are reduced ***(Option e)*** in hereditary type but MCV is often raised in acquired type.
- *Bone marrow examination* shows erythroid hyperplasia (***Option b***) with usually macronormoblastic erythropoiesis. Marrow iron stores are raised and pathognomonic ring sideroblasts are present.
- *Serum ferritin* levels are raised.
- *Serum iron* is usually raised with almost complete saturation of TIBC.
- There is increased *iron deposition* in the tissue.

2. Primary myelofibrosis true is/ are:

a. Dry tap on bone marrow aspiration
b. Increase myeloblastic in peripheral blood
c. Spleen size reduces after treatment
d. Only treatment option is stem cell transplant
e. Option not recalled

Ans. a. Dry tap on bone marrow aspiration; b. Increase myeloblastic in peripheral blood and d. Only treatment option is stem cell transplant *Ref: Williams Hematology,9e/p1323 Table 86-2. Harrison's Principles of Internal Medicine 19th/ed p676*

EXPLANATION

Diagnostic Findings in Primary Myelofibrosis (PMF)

Prefibrotic Stage

- Anemia may be absent or mild
- Leukocytosis may be absent or slight
- Thrombocythemia is invariable
- *BCR-ABL* fusion gene absent
- Presence of *JAK2, CALR, or MPL* mutations indicative of diagnosis of myeloproliferative disease (one of these mutations present in ~90% of patients)
- Cellular marrow with mild increase in granulopoiesis; increased megakaryocytes, clusters of very dysmorphic megakaryocytes and megakaryocytic nuclei; no to very slight increase in reticular fibers on silver stain
- Palpable splenomegaly infrequent
- Absent or slight anisopoikilocytosis including teardrop red cells

Fully Developed Stage

- Marrow reticulin fibrosis plus or minus collagen fibrosis (dry tap)
- *BCR-ABL* fusion gene absent
- *JAK2, CALR, or MPL* mutation in approximately 90% of patients
- Splenomegaly
- A blood smear will show the characteristic features of extramedullary hematopoiesis: teardrop-shaped red cells, nucleated red cells, myelocytes, and promyelocytes; myeloblasts may also be present (***Option b***)
- Increased CD34+ cells in blood
- Nucleated red cells in blood
- Marrow usually hypercellular but invariably has increased megakaryocytes, clusters of highly dysmorphic megakaryocytes, and megakaryocyte bare nuclei regardless of overall marrow cellularity. Marrow is usually inaspirable due to the myelofibrosis.(***Option a***)

Treatment

- No specific therapy exists for PMF
- Allogeneic bone marrow transplantation is the only curative treatment for PMF and should be considered in younger patients (***Option d***)
- Nonmyeloablative conditioning regimens may permit hematopoietic cell transplantation to be extended to older individuals, but this approach is currently under investigation.
- About splenomegaly (***Option c***) in PMF
    - Splenomegaly is by far the most distressing and intractable problem for PMF patients, causing abdominal pain, portal hypertension, easy satiety, and cachexia.
    - Surgical removal of a massive spleen is associated with significant postoperative complications including mesenteric venous thrombosis, hemorrhage, rebound leukocytosis and thrombocytosis, and hepatic extramedullary hematopoiesis with no amelioration of either anemia or thrombocytopenia when present.
    - For unexplained reasons, splenectomy also increases the risk of blastic transformation. Splenic irradiation is, at best, temporarily palliative and associated with a significant risk of neutropenia, infection, and subsequent operative hemorrhage if splenectomy is attempted.

3. Diagnostic of AML:

a. T(11:14)
b. T(8:14)
c. T(8:11
d. T (9:22)
e. T(15:17)

Ans. e. T(15:17) *Ref. Rodaks Hematology 5th/ed p608*

EXPLANATION

Acute myeloid leukemia with recurrent genetic abnormalities (2008 World Health Organization Classification)

- AML with t(8;21)(q22;q22); *RUNX1-RUNX1T1*
- AML with inv(16)(p13.1q22) or t(16;16)(p13.1;q22); *CBFB-MYH11*
- APL with t(15;17)(q22;q12); *PML-RARA*
- AML with t(9;11)(p22;q23); *MLLT3-MLL*
- AML with t(6;9)(p23;q34); *DEK-NUP214*
- AML with inv(3)(q21q26.2) or t(3;3)(q21;q26.2); *RPN1-EVI1*
- AML with t(1;22)(p13;q13) *RBM15-MKL1*

4. Erythropoietin is secreted from:

a. Peritubular capillary
b. JG apparatus
c. DCT
d. Glomerulus
e. Pars recta of PCT

Ans. a. Peritubular capillary *Ref. Rodaks Hematology 5th/ed p89*

EXPLANATION

EPO is a lineage-specific glycoprotein produced in the *renal peritubular interstitial cells*. In addition, a small amount of EPO is produced by the liver.

5. Both PT and APTT will be increased in:

a. Factor 2 deficiency
b. Factor 5 deficiency
c. Factor 10 deficiency
d. Factor 8 deficiency
e. Factor 12 deficiency
f. DIC

Ans. a. Factor 2 deficiency; b. Factor 5 deficiency; c. Factor 10 deficiency and f. DIC

Ref. Harsh Mohan—Textbook of Pathology p331

EXPLANATION

Following are the common causes for higher values in both these tests:

i. Hypofibrinogenemia (e.g. in DIC).
ii. Raised concentration of FDP.
iii. Presence of heparin.
Deficiency of common pathway factors-10, 5, prothrombin (factor 2), fibrinogen (factor 4)

6. What decreases during acute inflammation?

a. Ceruloplasmin
b. Transferrin
c. CRP
d. ESR
e. Albumin
f. Haptoglobin

Ans. e. Albumin *Ref. Dacie and Lewis Practical Hematology 11th/ed p101*

EXPLANATION

Inflammatory response to tissue injury includes alteration in serum protein concentration, especially **increases in fibrinogen, haptoglobin, ceruloplasmin, immunoglobulins and CRP**, and **decrease in albumin**.

7. Which of these is/are small vessel vasculitis?

a. Anti-GBM
b. Takayasu
c. Temporal
d. Kawasaki
e. Carcinoma induced vasculitis
f. Cutaneous

Ans. a. Anti-GBM; d. Kawasaki and e. Carcinoma induced vasculitis.

Ref. Robbins and Cotran Pathologic Basis of Diseases 9th/ed p505-513

EXPLANATION

- ❑ Small vessel vasculitis:
  - ▪ Granulomatosis with polyangiitis

- Churg-Strauss syndrome
- Polyarteritis nodosa
- Leucocytoclastic vasculitis (**cutaneous/carcinoma**),

❑ Buerger disease
❑ Behcet disease
❑ Immune complex mediated vasculitis [SLE, HSP, Cryoglobulin vasculitis, **Kawasaki disease, Goodpasture disease** (antiGBM)]

8. Antigen presenting cells:

a. Langerhan of skin
b. Kupffer
c. Macrophages
d. Monocytes
e. Thymic cells

Ans. a. Langerhan of skin; b. Kupffer and c. Macrophages

Ref. Robbins and Cotran Pathologic Basis of Diseases 9th/ed p195,825

EXPLANATION

Class II MHC molecules are mainly expressed on cells that present ingested antigens and respond to T-cell help (**macrophages**, B lymphocytes, and dendritic cells). Immature dendritic cells within the epidermis are called ***Langerhans cells.*** Antigens in the liver are taken up by Kupffer cells (antigen presenting cells).

9. Autosomal recessive polycystic kidney disease features include:

a. Can be diagnosed intrauterine
b. Proceeds to renal failure till children reaches school going age
c. Can be palpated abdominally
d. Hypertension doesn't develop until late stages of the disease
e. Enlarged kidney

Ans. a. Can be diagnosed intrauterine *Ref: Harrison's Principles of Internal Medicine 19th ed/p1853*

EXPLANATION

Clinical features of ARPKD (Autosomal recessive polycystic kidney disease) are:

❑ Classic ARPKD **is generally diagnosed in utero** or within the neonatal period and characterized by greatly enlarged echogenic kidneys in diseased fetuses. (***Option a***)
❑ Reduced fetal urine production may contribute to oligohydramnios and pulmonary hypoplasia.
❑ About 30% of affected neonates die shortly after birth due to respiratory insufficiency. Close to 60% of mortality occurs within the first month of life.
❑ In the classic group, **most patients are born with renal insufficiency and ESRD** (End stage renal disease). (***Option b***)
❑ However, infants often have a transient improvement in their GFR; death from renal insufficiency at this stage is rare.
❑ Some patients are diagnosed after the neonatal stage and form the older group. Morbidity and mortality in this group often involve systemic hypertension, progressive renal insufficiency, and liver manifestations.
❑ The hallmarks of ARPKD liver disease are biliary dysgenesis due to a primary ductal plate malformation with associated periportal fibrosis, namely congenital hepatic fibrosis (CHF) and dilatation of intrahepatic bile ducts (Caroli's disease). CHF and Caroli's disease can then lead to portal hypertension exhibiting hepatosplenomegaly, variceal bleeding, and cholangitis.

- ❑ Some patients with the diagnosis of ARPKD **at 1 year of age with nephromegaly** exhibit slowly declining renal function over 20 years with **only minimally enlarged kidneys at ESRD** (***Option c and e***) and markedly atrophic kidneys following renal transplantation.
- ❑ The slow progression of renal disease is likely due to increasing fibrosis rather than the development of cysts.
- ❑ Systemic hypertension is common in all ARPKD patients, even those with normal renal function. ***(option d)***

10. True statement/s among the following is/are:

a. In Hemophilia B factor 8 concentrate is used.
b. Both PT and aPTT are increased in DIC
c. IV Immunoglobulin is useful in Idiopathic thrombocytopenic purpura
d. In DIC thrombocytopenia is present in approximately 50% of cases

Ans. b. Both PT and aPTT are increased in DIC and c. IV Immunoglobulin is useful in Idiopathic thrombocytopenic purpura *Ref: Rodaks Hematology,5e p681,p705 and p720*

EXPLANATION

Option c: Idiopathic thrombocytopenic purpura (ITP)

- ❑ Most patients with acute ITP recover with or without treatment in about 3 weeks, although for some, recovery may take 6 months
- ❑ Most patients with acute ITP have relatively mild symptoms, and no treatment is needed.
- ❑ The most severe cases may need to be treated, however, and **intravenous immunoglobulin (IVIG)**, platelet transfusions, and splenectomy (or some combination of these) seem to offer the most immediate benefit.

***Option a*: Hemophilia**

- ❑ *Hemophilia A- Factor VIII deficiency*
  - Hemophilia A is the most common hereditary cause of serious bleeding.
  - It is an X-linked recessive disorder caused by reduced factor VIII activity.
  - Hemophilia A is treated with factor VIII infusions
- ❑ *Hemophilia B—Factor IX Deficiency*
  - Severe factor IX deficiency is an X-linked disorder that is indistinguishable clinically from hemophilia A but much less common.
  - The diagnosis is made using specific assays of factor IX.
  - It is treated by infusion of recombinant factor IX.

***Option b*: Common causes for higher values in both PT and APTT:**

- ❑ Hypofibrinogenemia (e.g. in DIC).
- ❑ Raised concentration of FDP (Fibrin degradation products).
- ❑ Presence of heparin.
- ❑ Deficiency of common pathway factors-10, 5, prothrombin (factor 2), fibrinogen (factor 1)

Option d: Disseminated intravascular coagulation (DIC). In DIC thrombocytopenia is present in almost all cases.

- ❑ Prolonged PT and aPTT reflect coagulation factor consumption.
- ❑ Fibrinogen concentrations may decrease in DIC, but because fibrinogen is an acute phase reactant that rises in inflammation, the fibrinogen concentration alone provides little reliable information and may exceed 400 mg/dL.
- ❑ The peripheral blood film platelet estimate confirms thrombocytopenia in nearly all cases (***Option d***), and the presence of schistocytes helps establish the diagnosis of DIC in about 50% of cases.

12. Pick the correctly matched pairs and inheritance patterns

a. Hypophosphatemic rickets—XLD
b. Duchene—CLR
c. Achondroplasia—AR
d. Sickle—AR
e. Osteogenesis imperfecta 1—AR

Ans. a. Hypophosphatemic rickets—XLD; b. Duchene—CLR and d. Sickle—AR

Ref. Harsh Mohan Textbook of Pathology, p260

EXPLANATION

Important Examples of Mendelian Disorders (Single Gene Defects):

I. Autosomal Recessive Inheritance

1. β-thalassemia
2. **Sickle cell anemia**
3. Hemochromatosis
4. Cystic fibrosis of pancreas
5. Albinism
6. Wilson's disease
7. Xeroderma pigmentosum
8. Inborn errors of metabolism (lysosomal storage diseases, glycogenosis, alkaptonuria, phenylketonuria)

II. Autosomal Codominant Inheritance

1. ABO blood group antigens
2. α1-antitrypsin deficiency
3. HLA antigens

III. Autosomal Dominant Inheritance

1. Familial polyposis coli
2. Adult polycystic kidney
3. Hereditary spherocytosis
4. Neurofibromatosis (von Recklinghausen's disease)
5. Marfan's syndrome
6. von Willebrand's disease
7. Hereditary hemorrhagic telangiectasia
8. Acute intermittent porphyria
9. Familial hypercholesterolemia
10. **Osteogenesis imperfect**
11. **Achondroplasia**

IV. Sex-(X-) Linked Recessive Inheritance

1. Hemophilia A
2. G6PD deficiency
3. Diabetes insipidus
4. Chronic granulomatous disease
5. Color blindness
6. Bruton's agammaglobulinemia
7. **Muscular dystrophies (Duchenne's)**

V. Sex-(X-) Linked Dominant Inheritance

1. **Hypophosphatemic rickets**
2. Incontinentia pigmenti

12. Which is not a tumor suppressor protein?

a. P53
b. RB
c. RAS
d. CD95
e. ST7

Ans. c. RAS and d. CD95 *Ref. Robbins and Cotran Pathologic Basis of Diseases 9th/ed p280*

EXPLANATION

- P53/Rb/ST7/ST11 are tumor suppressor genes
- RAS is a proto-oncogene
- CD 95 is an apoptosis associated gene

There are 4 groups of genes involved in cancer:

1. Proto-oncogene
2. Tumor suppressor gene
3. Apoptosis associated gene
4. Cyclins and CDK associated genes.

Four classes of normal regulatory genes—the growth promoting proto-oncogenes, the growth-inhibiting tumor suppressor genes, genes that regulate programmed cell death (apoptosis), and genes involved in DNA repair—are the principal targets of cancer causing mutations. APC, NF1, NF2, PTCH, PTEN, SMAD2, SMAD4, **RB**, CDKN2A, VHL, STK11, SDHB, SDHD, CDH1, TP53, BRCA1, BRCA2, MSH2, MLH1, MSH6, WT1, MEN1 are tumor suppressor genes.

13. Multiple myeloma causes:

a. Amyloidosis
b. Interstitial nephritis
c. Nephrocalcinosis
d. Cast nephropathy
e. Cryoglobulinemia

Ans. a. Amyloidosis; c. Nephrocalcinosis and d. Cast nephropathy

Ref. Harsh Mohan Textbook of Pathology p382

EXPLANATION

Myeloma kidney: Renal involvement in myeloma called myeloma nephrocalcinosis occurs in many cases. The main mechanism of myeloma kidney is by filtration of light chain proteins (Bence Jones proteins) which are precipitated in the distal convoluted tubules in combination with Tamm-Horsfall proteins as tubular casts. The casts may be surrounded by some multinucleate giant-cells and a few inflammatory cells. Systemic primary generalized amyloidosis (AL amyloid) may occur in 10% cases of multiple myeloma and involve multiple organs and systems.

14. Tumor marker for lung adenocarcinoma:

a. Cytokeratin 7
b. Cytokeratin 20
c. TTF1
d. Cytokeratin 5

Ans. a. Cytokeratin 7 and c. TTF1 *Ref. Rosai and Ackerman 10th/ed p372*

EXPLANATION

Lung adenocarcinoma: There is reactivity for low molecular weight keratins (sometimes in conjunction with vimentin), EMA, CEA, secretory components, and various members of the MUC family. Expression of **keratin** 7 has been taken as evidence of glandular differentiation in lung carcinoma. **TTF1** is usually positive. Napsin A is positive in most cases.

15. Which subtype has been included under squamous cell carcinoma of lung?

a. Basaloid type
b. Lymphoepitheliod type
c. Papillary
d. Clear cell
e. Nonkeratinizing

Ans. a. Basaloid type and e. Nonkeratinizing

Ref. The 2015 World Health Organization Classification of Lung Tumors Impact of Genetic, Clinical and Radiologic Advances Since the 2004 Classification/p1251

Explanation

The subtyping of squamous cell carcinoma was modified to consist of:

- Keratinizing
- Nonkeratinizing, and
- Basaloid subtypes.

16. Cancers caused by viruses:

a. Nasopharyngeal
b. Kaposi
c. Hepatocellular
c. Endometrial Ca
e. Basal cell carcinoma

Ans. a. Nasopharyngeal; b. Kaposi and c. Hepatocellular

Ref. Robbins and Cotran Pathologic Basis of Diseases 9th/ed p327

Explanation

Epstein-Barr Virus: EBV, a member of the herpesvirus family, has been implicated in the pathogenesis of several human tumors: the African form of Burkitt lymphoma; B-cell lymphomas in immunosuppressed individuals (particularly in those with HIV infection or undergoing immunosuppressive therapy after organ or bone marrow transplantation); a subset of Hodgkin lymphoma; **nasopharyngeal** and some gastric carcinomas; and rare forms of T-cell lymphoma and natural killer (NK) cell lymphoma.

HHV8 (Human Herpesvirus 8) causes **Kaposi's sarcoma**

HTLV-1 causes *adult T-cell leukemia/lymphoma.*

It is estimated that 70% to 85% of hepatocellular carcinomas worldwide are caused by infection with hepatitis B virus (HBV) or hepatitis C virus (HCV).

LIST OF QUESTIONS THAT WERE NOT RECALLED PROPERLY

Question: True statement about RAS was asked and options were like (a) It is a tyrosine kinase and other options were related to location and mechanism

Ref: Robbins and Cotran Pathologic basis of diseases, 9th/ed p286

Explanation

About RAS:

- **Point mutations of *RAS* family genes constitute the most common type of abnormality involving proto-oncogenes in human tumors.**
- Approximately 15% to 20% of all human tumors express mutated RAS proteins, but in some types of cancers the frequency of *RAS* mutations is much higher. For example:

- 90% of pancreatic adenocarcinomas and cholangiocarcinomas contain a *RAS* point mutation,
- 50% of colon, endometrial, and thyroid cancers and
- 30% of lung adenocarcinomas and myeloid leukemias.

❑ Its role in cell signaling
- Stimulation of receptor tyrosine kinases by growth factors leads to exchange of GDP for GTP and subsequent conformational changes that generate active RAS, which in turn stimulates both the MAPK and PI3K/AKT arms of the receptor tyrosine kinase signaling pathway

Question: True or false statements were asked about Gastric lymphoma and options were related to its incidence and types

Ref: Rosai and Ackerman,10th/ed p644

EXPLANATION

Gastric lymphoma:

❑ **Primary malignant lymphoma** of the stomach makes up only a small percentage (about 10%) of all malignant tumors of this organ, but there is evidence that its incidence is increasing.

❑ They are regarded as primary gastric tumors if the bulk of the disease is present in the stomach, with or without regional lymph node involvement.

❑ Nearly all of the cases are of non-Hodgkin type and the large majority is of B-cell derivation. As such, they show monotypic expression of immunoglobulin and rearrangements of the immunoglobulin genes.

❑ For practical purposes, they can be divided into two large categories:
1. Low-grade lymphomas, composed of small lymphoid cells
2. High-grade lymphomas, composed of large cells.
   - **Note:** Mixed small cell–large cell lymphomas also occur, but they constitute a distinct minority of the cases.

Question: Succinate Dehydrogenase (SDH) deficient variety of GIST was asked.

Ref: Enzinger and Weiss' Soft Tissue Tumor, 6th/ed p582

EXPLANATION

SDH- deficient GIST:

❑ **Germline mutations** have been identified in SDH-deficient GISTs in the genes for **four of the five protein subunits that comprise the SDH complex**: *SDHA, SDHB, SDHC,* and *SDHD.*

❑ SDH-deficient GISTs are also unusual with respect to clinical behavior. Unlike conventional GISTs, SDH-deficient GISTs have a **propensity to metastasize to lymph nodes**, which happens in approximately 50% of cases.

❑ Characterized by a predilection for **gastric location**

❑ Composed of epithelioid or mixed epithelioid and spindle cell morphology,

❑ Have a distinctive **multinodular/infiltrative growth pattern**, frequently are multoifocal

❑ Diffusely and strongly positive for KIT by immunohistochemistry

❑ All demonstrate loss of ***SDHB*** expression by immunohistochemistry

Question: Translocation in synovial cell sarcoma was asked

Ref: Rosai and Ackerman,10th/ed p2176

EXPLANATION

Question: Synovial sarcoma translocation:

- In over 90% of the cases the chromosomal translocation t(X;18)(p11.2;q11.2) is seen
- This results in the fusion of the *SS18* (formerly known as *SYT*) gene on chromosome 18 with either *SSX1* (in two-thirds of the cases) or *SSX2* (the other third) on chromosome X.

JIPMER Pattern Based

1. Protein involved in the pathology of dementia with lewy body?

a. Tau protein
b. Amyloid
c. Alpha synuclein
d. Neurofibrillary tangle

Ans. c. Alpha synuclein

Ref: Robbins and Cotran Pathologic basis of diseases,9e/ p836

EXPLANATION

Lewy Body

- Lewy bodies are seen in Lewy body dementia and Parkinson's disease.
- When dementia arises within 1 year of the onset of motor symptoms, it is referred to *Lewy body dementia* (LBD).
- Lewy bodies are also seen in Parkinson's disease, but dementia occurs 1 year after onset of motor symptoms.
- **Lewy bodies** are single or multiple, intracytoplasmic, eosinophilic, round to elongated inclusions that often have a dense core surrounded by a pale halo.
- On ultrastructural examination, Lewy bodies consist of fine filaments, densely packed in the core but loose at the rim, composed of α-synuclein (***Answer***) and other proteins, including neurofilaments and ubiquitin.

See below table for a glance on other neurodegenerative diseases and respective proteins involved.

Protein Inclusions in Degenerative Diseases

Disease	Protein	Location
Alzheimer disease	Aβ Tau	Extracellular Neurons
Frontotemporal lobar degeneration	Tau	Neurons
Progressive supranuclear palsy	Tau	Neurons and glia
Corticobasal degeneration	Tau	Neurons and glia
Parkinson disease	α–synuclein	Neurons
Multiple system atrophy	α–Synuclein	Glia and some neurons
Frontotemporal lobar degenerations	TDP–43	Neurons
Amyotrophic lateral sclerosis	TDP–43 SOD–I (familial disease)	Neurons Neurons

Protein Inclusions in Degenerative Diseases		
Huntington disease	Huntingtin	Neurons
Spinocerebellar ataxias	Ataxins (various)	Neurons
SOD–I, superoxide dismutase–I; TDP–43, TAR DNA–binding protien 43.		

2. Osteogenesis imperfecta associated with normal sclera, normal dentition and better prognosis is:

a. Type 1
b. Type 2
c. Type 3
d. Type 4

Ans. a. Type 1 *Ref. Robbins and Cotran Pathologic Basis of Diseases 9th/ed*

EXPLANATION

In various subtypes of OI the color of sclera is not a distinguishing features, it can be normal or blue in all subtypes except type 2.

Subtype	Collagen defect	Inheritance	Major clinical features	Prognosis
I	Decreased synthesis of pro-α1(1) chain Abnormal pro-α1(1) or pro-α2(1) chains	Autosomal dominant	Postnatal fractures, blue sclera Normal stature Skeletal fragility Dentinogenesis imperfecta Hearing impairment Joint laxity Blue sclerae	Compatible with survival
II	Abnormally short pro-α1(1) chain Unstable triple helix Abnormal or insufficient pro-α2(1)	Most autosomal recessive Some autosomal dominant New mutations	Death in utero or within days of birth Skeletal deformity with excessive fragility and multiple fractures Blue sclera	Perinatal lethal
III	Altered structure of propeptides of pro-α2(1) Impaired formation of triple helix	Autosomal dominant (75%) Autosomal recessive (25%)	Compatible with survival Growth retardation Multiple fractures Progressive kyphoscoliosis Blue sclera at birth that become white Hearing impairment Dentinogenesis imperfecta	Progressive, deforming
IV	Short pro-α2(1) chain Unstable triple helix	Autosomal dominant	Postnatal fractures, normal sclerae Moderate skeletal fragility Short stature Sometimes dentinogenesis imperfecta	Compatible with survival

3. Common antibody seen in antiphospholipid syndrome:

a. Anticardiolipin
b. Anti-β2GPI
c. ANA
d. Anti-Sm

Ans. a. Anticardiolipin *Ref. Williams Hematology 9th/ed p2241*

EXPLANATION

Anticardiolipin IgG and IgM assays are the most sensitive, but the least specific. Anti-β2GPI IgG and IgM assays are more specific but less sensitive.

4. MYD88 L265P mutation is seen in

a. Waldenstrom macroglobulinemia
b. Multiple myeloma
c. Burkitts lymphoma
d. B cell disorders

Ans. a. Waldenstrom macroglobulinemia *Ref: Williams hematology,9e/p1787; http://www.nejm.org/doi/full/10.1056/NEJMoa1200710#t=article*

EXPLANATION

MYD88L 265P is expressed in 90 to 95% of WM cases when more sensitive allele-specific PCR has been employed.

Waldenstrom's macroglobulinemia (WM):

- It is a IgM-secreting lymphoplasmacytic lymphoma (LPL).
- Clinical manifestations:
  - Cytopenia resulting from bone marrow infiltration by lymphoplasmacytic cells,
  - Paraprotein-related cryoglobulinemia,
  - The cold agglutinin syndrome,
  - Demyelinating neuropathy
  - Symptomatic hyperviscosity.
- Oncogenic basis: not been defined.
  - Familial clustering of Waldenstrom's macroglobulinemia and other B-cell disorders suggests that genetic factors play a role in certain patients.
  - IgM monoclonal gammopathy of unknown significance (MGUS) is characterized by the presence of a monoclonal IgM protein and the absence of bone marrow disease involvement on histologic examination. IgM MGUS can progress to Waldenström's macroglobulinemia or other B-cell lymphoproliferative disorders
- MYD88 L265P is a commonly recurring mutation in patients with Waldenström's macroglobulinemia that can be useful in differentiating Waldenström's macroglobulinemia and non-IgM LPL from B-cell disorders that have some of the same features.

5. Paraneoplastic syndrome with Ig-G antibodies to amphyphysin is:

a. Brainstem encephalitis
b. Stiff Person syndrome
c. Cerebellar degeneration
d. Striatal degeneration

Ans. b. Stiff Person syndrome *Ref: Harrison's Principles of Internal Medicine 19th/ed p614*

Explanation

Anti-amphiphysin is associated with stiff person syndrome and encephalomyelitis which are seen in breast cancer and SCLC.

- ❑ *See table below for other antibodies in various paraneoplastic syndromes*

Antibodies to intracellular antigens, syndromes, and associated cancers		
Antibody	Associated Neurologic Syndrome(s)	Tumors
Anti-Hu (ANNA1)	Encephalomyelitis, subacute sensory neuropathy	SCLC
Anti-Yo (PCA1)	Cerebellar degeneration	Ovary, breast
Anti-Ri (ANNA2)	Cerebellar degeneration, opsoclonus, brainstem encephalitis	Breast, gynecologic, SCLC
Anti-Tr	Cerebellar degeneration	Hodgkin's lymphoma
Anti-CRMP5 (CV2)	Encephalomyelitis, chorea, optic neuritis, uveitis, peripheral neuropathy	SCLC, thymoma, other
Anti-Ma proteins	Limbic, hypothalamic, brainstem encephalitis	Testicular (Ma2), other (Ma)
Anti-amphiphysin	Stiff-person syndrome, encephalomyelitis	Breast, SCLC
Recoverin, bipolar cell antibodies, others[a]	Cancer-associated retinopathy (CAR) Melanoma-associated retinopathy (MAR)	SCLC (CAR), melanoma (MAR)
Anti-GAD	Stiff-person, cerebellar syndromes, limbic encephalitis	Infrequent association (thymoma)

[a]A variety of target antigens have ben identified.
Abbreviations: CRMP, collapsing response-mediator protien; SCLC, small-cell lung cancer.

6. Gene mutation in AML with poor prognosis all *except*:

a. FLT3 gene
b. WT-1
c. NPM1
d. MLL

Ans. c. NPM1 *Ref. WHO Classification of Tumors of Hematopoietic and Lymphoid Tissue 4th/ed*

Explanation

- ❑ Associated with worse prognosis:
  - FLT3-ITD
  - KIT
  - MLL-PTD
  - WT-1
- ❑ Associated with favorable prognosis:
  - CEBPA
  - NPM1

7. Oral + skin lesions:

a. Desmoglein 3
b. Desmoglein 1
c. Antibodies against desmoglein
d. Antibodies against Hemidesmoglein

Ans. c. Antibodies against desmoglein

Ref. Robbins and Cotran Pathologic Basis of Diseases 9th/ed p1169

Explanation

All forms of pemphigus are autoimmune diseases caused by IgG autoantibodies against desmogleins that disrupt intercellular adhesions and result in the formation of blisters. The distribution of desmoglein 1 and 3 in the epidermis and the presence of autoantibodies to one or both proteins appear to explain the position and severity of the blisters. **For details refer Q no. 6 of AIIMS dermatology**

8. Velocardiofacial syndrome all true *except*:

a. 22q11.2
b. 21.q11.1
c. Long face, large nose, cardiac defects
d. Di George anomaly

Ans. b. 21.q11.1 *Ref. Robbins and Cotran Pathologic Basis of Diseases 9th/ed p164*

Explanation

Deletion of genes at chromosomal locus **22q11.2** gives rise to malformations affecting the face, heart, thymus, and parathyroids. The resulting disorders are recognized as:

- **DiGeorge syndrome** (thymic hypoplasia with diminished T-cell immunity and parathyroid hypoplasia with hypocalcemia) and
- **Velocardiofacial** syndrome [congenital heart disease involving outflow tracts, facial dysmorphism{ prominent nose, retrognathia), cleft palate and developmental delay].

9. A-15 year-old boy presented with anemia and jaundice. On examination his hemoglobin was 6 g/dL, USG showed gall stones and Peripheral smear showed the following. Most likely diagnosis is:

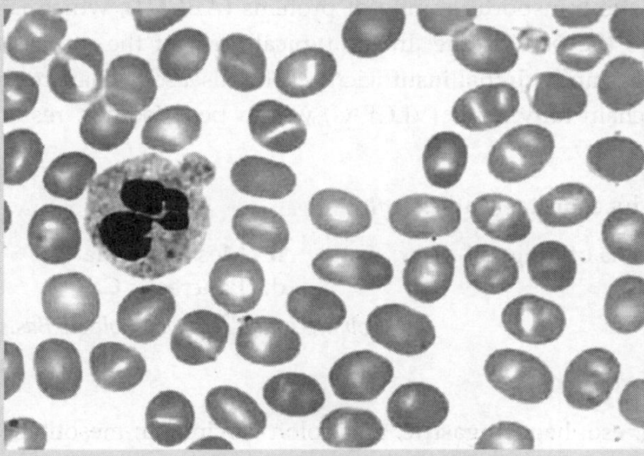

a. Hereditary acanthocytosis
b. Hereditary spherocytosis
c. Hereditary ovalocytosis
d. Hereditary xerocytosis

Ans. c. Hereditary ovalocytosis *Ref: Robbins Basic Pathology 9th/ed p409*

Explanation

History given in question is of hemolytic anemia

- Hereditary spherocytosis and ovalocytosis both can present with similar manifestations given in the question.
- Based on peripheral smear answer is hereditary ovalocytosis (oval shaped RBCs).

10. Myotonic dystrophy:

a. CTG trinucleotide repeats
b. Dystrophin 1
c. Dystrophin 2
d. CAG repeats

Ans. a. CTG trinucleotide repeats *Ref. Robbins and Cotran Pathologic Basis of Diseases 9th/ed p1244*

Explanation

Myotonic dystrophy is an autosomal dominant multisystem disorder associated with skeletal muscle weakness, cataracts, endocrinopathy, and cardiomyopathy. The disease is caused by expansions of CTG triplet repeats in the 3′-noncoding region of the myotonic dystrophy protein kinase (*DMPK*) gene.

11. ABCD l mutation is seen in:

a. Metachromatic leukodystrophy
b. Krabbe's disease
c. X- linked adrenoleukodystrophy
d. Canavan's disease

Ans. c. X- linked adrenoleukodystrophy
Ref. Robbins and Cotran Pathologic Basis of Diseases 9th/ed p1303

Explanation

Adrenoleukodystrophy is an X-linked recessive disease associated with mutations in a member of the ATP binding cassette transporter family of proteins **(ABCD1)**, which is involved in the transport of molecules into the peroxisome. In the typical form of the disease, young males present with behavioral changes and adrenal insufficiency. The disease is characterized by the inability to catabolize very-long-chain fatty acids (VLCFAs) within peroxisomes, resulting in elevated levels of VLCFAs in serum.

12. Cancers caused by asbestosis all *except*:

a. Adenocarcinoma of lung
b. Mesothelioma
c. Gastric Ca
d. Pancreatic Ca

Ans. d. Pancreatic Ca *Ref. Robbins and Cotran Pathologic Basis of Diseases 9th/ed p278*

Explanation

Asbestos causes lung, esophageal, gastric, and colon carcinoma; mesothelioma.

13. FLI1 translocation—is seen in:

a. Osteosarcoma
b. Ewing sarcoma
c. Chondrosarcoma
d. Option not recalled

Ans. b. Ewing sarcoma *Ref. Rosai and Ackerman 10th/ed p2049*

Explanation

About 95% of cases of Ewing sarcoma/PNET show on cytogenetic examination the reciprocal translocation t(11;22)(q24;q12) or t(21;22)(q22;q12), which results in the fusion of the *EWS* (Ewing sarcoma) gene at 22q12 with the ***FLI1*** or ***ERG gene***, respectively.

14. DAX 1 gene Mutation is associated with

a. Cushing's disease
b. Hashimoto's disease
c. Congenital adrenal hypoplaisa
d. Addison's disease

Ans. c. Congenital adrenal hypoplasia *Ref: Achermann JC, Meeks JJ, Jameson JL (Dec 2001). "Phenotypic spectrum of mutations in DAX-1 and SF-1". Molecular and Cellular Endocrinology*

Explanation

DAX1 mutation is seen in congenital adrenal hypoplasia.

DAX1 (dosage-sensitive sex reversal, adrenal hypoplasia critical region, on chromosome X, gene 1) is a nuclear receptor protein encoded by the NR0B1gene.

- DAX1 plays an important role in the normal development of several hormone-producing tissues.
  - The adrenal glands,
  - The pituitary gland and
  - Hypothalamus
  - The testes and ovaries
- Mutations in this gene result in both X-linked congenital adrenal hypoplasia and hypogonadotropic hypogonadism

15. Tumor lysis syndrome, all are true *except*:

a. Hypocalcemia
b. Hyperuricemia
c. Hypophosphatemia
d. Hyperkalemia

Ans. c. Hypophosphatemia *Ref. Harrisons Principle of Internal Medicine 19th/ed p1795*

Explanation

Tumor lysis syndrome (TLS) is characterized by hyperuricemia, hyperkalemia, hyperphosphatemia, and hypocalcemia and is caused by the destruction of a large number of rapidly proliferating neoplastic cells. Acidosis may also develop. Acute renal failure occurs frequently.

16. vWF is used as a marker for

a. Angiosarcoma
b. Polycythemia vera
c. Leukemia
d. Option not recalled

Ans. a. Angiosarcoma *Ref: Enzinger and Weiss's Soft Tissue Tumors,6e/p160*

Explanation

The vWF is the least sensitive of the vascular markers and is positive in 50% to 75% of vascular tumors.

von Willebrand factor (vWF):

- It is a glycoprotein produced uniquely by endothelial cells and megakaryocytes, is routinely used to identify vessels in tissue sections.
- Vessel density in tumor specimens, as determined by immuno-histochemical staining for vWF or other endothelial cell markers, is a negative prognostic factor for many solid tumors.
- vWF is heterogeneously distributed throughout the vasculature, transcriptional control in response to the tissue microenvironment being responsible for local variations in endothelial cell levels of vWF.

- ❑ Fibroblast growth factor-2 and vascular endothelial growth factor, potent angiogenesis inducers expressed in a variety of tumors, up-regulate expression of vWF mRNA and protein in cultured endothelial cells with a synergistic effect.
- ❑ Measurement of vWF mRNA in tumors detect activated endothelium or angiogenesis.

17. Sialylated Lewis glycoprotein is:

a. CEA
b. CA-125
c. CA19-9
d. Alpha-fetoprotein

Ans. c. CA19-9 *Ref. Rosai and Ackerman 10th/ed p47*

EXPLANATION

CA19-9. This is a carbohydrate antigen recognized by a monoclonal antibody produced by a hybridoma raised against a human colonic carcinoma cell line. It has been characterized as a monosialoganglioside related to the Lewis A blood group antigen. Its most common clinical application has been in the diagnosis and monitoring of pancreatic carcinoma.

18. CADASIL is caused due to::

a. NOTCH-1
b. NOTCH-2
c. NOTCH-3
d. NOTCH-4

Ans. c. NOTCH-3 *Ref. Robbins and Cotran Pathologic Basis of Diseases 9th/ed p1269*

EXPLANATION

Cerebral autosomal dominant arteriopathy with subcortical infarcts and leukoencephalopathy (CADASIL) is an autosomal dominant disorder caused by mutations in the *NOTCH3* gene that lead to misfolding of the extracellular domain of the **NOTCH3 receptor**. The disease is characterized clinically by recurrent strokes (usually infarcts, less often hemorrhages) and dementia. Imaging studies show that the first detectable changes are in white matter, usually by around the age of 35 years, whereas infarcts typically occur 10–15 years later. The diagnosis is made through the identification of these deposits in the walls of vessels in biopsies of other tissues, such as skin or muscle, or by sequencing of *NOTCH3*.

19. MOC 31 IHC is used to differentiate Adenocarcinoma from:

a. Malignant mesothelioma
b. Squamous cell carcinoma
c. Melanoma
d. Bronchial carcinoid

Ans. a. Malignant mesothelioma *Ref. Rosai and Ackerman 10th/ed p344*

EXPLANATION

Markers that are usually expressed in pulmonary adenocarcinoma but not in mesothelioma: carcinoembryonic antigen (CEA), CD15, B72.3, Ber-EP4, BG8, **MOC-31**, MUC4, thyroid transcription factor 1 (TTF-1), napsin A, and secretory component.

Markers that are usually expressed in mesothelioma but not in pulmonary adenocarcinoma: calretinin (especially when using the human recombinant antibody 120), WT1, keratin 5/6, thrombomodulin, D2-40/podoplanin, h-caldesmon, claudin-4 (a tight junction-associated protein), caveolin-1, and vimentin.

20. Wiskott Aldrich syndrome is due to mutation in gene located at:

a. 11p22
b. Xp11.23
c. 22q11
d. Option not recalled

Ans. b. Xp11.23 *Ref. Robbins and Cotran Pathologic Basis of Diseases 9th/ed p242*

Explanation

Wiskott-Aldrich syndrome is an X-linked disease characterized by thrombocytopenia, eczema, and a marked vulnerability to recurrent infection, resulting in early death. The Wiskott-Aldrich syndrome is caused by mutations in the gene encoding *Wiskott-Aldrich syndrome protein (WASP)*, which is located at **Xp11.23.**

LIST OF QUESTIONS THAT WERE NOT RECALLED PROPERLY

Question: Mastocytosis and CD marker expression.

Ref: Surrogate Markers of Disease in Mastocytosis Cem Akin Dean D. Metcalfe

Explanation

- Mastocytosis is a disorder characterized by an excessive and pathologic accumulation of mast cells in tissues.
- The clinical presentation in mastocytosis ranges from isolated cutaneous disease to more aggressive forms associated with hematologic abnormalities.
- Systemic forms of mastocytosis commonly involve the bone marrow, liver, spleen, lymph nodes and gastrointestinal tract.
- Surrogate disease markers can be

Surrogate disease markers of mastocytosis				
Marker	**Sample**	**Sensitivity**	**Specificity**	**Elevation in mast cell degranulation/ activation**
Tryptase (total)[1]	Serum/plasma	+++	+++	Yes
Histamine metbolties[1]	24-hour urine	++	++	Yes
Soluble CD117 (kit)	Serum/plasma	++	++	No
Soluble CD25	Serum/plasma	+	+	No
PGD-M	24-hour urine	++	?	Likely
Thromboxane B_2 (or its metabolites)	Plasma/24-hour urine	++	?	Likely

[1]Tests available through commercial diagnostic laboratories.

Question: Amyloidosis and multiple myeloma

Ref: http://theoncologist.alphamedpress.org/content/11/7/824.full.html

Explanation

- Amyloidosis is a rare systemic disorder of protein metabolism with progressive **extracellular deposition of insoluble fibrillary protein**, disorganization of tissue architecture, and subsequent organ dysfunction.
- In AL amyloidosis, fibrils derive mostly from the **N-terminal amino acid residues of LC immunoglobulin variable regions**, which are synthesized by a monoclonal plasma cell population. bone marrow (BM) infiltration is present.

- AL amyloidosis shares **numerical chromosomal changes with monoclonal gammopathy of undetermined significance (MGUS) and multiple myeloma (MM), particularly 13q14 deletions and t(11;14), and belongs to the spectrum of clonal plasma proliferative disorders.**
- A number of deregulated genes and pathways in AL plasma cells have been described, that appear to feed into a common loop related to **protein processing and folding, suggesting an association with deregulated protein clearance, degradation, intercellular folding, and increased fibrillogenesis.**
- The exact mechanisms of pathogenesis, along with specific differences between MM with and without amyloidosis, have not yet been clearly elucidated.

Question: CYFRA 21

Explanation

- CYFRA 21-1 is a **cy**tokeratin-19 **fra**gment that is soluble in serum and may be a useful circulating tumor marker
- Measurement of serum CYFRA-21 level is a useful auxiliary test in diagnosis of non small cell lung cancer. And particularly high specificity for Squamous cell carcinoma of lung.
- Cytokeratins are structural proteins forming the subunits of epithelial intermediary filaments.
- Fragments of cytokeratin-19 (CYFRA 21-1) are frequently released into the blood of cancer patients.
- Due to the high specificity relative to benign lung diseases, it is suitable for use as a differentiation marker in tumor pathology especially in lung cancer.
- CYFRA 21-1 in lung cancer Differential diagnosis of suspicious lung masses is essential for appropriate therapy selection. Whereas early stages of non-small cell lung cancer (NSCLC) and single lung metastases from other cancers are mostly resected by surgery, late stage NSCLC, small cell lung cancers (SCLC) and multiple lung metastases are treated by chemo- and/or radiotherapeutic approaches.
- It is not always possible to take a biopsy for histopathological subtyping due to multimorbidity, instable clinical conditions of the patients or unfavorable localization of the tumor.
- The main indication for CYFRA 21-1 is monitoring the course of NSCLC and detection of recurrent disease after primary therapy.
- Successful therapy is accompanied by a rapid fall in the serum level into the normal range.
- Progression is often shown earlier by increasing values than by clinical symptoms or imaging procedures.
- An unclear focus in the lung together with values > 30 ng/mL indicate the existence of primary bronchial carcinoma with high probability.
- CYFRA 21-1 has a clear prognostic value in both early and late stages of NSCLC and high serum levels indicate an advanced tumor stage and a poor prognosis.
- During the initial treatment phase CYFRA 21-1 is able to predict the response to therapy later on.
- CYFRA 21-1 is a valuable marker in the prediction of the response to cytotoxic therapies (such as selective internal radiation therapy (SIRT) or transarterial chemoembolization (TACE)) in diverse cancers such as hepatic cancer or hepatic metastases from other cancers.
- CYFRA 21-1 is also elevated in sera of patients with urological, gastrointestinal and gynaecological cancers.

Question: Bi T cell enhancers

EXPLANATION

- Bi-Specific T-Cell Enhancer (BiTE)
    - Monoclonal antibodies may also be engineered to combine the antibody with a toxin (immunotoxin) or a radioactive isotope (radioimmunoconjugates), or to contain a second specificity (bispecific antibodies).
    - For example, it is possible to conjugate an antibody with specificity to B-cell lymphomas with an antibody against CD3, which binds to and activates normal T cells, so as to enhance T-cell–mediated lysis of the lymphoma cell.
    - One such example of a bispecific antibody (Bispecific T-cell engager) **blinatumomab** contains anti-CD3 and anti-CD19 specificity.
    - Monoclonal antibodies raised against the immunoglobulin idiotype on a B-cell lymphoma represent another therapeutic strategy.

Author: Bahram Gor

AIIMS May 2017

1. Storage of drug in the tissues is suggested by:

a. Small volume of distribution
b. Large volume of distribution
c. Excretion in urine
d. Excretion in saliva

Ans. b. Large volume of distribution *Ref: Essentials of Medical Pharmacology by KD Tripathi 7th/ed, p21*

Explanation

- **Volume of distribution** is the apparent volume required to contain the amount of drug homogeneously at the concentration found in the plasma.
- Drugs having high volume of distribution get sequestrated in various tissues and are unequally distributed and tend to have longer duration of action.
- Due to sequestration may exert local toxicity, e.g. **tetracyclines** on bone and teeth, chloroquine on retina, **streptomycin** on vestibular apparatus, **emetine** on heart and skeletal muscle.

Option a: small volume of distribution means drug stays in vascular compartment either due to high plasma protein binding or due to less lipid solubility, therefore less is distributed to tissues.

2. A patient was administered 200 mg of a drug. 75 mg of the drug is eliminated from the body in 90 minutes. If the drug follows first order kinetics, how much drug will remain after 6 hrs?

a. 30 mg
b. 12.5 mg
c. 25 mg
d. 50 mg

Ans. a. 30 mg *Ref: Essentials of Medical Pharmacology by KD Tripathi 7th/ed, p30*

Explanation

This question can be solved easily by the fact that in first order kinetic **"constant fraction of drug is eliminated per unit time"**.

Step 1:

- In the question 75 mg out of total 200 mg is eliminated in 90 minutes. Means 75/200*100 = 37.5%
- 37.5% (fraction) of drug will be eliminated every 90 minutes.

Step 2:

- We have to find out how much drug remains in the body at the end of 6 hours (4 times 90 mins)
- At the end of 1st 90 mins: 200–75 = 125 mg is the remaining amount
- **2nd 90 min:** Now 37.5% of 125 will be eliminated = 37.5/100*125 = 47
  Drug remaining at the end of 2nd 90 min (3 hours) = 125–47 = 78
- **3rd 90 min:** 37.5% of 78 = 29.25
  Drug remaining at the end of 3rd 90 min (4 and half hour) = 78–29.25 = 48.75

- **4th 90 min:** 37.5% of 48.75 = 18.3
  Drug remaining at the end of 4th 90 min (6 hour) = 48.7–18.3 = 30.4 = 30 mg
  Thus the answer.

3. A drug X was administered by continuous IV infusion at the rate of 1.6 mg/min. Clearance of drug X is 640 mL/min. If the T½ of the drug is 1.8 hours, what would be the plasma concentration of drug after achieving steady state?

a. 2.5 mg/L
b. 5 mg/L
c. 7.5 mg/L
d. 10 mg/L

Ans. a. 2.5 mg/mL *Ref: Essentials of Medical Pharmacology by KD Tripathi 7th/ed, p32*

Explanation

- Plasma steady state concentration (Cp_{ss}) is achieved after repeated administration of drug leading to a balance between drug input and elimination.
- Cp_{ss} is directly proportional to the dose rate and inversely to the clearance of the drug and the relation is as follows:
  Cp_{ss} = Dose rate/Clearance
  Dose rate = 1.6 mg/mL, Clearance = 640 mL/min
  Cp_{ss} = 1.6/640 = 0.0025 mg/mL = 2.5 mg/L

4. Which of the following is a P-glycoprotein inducer?

a. Ketoconazole
b. Rifampicin
c. Erythromycin
d. Itraconazole

Ans. b. Rifampicin *Ref: Essentials of Medical Pharmacology by KD Tripathi 7th/ed, p13, 14 and 15*

Explanation

- Transport of drugs across membranes can occur through various pathways, one of them being primary active transport which involves transport of solutes against electrochemical gradient. **P-glycoprotein** is most well known primary active transporter.
- **P-glycoprotein:**
  - **Location:** Intestinal mucosa, renal tubules, bile canaliculi, choroidal epithelium, astrocyte foot processes around brain capillaries (the blood-brain barrier), testicular and placental microvessels.
  - Pgp is a non-selective transporter developed by body to deal with xenobiotics.
  - **Function:** Pumps out many drugs/metabolites and thus limits their intestinal absorption, penetration into brain, testes and fetal tissues as well as promotes biliary and renal elimination.
  - **E.g.:** Digoxin and cyclosporine have low oral bioavailability in spite of good oral absorption because of Pgp. Pgp pumps out the drug from epithelium back into the lumen.
- **Inducers and inhibitors:** It acts in synergy with CYP3A4. Usually the xenobiotics inducing and inhibiting CYPs also induce and inhibit Pgp.
- **Inhibitors** of Pgp quinidine, verapamil, erythromycin, etc. enhance oral bioavailability
- **Inducers** of Pgp like rifampin and phenobarbitone reduce the oral bioavailability of these drugs.

Remaining ***options (a, c, d)*** are Pgp inhibitors.

5. In an animal model how will you show Vasomotor reversal of Dale?

a. Block of α1 followed by stimulation of β1
b. Block of α1 followed by stimulation of β2
c. Block of β1 followed by block of α1
d. Block of β1 followed by block of β2

Ans. b. Block of α1 followed by stimulation of β2 *Ref: Essentials of Medical Pharmacology by KD Tripathi 7th/ed, p131*

EXPLANATION

- **Concept:** Adrenaline acts on all **α and β (α1, α2, β1, β2)**
  - At low concentration: β2 are more sensitive (vasodilation)
  - At high concentration: **α** activity predominates (vasoconstriction)
  - When Adrenaline given by iv: initially → high concentration → **α** activity predominates → increase vascular resistance → ↑BP with time as the concentration falls → no action on **α** receptors but due to β2 activity (vasodilation) → ↓BP
  - Thus normal response is ↑BP followed by ↓BP
  - In other words: **α1** mediated vasoconstriction is followed by β2 mediated vasodilation.
- **What is *'vasomotor reversal of Dale'*?**
  - When adrenaline is given after administration of nonselective **α** blocker → no rise in BP (because **α** blocked) → only fall in BP is seen (because of **β2** mediated vasodilation)
  - Response: Only ↓BP
  - In other words: block of **α1** followed by β2 (**answer**).

6. Which of the following disease modifying anti-rheumatoid drugs acts by increasing extracellular adenosine?

a. Methotrexate
b. Leflunomide
c. Sulfasalazine
d. Chloroquine

Ans. a. Methotrexate *Ref: Harrison's Principles of Internal Medicine 19th/ed, p2145*

EXPLANATION

This is a direct line from harrison's *"At the dosages used for the treatment of RA, methotrexate has been shown to stimulate adenosine release from cells, producing an anti-inflammatory effect."*

Other salient points from the above text are as follows:

- Conventional DMARDs include → hydroxychloroquine, sulfasalazine, methotrexate, and leflunomide
- Onset of action is delayed by ⇒ 6 to 12 weeks
- **DMARD of choice for rheumatoid arthritis is** → Methotrexate
- **Methotrexate** → stimulates adenosine release → anti-inflammatory effect
- **Leflunomide** → inhibitor of pyrimidine synthesis → equally effective as methotrexate as both monotherapy and combination therapy
- **Hydroxychloroquine** → does not delay radiographic progression of disease; therefore not a true DMARD. (Disease Modifying Anti Rheumatic Drugs DMARDs by definition reduce the disease activity and retard the progression)
- **Sulfasalazine** → delays radiographic progression of disease
- Other drugs that are rarely used include: Minocycline, gold salts, penicillamine, azathioprine, and cyclosporine.

7. A 70-year-old patient has diabetes mellitus and hypertension. He presents with renal failure and does not want to take insulin. Which antidiabetic drug will you prefer in this patient that does not require dose modification in renal disease?

a. Exenatide
b. Repaglinide
c. Linagliptin
d. Vildagliptin

Ans. c. Linagliptin *Ref: CMDT 2017 p1227, Harrison's Principles of Internal Medicine 19th/ed, p2414 Table 418–5*

EXPLANATION

Question asks about antidiabetic drug to be used in renal failure. The preferred agent in renal failure patient is insulin with reduced dosage. As the question mentions that patient does not wish to take insulin and alternate agent preferred among given options is linagliptin.

Option a: Exenatide. All GLP-1 agonist are contraindicated in renal disease.

Option b: Repaglinide. All secretagogues (Both Sulfonylureas and non-sulfonylureas) are contraindicated in renal and liver disease.

Options c and d: All DPP4 inhibitors require dose reduction in renal failure except linagliptin, which is excreted in bile. *Ref: CMDT 2017, p1227*

DPP-4 inhibitors approved in US are:

1. Sitagliptin
2. Saxagliptin
3. Alogliptin
4. Linagliptin

- Vildagliptin ***(option d)*** is approved only in Europe not in US
- All are for oral use
- All require dose reduction based on creatinine clearance except Linagliptin which is excreted in bile unmetabolized ***(option and answer)***
- Unique side effect profile
  - Nausea and vomiting are not a side effect of this class
  - Are well tolerated and do not cause hypoglycemia
  - Upper respiratory tract infections (Nasopharyngitis)
  - Allergic reactions: sitagliptin
  - Pancreatitis
  - Risk of heart failure (saxagliptin >alogliptin)
  - Hepatic dysfunction (alogliptin, vildagliptin)

Also see table below which is compiled from *Harrison's 19th/ed, p2414, Table 418–5.*

Contraindications of various antidiabetic agents is as follows:

Condition where use is contraindicated	Agent class contraindicated	Examples
Renal/liver disease	Insulin secretagogues: Sulfonylureas	Glibornuride, gliclazide, glimepiride, glipizide, glyburide, glyclopyramide
Renal/liver disease	Insulin secretagogues: Nonsulfonylureas	Nateglinide, repaglinide ***(option b)***, mitiglinide
Renal/liver disease	α-Glucosidase inhibitors	Acarbose, miglitol, voglibose

Contd...

Contd...

Condition where use is contraindicated	Agent class contraindicated	Examples
Renal disease	GLP-1 receptor agonists	Exenatide ***(option a)***, liraglutide, dulaglutide
Renal disease	Biguanides	Metformin
Liver disease	Thiazolidinediones	Rosiglitazone, pioglitazone

8. Components of lente insulin are:

a. 30% amorphous + 70% crystalline
b. 30% crystalline + 70 % amorphous
c. Same as NPH insulin
d. Only 70% amorphous

Ans. a. 30% amorphous + 70% crystalline

Ref: Essentials of Medical Pharmacology by KD Tripathi 7th/ed, p264

Explanation

Lente insulin is a combination of 30% semilente (amorphous) and 70% ultralente (crystalline) insulin zinc suspension.

- One of the problems with regular insulin is it peaks 2 to 3 hours after administration and sustains over 6 to 8 hours, which does not mimic the physiological insulin response. This leads to postprandial hyperglycemia and intermittent hypoglycemia. To overcome this, long-acting 'modified' or 'retard' preparations of insulin were developed.
- Retard preparations, are obtained by making insulin insoluble either by:
  - Complexing it with protamine (isophane) or
  - By precipitating it with excess zinc and increasing the particle size (ultralente, semilente, lente).

<table>
<tr><th colspan="2">Insulin-zinc suspension</th><th>Isophane (Neutral Protamine Hagedorn or NPH) insulin</th></tr>
<tr><td colspan="2">Two types of insulin-zinc suspensions have been produced</td><td rowspan="2">• Protamine is added in a quantity just sufficient to complex all insulin molecules
• Neither of the two is present in free form
• On S.C. injection, the complex dissociates slowly to yield an intermediate duration of action
• Mostly used in combination with regular insulin (70:30 or 50:50)</td></tr>
<tr><td>1. Ultralente
▪ Large particles
▪ Crystalline
▪ Long-acting
▪ Insoluble in water</td><td>2. Semilente
▪ Smaller particles
▪ Amorphous
▪ Short acting</td></tr>
<tr><td colspan="2">• Lente = ultralente + semilente in the ratio of 7:3</td><td></td></tr>
</table>

(It can be remembered like this: 70% bigger particle and 30% smaller particle)

- Therefore lente insulin which is 70% ultralente + 30% semilente can be written in different ways as follows:
  - 70 % large particle + 30% small particle
  - 70 % crystalline + 30% amorphous *(Answer)*
  - 70 % long acting + 30% short acting
- Apart from the above mentioned retard preparations, recently other insulin analogs like rapidly acting (lispro, aspart, glulisine) peakless and long-acting (glargine and detemir) have become available.

9. An epileptic adult man is on levetiracetam therapy 1 gram BD. He is seizure free for 2 years. Now, he started developing irritability and lability of mood that is affecting his daily life. What should the doctor do?

a. Stop levetiracetam therapy suddenly
b. Taper the drug over 6 months
c. Continue the medication for another 3 years
d. Stop Levetiracetam and start another antiepileptic
e. Wait till 5 year clearance period of seizure

Ans. b. Taper the drug over 6 months *Ref: Katzung's Basic and Clinical Pharmacology 13th/ed, p408 and Harrison's Principles of Internal Medicine 19th/ed, p2556*

EXPLANATION

This question is about whether to stop levetiracetam or to switch to different antiepileptic due to adverse effects of levetiracetam.

Levetiracetam is a well tolerated antiepileptic with very few adverse effects.

- The usual adverse effects include: somnolence, asthenia, ataxia, and dizziness.
- Less common but important: mood and behavioral changes.
- Rare: Psychotic reaction.

STOPPING an antiepileptic:

- Stopping or switching an antiepileptic is mandated based on 2 parameters:
  1. Seizure free period and 2. Compliance or adverse effect of the drug
- The appropriate seizure free interval is unknown and undoubtedly varies for different forms of epilepsy. It is reasonable to attempt withdrawal of antiepileptic after 2-years seizure free period if the patient meets the following criteria:
  - Complete medical control of seizures for 1–5 years;
  - Single seizure type, either focal or generalized;
  - Normal neurologic examination, including intelligence; and
  - Normal EEG.
- Withdrawal of therapy should be gradual over a period of 2 to 3 months.

Switching to different antiepileptic:

- If seizure free period is not sufficient to withdraw or seizures are not controlled by the drug or if there is significant toxicity then switching to another antiepileptic may be considered.
- "This is usually done by maintaining the patient on the first drug while a second drug is added. The dose of the second drug should be adjusted to decrease seizure frequency without causing toxicity. Once this is achieved, the first drug can be gradually withdrawn (usually over weeks unless there is significant toxicity). The dose of the second drug is then further optimized based on seizure response and side effects. Monotherapy should be the goal whenever possible".

Based on above explanation ***option a*** and ***option c*** are wrong.

Option b: Tapering is usually 2 to 3 months but may vary with different drugs and different scenarios. Therefore over 6 months can be regarded as true.

Option d: The patient is seizure free for 2 years, but other criteria like type of seizure, neurologic examination and EEG has not been mentioned in question. Remember that all the criteria needs to be met to stop the drug. This could have been the answer if tapering of levetiracetam over a period and then gradually shifting to other antiepileptic would have been mentioned.

10. All are idiosyncratic reactions to carbamazepine *except*:

a. Rash
b. Stevens-Johnson syndrome
c. Blurred vision
d. Agranulocytosis

Ans. c. Blurred vision *Ref: Katzung's Basic and Clinical Pharmacology 13th/ed, p402 and Harrison's Principles of Internal Medicine 19th/ed, p383*

Explanation

- **MC drugs causing Stevens-Johnson syndrome** are (Harrison's 19th pg 383): sulfonamides, nevirapine, allopurinol, lamotrigine, aromatic anticonvulsants (including phenytoin, carbamazepine, and barbiturates), and NSAIDs, specifically oxicam.
- **Unpredictable reactions or type B or Bizarre reactions** varies from patient to patient and are not due to drug as such. These include idiosyncratic reactions (IR) and allergy.
- Unpredictable reactions are rare. Carbamazepine is known for unpredictable reactions.
- **Adverse drug effects** are due to drug's off target actions and on contrary reason for IRs is unpredictable and is considered to be related to patient.
- **Idiosyncratic reactions due to carbamazepine are:**
  - **MC IR** is: Erythematous skin rash (SJS)
  - **Dangerous IRs** but rare include: aplastic anemia and agranulocytosis.
  - **Other IRs** leukopenia (common idiosyncratic blood dyscrasia) and hepatic dysfunction (rare).
- **Adverse effects of carbamazepine are as follows:**
  - **MC dose-related adverse effects of carbamazepine** are diplopia and ataxia.
  - Other dose-related complaints include mild gastrointestinal upsets, unsteadiness, and, at much higher doses, drowsiness.
  - Hyponatremia and water intoxication are rare and may be dose related.

About ***option c*** blurred vision: Diplopia (not blurred vision) is a adverse effect of carbamazepine not an idiosyncratic reaction.

11. A 60-year-old patient who had myocardial infarction 2 weeks back with TG-262 mg/ dl, LDL-124 mg/dl, HDL - 32 mg/dl. Which of the following will you use?

a. Atorvastatin 80 mg
b. Rosuvastatin 10 mg
c. Rosuvastatin + Fenofibrate
d. Fenofibrate

Ans. a. Atorvastatin 80 mg *Ref: CMDT 2017 p1263-64*

Explanation

- When lipid lowering agents are indicated the treatment is started with HMG Co-A reductase inhibitors (statins).
- ***(Option c)*** Combination therapy is rarely indicated. Only ezetimibe plus simvastatin has shown benefit in trials even though very small. Gemfibrozil and HMG-CoA reductase inhibitors increases the risk muscle and liver disease more than either drug alone.
- ***(Option d)*** Fibrates are used to reduce triglycerides and increase HDL levels, which is not the case here and also first line therapy is always statins.

This table serves as a guide to type of therapy to be used under specific conditions.

Indications	Treatment recommendation
Presence of clinical atherosclerotic cardiovascular disease	High intensity statin or Moderate intensity statin if > 75 years
Primary elevation of LDL cholesterol ≥ 190 mg/dL (4.91 mmol/L)	High intensity statin
Age 40–75 Presence of diabetes LDL ≥ 70 mg/dL (1.81 mmol/L)	Moderate intensity statin or High intensity statin if 10-year CVD risk 7.5% or higher

Contd...

Contd...

Indications	Treatment recommendation
Aged 40–75 No clinical atherosclerotic cardiovascular disease or diabetes LDL 70–189 mg/dL (1.81–4.91 mmol/L) Estimated 10-year CVD risk 7.5% or higher	Treat with moderate-to-high intensity statin

As per the table above patient comes under 1st category (presence of clinical cardiovascular disease). It is also important to point out that even if the patient is not having deranged lipid profile he may be started with statin therapy.

- ❑ High intensity statin therapy: lowers LDL cholesterol by approximately 50%.
  - Atorvastatin 40–80 mg ***(option a)*** and rosuvastatin 20–40 mg/day
- ❑ Moderate intensity statins lower LDL cholesterol by approximately 30–50%.
  - Atorvastatin 10–20 mg, rosuvastatin 5–10 mg ***(option b)***, simvastatin 20–40 mg, pravastatin 40–80 mg, and lovastatin 40 mg.

12. Antidote for overdose of fibrinolytic therapy is:

a. Heparin
b. Epsilon aminocaproic acid
c. Protamine
d. rtPA

Ans. b. Epsilon aminocaproic acid *Ref: Essentials of Medical Pharmacology by KD Tripathi 7th/ed, p628*

EXPLANATION

- ❑ Fibrinolysis (clot dissolution) occurs by activation of plasminogen to plasmin
- ❑ Drugs that inhibit plasmin act as antifibrinolytics and thereby prevent excess bleeding.
- ❑ Anti-fibrinolytic drugs are:
  - **Epsilon aminocaproic acid (EACA)**
    - Binds to plasminogen and plasmin so that it cannot bind to fibrin
    - It is a specific antidote for fibrinolytic agents
    - Less preferred agent because requires high doses.
  - **Tranexamic acid**
    - Acts by same mechanism as EACA
    - 7 times more potent than EACA
    - Preferred for prevention/control of excessive bleeding due to:
      - » Fibrinolytic drugs.
      - » Cardio-pulmonary bypass surgery.
      - » Tonsillectomy, prostatic surgery, tooth extraction in hemophiliacs.
      - » Menorrhagia, especially due to IUCD.
      - » Recurrent epistaxis, hyphema due to ocular trauma, peptic ulcer.
- ❑ Other options:
  - ***Heparin*** is anticoagulant (indirect thrombin inhibitor).
  - ***Protamine sulphate*** is heparin antagonist, used to terminate heparin action rapidly.
  - ***Recombinant tissue plasminogen activator*** (Alteplase) is fibrinolytic drug.

13. Drug of choice for prophylaxis of *Pneumocystis jirovecii* in an immunocompromised patient is:

a. Cotrimoxazole
b. Amoxicillin
c. Dexamethasone
d. Cephalosporin

Ans. a. Cotrimoxazole *Ref: Essentials of Medical Pharmacology by KD Tripathi 7th/ed, p706-708 and Katzung's Basic and Clinical Pharmacology 13th/ed, p 884*

Explanation

- Cotrimoxazole is **drug of choice for both treatment and prophylaxis of *P. jirovecii*** (previously known as *P. carinii*) infection.
- Cotrimoxazole is a fixed dose combination of trimethoprim and sulfamethoxazole.
- The required **plasma concentration ratio** of sulfamethoxazole: trimethoprim is **20:1**, which shows synergistic activity against most organisms. This is achieved by **dose ratio** of **5:1**, because trimethoprim has high tissue distribution. For e.g., 1 Double Strength (DS) tablet = sulfamethoxazole 800 mg + trimethoprim 160 mg.
- **For curative treatment of PCP →** high dose cotrimoxazole (4–6 DS tablets per day) + prednisone or methyl prednisolone as adjunctive.
- **For prophylaxis of PCP** low dose is used (1 DS tablet daily).

Other important chemoprophylaxis is as follows *(Katzung's 13th/884)*

Infection	Drug of choice for chemoprophylaxis
PCP pneumonia	Cotrimoxazole
Toxoplasmosis	Cotrimoxazole
Recurrent UTI	Cotrimoxazole
Cholera	Tetracycline
Diphtheria	Penicillin or erythromycin
Anthrax	Ciprofloxacin or doxycycline
Tuberculosis	Isoniazid alone or with rifampicin
Mycobacterium avium complex	Azithro/ clarithro/ ceftriaxone
Influenza A and B	Oseltamivir
H. influenza type B	Rifampin
Meningococcal meningitis	Rifampin/azithro/ceftriaxone
Endocarditis	Amoxicillin/clindamycin
Rheumatic fever	Benzathine penicillin
Pertussis	Azithromycin
Plague	Tetracycline
Malaria	Chloroquine (if susceptible) Mefloquine/doxycycline (areas endemic for chloroquine resistant disease)

14. A 40-year-old patient came with complaints of spikes of fever and difficulty in breathing. Transesophageal echo found out vegetations in the heart. The culture showed positive for *Burkholderia cepacia*. Which of the following is the first line management?

a. Aminoglycosides and colistin
b. Carbapenems and 3rd generation cephalosporins
c. Tigecycline and cefepime
d. Cotrimoxazole with 3rd generation cephalosporin

Ans. d. Cotrimoxazole with 3rd generation cephalosporin

Ref: Katzung's Basic and Clinical Pharmacology 12th/ed, p802 and 904 and *Harrison's Principles of Internal Medicine 19th/ed, p1048*

Explanation

- What *Harrison's* says on page 1048
  - B cepacia is intrinsically resistant to most antimicrobials.
  - TMP-SMX, meropenem, and doxycycline **are most effective drugs.**
  - **Empirical treatment of choice is** TMP-SMX or Meropenem
  - Some strains are susceptible to third-generation cephalosporins and fluoroquinolones
  - When serious pulmonary infection is there, for e.g. cystic fibrosis then combination therapy is suggested, but combination of meropenem and TMP-SMX is antagonistic.
  - Resistance to all agents has been reported.
- What *Katzung* says on page 904
  - **DOC for B. cepacia** is TMP-SMX **and alternative agents are** Ceftazidime, chloramphenicol.

15. A patient came with complaints of high grade fever and altered sensorium. He was diagnosed to be suffering from meningococcal meningitis. Empirical drug of choice for treatment of meningococcal meningitis is:

a. Ceftriaxone
b. Cefotetan
c. Gentamicin
d. Cefoxitin

Ans. a. Ceftriaxone

Ref: Harrison's Principles of Internal Medicine 19th/ed, Table 147-1, p780, 889.

Explanation

Meningitis can be broadly classified into community acquired (usual case) or hospital acquired. The empirical therapy for both of these is discussed in the table below.

Type of meningitis	MC cause	Empirical treatment	Addition to empirical R_x	Rationale
Community acquired Meningitis	S. pneumonia (50%) and N. Meningitidis (25%)	3rd/4th gen cephalosporin (ceftriaxone, cefotaxime, cefepime) + Vancomycin + Acyclovir + Dexamethasone	+ Ampicillin	3 months of age, those >55, or immunocompromised (to cover Listeria monocytogenes)
			+ metronidazole	In patients with otitis, sinusitis, or mastoiditis (to cover gram-negative anaerobes)
			+Doxycycline	In tick season (tick-borne bacterial infections)

Contd...

Contd...

Hospital acquired meningitis	Staphylococci and gram -ve organisms (P. aeruginosa)	Vancomycin + ceftazidime or cefepime or meropenem	Ceftriaxone and cefotaxime do not provide activity against central nervous system (CNS) infection with pseudomonas therefore replaced by active agents.

All that should be known about treatment of meningococcal meningitis.

Specific type	Empirical Rx	DOC if susceptible	DOC if resistance to Penicillin G	Chemoprophylaxis for adults and children >1yr	Alternate chemoprophylaxis for adults
Meningococcal meningitis	Ceftriaxone or Cefotaxime	Penicillin G	Ceftriaxone or Cefotaxime	2-day regimen of rifampin (not recommended in pregnancy)	1 dose of azithromycin (500 mg) or 1 im dose of ceftriaxone (250 mg)

16. Which of the following is a bactericidal drug for *Mycobacterium leprae*?

a. Ofloxacin
b. Ciprofloxacin
c. Amoxicillin
d. Erythromycin

Ans. a. Ofloxacin *Ref: Essentials of Medical Pharmacology by KD Tripathi 7th/ed, p782,783*

EXPLANATION

- Among the given options ofloxacin, ciprofloxacin and amoxicillin have bactericidal activity, but only ofloxacin is anti-leprosy drug. Erythromycin is a bacteriostatic drug and not used in leprosy.
- **Commonly used** anti-leprosy drugs include: Dapsone, Clofazimine, Rifampin, Ethionamide.
- **Other antibiotics** effective against M leprae are: Ofloxacin, Moxifloxacin, Minocycline and Clarithromycin
- Bactericidal activity of anti-leprosy drugs is as follows:
  - Rifampicin: up to 99.99% *M. leprae* are killed in 3–7 days by 600 mg/day dose.
  - Ofloxacin: over 99.9% bacilli were found to be killed by 22 daily doses of ofloxacin monotherapy
  - Clarithromycin: monotherapy with 500 mg daily caused 99.9% bacterial killing in 8 weeks.

17. Mechanism of action of protease inhibitor is:

a. It inhibits translation
b. It inhibits assembly of virus protein
c. It inhibits proviral RNA synthesis
d. Inhibits conversion of RNA to DNA

Ans. b. Inhibits assembly of virus proteins

Ref: Goodman & Gilman's The Pharmacological Basis of Therapeutics 12th/ed, p1628-1659

EXPLANATION

Option d: NRTI & NNRTI inhibit Reverse transcriptase thereby inhibiting conversion of RNA to DNA.

Option a and ***option c:*** Translation and transcription of HIV viral DNA is by using host (human) enzymes so as of now no drugs target this system

Option b: Function of HIV protease is cleavage of gag and pol precursor polypeptides and other precursor proteins to final structural proteins of mature virion.

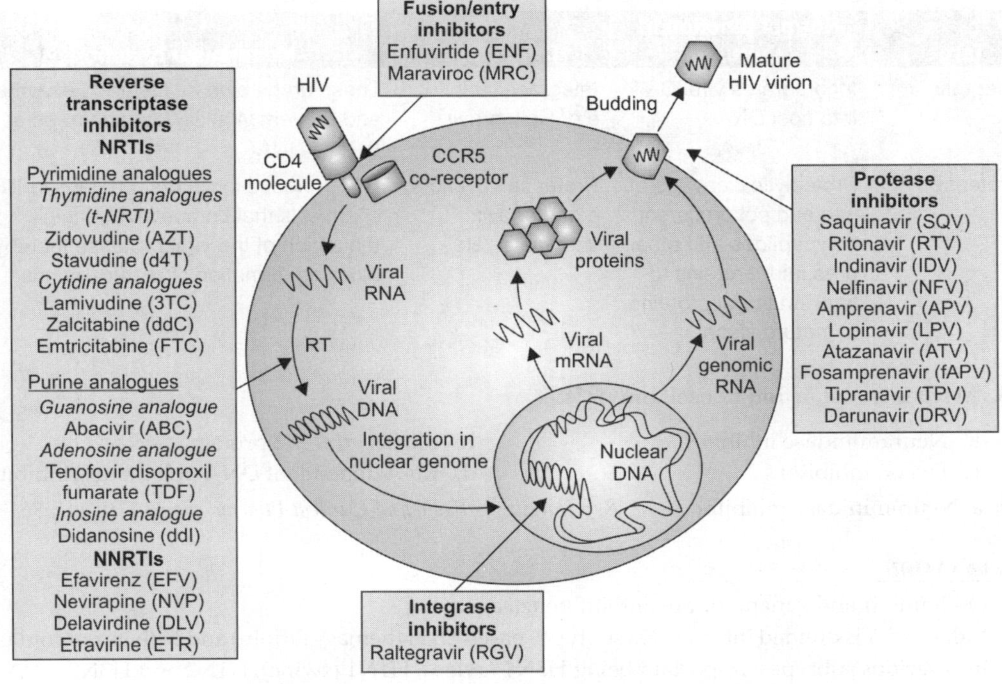

Fig. 1: Pathogenesis and targets of antiretroviral drugs.

Targets and mechanism of antiretroviral drugs is as below:

Target	Normal function in virus	Drug class	Mechanism of action
gp41	HIV attaches through gp160 (which includes gp120 and gp41) → gp 41 fuses viral envelop	Enfuvirtide (Entry inhibitor)	Binds to gp41 → does not allow conformational changes that allow fusion of virus → blocks entry of virus into host cell.
CCR5	To host membrane → entry of virus	Maraviroc (Entry inhibitor)	Binds specifically to host protein ccr5 → blocks entry
RT (reverse transcriptase)	RT then converts viral RNA to DNA	NRTI [Nucleoside/ Nucleotide (tenofovir)] e.g. zidovudine, lamivudine, etc.	These drugs are purine or pyrimidine analogues that enter cells get phosphorylated and then blocks replication by 2 ways: 1. Competitively inhibits incorporation of native nucleotides. 2. Once incorporated terminates elongation of nascent DNA because NRTI lack 3' hydroxyl group
		NNRTI (Nonnucleoside) e.g. nevirapine	Bind to NNRTI binding pocket in enzyme RT which is separate from catalytic site and cause change in 3D structure of the enzyme → reducing its activity

Contd...

Contd...

Target	Normal function in virus	Drug class	Mechanism of action
Integrase	Incorporates viral DNA into host DNA.	Integrase inhibitor, e.g. Raltegravir	These drugs bind to integrase enzyme and prevent viral DNA strand transfer to host DNA
Protease	Proteolytic cleavage of gag and pol precursor polypeptides and other precursor proteins to final structural proteins of mature virion	Protease inhibitors, e.g. ritonavir, saquinavir, etc.	HIV protease inhibitors are peptide-like chemicals that competitively inhibit the action of the viral protease thereby blocking formation of mature virions.

18. Mechanism of action of oseltamivir is:

a. Neuraminidase inhibitor
b. Blocks viral M2 protein
c. Fusion inhibitor
d. RNA dependent DNA polymerase inhibitor

Ans. a. Neuraminidase inhibitor *Ref: Katzung's Basic and Clinical Pharmacology 13th/ed, p861-62*

Explanation

- Oseltamivir and zanamivir are anti influenza agents
- Influenza A is divided into various subtypes based on H (hemagglutinin) and N (Neuraminidase) into various subtypes. Important being H5N1 (avian), H1N1 (swine), H1N2 and H3N2.
- Neuraminidase inhibitors: **Oseltamivir** and **Zanamivir**
  - Influenza virus requires neuraminidase to sialic acid residues in host membrane to get released from the cell.
  - Neuraminidase inhibitors interfere with release of progeny influenza virus from infected host cells, thus halting the spread of infection within the respiratory tract.
  - Inhibition of viral neuraminidase results in clumping of newly released influenza virions to each other and to the membrane of the infected cell.
  - Active against both Influenza A and B.
- **Amantadine** and its α-methyl derivative **rimantadine**, block the M2 proton ion channel ***(option b)*** of the virus particle and inhibit uncoating of the viral RNA within infected host cells, thus preventing its replication.
  - Active against influenza A only.
- ***Options c and d*** are examples of antiretroviral agents discussed above.

PGI May 2017

1. True about first order kinetics is/are:

a. Very few drugs follow it
b. Option not recalled but was related to t1/2
c. Salicylates follow it throughout therapeutic ranges
d. Rate of elimination increases with increase in concentration of drug and decreases with decrease in concentration of drug

Ans. d. Rate of elimination increases with increase in concentration of drug and decreases with decrease in concentration of drug *Ref: Essentials of Medical Pharmacology by KD Tripathi 7th/ed, p30,31*

Explanation

- ❑ Clearance (CL): defined as *"the theoretical volume of plasma from which the drug is completely removed in unit time"*.
- ❑ CL = rate of elimination/plasma concentration .... (equation)
- ❑ Drug elimination is the sum-total of metabolic inactivation and excretion.
- ❑ Elimination of drug depends on the availability of metabolic or excretion pathway.
- ❑ **For majority of drugs,** the processes involved in elimination (transporters, enzymes, blood flow, etc.) are not saturated over the clinically obtained concentrations, thus they follow first order kinetics ***(option a).***

First order kinetics (linear kinetics)	Zero order kinetics (nonlinear kinetics)
• **Rate of elimination** is directly proportional to the drug concentration ***(option d)*** • ***CL*** remains constant • See equation above	• **Rate of elimination** remains constant irrespective of drug concentration • ***CL*** ↓ with increase in concentration • See equation above
• **Constant '*fraction*'** of the drug present in the body is eliminated in unit time.	• **Constant '*amount*'** of the drug is eliminated in unit time.
• **t½** remains **constant** because *CL* does not change with dose.	• **t½ increases** with dose because *CL* progressively decreases as dose is increased.
• **Most drugs** follow first order elimination ***(option a)*** • Low dose aspirin	• Example: Alcohol and **very few drugs** follow this in therapeutic range; e.g.warfarin, theophylline, tolbutamide and phenytoin. • Aspirin at high dose ***(option c)***
• Relationship between dose rate and steady state plasma concentration (Cp_{ss}) is **linear.**	• Increase in dose beyond saturation levels causes an increase in Cp_{ss} which is **out of proportion** to the change in dose rate.

- ❑ Zero order kinetics is also known as 'capacity limited elimination' or 'Michaelis-Menten elimination'.
- ❑ **Options c and e were t1/2 related but not recalled.**

2. Long acting beta agonist used once a day:

a. Salmeterol
b. Formoterol
c. Indacaterol
d. Terbutaline
e. Arformoterol

Ans. c. Indacaterol *Ref: Katzung's Basic and Clinical Pharmacology 13th/ed, p340*

Explanation

β_2 agonist	Features
• Albuterol (salbutamol) • **Terbutaline** • Metaproterenol • Pirbuterol	• Metered-dose inhalers • Bronchodilation is maximal within 15–30 minutes and persists for 3–4 hours. Frequent administrations required based on clinical status. • Can be given by nebulizer if using metered dose is not possible. • Albuterol and terbutaline are also available in tablet form (2 to 3 times daily) ***(option d)***, no added advantage therefore prescribed rarely.

Contd...

Contd...

β_2 agonist	Features
	• Only terbutaline is available for subcutaneous injection; useful in severe asthma requiring emergency treatment when aerosolized therapy is not available or has been ineffective; CAUTION: Due to its longer duration of action cumulative effects may be seen after repeated injections.
Bambuterol	• It is prodrug of terbutaline. • Slowly hydorlyzed by pseudocholinesterase to release the active drug over a period of 24 hours. • Available in tablet form and given once daily.
Long acting: Salmeterol • **Formoterol** • **Arformoterol** • Carmoterol	• Salmeterol a partial agonist and formoterol a full agonist. • Duration of action: 12 hours or more; **used 2 times daily *(options a,b,e)***. • In asthma should not be used as monotherapy; interact with inhaled corticosteroids to improve asthma control.
Indacaterol	• **Ultra long acting** β_2 agonist; **used once daily *(Answer)*** • Approved for once daily long-term treatment of COPD and not for asthma and not for acute exacerbations of COPD.

3. About codeine true is/are:

a. Acts as antitussive
b. Is less potent than morphine in suppressing cough
c. Partly metabolized to morphine
d. Has same effect as morphine in analgesia
e. Causes no constipation

Ans. a. Acts as antitussive; b. Is less potent than morphine in suppressing cough and c. Partly metabolized to morphine *Ref: Essentials of Medical Pharmacology by KD Tripathi 7th/ed, p218,474*

EXPLANATION

- **Antitussives:** These are drugs that act in the CNS to raise the threshold of cough center or act peripherally in the respiratory tract to reduce tussal impulses, or both these actions.
  - *Opioids:* Codeine, Ethylmorphine, Pholcodine.
  - *Nonopioids:* Noscapine, Dextromethorphan, Chlophedianol.
  - *Antihistamines:* Chlorpheniramine, Diphenhydramine, Promethazine.
  - *Peripherally acting:* Prenoxdiazine.
- **Codeine:**
  - It is **methyl-morphine**, occurs naturally in opium.
  - It is partly converted in the body to morphine (demethylation by CYP2D6). This metabolite (morphine) is responsible for its analgesic activity. Codeine itself has very low affinity to opioid receptors and if CYP2D6 polymorphism is there then it will not have any analgesic activity ***(options c and d).***
  - It is less potent (1/10th) and less efficacious than morphine for analgesia ***(option d).***
  - Codeine is more selective cough suppressant (1/3rd as potent as morphine) ***(option b).*** It suppresses cough at subanalgesic doses (10–30 mg).
  - Codeine is less potent compared to morphine for both analgesic (1/10th) and cough suppressant (1/3rd).

- Has good activity by the oral route (oral: parenteral ratio 1:2).
- Side effect profile:
  - Abuse liability is present but is low.
  - **Constipation** is a prominent side effect. Also used for diarrhea treatment ***(option e).***
  - Respiratory depression and drowsiness at higher doses.
  - **Contraindicated in** asthmatics and in patients with diminished respiratory reserve; should be avoided in children.
- Ethylmorphine similar to codeine (methyl morphine) but less constipating.
- Pholcodine similar to codeine but no addicting or analgesic property and is longer acting (12 hours) compare to codeine (6 hours).

4. Long acting insulin:

a. Lispro
b. Aspart
c. Glargine
d. Zn suspension of insulin
e. Isophane

Ans. c. Glargine *Ref: Essentials of Medical Pharmacology by KD Tripathi 7th/ed, p263*

Explanation

See table below and for further details refer explanation of AIIMS question number 8

Type	Example
Rapid acting	Lispro Aspart Glulisine
Short acting	Regular (soluble) insulin
Intermediate acting	Lente NPH or isophane
Long acting	Insulin glargine Insulin detemir

5. Which is not a prodrug?

a. Captopril
b. Enalapril
c. Lisinopril
d. Perindopril
e. Ramipril

Ans. a. Captopril and c. Lisinopril *Ref: Essentials of Medical Pharmacology by KD Tripathi 7th/ed, p502*

Explanation

This is a commonly tested question. Remember **all ACE inhibitors are prodrugs except captopril and lisinopril.**

Other commonly tested part in ACE inhibitors include drug interactions with ACE inhibitors.

- ❑ Diuretics + ACE inhibitors = Synergistic hypotensive action, therefore may precipitate profound hypotension. In diuretic treated patient, ACE inhibitor should be started with low doses.
- ❑ NSAIDs + ACE inhibitors = NSAIDs attenuate the hypotensive action by retaining salt and water. Patient on ACE inhibitor + Diuretic → takes NSAID = chance of renal failure.
- ❑ Potassium supplements or K^+ sparing diuretics + ACE inhibitor = Hyperkalemia.
- ❑ Antacids + Captopril = Antacids reduce bioavailability of captopril.
- ❑ Lithium + ACE inhibitor = ACE inhibitors reduce Li^+ clearance and predispose to lithium toxicity.

6. Drug/s causing QT_c prolongation:

a. Amiodarone
b. Cisapride
c. Calcium gluconate
d. Lignocaine
e. Ketoconazole

Ans. a. Amiodarone; b. Cisapride and e. Ketoconazole

Ref: Harrison's Principles of Internal Medicine 19th/ed, p1457 and Goodman and Gilman's Pharmacological Basis of Therapeutics 12th/ed, p821.

EXPLANATION

- QT interval: Start of 'q' wave to end of 't' wave, it includes time for both ventricular depolarization and repolarization and varies inversely with the heart rate (HR).
- QT interval is prolonged if HR is low and short at higher heart rates.
- Therefore the drugs that increase ventricular action potential duration (APD) prolong the QT interval.
- Class 1a and class 3 ***(amiodarone)*** antiarrhythmics prolong APD thus cause QT prolongation and class 1b shorten APD and cannot cause QT prolongation ***(lignocaine ruled out).***
- Hypocalcemia prolongs QT interval and hypercalcemia shortens it ***(option c—calcium gluconate-ruled out).***
- There is a exhausting list of drugs that can cause QT prolongation see 2nd table below.
- Have a look at antiarrhythmic drugs that may help in solving MCQs related to QT prolongation.

Anti-arrhythmic class	Mechanism of action	Ability to cause QT prolongation (TDP)	Examples
Class 1a	Na^+ and K^+ channel blockade	Prolong APD, therefore **can cause QT prolongation**	Quinidine, disopyramide, procainamide, tricyclic antidepressants (amitriptyline and other) , phenothiazines
Class 1b	Na^+ channel blockade and K^+ channel opening property	Shorten APD, therefore cannot cause QT prolongation	Lignocaine ***(option d)***, mexiletine, tocainide and phenytoin
Class 1c	Na^+ channel blockade only	No effect on APD	Encainide, moricizine, flecainide and propafenone
Class 2	Beta blockers	Reduce the automaticity and are used in TDP treatment	Esmolol, propranolol, and metoprolol
Class 3	Potassium channel blockers	Prolong the APD therefore **can cause QT prolongation**	Amiodarone, ***(option a)*** dofetilide, dronedarone, sotalol, ibutilide
Class 4	Calcium channel blockers	Reduce the automaticity of SAN and conduction through AVN	Verapamil and diltiazem

- Apart from drugs prolonging APD mentioned above; other drugs that can cause QT prolongation or Torsades de pointes include as follows:

Antibacterials	Erythromycin, most quinolone antibiotics (Sparfloxacin, moxifloxacin, levofloxacin)
Antifungals	Voriconazole and fluconazole ***(option e ketoconazole also)***
Antiretrovirals	Efavirenz

Contd...

Contd...

Antimalarials	Quinine, mefloquine, artemisinin, halofantrine
Antipsychotics	Thioridazine, ziprasidone, risperidone, and quetiapine
Analgesics	Notably methadone and celecoxib
Antiemetics	Droperidol, dolasetron
Antihistamines	Terfenadine, astemizole, ebastine
Bronchodilators	Albuterol, formoterol, and salmeterol
Some 5-HT1 antagonists	Sumatriptan, zolmitriptan
SSRIs (selective serotonin reuptake inhibitors)	Citalopram, fluoxetine, paroxetine, sertraline, and venlafaxine
Other important drugs	Prednisone, cisapride, famotidine, tacrolimus Haloperidol, trazodone Tizanidine, and certain tricyclic antidepressants.

7. Not a 5th generation cephalosporin:

a. Cefoxitin
b. Ceftolozane
c. Ceftobiprole
d. Cefotetan
e. Cefaclor

Ans: a. Cefoxitin; d. Cefotetan and e. Cefaclor *Ref: Harrison's Principles of Internal Medicine 19th/ed, p941*

Explanation

See table below

1st generation	2nd generation	3rd generation	4th generation	5th generation
Cef + a and ceph	Random	Cef + t + me	Cef + pi	Ceft + ol
Cef**a**zolin	Cefamandole	Cefoperazone	Cef**pi**me	**Ceftarol**ine
Cef**a**droxil	Cefuroxi**me**	Cefotaxi**me**	Cef**pi**rome	**Ceftol**ozane (option)
Cephalexin	**Cefaclor (option)**	Ceftazidi**me**		**Ceft**obip**rol**e (option)
Cepharadine	Cefprozil	Cef**t**riaxone		
	Cefuroxime axetil	Cefdinir		
	Cefoxitin (option)	Cefixi**me**		
	Cefo**t**etan (option)	Cefpodoxi**me**		

8. Drug of choice for non-gonococcal urethritis:

a. Penicillin
b. Ceftriaxone
c. Cefixime
d. Doxycycline
e. Azithromycin

Ans. e. Azithromycin *Ref: API Textbook of Medicine 9th/ed, p543*

Explanation

If single best answer to be selected then azithromycin will be the answer. Single dose azithromycin is preferred over 7 day course of doxycycline. See table on next page:

Gonococcal urethritis	Non-gonococcal urethritis
• Caused by *Neisseria gonorrhoeae;* treated by single dose of following: ▪ Ceftriaxone 125 mg IM or ▪ Cefixime 400 mg oral or ▪ Ciprofloxacin 500 mg oral or ▪ Ofloxacin 400 mg oral or ▪ Levofloxacin 250 mg oral	• Caused by variety of organisms, ***Chlamydia trachomatis*** **(MCC)**. Treated as Chlamydial infection: ▪ Azithromycin 1 g oral single dose or ▪ Doxycycline 100 mg bid for 7 days or ▪ Erythromycin 500 mg qid for 7 days or ▪ Fluoroquinolone (ofloxacin, 300 mg twice daily; or levofloxacin, 500 mg/d)

9. Following is/are true about aminoglycoside associated acute renal failure:

a. Seen in 10% of population
b. Develops after 72 hours
c. Therapeutic dose can also cause acute renal failure
d. Option not recalled

Ans. a. Seen in 10% of population and c. Therapeutic dose can also cause acute renal failure

Ref: Harrison's Principles of Internal Medicine 19th/ed, p1803

EXPLANATION

Antimicrobials causing acute kidney injury (AKI) (previously called acute renal failure) are:

- **Aminoglycosides:**
  - Nonoliguric AKI occurs in **10–30%** of courses ***(option a)***.
  - AKI may occur even when plasma levels are in the **therapeutic range** ***(option c)***.
  - AKI typically manifests **after 5–7 days of therapy** ***(option b)*** and can present even after the drug has been discontinued.
  - Mechanism of toxicity: Aminoglycosides → **freely filtered** across the glomerulus → accumulate within the **renal cortex** → concentrations in cortex is much more than plasma → **Tubular necrosis.**
  - Hypomagnesemia is a common finding.
- **Amphotericin B:**
  - AKI develops because of 2 mechanisms:
    - Renal vasoconstriction due to increase in tubuloglomerular feedback.
    - Direct tubular toxicity mediated by reactive oxygen species. It also binds to tubular membrane cholesterol and introduces pores.
  - AKI is due to **tubular necrosis.**
  - Nephrotoxicity is **dose and duration dependent**.
  - Clinical features: Polyuria, hypomagnesemia, hypocalcemia, and non-gap metabolic acidosis.
- **Vancomycin:**
  - Associated with AKI, when trough levels are high
  - Causal relationship with AKI has not been established.
- **Acyclovir:**
  - Gets precipitated in tubules and cause **tubular obstruction**, particularly when given as an intravenous bolus at high doses in the setting of hypovolemia.
- **Other drugs causing AKI secondary to tubular toxicity** are:
  - *Foscarnet, pentamidine, tenofovir,* and *cidofovir.*
- **Drugs causing AKI secondary to acute interstitial nephritis** are
  - *Penicillins, cephalosporins, quinolones, sulfonamides,* and *rifampin.*

10. Drugs used in mycoplasma infection:

a. Doxycycline
b. Penicillin
c. Fluconazole
d. Azithromycin
e. Fluoroquinolones

Ans. a. Doxycycline; d. Azithromycin and e. Fluoroquinolones

Ref: Harrison's Principles of Internal Medicine 19th/ed, p1163

EXPLANATION

Mycoplasma species has few typical features:

- Its size is closer to virus than to bacteria.
- But differs from virus in that it can be cultured in cell free media, it is the smallest organism capable of independent replication.
- Its genome is smallest of all prokaryotes, in fact its genome is used to define the minimal set of genes necessary for cellular life.
- It contains no genes for amino acid synthesis, fatty acid metabolism and cholesterol, thus parasitic or saprophytic nature and hence requires a complex fastidious media for culture.
- It has no cell wall, therefore **penicillins** and cephalosporins are ineffective ***(option b).***
- Species that are pathogenic to humans:
  - *M. pneumonia* (Respiratory infection)
  - *M. hominis* (genitourinary and neonatal infections)
  - *U. urealyticum* (genitourinary and neonatal infections)
  - *U. parvum* (genitourinary and neonatal infections)
  - *M. genitalium* (genitourinary).

Organism	Drugs useful
M. pneumoniae	Macrolides (**Azithromycin**, clarithromycin, erythromycin) **Doxycycline** **Fluoroquinolones** (levofloxacin, moxifloxacin, gemifloxacin *not* ciprofloxacin or ofloxacin)
U. urealyticum, U. parvum	Macrolides (Azithromycin, clarithromycin, erythromycin) Doxycycline
M. hominis	**Doxycycline**, clindamycin
M. genitalium	Moxifloxacin, doxycycline, azithromycin

11. Which of the following is/are true?

a. Echinocandins have least side effects
b. Amphotericin B is fungistatic
c. Fluconazole has 100 % bioavailability
d. Fluconazole is drug of choice in invasive aspergillosis
e. Amphotericin B causes dose dependent nephrotoxicity

Ans. e. Amphotericin B causes dose dependent nephrotoxicity

Ref: Essentials of Medical Pharmacology by KD Tripathi 7th/ed, p787-794

EXPLANATION

Option a: Echinocandins are newest class developed in antifungal drugs. These are semisynthetic antifungal antibiotics and outstanding feature of this class is low toxicity compared to amphotericin B (Amp-B).

- Not sure whether least toxic among all antifungals. Organ toxicity noted with Amp-B (nephrotoxicity, CNS, marrow depression → anemia) is not seen with echinocandins.
- Following is a comparison between various available antifungal antibiotics.

Antifungal antibiotics	Polyenes	Echinocandins	Heterocyclic benzofuran
Examples	Amphotericin B (Amp-B), Nystatin, Hamycin	Caspofungin, Micafungin, Anidulafungin	Griseofulvin
Source of drug	Obtained from different species of streptomyces	Semisynthetic	Obtained from *Penicillium griseofulvum*.
Route of administration	IV infusion (orally not absorbed)	IV infusion (orally not absorbed)	Orally used
Mechanism of action	Bind with ergosterol and form pore in the fungal membrane	Inhibits the synthesis of a component of fungal cell wall (β-1, 3-glucan).	Interferes with mitosis (binds to polymerized microtubules and interferes with their function)
Toxicity profile	Highly toxic	Most well tolerated	Low toxicity and usually well tolerated
Static or cidal	Fungicidal at high dose and static at low dose ***(option b)***	Both static and cidal	Fungi-static (therefore treatment is very long; till the fungus sheds off)

Option e: Nephrotoxicity due to Amp-B is dose dependent.

- **Amphotericin B (Amp-B)**
- Antifungal spectrum: Active against most fungal infections; **ineffective against dermatophytes**; gold standard therapy for systemic mycosis; also effective against **leishmaniasis.**
- Adverse effects:
  - Acute reaction on iv infusion (chills, fever, aches and pain all over, nausea, vomiting and dyspnea).
  - Organ toxicity:
    - Nephrotoxicity—dose related
    - Bone marrow depression → anemia—reversible
    - CNS toxicity—on intrathecal administration only.

Options c and d: Oral bioavailability of fluconazole is good (not 100% but 94% of the oral dose is absorbed).

- **Fluconazole:**
  - Oral bioavailability—94% **(option c)**.
  - More selective for fungal cyp450 than cyp450 of human, therefore less inhibition compared to ketoconazole.
  - Does not have endocrine side effects.
  - Antifungal spectrum:
    - Preferred drug for fungal meningitis, because of good CSF penetration
    - First line treatment for candida esophagitis
    - Most tinea infections and cutaneous candidiasis
    - Disseminated candidiasis, cryptococcal/coccidioidal meningitis and other systemic fungal infections
    - **Ineffective in** aspergillosis and mucormycosis, and **inferior to itraconazole for** histoplasmosis, blastomycosis and sporotrichosis, as well as in tinea unguium ***(option d)***
    - **DOC for aspergillosis is** Amp B or voriconazole.

❑ **Drug of first choice in fungal infections is as follows:**

Fungal infection	Drugs of first choice
Candidiasis	Oral—Fluconazole Vaginal—Fluconazole Cutaneous—Clotrimazole Deep/invasive—Amp-B/Voriconazole
Cryptococcosis	Amp-B
Histoplasmosis	Itraconazole/Amp-B
Coccidioidomycosis	Amp-B/Fluconazole
Blastomycosis	Itraconazole/AMB
Sporotrichosis (disseminated)	Amp-B
Paracoccidioidomycosis	Itraconazole
Aspergillosis	Voriconazole / Amp-B
Mucormycosis	Amp-B
Chromomycosis	Itraconazole

12. True about mechanism of action of following drugs is/are:

a. Protease inhibitor—Darunavir
b. Reverse transcriptase inhibitor—Nevirapine
c. Integrase inhibitor—Maraviroc
d. Protease inhibitor—Tenofovir
e. Entry inhibitor—Raltegravir

Ans. a. Protease inhibitor—Darunavir and b. Reverse transcriptase inhibitor—Nevirapine

Ref: Essentials of Medical Pharmacology by KD Tripathi 7th/ed, p798

Explanation

See table below

Reverse transcriptase inhibitors		Protease inhibitors	Entry (fusion) inhibitor	CCR5 receptor inhibitor	Integrase inhibitor
NRTI	NNRTI				
Named drugs	**'vir'** in middle of name	**'navir'** at end of name	**En-Fu**-virtide		**'gra'**
Nucleoside RTI Zidovudine Didanosine Stavudine Lamivudine Abacavir Emtricitabine ***Nucleotide RTI*** Tenofovir ***(option d)***	Nevi**rapine** ***(option b)*** Efa**vir**enz, Dela**vir**dine	Rito**navir** Ataza**navir** Indi**navir** Nelfi**navir** Daru**navir** ***(option a)*** Saqui**navir** Ampre**navir** Lopi**navir**	**Enfu**virtide	Maraviroc ***(option c)***	Ralte**gra**vir ***(option e)***

❑ For further details refer question number 17 in AIIMS pharmacology.

13. Drug of Choice for strongyloides infection:

a. Mebendazole
b. Albendazole
c. Ivermectin
d. Levamisole
e. DEC

Ans. c. Ivermectin *Ref: Katzung's Basic and Clinical Pharmacology 13th/ed, p909*

EXPLANATION

- If the question is drug of choice the answer will be ivermectin.
- If the question is which are effective then answer will be albendazole and ivermectin. See table below:

Helminths common in India	Also known as	Drug of choice	Alternate agents	How to remember?
Ascaris lumbricoides	Roundworm	Albendazole Mebendazole Pyrantel	Piperazine, Levamisole Ivermectin	Albendazole, mebendazole and pyrantel are the usual drug of choice for nematodes. Exceptions include ivermectin (for *S. stercoralis*), DEC (for *filariasis*) and Metronidazole for (*D. medinensi*)
Ancylostoma duodenale and Necator americanus	Hookworm	Albendazole Mebendazole Pyrantel	Levamisole	
Enterobius (Oxyuris) Vermicularis	Pin worm	Mebendazole Pyrantel	Albendazole	
Strongyloides stercoralis	**Thread worm**	**Ivermectin**	**Albendazole, thiabendazole**	
Trichuris trichiura	Whipworm	Mebendazole Albendazole	Ivermectin	
Trichinella spiralis	Trichinosis	Mebendazole Albendazole		
Wuchereria bancrofti *Brugia malayi*	Filariasis	Diethyl carbamazine	Ivermectin	
Dracunculus medinensi	Guinea worm	Metronidazole	Thiabendazole, Mebendazole	
Taenia saginata	*Beef* tape-worm (tw)	Praziquantel, Niclosamide	Mebendazole	Praziquantel is the usual drug of choice for cestodes. Exception include Albendazole (for cysticercosis and *echinococcus*)
Taenia solium	*Pork tw*	Praziquantel		
Hymenolepis nana	Dwarf tw	Praziquantel		
Neurocysticercosis	Pork tw	Albendazole	Praziquantel	
Echinococcus granulosus	Hydatid disease	Albendazole	Mebendazole	
E. multilocularis		Albendazole		

14. Which of the following anti-tumor drug is gonadotoxic?

a. Vinblastine
b. Adriamycin
c. Actinomycin
d. Busulfan
e. Ifosfamide

Ans. d. Busulfan and e. Ifosfamide *Ref: Harrison's Principles of Internal Medicine 19th/ed p103 e-8.*

EXPLANATION

See table below

Alkylating agents	Toxicity shared by all drugs of group
• Cyclophosphamide, **Ifosfamide**, Mechlorethamine, Chlorambucil, Melphalan • ThioTEPA • Altretamine • **Busulfan** • Carmustine, Lomustine • Dacarbazine, Temozolomide • Procarbazine • Cisplatin, Carboplatin, Oxaliplatin	• Myelosuppression • Alopecia • **Gonadal dysfunction** • Mucositis • Pulmonary fibrosis • "Second" neoplasms, particularly leukemia

15. Drugs affecting purine synthesis:

a. Azathioprine
b. Methotrexate
c. Cytarabine
d. 6-thioguanine
e. 5-fluorouracil

Ans. a. Azathioprine and d. 6-thioguanine

Ref: Essentials of Medical Pharmacology by KD Tripathi 7th/ed, p858

EXPLANATION

- ❑ Antimetabolites are analogues related to the normal components of DNA or of coenzymes involved in nucleic acid synthesis.
- ❑ Competitively inhibit utilization of the normal substrate or get themselves incorporated forming dysfunctional macromolecules.
- ❑ Antimetabolites can be folate, purine or pyrimidine antagonists. See table below:

Antimetabolites	Examples
Folate antagonist	Methotrexate (MTX) ***(option b)*** Pemetrexed
Purine antagonist	6-Mercaptopurine (6-MP) 6-Thioguanine (6-TG) ***(option d)*** Azathioprine ***(option a)*** Fludarabine
Pyrimidine antagonist	5-Fluorouracil (5-FU) ***(option e)*** Capecitabine Cytarabine (cytosine arabinoside) ***(option c)***

JIPMER Pattern Based

1. A patient presented with dry mouth, dry hot skin and dilated pupils, cause could be:

a. Anticholinergic poisoning
b. Cholinesterase inhibitor poisoning
c. Organophosphate poisoning
d. Option not recalled

Ans. a. Anticholinergic poisoning

Ref: Harrison's Principles of Internal Medicine 19th/ed, Table 473-e2 and e4

EXPLANATION

- ❑ Dry mouth, dry hot skin and dilated pupils (mydriasis), all are features of anticholinergic poisoning.
- ❑ Understanding of sympathetic and parasympathetic actions is of prime importance in understanding cholinergic or anti cholinergic poisoning.
- ❑ In cholinergic poisoning → symptoms resembling parasympathetic activity appear.
- ❑ In anticholinergic poisoning → parasympathetic activity is inhibited and as you know each organ has both sympathetic and parasympathetic innervations; inhibition of parasympathetic actions leads over expression of uninhibited sympathetic activity, in other words symptoms of sympathetic over-activity are seen.
- ❑ Features of cholinergic and anticholinergic poisoning is as follows:

	Anticholinergic poisoning	Cholinergic poisoning
Mechanism	Inhibition of central and postganglionic parasympathetic muscarinic cholinergic receptors	Inhibition of AChE leading to increased synaptic ACh at muscarinic and nicotinic cholinergic receptor sites
Examples	Atropine, hyoscyamine, scopolamine	• Carbamates (aldicarb, carbaryl, etc.) • Drugs (neostigmine, tacrine, etc.) • Nerve gases (sarin, soman, tabun) • Organophosphates (diazinon, chlorpyrifos, malathion)
Features	1. **Physiologic stimulation: Grade 1** Anxious, irritable, tremulous; vital signs normal; diaphoresis, flushing or pallor, **mydriasis**, and hyperreflexia sometimes present. **Grade 2** Agitated; may have confusion or hallucinations but can converse and follow commands; vital signs mildly to moderately increased. **Grade 3** Delirious; unintelligible speech, uncontrollable motor hyperactivity; moderately to markedly increased vital signs; tachyarrhythmias possible. **Grade 4** Coma, seizures, cardiovascular collapse.	1. **Physiologic depression:** **Grade 1** Awake, lethargic, or sleeping but arousable by voice or tactile stimulation; able to converse and follow commands; may be confused. **Grade 2** Responds to pain but not voice; can vocalize but not converse; spontaneous motor activity present; brainstem reflexes intact. **Grade 3** Unresponsive to pain; spontaneous motor activity absent; brainstem reflexes depressed; motor tone, respirations, and temperature decreased. **Grade 4** Unresponsive to pain; flaccid paralysis; brainstem reflexes and respirations absent; cardiovascular vital signs decreased.

Contd...

Contd...

	Anticholinergic poisoning	Cholinergic poisoning
	2. **Dry skin and mucous membranes,** decreased bowel sounds, flushing, and urinary retention; myoclonus and picking activity. 3. Central effects may occur without significant autonomic dysfunction.	2. **Muscarinic signs and symptoms:** Seizures, excessive secretions (lacrimation, salivation, bronchorrhea and wheezing, diaphoresis), and increased bowel and bladder activity with nausea, vomiting, diarrhea, abdominal cramps, and incontinence of feces and urine. 3. **Nicotinic signs and symptoms:** Hypertension, tachycardia, muscle cramps, fasciculations, weakness, and paralysis. Death is usually due to respiratory failure.
Treatment	Physostigmine, (AChE inhibitor), for delirium, hallucinations, and neuromuscular hyperactivity. C/I are asthma and non-anticholinergic cardiovascular toxicity (e.g., cardiac conduction abnormalities, hypotension, and ventricular arrhythmias).	Atropine for muscarinic signs and symptoms; 2-PAM, a cholinesterase reactivator, for nicotinic signs and symptoms due to organophosphates, nerve gases, or an unknown anticholinesterase.

2. Cardioselective beta-blocker is:

a. Labetalol
b. Pindolol
c. Carvedilol
d. Metoprolol

Ans. d. Metoprolol *Ref: Essentials of Medical Pharmacology by KD Tripathi 7th/ed, p144,148*

Explanation

- **Beta-blockers are divided into:**
  - **1st generation:** Older and non-selective (β1 and β2)
    Propranolol, sotalol, timolol, (without intrinsic sympathomimetic activity) and pindolol (with intrinsic sympathomimetic activity).
  - **2nd generation:** β1 selective or cardioselective β-blockers:
    Nebivolol, betaxolol, bisoprolol, acebutolol, esmolol, atenolol, metoprolol, celiprolol.
  - **3rd generation:** With additional α blocking and/or vasodilatory properties:
    Labetalol, carvedilol, celiprolol, nebivolol and betaxolol.
- Other properties shared in common by β-blockers is as follows:
- β-blockers with partial **agonist activity** at β_1 receptors
  - Preferred in patients who are prone for bradycardia:
  - **Pindolol >> Acebutolol, Labetalol > Celiprolol,** oxprenolol, penbutolol, alprenolol
- β-blockers with **Membrane stabilizing activity**
  - Due to Na^+ channel blockade and posses antiarrhythmic activity:
  - Propranolol>> acebutolol, **L**abetalol > Oxprenolol, **M**etoprolol, **P**indolol
- **Lipid insoluble** β-blockers:
  - Incompletely absorbed orally, but do not undergo first pass metabolism and are primarily excreted unchanged in urine.
  - Atenolol, celiprolol, bisoprolol, sotalol.

3. Drug with NO releasing property is:

a. Labetalol
b. Carvedilol
c. Celiprolol
d. Nebivolol

Ans. d. Nebivolol *Ref: Essentials of Medical Pharmacology by KD Tripathi 7th/ed, p144*

EXPLANATION

- **3rd generation:** With additional α blocking and/or vasodilatory properties: labetalol, carvedilol, celiprolol, nebivolol and betaxolol. See table below
  - **Nitric oxide release: Nebivolol >>> Celiprolol (thus answer)**

3rd gen β blocker	Receptors blocked	Vasodilation is due to	Other relevant points
Labetalol	**β** (β1 + β2) + **α** [weak β2 agonist]	α1 + β1 blockade as well as β2 agonism	5 times more potent in blocking β than α
Carvedilol	**β** (β1 + β2) + **α**	α1 + calcium channel blockade	Also has antioxidant property
Celiprolol	Selective **β1** + weak β2 agonistic activity	β2 agonism + **NO release**	
Nebivolol	Selective **β1**	**NO release**	Due to NO release it improve endothelial function
Betaxolol	Selective **β1**	Calcium channel blockade	Protective effect on retinal neurones apart from lowering IOP.

4. Following is a specific antidote for poisoning due to metoprolol:

a. Atropine
b. Isoproterenol
c. Glucagon
d. Verapamil

Ans. c. Glucagon *Ref: Goodman & Gilman's The Pharmacological basis of Therapeutics 12th/ed, p317*

EXPLANATION

β blocker overdosage	Treatment
• Common manifestations ▪ Bradycardia **(MC)** ▪ Hypotension ▪ Prolonged AV conduction times, and widened QRS complexes • Other manifestations ▪ Seizures and depression ▪ Hypoglycemia and bronchospasm.	• Significant bradycardia: initially **atropine *(option a)*** → cardiac pacemaker often required • Hypotension: Large doses of **isoproterenol *(option b)*** or an α agonist • **Glucagon *(option c)*:** Acts through its own GPCR and independently of the β-adrenergic receptor, has positive chronotropic and inotropic effects on the heart and is used as antidote in β-blocker overdosage.

If question was like this: Following are used for poisoning due to metoprolol *except*:

a. Atropine
b. Isoproterenol
c. Glucagon
d. Verapamil

Ans. d. Verapamil

- ❑ Adverse effects depend on various properties of drug like receptor selectivity, membrane stabilizing property, etc. as follows:

Adverse effects depend on the following properties of the drug	Caution to be exercised
Non-selective β blocker	• Worsening of asthma, COPD: β1 selective blockers preferred but should be used with caution • Worsening peripheral vascular disease: β1 blockers well tolerated in mild to moderate PVD, used with caution in severe disease
β blocker with intrinsic sympathomimetic activity	• Preferred in patients prone to develop severe bradycardia with β blocker therapy • Are less useful in angina patients because of stimulation of heart
β blocker with membrane-stabilizing properties	• Avoid in glaucoma due to risk of cornell anesthesia
β blocker with low lipid solubility	• Have less CNS adverse effects compared to more lipid soluble • C/I in renal failure, because are excreted primarily by kidney

5. True about combination therapy with anakinra and infliximab in rheumatoid arthritis patients is:

a. Combination should be avoided
b. Combination is superior to methotrexate plus etanercept
c. Combination is superior to methotrexate alone
d. Combination is equally effective as oral triple therapy

Ans. a. Combination should be avoided *Ref: Harrison's Principles of Internal Medicine 19th/ed, p2147*

EXPLANATION

- ❑ ***Option a:*** Anakinra (IL 1 antagonist) and infliximab (anti-TNF) should not be combined.
- ❑ Both agents restrict inflammatory process markedly and lead to high rate of serious infections.
- ❑ This finding is observed in trials that used this regimen.
- ❑ New strategy in treatment of RA focuses on several goals:
  1. Early, aggressive therapy to prevent joint damage and disability.
  2. Frequent modification of therapy and use of combination therapy where appropriate.
  3. Individualization of therapy, to maximize response and minimize side effects;
  4. Achieving, remission of clinical disease activity.
- ❑ **Preferred first line drug as monotherapy** in moderate to severe RA: Methotrexate
- ❑ **Effective combinations** include:
  - Methotrexate, sulfasalazine, and hydroxychloroquine (oral triple therapy);
  - Methotrexate and leflunomide;
  - Methotrexate plus a biological (e.g. methotrexate and infliximab an anti-TNF agent; methotrexate + Etanercept is equivalent to oral triple therapy ***options b and d***)
- ❑ Early RA (<6 months of disease duration)
  - Started with methotrexate → switch or add DMARD therapy after 3 months of worsening or persistent moderate/high disease activity → If disease still persists after 3 months of intense DMARD therapy, add a biologic agent.

- Oral triple therapy (hydroxychloroquine, methotrexate, and sulfasalazine) is a reasonable first step for the treatment of early RA, including its use as a step-up strategy where treatment is initiated with methotrexate alone and then combined at 6 months with hydroxychloroquine and sulfasalazine if the disease is not adequately controlled.

❑ Patients with established RA.

- Treatment with a biologic agent or aggressive combination DMARD therapy was also recommended as initial therapy in certain patients with high disease activity and poor prognosis.

6. True about anastrozole is:

a. Reversible aromatase inhibitor
b. Irreversible aromatase inhibitor
c. Irreversible steroidal aromatase inhibitor
d. Irreversible nonsteroidal aromatase inhibitor

Ans. a. Reversible aromatase inhibitor

Ref: Essentials of Medical Pharmacology by KD Tripathi 7th/ed, p306-320

EXPLANATION

❑ **Mechanism of action:** Locally produced estrogens appear to play an important role in the development of breast cancer. Aromatase inhibitors inhibit aromatization of 'A' ring of testosterone and androstenedione, the final and key step in the production of estrogens (estradiol/estrone) in the body.

❑ Till recently tamoxifen has been the standard hormonal treatment of breast cancer in both pre and post-menopausal women, but aromatase inhibitors have now gained prominence. Available inhibitors are orally active

❑ **Adverse effects:**

- Due to absence of estrogen at all sites in the body like hot flushes, thinning of hair and accelerated bone loss (not seen with tamoxifen), vaginal dryness, vaginal bleeding,
- Nausea, diarrhea and dyspepsia.
- Risk of endometrial Ca, thromboembolism, deterioration of lipid profile is associated with use of Tamoxifen, but not with aromatase inhibitors.

❑ Aromatase inhibitors in use are discussed in table below:

Aromatase inhibitor	Characteristics	Uses
Letrozole	• **Nonsteroidal and reversible inhibitor** of aromatase (Type 2 compound) • Inhibits aromatization all over the body	1st line drug for adjuvant therapy after mastectomy in ER +ve postmenopausal women.
Anastrozole ***(answer)***	• **Nonsteroidal and reversible** inhibitor of aromatase (Type 2 compound) • More potent than letrozole and suitable for single daily dosing.	Adjuvant therapy in early ER +ve breast ca. as well as for palliation of advanced cases in postmenopausal women.
Exemestane	• **Steroidal and Irreversible inhibitor** of aromatase (Type 1 compound) • Also has weak androgenic activity similar to androstenedione	Found to be beneficial in both early and advanced breast Ca.

Other drugs in the class of estrogens and progestins and important uses are given in table below:

Class of drug	Examples	Uses
Synthetic estrogens	• Steroidal: Ethinylestradiol Mestranol Tibolone • Nonsteroidal: Diethylstilbestrol (stilbestrol) Hexestrol Dienestrol	1. Hormone replacement therapy (HRT) 2. Senile vaginitis 3. Delayed puberty in girls 4. Dysmenorrhea 5. Acne 6. Dysfunctional uterine bleeding 7. Carcinoma prostate (not preferred uses are 4, 5, 6 and 7)
Antiestrogens	Clomiphene citrate	Infertility due to failure of ovulation aid in vitro fertilization Oligozoospermia: In men
Selective estrogen receptor modulators' (SERMs)	Tamoxifen citrate, and Toremifene (new congener of Tamoxifen)	Breast cancer in both pre and post-menopausal women.
	Raloxifene	Prevents bone loss and reduces LDL cholesterol in postmenopausal women.
Progestins (Progestin = favoring pregnancy) • Natural progestin: Progesterone	**Synthetic progestins progesterone derivatives (21 C):** Medroxyprogesterone acetate Megestrol acetate Dydrogesterone Hydroxyprogesterone caproate Nomegestrol acetate (Newer compound) **19-nortestosterone derivatives, (a/k/a 'estranes' -18 C):** *Older compounds* • Norethindrone(Norethisterone) • Lynestrenol (Ethinylestrenol) • Allylestrenol • Levonorgestrel (Gonane) *Newer compounds (Gonanes)* • Desogestrel • Norgestimate • Gestodene	1. As contraceptive 2. HRT 3. DUB 4. Endometriosis 5. Premenstrual syndrome/tension 6. Threatened/habitual abortion 7. Endometrial carcinoma
Antiprogestin	Mifepristone	1. Termination of pregnancy 2. Cervical ripening 3. Postcoital contraceptive 4. Once-a-month contraceptive 5. Induction of labour 6. Cushing's syndrome (Mifepristone is not preferred treatment for 4,5,6)
Selective progesterone receptor modulator' (SPRM)	Ulipristal	Emergency contraception *advantage of being effective up to 5 days post coitus, if woman misses to take LNG in first 3 days (LNG is effective in first 72 hours).

7. Blood therapeutic levels of antiepileptics all are correct *except*:

a. Phenobarbitone 5–10 μg/mL
b. Phenytoin 10–20 μg/mL
c. Carbamazepine 6–12 μg/mL
d. Valproate 40–120 μg/mL

Ans. a. Phenobarbitone 5–10 μg/mL *Ref: Harrison's Principles of Internal Medicine 19th/ed, p2553-4*

Explanation

- Important points regarding monitoring levels of antiepileptic drugs are:
  - Useful for establishing the initial dosing schedule and during modification of therapy and should not be used for exact dosing in a particular patient.
  - Monitoring drug levels is **most useful for documenting adherence.**
  - Therapeutic ranges are approximate guide for determining the proper dose for a given patient. The key determinants are:
    - Clinical measures of seizure frequency and
    - Presence of side effects, not the laboratory values.
- Therapeutic range and adverse effects of first line drugs is discussed in table below:

Drug	Therapeutic range	Adverse effects	
		Neurologic	**Systemic**
Carbamazepine	4–12 µg/mL ***(option c)***	Ataxia Dizziness Diplopia Vertigo	Aplastic anemia Leukopenia Gastrointestinal irritation Hepatotoxicity Hyponatremia
Oxcarbazepine	10–35 µg/mL	Fatigue Ataxia Dizziness Diplopia Vertigo Headache	Same as carbamazepine
Phenytoin	10–20 µg/mL ***(option b)***	Dizziness Diplopia Ataxia Incoordination Confusion	Gingival hyperplasia Lymphadenopathy Hirsutism Osteomalacia Facial coarsening Skin rash
Ethosuximide	40–100 µg/mL	Ataxia Lethargy Headache	Gastrointestinal irritation Skin rash Bone marrow suppression
Lamotrigine	2.5–20 µg/mL	Dizziness Diplopia Sedation Ataxia Headache	Skin rash Stevens-Johnson syndrome
Levetiracetam	5–45 µg/mL	Sedation Fatigue Incoordination Mood changes	Anemia Leukopenia
Phenobarbital	10–40 µg/mL ***(option a)***	Sedation Ataxia Confusion Dizziness Decreased libido Depression	Skin rash

Contd...

Contd...

Drug	Therapeutic range	Adverse effects	
		Neurologic	Systemic
Topiramate	2–20 μg/mL	Psychomotor slowing Sedation Speech or language problems Fatigue Paresthesias	Renal stones (avoid use with other carbonic anhydrase inhibitors) Glaucoma Weight loss Hypohidrosis
Valproic acid	50–125 μg/mL ***(option d)***	Ataxia Sedation Tremor	Hepatotoxicity Thrombocytopenia Gastrointestinal irritation Weight gain Transient alopecia Hyperammonemia

8. Risk for carbamazepine induced Stevens-Johnson syndrome is:

a. HLA B 1502
b. Male sex
c. Pre-existing psoriasis
d. Pre-existing atopic dermatitis

Ans. a. HLA B 1502 *Ref: Fitzpatrick's Color Atlas and Synopsis of Clinical Dermatology 7th/ed, p137*

EXPLANATION

- Two life threatening skin disorders associated with drugs are:
  - Epidermal necrolysis (SJS, SJS/TEN and TEN) and
  - Exfoliative erythroderma syndrome (EES)
- Stevens–Johnson syndrome *(SJS) can be considered less severe form of Toxic epidermal necrolysis (TEN).*

SJS	<10% epidermal detachment
SJS/TEN overlap	10–30% epidermal detachment
TEN	>30% epidermal detachment

- Features of SJS or SJS/TEN and TEN are as follows:

	Epidermal necrolysis	EES
Age/sex	• Any age, but MC in adults >40 years • Equal sex incidence ***(option b)***	• Usually >50 years (In children—results from atopic dermatitis) • Males > females ***(option b)***
Risk factors	• Systemic lupus erythematosus • HLA-B12, **HLA-B1502 *(option a)***, and HLA-B5801 in Han Chinese • HIV/AIDS.	See etiology
Etiology	• Polyetiology but drugs are the leading causative factor. • Drugs with high risk are: Allopurinol, Sulfamethoxazole, Sulfadiazine, Sulfapyridine, Sulfadoxine, Sulfasalazine, Sulfasalazine, Lamotrigine, Phenobarbital, Phenytoin, Phenylbutazone, Nevirapine, Oxicam NSAIDs, Thiacetazone	• Pre-existing dermatosis is the leading cause [psoriasis ***(option c)***, atopic dermatitis ***(option d)***, adverse cutaneous drug reactions, cutaneous T-cell lymphoma (CTCL), allergic contact dermatitis, and pityriasis rubra pilaris] • Drugs most commonly implicated are: Allopurinol, Calcium channel blockers, Carbamazepine, Cimetidine, Gold, Lithium, Quinidine, Sulfonamides
Prognosis	• SCORTEN prognostic scoring system	

9. Olcegepant, mechanism of action is:

a. $5HT_{1D/1B}$ agonist
b. Inhibits the release of vasodilating peptides
c. CGRP antagonist
d. Decreases the excessive firing of vasoconstrictor nerve fibers

Ans. c. CGRP antagonist *Ref: Katzung's Basic and Clinical Pharmacology 13th/ed, p308*

EXPLANATION

- Calcitonin family of peptides includes:
  - Calcitonin
  - Calcitonin gene-related peptide **(CGRP)**
  - Adrenomedullin
  - Amylin
- CGRP
  - Widely distributed: Largely in the C-cells of the thyroid gland, also found in CNS (central nervous system), PNS (peripheral nervous system), CVS (cardiovascular system), RS (respiratory system) and GIT (gastrointestinal tract).
  - CGRP-containing neuronal fibers are more abundant around arteries than around veins and in atria than in ventricles.
  - This peptide has vasodilatory property, in fact CGRP is the **most potent vasodilator yet discovered**.
  - When injected in systemic circulation, it causes hypotension and tachycardia.
  - When injected into CNS, it causes hypertension and suppression of feeding.
  - Release of CGRP from trigeminal nerves **plays a central role in the pathophysiology of migraine**. Selective serotonin agonist (*triptans*) normalizes CGRP levels.
  - CGRP antagonists though have not yet received FDA approval have shown promising results in trials for migraine. Antagonists developed are:
    - **Olcegepant**
    - **Telcagepant**
  - Note the name ol**cegepant**: **C**alcitonin **ge**ne-related **p**eptide **ant**agonist.
  - These drugs are non-peptide antagonist.
- Two primary hypotheses to explain the actions of antimigraine drugs are:
  - First, The triptans, ergot alkaloids, and antidepressants may activate $5\text{-}HT_{1D/1B}$ receptors on presynaptic trigeminal nerve endings, thereby inhibiting the release of vasodilating peptides, ***(option b)*** and antiseizure agents may suppress excessive firing of these nerve endings ***(option d)***.
  - Second, the vasoconstrictor actions of direct 5-HT agonists (the triptans and ergot) may prevent vasodilation and stretching of the pain endings. It is possible that both mechanisms contribute in the case of some drugs.
- ***Option a:*** Triptans (sumatriptan is 5 HT agonist).
- ***Option b:*** CGRP itself is vasodilating peptide and olcegepant is CGRP antagonist. The triptans, ergot alkaloids, and antidepressants act by inhibiting the release of vasodilating peptides.
- ***Option d:*** Antiseizure drugs like valproic acid and topiramate are useful in treatment of migraine, they reduce the excessive firing by trigeminal neurons.

10. True about buspirone:

a. No dependence or withdrawal
b. Tremors
c. Anxiolytic
d. Extrapyramidal effects

Ans. c. Anxiolytic *Ref: Essentials of Medical Pharmacology by KD Tripathi 7th/ed, p465*

Explanation

- Buspirone a 5 HT_{1A} agonist is used as antianxiety drug. By stimulating presynaptic 5-HT1A autoreceptors, it reduces the activity of dorsal raphe serotonergic neurons, thereby producing anti-anxiety or anxiolytic effect ***(option c)***.
- General features of antianxiety drugs (BZDs (Benzodiazepines), azapirones, hydroxyzine an antihistaminic and propranolol) are:
  - Have no therapeutic effect to control thought disorder of schizophrenia.
  - Do not produce extrapyramidal side effects ***(option d)***.
  - Have anticonvulsant property.
  - Produce physical dependence and carry abuse liability.
  - Do not selectively block conditioned avoidance response in animals.
- Azapirones (Buspirone, Gepirone, Ipsapirone) differs significantly from benzodiazepines as follows:
  - **Does not produce significant sedation** or cognitive/functional impairment.
  - Does not interact with BZD receptor or modify GABAergic transmission.
  - **Does not produce tolerance or physical dependence *(option)***.
  - Does not suppress BZD or barbiturate withdrawal syndrome.
  - **Has no muscle relaxant or anticonvulsant activity**.
- Therefore, if anxiolytic ***(option c)*** was not there, then ***option a*** (no dependence) would have been the answer.
- Anxiety treatment:
  - For quick relief or short term treatment or acute anxiety disorder: BZDs are the preferred agents.
  - For chronic use: SSRI or SNRI (serotonin norepinephrine reuptake inhibitor) or Buspirone are used, because BZDs have abuse potential on long term use.
  - SSRIs are now **drugs of choice** for social anxiety, OCD, eating disorders and PTSD.
  - Buspirone is used for mild to moderate chronic anxiety states because of its non-sedating nature.

11. True about sacubitril is:

a. Available as a fixed dose combination with valsartan
b. It is a recombinant brain natriuretic peptide
c. Reduces hospitalization but not cardiovascular death in heart failure patients
d. It is a recombinant atrial natriuretic peptide

Ans. a. Available as a fixed dose combination with valsartan

Ref: Katzung's Basic and Clinical Pharmacology 13th/ed, p219

Explanation

- Vasodilators are effective in acute heart failure because of:
  - Reduction in preload (through venodilation) or
  - Reduction in afterload (through arteriolar dilation), or both.

- Currently in-use vasodilators for heart failure patients are:
  - Nitroglycerin
  - Nesiritide (recombinant BNP analogue)
  - Nitroprusside
- In heart failure vasodilators are used in:
  - Acute decompensated heart failure (ADHF)
  - If pulmonary congestion is there these provide rapid relief
  - And with preserved blood pressure
- Disadvantages of available vasodilators:
  - Nesiritide—Its efficacy is clinically insignificant and hypotension is a major side-effect.
  - Nitroglycerin—Higher doses are required to produce effect, tolerance is a major issue with this.
  - Nitroprusside—Requires arterial line placement for titration of precise BP; thiocyanate toxicity may precipitate in patients with renal insufficiency.
- Newer vasodilators being developed for ADHF include the following:

Newer vasodilators	Features of the drug
Sacubitril	• Nesiritide is a synthetic BNP (Brain natriuretic peptide analogue) ***(option b)*** • Endogenous BNP is degraded by a peptidase known as neprilysin • There are many **neprilysin inhibitors** in pipeline, but Sacubitril has received approval in 2015 • The combination **Sacubitril + Valsartan (Entresto™)** has been approved, i.e. a neprilysin inhibitor and a angiotensin receptor blocker • Administered in conjunction with other heart failure therapies, in place of an ACE inhibitor or other ARB • Reduces the risk of cardiovascular death and hospitalization in CHF patients (NYHA Class II-IV) with reduced ejection fraction ***(option c)***
Serelaxin	• A **recombinant human relaxin-2** • Showed successful result in phase 1 and 2 trial • Recently (March 2017) the result of phase 3 trials were said to be unsuccessful
Ularitide	• **Synthetic urodilatin** (a natriuretic peptide produced by kidney) • Has received FDA fast track status for ADHF • Currently in phase 3 trial
Carperitide	• **Synthetic ANP** (Atrial natriuretic peptide) ***(option d)*** • Approved in Japan (PMDA)

12. Male with erythematous patch over penis after taking an over the counter medicine. Causal drug is:

a. Azithromycin b. Ofloxacin
c. Doxycycline d. Aceclofenac

Ans. d. Aceclofenac *Ref: Fitzpatrick's Color Atlas and Synopsis of Clinical Dermatology, 7th/ed p498-99*

Explanation

- Findings given in question are suggestive of 'fixed drug eruptions (FDE)'.
- Among the ***given options*** ofloxacin, doxycycline and azithromycin are prescription only drugs hence most probably the answer is aceclofenac.

- ❑ **If in question 'over the counter' has not been mentioned then the answer will be doxycycline.**
- ❑ A FDE is an adverse cutaneous reaction to an ingested drug, characterized by the formation of a solitary (but at times multiple) erythematous patch or plaque.
- ❑ If the patient is rechallenged with the offending drug, the FDE occurs repeatedly at the identical skin site (i.e., fixed) within hours of ingestion.
- ❑ Usually asymptomatic. May be pruritic, painful, or burning.
- ❑ *Time to onset of lesion(s)*: Occur from 30 min to 8 h after ingestion of drug in previously sensitized individual.
- ❑ *Duration of lesion(s)*: Lesions persist if drug is continued. Resolve days to few weeks after drug is discontinued.

Drugs most commonly implicated in FDE
• Tetracyclines (tetracycline, **doxycycline**, minocycline)
• Sulfonamides, other sulfa drugs
• Metronidazole, nystatin, salicylates, **NSAIDs**, phenylbutazone, phenacetin
• Barbiturates
• Oral contraceptives
• Quinine (including quinine in tonic water), quinidine
• Phenolphthalein
• Food coloring (yellow): in food or medications

13. MRSA is resistant to action of methicillin because of:

a. Drug efflux mechanism
b. Altered PBP
c. Beta lactamase
d. Decreased penetration

Ans. b. Altered PBP *Ref: Katzung's Basic and Clinical Pharmacology 13th/ed, p772*

Explanation

Resistance to β-lactam group of antibiotics is by 4 different mechanisms:

Mechanism of resistance	Organisms showing the said mechanism	Resistance develops to following antimicrobials	Other relevant information
1. Inactivation by β lactamase (MC mechanism of penicillin resistance)	*Staph. aureus, H. influenza* and *E. coli*	Hydrolyze penicillins >> cephalosporins	Carbapenems are highly resistant to hydrolysis by penicillinases and cephalosporinases, but they are hydrolyzed by metallo-β lactamase and carbapenemases
	Pseudomonas aeruginosa and *Enterobacter* sp.	hydrolyze both cephalosporins and penicillins, e.g. AmpC β-lactamase	
2. **Modification of target PBPs**	**Staphylococci**	**Methicillin** resistance	These resistant organisms produce **altered PBPs** that have low affinity for binding β-lactam antibiotics
	pneumococci and *enterococci*	penicillin resistance	
3. Impaired penetration	Only in gram-negative species	Penicillins active against Gram –ve (e.g. ampicillin)	Absence of the 'porin' or downregulation of its production can greatly impair drug entry into the cell
4. Drug efflux	Gram-negative organisms	Penicillins active against Gram –ve organisms	Transport some β-lactam antibiotics from the periplasm back across the outer membrane.

14. Anti-mycobacterial agent that causes anterior uveitis when used along with clarithromycin is:

a. Ethambutol
b. Rifabutin
c. Ethionamide
d. Thiacetazone

Ans. b. Rifabutin *Ref: Goodman & Gilman's The Pharmacological basis of Therapeutics 12th/ed, p1553*

EXPLANATION

This direct line from the text clarifies the answer *"Uveitis and arthralgias have occurred in patients receiving rifabutin doses >450 mg daily in combination with clarithromycin or fluconazole."* However it alone can also cause anterior uveitis.

- Adverse effect profile of rifabutin is as follows:
  - **Unique side effects of Rifabutin** include: polymyalgia, pseudojaundice, and anterior uveitis.
  - **Reasons for discontinuation of rifabutin therapy** include: rash (4%), GI intolerance (3%), and neutropenia (2%).
  - Uveitis and arthralgias: rifabutin doses >450 mg daily + clarithromycin or fluconazole.
  - Rifabutin causes an orange-tan discoloration of skin, urine, feces, saliva, tears, and contact lenses, like rifampin.
  - Rarely, thrombocytopenia, a flu-like syndrome, hemolysis, myositis, chest pain, and hepatitis may develop.
- **Other options: Ethambutol** and **ethionamide** both can cause optic neuritis. **Thioacetazone** has no adverse effects on eye.

15. Amantadine. True are all *except*:

a. Prophylaxis of Influenza B
b. Treatment of H1N1
c. Acts through M2 protein
d. Useful in Parkinson's disease

Ans. a. Prophylaxis of Influenza B

Ref: Essentials of Medical Pharmacology by KD Tripathi 7th/ed, p432,801

EXPLANATION

Option a: It is effective against influenza A and not effective against influenza B.

Amantadine

- Inhibits replication of influenza A virus (a myxovirus).
- Active only against influenza A, no activity against influenza B ***(option a)***.
- In most areas H5N1 (avian) and H1N1 (swine) strains of influenza A are resistant, but it can be used if susceptible ***(option b)***.
- A protein designated 'M2' which acts as an ion channel has been identified as one of its targets of action ***(option c)***.
  - Acts at an early step (possibly uncoating) as well as at a late step (viral assembly) in viral replication.
  - Resistance to amantadine develops by mutation causing amino acid substitutions in the M2 protein.
- **Side effects** are rare but unique due to its CNS effects: anorexia, insomnia, dizziness, nightmares, lack of mental concentration, rarely hallucinations. Ankle edema occurs due to local vasoconstriction.
- **Uses:**
  - Prophylaxis of influenza A2 during an epidemic (generally lasts 2 months)

- Amantadine does not interfere with antibody response to influenza vaccination; both may be given together.
- Treatment of influenzal (A2) illness
- Parkinsonism *(option d)*
  - Due to its antagonistic action on NMDA type of glutamate receptors, through which the striatal dopaminergic system exerts its influence.
  - Acts rapidly but has lower efficacy than levodopa.
  - Tolerance develops over months and the efficacy is gradually lost.
  - Used in milder cases, or in short courses to supplement levodopa for advanced cases.
  - Fixed dose of 100 mg BD is used (not titrated according to response).

16. Famciclovir is a prodrug of:

a. Acyclovir
b. Valganciclovir
c. Ganciclovir
d. Penciclovir

Ans. d. Penciclovir *Ref: Essentials of Medical Pharmacology by KD Tripathi 7th/ed, p23,799*

Explanation

- Few drugs are inactive as such and need conversion in the body to one or more active metabolites. Such a drug is called a *prodrug*.
- Acyclovir gets converted to acyclovir triphosphate by viral specific enzymes, therefore effective in virus infected cells. The active metabolite, acyclovir triphosphate inhibits viral DNA synthesis and replication.
- Valacyclovir is prodrug of acyclovir ***(option a)***.
- Famciclovir is prodrug of 6-deoxypenciclovir (or simply penciclovir).
- The active component penciclovir is available for topical use.
- Ganciclovir: is activated intracellularly by virus specific enzymes to ganciclovir triphophate, this active metabolite attains much higher concentration inside CMV infected cells and inhibits viral replication,
- Valganciclovir is prodrug of ganciclovir ***(options b and c)***.

Drug	Active metabolite	Antiviral spectrum
Acyclovir	Acyclovir triphosphate	HSV-1 > HSV-2 > VZV = EBV. CMV not affected Oral bioavailability is only 20%
Valacyclovir	Acyclovir → acyclovir triphosphate	Higher plasma levels of acyclovir are achieved. DOC for Herpes zoster
Famciclovir	**Penciclovir**	**HSV, VZV some activity against HBV**
Ganciclovir	Ganciclovir triphos-phate	Use restricted to severe CMV in immunocompromised states because of high systemic toxicity < 10% oral bioavailability
Valganciclovir	Ganciclovir → ganci-clovir triphosphate	8 times higher bioavailability

17. True about Ibrutinib:

a. Used in solid tumors like renal cell carcinoma
b. Is a small molecule kinase inhibitor
c. Useful in B cell neoplasms
d. Janus kinase inhibitor

Ans. c. Useful in B cell neoplasms *Ref: Harrison's Principles of Internal Medicine 19th/ed, p103 e-19*

EXPLANATION

- *Agents targeting oncogenically activated pathways*: These agents target specific regulatory molecules in tumor cells. The targeted specific regulatory molecules, promotes the survival of tumor cells. Agents included here are:
  - 'Multitargeted' kinase antagonists: *Sorafenib, regorafenib, pazopanib, sunitinib*
  - mTOR inhibitors: *Temsirolimus and Everolimus*
  - Proteasome inhibitors: *Bortezomib, carfilzomib*
  - Novel class of inhibitors:
    - **Bruton's tyrosine kinase inhibitor—*Ibrutinib***
    - Janus kinase inhibitor—*ruxolitinib* ***(option d)***
  - Inhibitor of histone deacetylases (*Vorinostat, romidepsin*)
  - DNA methyltransferase inhibitors [*5-aza-cytidine and 2´-deoxy-5-azacytidine (decitabine)*]

  Agents targeting oncogenically activated pathways include:

MOA of drug class	Agents and target	Approved use	Adverse effects
'Multitargeted' kinase antagonists			
Small-molecule ATP site directed antagonists that inhibit more than one protein kinase and have value in the treatment of several solid tumors. ***(options a and b)***	Sorafenib (VEGFR, PDGFR, RAF kinase)	Advanced RCC and HCC (hepatocellular)	• Anti-VEGFR effect—hypertension, proteinuria, rarely bleeding and clotting disorders and perforation of scarred GI lesions. • Other effects fatigue, diarrhea and the hand-foot syndrome (particularly with sorafenib)
	Regorafenib (similar to sorafenib)	Relapsed advanced colon cancer	
	Pazopanib (VEGFR> PDGFR)	RCC and soft tissue sarcomas	
	Sunitinib (VEGFR, PDGFR and c-kit)	RCC and GIST	
Mammalian target of Rapamycin (mTOR) inhibitors			
mTOR inhibition useful in RCC	Temsirolimus	RCC Ca breast Certain neuroendocrine and brain tumors	Stomatitis, fatigue, and some hyperlipidemia (10%), myelosuppression (10%), and rare lung toxicity
	Everolimus	RCC	
Proteasome inhibitors (answer for question number 18 of JIPMER pattern)			
Proteasome (multiple proteases joined together) selectively degrade proteins that regulate activation of transcription factors (NF-κB) and proteins regulating cell cycle progression. Proteasome inhibitors act by inhibiting these proteases	Bortezomib	Multiple myeloma and certain lymphomas	neuropathy, orthostatic hypotension with or without hyponatremia, and reversible thrombocytopenia
	Carfilzomib	Multiple myeloma	Neuropathy not a feature, cytokine release syndrome, which can be a cardiopulmonary stress.

Contd...

Contd...

MOA of drug class	Agents and target	Approved use	Adverse effects
Novel class of inhibitors			
Bruton's tyrosine kinase has important role in the function of B-cells.	Ibrutinib	Mantle cell lymphoma (received accelerated approval by FDA based on response rates). Potentially applicable to a number of B cell neoplasms ***(option c)***	Thrombocytopenia, neutropenia, diarrhea, anemia, fatigue, musculoskeletal pain, bruising, nausea, upper respiratory tract infection, and rash
Janus kinases function downstream of a variety of cytokine receptors to amplify cytokine signals	Ruxolitinib ***(option d)***	Myelofibrosis (ameliorate splenomegaly and systemic symptoms).	Thrombocytopenia and anemia bruising, dizziness and headache
Inhibitor of histone deacetylases			
Histone deacetylases, maintain the proper orientation of histones on DNA. If acetylated may allow access of transcription of repressed genes.	Vorinostat	In cutaneous T-cell lymphoma	Dramatic skin clearing and very few side effects.
	Romidepsin	Cutaneous T-cell lymphoma	
DNA methyltransferase inhibitors			
These inhibitors increase transcription of genes "silenced" during the pathogenesis of a tumor by causing demethylation of the methylated cytosines that are acquired as an "epigenetic" (i.e., after the DNA is replicated) modification of DNA.	5-aza-cytidine	These drugs were originally considered antimetabolites but have clinical value in myelodysplastic syndromes and certain leukemias when administered at low doses.	
	2′-deoxy-5-azacytidine (decitabine)		

18. Mechanism of action of bortezomib in multiple myeloma is:

a. Inhibitor of proteasome
b. Tyrosine kinase antagonist
c. Inhibits histone deacetylase
d. Demethylates DNA

Ans. a. Inhibitor of proteasome

Explanation

Refer question number 17 of JIPMER pattern based question

19. Anti-cancer drug causing non-cardiac pulmonary edema:

a. Methotrexate
b. Azathioprine
c. Asparaginase
d. Cytosine arabinoside

Ans. d. Cytosine arabinoside *Ref: Harrison's Principles of Internal Medicine 19th/ed, Table 103e-4*

Explanation

- Among the toxicity list of anticancer drugs, noncardiogenic pulmonary edema is mentioned only with cytosine arabinoside.
- Toxicities of other options is mentioned in table below:

Drug	Toxicity
Cytosine arabinoside (AraC) or cytarabine	Marrow toxicity, Mucositis Neurologic and Conjunctivitis (high dose) Noncardiogenic pulmonary edema
Methotrexate	Marrow, liver/lung toxicity Renal tubular Mucositis
Asparaginase	Protein synthesis; indirect inhibition of DNA synthesis by ↓histone synthesis Clotting factors, Glucose, Albumin Hypersensitivity, CNS toxicity, Pancreatitis, Hepatic toxicity
Azathioprine	Marrow and Liver toxicity Nausea

Microbiology

Author: Bahram Gor, Co-author: Rashmi M Sangolikar

AIIMS May 2017

1. Which of the following is not associated with Zika virus?

a. Petechial rash
b. Conjunctivitis
c. Gullain-Barre syndrome
d. Fever with arthralgia

Ans. a. Petechial rash *Ref: Literature Review of Zika Virus, Vol 22, Number 7, July 2016, CDC*

Explanation

Zika virus causes maculopapular rash, not petechial rash.

- **Important points on Zika virus:**
  - Zika virus is a mosquito-borne flavivirus.
  - First isolated in 1947 from febrile rhesus macaque monkey in the Zika forest of Uganda.
  - It is positive-sense, single-stranded RNA virus.
- **Transmission:**
  - Bite of Aedes mosquito *(Ae. aegypti, Ae. africanus, Ae. hensilii, and Ae. albopictus).*
  - Congenital, perinatal, sexual.
  - Laboratory exposure, blood transfusion.
  - Animal bite.
- **Clinical features:**
  - Incubation period is 3–12 days.
  - Maculopapular rash, which is pruritic in most cases ***(option a).***
  - Low grade fever, myalgia, arthralgia, fatigue, headache, conjunctivitis ***(option b and d)***
  - Microcephaly
  - Neurological sequelae-meningitis, meningoencephalitis, Guillain-Barre syndrome ***(option c)***
  - Non-neurological sequelae-transient hearing loss, hypotension, genitourinary symptoms.
- **Diagnosis:** Clinically cannot be diagnosed, clinical features overlap with other arboviruses.
  - Diagnosis relies on laboratory testing.
  - History of travel to an area of ongoing Zika virus transmission should be taken.
  - RT-PCR is the ***most specific diagnostic approach.***
  - Detection of IgG and IgM antibodies are cross reactive with other flaviviruses like Dengue virus, hence limits their specificity.
- **Management and prevention:** No specific treatment nor vaccine is available.
  - Supportive management like rest, fluids, antipyretics, analgesics.
  - Prevention of mosquito bites, insect repellants, bed net, community-level strategies to prevent mosquito breeding.
  - Avoid travelling to areas with ongoing Zika virus infection.

2. Which of the following Staphylococcal infection is not toxin mediated?

a. Toxic shock syndrome
b. Scalded skin syndrome
c. Food poisoning
d. Septic shock

Ans. d. Septic shock

Ref: Essentials of Medical Microbiolgoy 1st/ed by Dr. Apurba Sankar Sastry, p212-15

EXPLANATION

Septic shock is a complication of bacteremia and is not toxin mediated.

Review of *Staph. aureus:*

- *Staphylococcus aureus* is gram positive cocci, arranged in grape like clusters, coagulase and catalase test positive, non-motile, non-sporing, occasionally capsulated.
- Virulence factors of *Staphylococcus aureus*:

1. Cell-wall associated factors
• Peptidoglycan • Teichoic acid • Cell surface adhesin, e.g. clumping factor • Protein A
2. Toxins
• Membrane active toxins: ▪ Hemolysins ▪ Leukocidin (for Panton valentine toxin) • Epidermolytic toxin (exfoliative toxin) • Enterotoxins • Toxic shock syndrome toxin
3. Extracellular enzymes
• Coagulase, heat stable thermonuclease, deoxyribonuclease, staphylokinase, lipase, protease.

- Clinical spectrum of ***Staphylococcus aureus*** infections:

1. Skin and soft tissue infections:
Folliculitis, furuncle, carbuncle, mastitis, breast abscess, impetigo, surgical site infections, cellulitis, botryomycosis, hidradenitis suppurativa.
2. Musculoskeletal infections:
Septic arthritis, osteomyelitis, pyomyositis, psoas abscess, epidural abscess.
3. Respiratory tract infections:
Ventilator associated pneumonia, septic pulmonary emboli, post viral pneumonia, empyema, pneumothorax, pneumatocele.
4. Bacteremia and its complications:
Sepsis, septic shock ***(option d***, bloodstream infections, infective endocarditis, intravenous drug use associated endocarditis.

Contd...

Contd...

5. Urinary tract infection
6. Toxin mediated illness ***(Question):***
Toxic shock syndrome ***(option a)***, food poisoning ***(option c)***, staphylococcal scalded skin syndrome ***(option b)***.
7. Community associated MRSA infections-necrotizing pneumonia etc.

3. A corneal swab from a hydrophobic patient of suspected case of rabies is taken. Choice of test to be performed from the following options is:

a. Seller stain for Negri body
b. Immunofluorescence
c. RT PCR
d. RFFIT

Ans. b. Immunofluorescence *Ref: Essentials of Medical Microbiology by Dr Apurba Sankar Sastry, p499*

Explanation

All options given are tests for rabies. ***Seller stain for Negri body*** *is done for postmortem diagnosis of rabies (the patient is hydrophobic and alive hence ruled out).* ***RFFIT*** *detects antibodies in CSF and serum.* ***RT PCR*** *amplifies genes of rabies virus RNA from brain tissue. The sample in the question is corneal swab, hence direct* ***immunofluorescence*** *test is done.*

Review of rabies

- ***Option a:*** Negri body: It is an intracytoplasmic eosinophilic inclusion body with characteristic basophilic inner granules.
  - Common site of Negri bodies: Neurons of cerebellum/hippocampus.
  - Less common sites: cortical and brainstem neurons.
  - Stains used: H&E, **Sellers stain**.
  - Negri body detection is **pathognomonic of rabies** virus, but it is not detected in 20% of cases and its absence doesn't rule out rabies.
- ***Option c:*** RT PCR- to amplify genes of rabies virus RNA from BRAIN TISSUE. **Most sensitive and specific for diagnosis of rabies**.
- ***Option d:*** RFFIT (Rapid fluorescent focus inhibition test). It detects antibodies in CSF and serum.

CSF antibodies	Serum antibodies
• More significant • Appears early • Present only in rabies infected individuals	• Less significant • Appears late • Present after vaccination

Other tests for antibody detection:

- MNT: Mouse neutralization test
- FAVN: Fluorescent antibody virus neutralization test
- IFA: Indirect fluorescence assay
- HAI: Hemagglutination inhibition test
- CFT: Complement fixation test.

- ***Option b:*** Direct immunofluorescence test. The sample in the question is corneal swab, hence direct immunofluorescence test is done.
  1. Detects rabies nucleoprotein antigen in specific by using monoclonal antibodies tagged with fluorescent dye (fluorescein isothiocyanate).

2. Best specimen is hair follicle of nape of neck **(most sensitive).**
3. Corneal impression smear is positive in late stage of disease (30% sensitive).

4. The following is a picture of genital ulcer scraping. Diagnosis is:

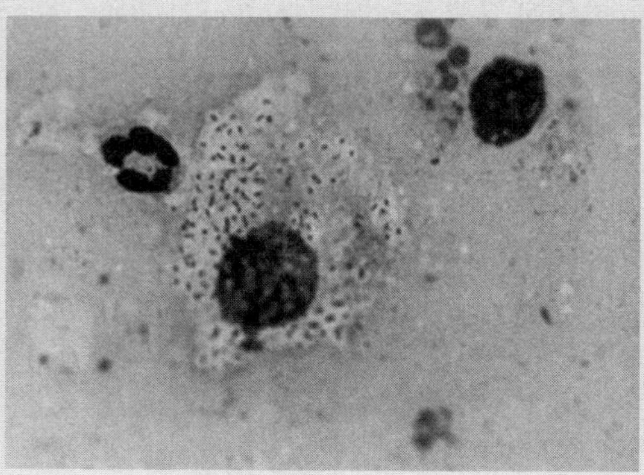

a. *Klebsiella granulomatis*
b. *Haemophilus ducreyi*
c. *Neisseria gonorrhea*
d. *Chlamydia trachomatis*

Ans. a. *Klebsiella granulomatis*

Ref: Essentials of Medical Microbiolgy by Dr. Apurba Sankar Sastry p603-04

EXPLANATION

Given figure shows donovan bodies (macrophage filled with bipolar stained bacilli) which is characteristic of *Klebsiella granulomatis.*

- ❑ Quick overview of sexually transmitted infections.
- ❑ STIs—a group of communicable diseases which are transmitted by sexual contact, these infections can be divided into those causing local disease and/or systemic manifestations.

<table>
<tr><th>Agents causing local manifestations</th><th>Agents causing systemic manifestations</th></tr>
<tr><td>• Genital ulcers
▪ Syphilis (Treponema pallidum)
▪ Herpes genitalia (HSV type 2 and 1)
▪ Chancroid (Haemophilus ducreyi)
▪ Lymphogranuloma venereum (Chlamydia trachomatis)
▪ Donovanosis (Klebsiella granulomatis)</td><td>• Pelvic inflammatory disease
▪ Neisseria gonorrhoeae,
▪ Chlamydia trachomatis.</td></tr>
<tr><td>• Urethral discharge
▪ Gonorrhea (N. gonorrhoeae)
▪ Non-gonococcal urethritis [C. trachomatis (D-K), ureaplasma urealyticum, Mycoplasma genitalium, Mycoplasma hominis, Herpes simplex virus, Candida albicans, Trichomonas vaginalis]</td><td rowspan="3">• No genital lesions but only systemic manifestations
▪ HIV
▪ HBV
▪ HCV</td></tr>
<tr><td>• Vaginal discharge
▪ Vulvovaginal candidiasis (candida species)
▪ Bacterial vaginosis (Gardnerella vaginalis, Mobiluncus sp.)
▪ Trichomonal vaginitis (Trichomonas vaginalis)</td></tr>
<tr><td>• Genital warts
▪ Condyloma acuminate (Human papilloma viruses)</td></tr>
</table>

- **Laboratory diagnosis of STIs:**
  1. Sample collection:
     - Vaginal/urethral discharge in sterile container
     - Sterile swabs (charcoal impregnated swabs for suspected gonococcal cases)
     - Fluid from vesicles (genital herpes).
  2. Microscopy
     - Wet mount examination:
       - Done for vaginal discharge
       - In trichomoniasis: Pus cells along with motile trophozoites seen.
       - In candidiasis: Yeast cells along with pseudohyphae seen.
     - Gram stain:
       - Bacterial vaginosis: CLUE CELLS seen (vaginal epithelial cells studded with gram variable pleomorphic coccobacilli).
       - Gonorrhea: Intracellular kidney shaped diplococci seen ***(option c)***.
       - Candidiasis: Gram positive budding yeast cells along with pseudohyphae seen.
     - Giemsa stain
       - *Klebsiella granulomatis*: To detect Donovan bodies (Macrophage filled with bipolar stained bacilli) ***(answer)***
       - *Chlamydia trachomatis*: Inclusion bodies ***(option d)***.
     - Dark field microscopy: Silver impregnation method is done for Syphilis, spirally coiled bacilli is seen.
  3. Culture:
     - Thayer-Martin medium—*N. gonorrhoeae*
     - Chocolate agar added with IsoVitaleX and vancomycin—*H. ducreyi.*
     - McCoy cell line—*C. trachomatis*
     - Sabouraud's dextrose agar—Candida sp.
     - Cell lines (vero, monkey kidney cell lines)—Herpes simplex virus.
  4. Serology—VDRL and RPR for primary syphilis.
  5. Molecular test—Multiplex PCR assays.

5. Papain cleaves the immunoglobulin molecule into:

a. 1 Fc and 1 Fab
b. 1 Fc and 2 Fab
c. 2 Fc and 1 Fab
d. 2 Fc and 2 Fab

Ans. b. 1Fc and 2 Fab *Ref: Essentials of Medical Microbiolgy by Dr. Apurba Sankar Sastry p112*

EXPLANATION

Papain cleaves Ig molecule at a point above disulfide bridge of hinge region, resulting in 3 fragments: two Fab fragments and one Fc fragment.

- When immunoglobulin molecule is subjected to enzymatic digestion, it generates various fragments.
- **Papain digestion**
  - Papain cleaves Ig molecule at a point above disulfide bridge of hinge region, resulting in 3 fragments each having a sedimentation coefficient of 3.5.
  - Two Fab fragments and one Fc fragment ***(answer)***.
  - Fab are soluble fragments which bind to antigen.
  - Fc is insoluble fraction which gets crystallized in cold.

❑ Figure below shows papain and pepsin digestion:

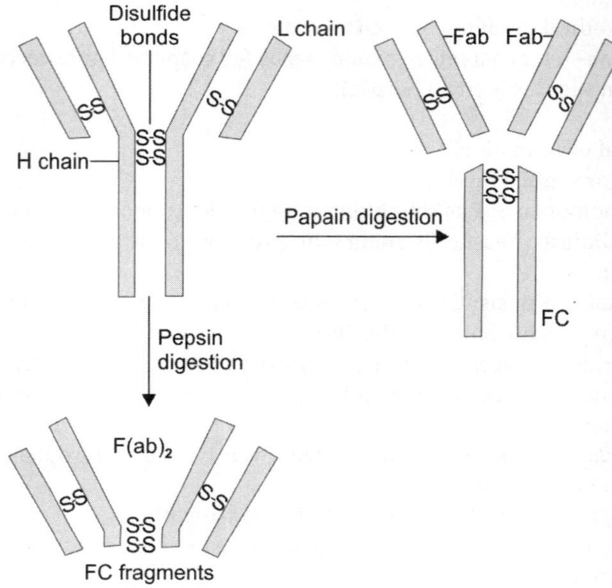

❑ Pepsin digestion
- Pepsin cleaves Ig molecule at a point below the disulfide bridge of hinge region resulting in one F $(ab')_2$ fragment and many smaller fragments.
- One F $(ab')_2$ – the sedimentation coefficient is 5S, and is composed of two Fab sub units bound together.
- Many smaller fragments are due to digestion of Fc portion of Ig.

❑ **Mercaptoethanol reduction of Ig molecule**
- Generates 2 H and 2 L chains.
- Cleaves only disulfide bonds and spares peptide bonds.

6. A 20-year-old male with history of fever and enlarged lymph nodes and sore throat was suspected to have infectious mono nucleosis and was ordered a Paul-Bunnel test. Which of the following is the principle of the test?

a. Heterophile agglutination test
b. Neutralization test
c. Complement mediated cell damage
d. Agglutination reaction

Ans. a. Heterophile agglutination test

Ref: Essentials of Medical Microbiolgy by Dr. Apurba Sankar Sastry p443

Explanation

Paul-Bunnel test is a tube **agglutination** test that uses sheep RBCs to detect **heterophile** antibody in patients serum.

❑ More about Paul-Bunnel-test:
- **Procedure**: Serial dilutions of inactivated (56°C for 30 minutes) patient's serum are mixed with equal volumes of 1 sheep RBCs and then tubes are incubated at 37°C for 4 hours.
- **Result:** Agglutination titer > 256 is considered as significant.
- **False positive:** In normal individuals and after serum therapy.

- ❑ **Differential absorption test** is done for confirmation.
- ❑ **Monospot test** is modified heterophile agglutination test available commercially (uses horse RBCs instead of sheep RBCs, its simple slide agglutination test).
- ❑ Heterophile antibodies appear early (40% in first week, 80–90% in third week of illness, disappears within 3 months).
- ❑ Heterophile antibodies not detected in children <5 years, in elderly, patients with atypical symptoms.
- ❑ Examples of other heterophile agglutination test are Typhus fever (Weil-Felix reaction) and *Mycoplasma pneumonia* (cold agglutination test).

7. Rhinosporidium seeberi belongs to:

a. Fungus
b. Bacteria
c. Aquatic protistan protozoa
d. Virus

Ans. c. Aquatic protistan protozoa

Ref: Essentials of Medical Microbiolgy by Dr. Apurba Sankar Sastry p562

Explanation

See below

Rhinosporidiosis

- ❑ Rhinosporidiosis is a chronic granulomatous disease characterized by large friable polyps in the nose **(most common site)**, conjunctiva, ears, larynx, bronchus, genitalia.
- ❑ Agent: Rhinosporidium seeberi, a lower aquatic fungus, taxonomic status is controversial; some believe that it may be a hydrophilic protist ***(Answer)***.
- ❑ Source: Stagnant water. Fungal spores are inhaled while taking bath in contaminated ponds and rivers.
- ❑ Distribution: Tropical countries like India (Tamil Nadu, Orissa, Kerala, and Andhra Pradesh) and Sri lanka.
- ❑ **Diagnosis:**
  - Histopathology of polyps—Spherules (large sporangia up to 350 μm which contains numerous endospore, ach 6–9 um).
  - Stained better with mucicarmine stain.

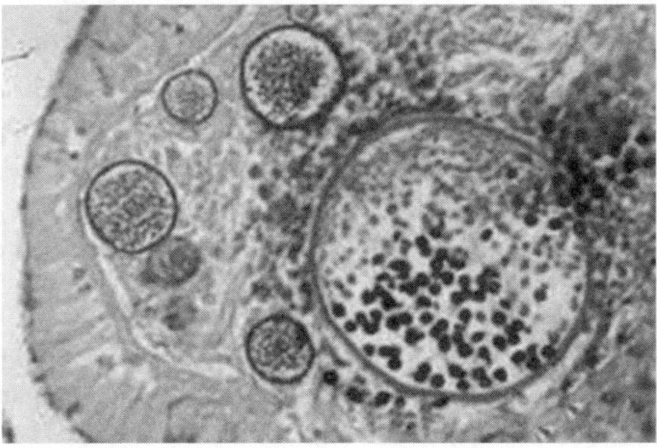

- ❑ It has not been cultivated yet.

8. Gene for thymic selection mechanism:

a. RAG 1/2
b. NOTCH 1
c. AIRE
d. GATA-2

Ans. c. AIRE

Ref: Kuby's Textbook of Immunology p27 and 132; US NATIONAL Library of Medicine; Genetics Home Reference

EXPLANATION

- ❑ *Option c:* AIRE GENE
  - It provides instructions for a protein called Autoimmune regulator.
  - This protein is active in thymus.
  - Thymus prepares immune cells called T cells for their role in fighting infection, this is called thymic education.
  - In a healthy person, T cells identify and destroy potentially harmful invaders (like bacteria, virus, fungi) while sparing body's normal tissues.
  - AIRE protein plays a role in helping T cells to distinguish body's own proteins from those of foreign invaders.
  - When this system, malfunctions, the immune system cannot distinguish between foreign invaders and body's own proteins.
  - Body's own tissues and organs are attacked.
  - This leads to autoimmunity.
  - In thymus AIRE protein destroys T cells that otherwise would cause autoimmune damage.
- ❑ *Option b:* NOTCH1 GENE
  - This gene instructs to make a protein called NOTCH1.
  - When ligand attaches to Notch1 receptor, it signals the normal development of many tissues before and after birth.
  - It determines specialization of cells into certain cell types that perform particular functions in the body (cell fate determination).
  - It plays role in cell growth, division, maturation and apoptosis.
- ❑ *Option d:* GATA-2 GENE
  - This gene specifies the transcription factor, which is essential for development of lymphoid, erythroid, myeloid lineages.
- ❑ *Option a:* RAG 1/2
  - Recombinase activating genes 1 and 2.

9. Patient gives presents with diarrhea, associated with blood, stool, mucus and fever. What is your likely diagnosis?

a. *Giardia lamblia*
b. *E. histolytica*
c. *Salmonella typhi*
d. Isospora species

Ans. b. *E. histolytica*

Ref: Paniker's Textbook of Parasitology p18,32,94 and Harrisons Textbook of Medicine 17th/ed p960

EXPLANATION

Among the options given, only *E. histolytica* produces diarrhea with blood streaked mucus.

- ❑ *Option a: Giardia lamblia* causes diarrhea associated with mucus, steatorrhea, epigastric pain but never blood *(Panikers Textbook of Parasitology p32).*
- ❑ *Option d:* Coccidian parasites like Isospora species, Cyclospora species, Cryptosporidium species causes watery diarrhea but without blood *(Panikers Textbook of Parasitology p94).*

- ❑ ***Option c:*** *S. typhi* does not cause bloody diarrhea, whereas non-typhoidal salmonellosis causes diarrheal stools which are usually loose, non-bloody, and of moderate volume. However, large-volume watery stools, bloody stools, or symptoms of dysentery may occur *(Harrison's Textbook of Medicine 17th/ed p960).*

10. Which of the following fits to the life cycle in the diagram given below?

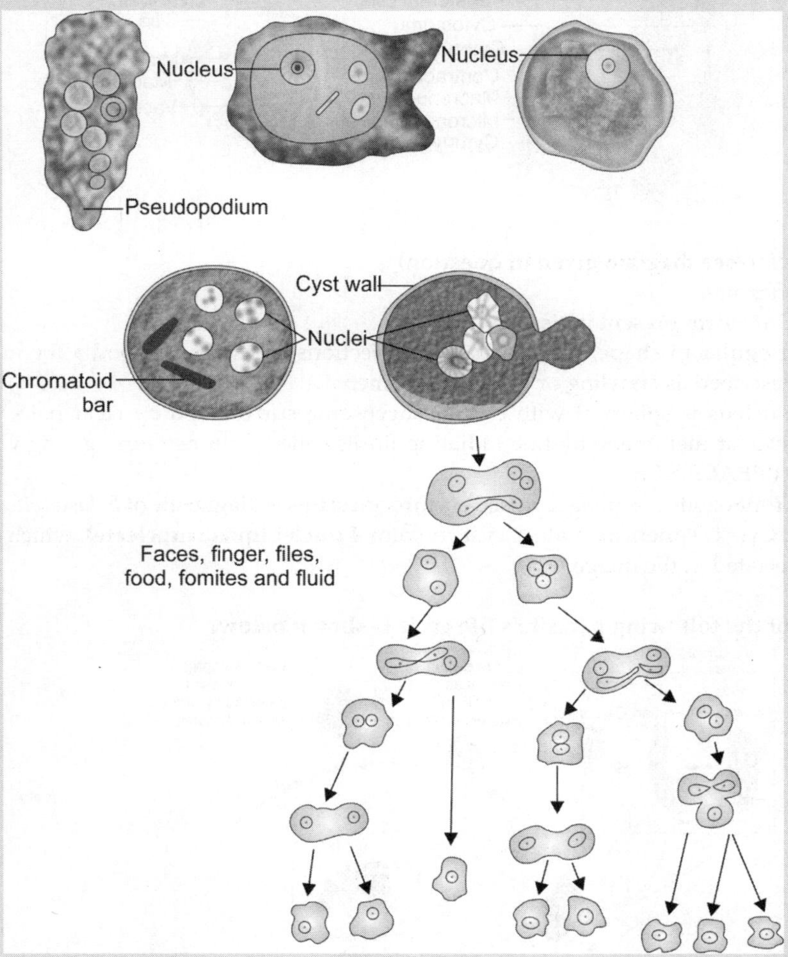

a. *B. coli*
b. *E. histolytica*
c. *A. duodenale*
d. *E. vermicularis*

Ans. b. *E. histolytica* *Ref: Paniker's Textbook of Parasitology p18*

Explanation

The above life cycle shows trophozoite and cyst form. Among the above options, only *Balantidium coli* and *E. histolytica* have trophozoite and cyst forms. Hence, *A. duodenale* and *E. vermicularis* can be ruled out. In the figure, it can be seen that cyst is having 4 nuclei, which is seen in *E. histolytica*

- *Balantidium coli*-some peculiar features are *(See figure below)*:
  - Only ciliate protozoan parasite of humans.
  - Largest protozoan parasite of humans.
  - It has cilia.
  - It has kidney shaped macronucleus and micronucleus.

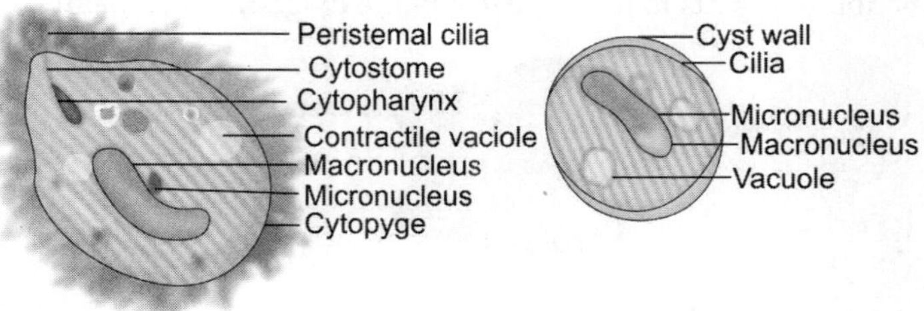

- *E. histolytica* **(see diagram given in question)**
  - Trophozoite:
    - Only form present in tissues.
    - Irregular in shape, has finger-like projections called pseudopodia for its locomotion, described as crawling or gliding movement.
    - Nucleus is spherical with central karyosome surrounded by clear halo, anchored by nuclear membrane by fine radiating fibrils called linin network, giving CARTWHEEL APPEARANCE.
    - Trophozoite has phagocytosed erythrocytes; this is diagnostic of *E. histolytica* trophozoite.
  - Cyst: Cyst is spherical, mature cyst contains **4 nuclei (quadrinucleate)**, which can be easily appreciated in the image.

11. Which of the following parasite's life cycle is shown below?

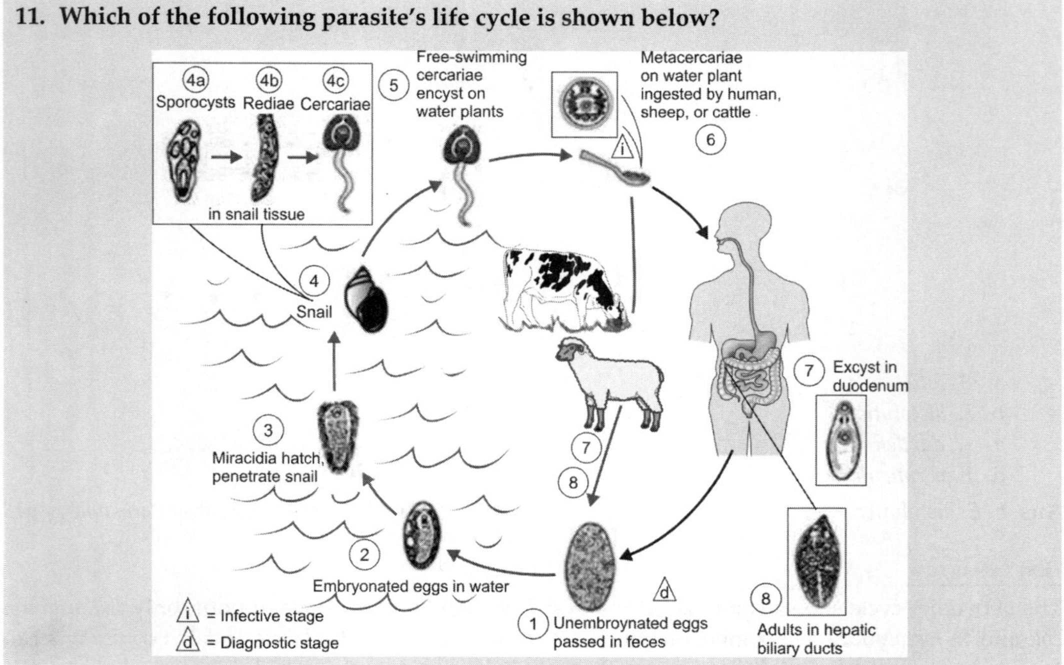

a. *Fasciola buski*
b. *Fasciola hepatica*
c. *Paragonimus westermani*
d. *Clonorchis sinensis*

Ans. b. *Fasciola hepatica* *Ref: Panikers Textbook of Parasitology 7th/ed p151*

EXPLANATION

Differentiating features of the four options in the question are given below:

Fasciola hepatica	Fasciola buski	Paragonimus westermani	Clonorchis sinensis
Common name is sheep liver fluke	Common name is giant intestinal fluke	Common name is oriental lung fluke	Common name is the chinese liver fluke, oriental liver fluke
Eggs are ovoid and operculated	Eggs are similar to F. hepatica	Eggs are operculated	Eggs are operculated at one side and small hook like spine on another
Definitive host: Sheep, cow and man	Definitive host: Man and pigs	Definitive host: Man, cats, tigers, leopards, foxes, dogs, beavers, other crab eating mammals and domestic animals	Definitive host: Man but dogs and other fish eating canines act as reservoir hosts
1st intermediate host: Fresh water snail	1st intermediate host: Snail	1st intermediate host: Fresh water snail	1st intermediate host: Snail
2nd intermediate host: Aquatic vegetation	2nd intermediate host: Aquatic plants, roots of lotus, bulb of the water chestnut	2nd intermediate host: Fresh water crab or cray-fish	2nd intermediate host: Fish
Infective form: Metacer-ceriae encysted on raw aquatic vegetations.	Infective form: Metacer-ceriae encysted on raw aquatic vegetations.	Infective form: Metacerceriae encysted in crab or crayfish.	Infective form: Metacer-caria larva.

12. Identify the organism from its egg in the picture:

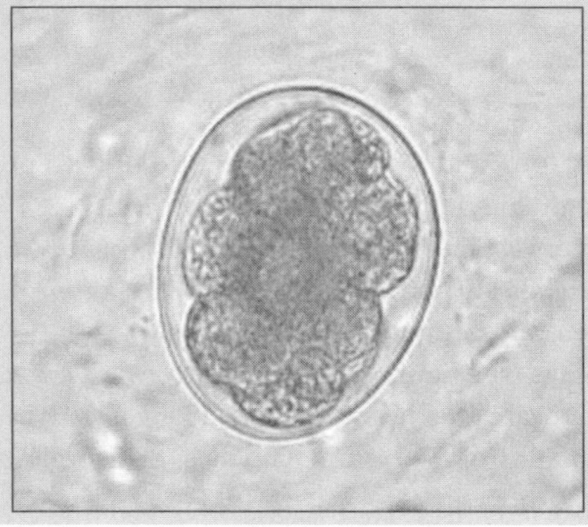

a. Enterobius vermicularis
b. Trichuris trichiura
c. Ascaris lumbricoides
d. Necator americanus

Ans. d. Necator americanus *Ref: Panikers Textbook of Parasitology 7th/ed p173,183,191 and 196*

Explanation

- ❑ Egg of Necator americanus **(see figure given in question)** *(Panikers Textbook of Parasitology 7th/ed, p183)*
  - Oval/elliptical (60 μm × 40 μm).
  - Colorless, non-bile stained, surrounded by a thin transparent hyaline shell membrane.
  - When released by worm, in intestine, egg contains unsegmented ovum.
  - During its passage, down the intestine, ovum develops.
  - In feces, egg contains a segmented ovum with 4–8 blastomeres, with clear space present between segmented ovum and egg shell.
  - Floats in saturated salt solution.
- ❑ Egg of A. duodenale is same as egg of N. americanus morphologically *(Panikers Textbook of Parasitology 7th/ed p183).*
- ❑ Egg of Trichuris trichiura **(see figure below)** *(Panikers Parasitology 7th/ed p173)*

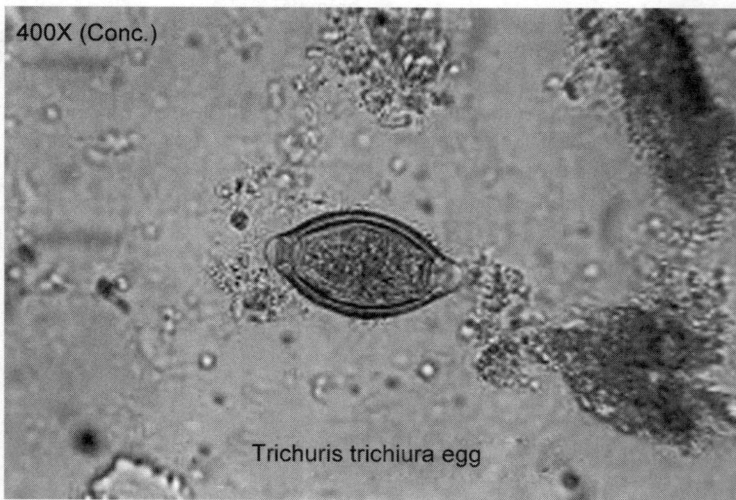

  - Barrel-shaped (50 μm long and 25 μm wide in middle) with projecting mucus plug at each pole containing unsegmented ovum, plugs are colorless.
  - Triple shell, outer layer is stained brown.
  - Egg is brown in color, bile stained.
  - Egg floats in saturated salt solution.
- ❑ Egg of Ascaris lumbricoides **(see figure)** *(Panikers Textbook of Parasitology 7th/ed p196)*
  - **Unfertilized egg**: Elliptical in shape, narrower and longer (80 × 55 μm), thin shell with irregular coating of albumin, small atrophied ovum with mass of disorganized highly refractile granules, doesn't float in salt solution.

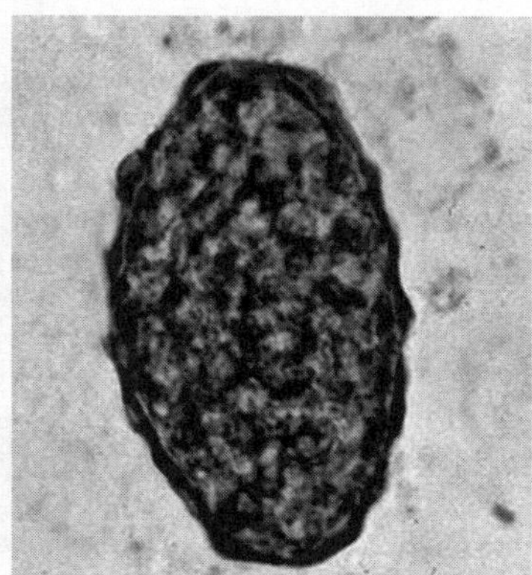

- **Fertilized egg**: Round/oval (60–75 μm), bile stained, golden brown in color, surrounded by thick smooth translucent shell with outer coarsely mammilliated albuminous coat, thick transparent middle layer and inner lipoidal vitelline membrane floats in salt solution.

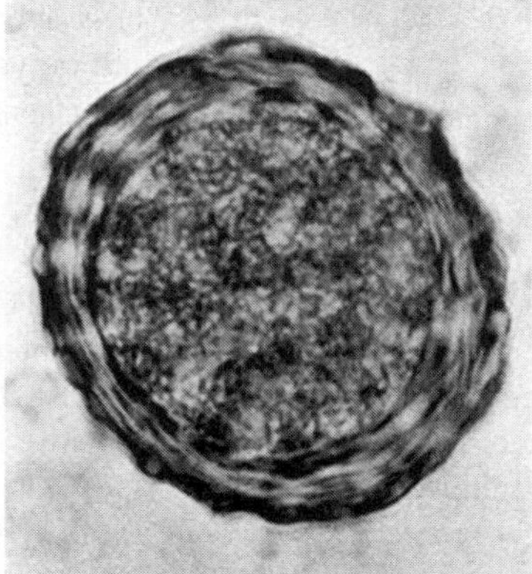

- Egg of Enterobius vermicularis **(see figure below)** (*Panikers Textbook of Parasitology 7th/ed, p191*)
  - Egg is colorless and not bile stained.
  - It floats in saturated salt solution.
  - Its planoconvex, flattened on one side, convex on other (50–60 μm by 20–30 μm).
  - Egg shell is double layered, thick, transparent, outer albuminous layer makes egg stick to each other and clothing.
  - Egg contains tadpole shaped coiled embryo, which is fully formed.

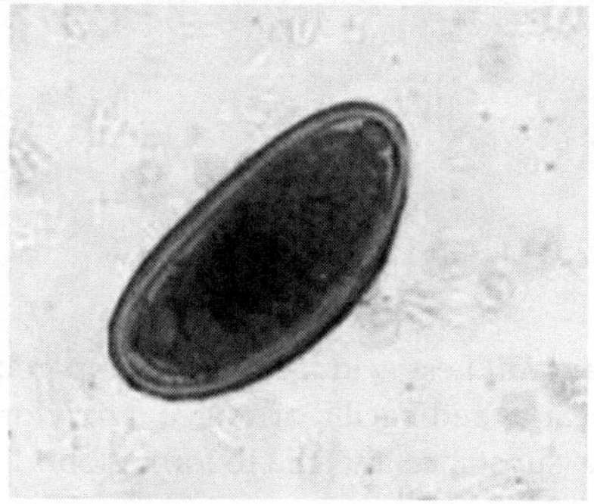

13. Identify the organism in the slide:

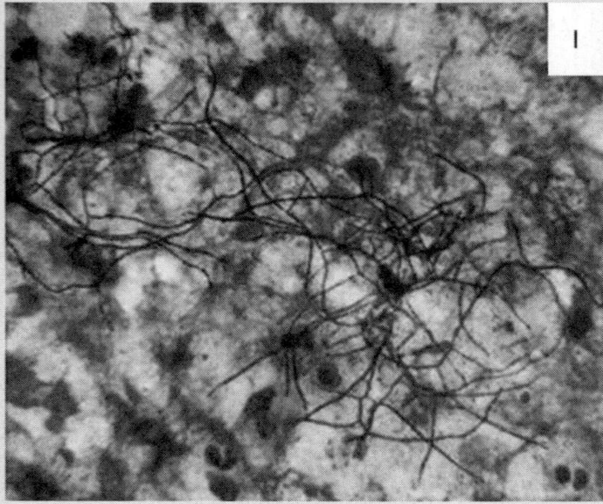

a. Nocardia species
b. *Mycobacterium tuberculosis*
c. *Mycobacterium leprae*
d. Actinomyces species

Ans. a. Nocardia species *Ref: Essentials of Medical Microbiolgy by Dr. Apurba Sankar Sastry p562*

Explanation

See below

- ❑ ***Option a:*** Nocardia species **(see diagram given in question)**: On modified acid fast stain, bacilli are seen red colored branching and filamentous, as appreciated in the image.
- ❑ ***Option b:*** *M. tuberculosis*: **(see diagram below)** on acid fast stain, they appear as long slender, beaded, less uniformly stained, red colored acid fast bacillus. (*M. bovis* appears as short, stout, uniformly stained acid fast bacillus).

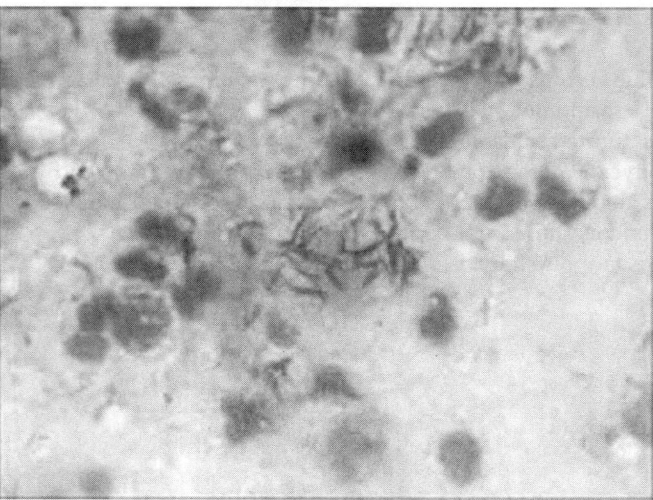

- ❑ ***Option c:*** *M. leprae*: **(see diagram)** Less acid fast when compared to *M. tuberculosis*, they appear on acid fast stain they appear as red bacilli, arranged singly or in groups, (cigar like bundles), bound together by lipid like substance, the glia to form globi.

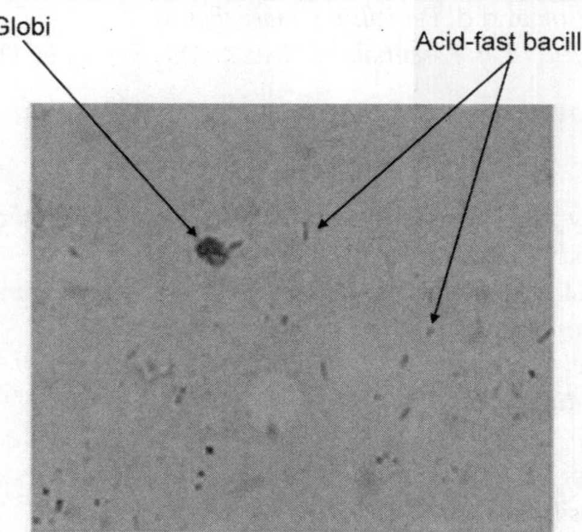

- Actinomyces species: They are non acid fast.

14. 1-3 beta-d-glucan assay for fungi is not used for:

a. Aspergillus species
b. Candida species
c. Cryptococcus species
d. *Pneumocystis jirovecii*

Ans. c. Cryptococcus species *Ref: Parija's Textbook of Microbiology and Immunology p596*

EXPLANATION

1-3 beta-d-glucan (BDG) is produced in the cell walls of many medically important fungi. Certain species like *Cryptococcus neoformans* and Zygomycetes either they lack glucan entirely or produce at minimal levels. Thus the answer.

- Its secretion in circulation during its life cycle, indicates presumptive diagnosis of invasive fungal diseases like Candidiasis, Aspergillosis, Pneumocystis infection ***(Options a, b and d).***
- 1-3 beta-d-glucan assay is based on ability to activate a coagulation cascade within amebocytes derived from hemolymph of horseshoe crabs.
- This uses different cascade than endotoxin to cause coagulation, hence is specific for fungi.
- This test does not detect certain species like *Cryptococcus neoformans* and Zygomycetes either they lack glucan entirely or produce at minimal levels ***(option c).***
- PLEASE NOTE, recent study reveals in HIV infected Ugandan and South african people with suspected meningitis, higher concentration of BDG were detected in CSF of individuals with Cryptococcal meningitis *(www.thelancet.com/infection vol 15 oct 2015).*
- Therefore among given options cryptococcus is the best answer.
- If options have both cryptococcus and zygomycetes, then answer will be zygomycetes.

PGI May 2017

1. Which of the following is/are dimorphic fungi?

a. *Cryptococcus neoformans*
b. *Histoplasma capsulatum*
c. Aspergillus species
d. *Penicillium marneffei*
e. Rhizopus species

Ans. b. *Histoplasma capsulatum* and d. *Penicillium marneffei*

Ref: Essentials of Medical Microbiolgy by Dr. Apurba Sankar Sastry p550

EXPLANATION

Dimorphic fungi

- They exist as molds (hyphal form) in the environment at ambient temperature (25°C) and yeasts in human tissues at body temperature (37°C).
- Examples of dimorphic fungi are: *(Mnemonic: His Pen can Blast Spores of coccido and paracoccido)*
  - *Histoplasma capsulatum* **(option b)**
  - *Penicillium marneffei* **(option d)**
  - *Blastomyces dermatitidis*
  - *Sporothrix schenckii*
  - *Coccidioides immitis*
  - *Paracoccidioides brasiliensis.*

2. Which of the following is/are true about actinomyces?

a. Causes actinomycetoma
b. Most commonly causes cervicofacial actinomycosis
c. Can be detected directly from sample by FISH
d. Drug of choice is penicillin
e. It is aerobic and acid fast

Ans. b. Most commonly causes cervicofacial actinomycosis; c. Can be detected directly from sample by FISH and d. Drug of choice is penicillin

Ref: Essentials of Medical Microbiolgy by Dr. Apurba Sankar Sastry p293

EXPLANATION

See below

- Actinomyces is a soil saprophyte and commensal of oral cavity.
- Causes actinomycosis in humans.
- *A. israelii* is common species; *A. naeslundii* and *A. odontolyticus* are rare pathogens.
- **Pathogenesis:** It causes chronic suppurative granulomatous infection characterized by multiple abscesses with formation of sinuses, discharge containing granules and later fibrosis and tissue destruction.
- The organism appears ray-like in granules.
- Endogenous infection following dental extraction.
- **Clinical features: (1)** Cervicofacial actinomycosis-**most common form *(option b)***, painless slow-growing, hard mass with cutaneous fistulas, causing lumpy jaw.
  (2) Other forms are abdominal, pelvic, disseminated form to organs like liver, lungs.
- **Lab diagnosis:**
  - **Specimen collection:** Discharge from sinuses of fistulas, rarely bronchoalveloar lavage, sputum, tissue sections.
  - **Direct microscopy:** Pus discharged washed in saline in test tube, and sediment collected contains gritty white yellowish sulfur granules < 5 mm in size.
  - **Gram staining** (Brown-Brenn modification): Central mass of gram-positive filamentous bacilli, radiating peripherally with hyaline, club-shaped ends.
  - It can be also detected from direct samples by **FISH** (Fluorescent in situ hybridization) using species specific probes ***(option c).***

- Histopathological staining: **H&E and Gomori's** granules composed of eosinophilic clubs surrounding basophilic filaments and inflammatory cells such as neutrophils and foamy macrophages **(sun-rays appearance)**.
- Culture: Sulfur granules cultured anaerobically at 37°C on Thioglycollate broth (A. israelli produces **fluffy balls** at bottom of test tube, A. bovis produces uniform turbidity) and Brain heart infusion agar (**spidery colonies** at 48 hrs which becomes enlarged and heaped up in 10 days).
- Species identification: Gas liquid chromatography, biochemical reactions, PCR-RFLP.

❑ **Treatment: DOC** penicillin for 6–12 months ***(option d)***.
- Erythromycin/tetracycline for people with penicillin allergy.
- Surgical removal of affected tissues.

❑ *Option a:* Actinomycetoma is caused by nocardia

3. Which of the following has barrel-shaped eggs?

a. E. vermicularis
b. Ascaris lumbricoides
c. A. duodenale
d. N. americanus
e. Trichuris trichiura

Ans. e. Trichuris trichiura *Ref: See Question Number 12 of AIIMS Micro*

4. Which is/are true about Donovanosis?

a. Caused by Leishmania donovani
b. Amphotericin B is drug of choice
c. Sodium stibogluconate is drug of choice
d. Caused by *Klebsiella granulomatosis*
e. Causes psudobubo

Ans. d. Caused by *Klebsiella granulomatosis* and e. Causes psudobubo

Ref: Essentials of Medical Microbiolgy by Dr. Apurba Sankar Sastry p366

EXPLANATION:

Donovanosis

❑ Also known as Granuloma inguinale

❑ It's a sexually transmitted disease caused by *Klebsiella granulomatis* (old name is *Calymmatobacterium granulomatis*) ***(Option a and d)***

❑ Disease was *first described in Calcutta* by McLeod in 1882.

❑ Characteristic *Donovan bodies* in genital lesion recognized by Charles Donovan in Madras in 1905.

❑ Donovanosis is prevalent in India. Brazil, Papua New Guinea and parts of South Africa.

❑ Risk factors → poor hygiene, low socio-economic status, multiple sex partners.

❑ Clinical features →
- *Incubation period*:1-4 weeks (up to 6 months),
- Painless papule → beefy red ulcer, which bleeds on touch,
- Lymph node enlargement is rare, however pseudobubos ***(Option e)*** seen in the inguinal region in 10% cases due to subcutaneous abscess,
- *Site affected are* genitals, mainly prepuce, frenulum and glans in males, and labia minora in women.

❑ Clinical diagnosis by characteristic lesion

❑ Laboratory diagnosis →
- Sample-swab rolled on the ulcer (alternatively piece of granulation tissue crushed and spread between two slides)

- Direct microscopy- Giemsa/Wright stain- Donovan bodies seen as large cyst like macrophages filled with deeply stained capsulated bacilli having a safety pin appearance.
- Culture-egg yolk medium and HEp-2 cell lines
- Molecular methods :PCR.

❑ Treatment→ **DOC-** Macrolides,azithromycin 1g on day 1,then 500 mg daily for 7 days. ***(Option b and c)***

- Alternatively, doxycycline (100 mg twice a day) OR tetracycline (500 mg twice a day) for 14 days
- Both sexual partners to be treated.

5. Cholera patient having stool output 1000–1500 mL/day is known as:

a. Cholera mitis
b. Cholera dumdum
c. Cholera magna
d. Cholera gravis
e. Cholera intermedius

Ans. d. Cholera gravis *Ref: Essentials of Medical Microbiolgy by Dr. Apurba Sankar Sastry p328*

EXPLANATION

❑ ***Vibrio cholera***

❑ They are curve (comma-shaped) gram negative, bacilli that are actively motile (single polar flagellum).

❑ **Classification:**

1. Based on salt requirement
   a. **Halophilic vibrios:** They can't grow in the absence of salt. They can tolerate salt at 7–10%. examples are *V. parahaemolyticus, V. alginolyticus, V. vulnificus.*
   b. **Non-halophilic vibrios:** They can grow without salt but 1% salt is needed. Examples are *V. cholerae, V. mimicus.*
2. Heiberg classification (1934)
   EIGHT GROUPS based on fermentation of mannose, arabinose and sucrose. *V. cholerae* placed in GROUP I.
3. Gardner and Venkatraman classification.

Based on serogrouping, biotyping, serotyping and phage typing.

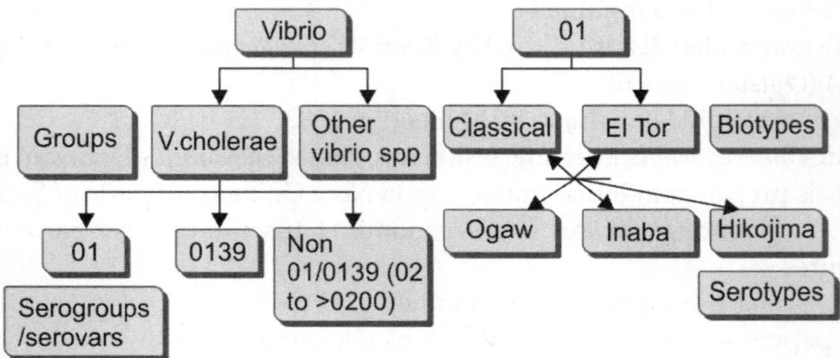

❑ **Pathogenesis of cholera:** Toxin mediated

- Mode of transmission: Ingestion of contaminated water and food.
- Infective dose: extremely acid labile, hence high infective dose is needed to bypass gastric barrier (10^8 bacilli).
- Factors promoting transmission: Hypochlorhydria, use of antacids.
- The bacilli penetrates mucous layer → Adheres to the epithelium → Cholera toxin is produced → Toxin has fragment B and fragment A → Fragment B is binding fragment, that binds to GM1

Ganglioside receptors → Fragment A, causes ADP-ribosylation of G protein → Upregulates the activity of adenylate cyclase → Intracellular accumulation of camp → water moves out due to osmolality, which leads to watery diarrhea → Loss of fluids and electrolytes leads to shock.

- Clinical features of cholera:
  - Asymptomatic infection (75% cases)
  - Mild diarrhea or cholera (20% cases)
  - Sudden onset of explosive and life threatening diarrhea (**Cholera gravis, in 5% of cases**).
  - Watery diarrhea, rice water stools, vomiting, fever usually absent, muscle cramps due to electrolyte imbalance.
- **Complications of cholera:**

Loss of body weight by	Symptoms
<5%	Increased thirst
5–10%	• Postural hypotension • Weakness • Tachycardia • Decreased skin turgor
>10%	Renal failure (acute tubular necrosis) and fluid loss results in: • Oliguria • Weak or absent pulse • Sunken eyes • Sunken fontanelles in infants • Wrinkled skin • Somnolence • Coma

- Epidemiology
  - History of pandemics:
    - Home land is DELTA REGION of Ganges and Brahmaputra in West Bengal. And Bangladesh.
    - First 6 pandemics caused by classical biotype of V.cholerae, had spread from Bengal to all over world.
    - Seventh pandemic-only pandemic originated outside india(in Indonesia),caused by El Tor biotype.
    - 0139 (Bengal strain)—first isolated in Chennai in 1992
    - It was not agglutinated by antisera (01 to 0138), hence designated as 0139.
    - It is capsulated, invasive causes bacteremia and extraintestinal manifestations.
  - **Cholera is a notifiable disease.**
    - National reference center for cholera is located at national institute of cholera and enteric diseases (NICED), Kolkata.
  - **Reservoir:** Humans.
  - **Source:** Asymptomatic cases or carriers.
  - **Carriers:** (1) Incubatory carriers (1–2 days), (2) Convalescent carriers (2–3 weeks), (3) Contact or healthy carriers (<10 days), (4) Chronic carriers.
  - **Factors determining severity:** People with O blood group, malnutrition, lack of pre-existing immunity.
  - **Habitat:** Natural habitat of coastal sea salt water and brackish estuaries, associated with crustaceans, copepods, crabs, plankton.

❑ Lab diagnosis

Specimens: Watery stool or rectal swab for carriers.

Transport media: Venkataramana Ramakrishna media, Cary-Blair medium.

Direct microscopy:
- Gram-negative rods, short curved, comma shaped (**fish in stream appearance**)
- Hanging drop demonstrates darting motility.

Culture:
- **Enrichment broth**: Alkaline peptone water, Monsur's taurocholate tellurite peptone water.
- **Selective media:** Bile salt agar, Monsur's GTTT agar, TCBS agar (yellow colonies)
- MacConkey agar-translucent non-lactose fermenting colonies.

Culture smear and motility testing to be done.

Biochemical identification:
- Catalase and oxidase positive.
- **ICUT:** Indole (+), Citrate (+/–), Urease (–), TSI: A/A, gas (-), H_2S (–)
- Cholera red reaction is positive
- **String test** is positive
- Salt tolerance test is positive
- Ferments glucose and sucrose

Biotyping: To differentiate Classical and El Tor

Serogrouping: To differentiate 01 and 0139.

Serotyping: To differentiate Ogawa, Inaba, Hikojima serotypes of serogroup 01

❑ Treatment

Fluid replacement: ORS solution, ringer's lactate

Antibiotics has minor role, WHO recommends antibiotic use only in severely dehydrated cases.

Adults: doxycycline or tetracycline

Children/pregnancy erythromycin/azithromycin.

❑ Prevention:

- **General measures:** Safe water, improved sanitary disposal of feces, notification, health education.
- **Chemoprophylaxis:** Tetracycline
- Vaccine:
  - Injectable killed vaccines: No longer in use
  - Oral cholera vaccines (OCV)
  - Killed whole-cell vaccine
  - Oral live-attenuated vaccine.

Killed whole-cell vaccine	Oral live-attenuated vaccine
1. Whole-Cell (WC) vaccine: Composed of killed whole cells of V. cholerae 01 (Classical and El Tor Inaba and Ogawa)	They use mutant strains that lack gene encoding for cholera toxin.
2. Whole-cell recombinant B subunit cholera vaccine (WC/RBS) (Dukoral): Same composition as above plus recombinant cholera toxin B subunits.	1. CVD103-hgr, (Orochol-contains live attenuated strain derived from reference strain 569B < classical, 01, inaba > Schedule-single dose) 2. Peru-15 3. V. cholerae 638 for classical and/or El Tor for biotypes of V. cholerae 1.
Schedule 2 oral dose, at 7 days gap • 3 doses for 3-5 years children • Not given for <2 years.	CVD-112 and Bengal-15 vaccine trials for V. cholerae 0139

6. Which is true about syphilis?

a. VDRL test detects antibodies
b. Jarisch herxheimer - IgE mediated
c. Primary and secondary treatment preferred is penicillin
d. RPR is done for CSF
e. T. pallidum can be easily cultivated in artificial culture media

Ans. a. VDRL test detects antibodies; b. Jarisch herxheimer - IgE mediated and c. Primary and secondary treatment preferred is penicillin

Ref: Essentials of Medical Microbiolgy by Dr. Apurba Sankar Sastry p372; Harrisons Textbook of Internal Medicine, 17th/ed p1084

Explanation

See below

- **SYPHILIS**
- An ancient sexually transmitted disease caused by Treponema pallidum.
- They are flexible, coiled bacilli, having 3–4 endoflagella.
- Pathogenesis:
  - Mode of transmission: Sexual contact, direct contact, blood transfusion, transplacental transmission.
  - Spread: Penetrates through minor abrasions → enters lymphatics and blood to produce systemic infection.
  - Incubation period: 9–90 days.
- Clinical features:
  - Primary syphilis: Hard chancre, inguinal lymphadenopathy.
  - Secondary syphilis: Skin rashes, condylomata lata, mucous patches generalized lymphadenopathy.
  - Latent syphilis: Absence of clinical manifestations with positive serological tests
  - Late or tertiary syphilis: Gumma, neurosyphilis, cardiovascular syphilis.
  - Congenital syphilis: Rhinitis, mucocutaneous lesions, hepatosplenomegaly, lymphadenopathy, interstitial keratitis, 8th nerve deafness, clutton's joints, mulberry molars, saddle nose, saber shins, Hutchinson's teeth.
- **Lab diagnosis:**

Microscopy
• Dark ground microscopy • Direct immunofluorescent antibody staining for T.pallidum • Silver impregnation method
Culture
• **Not cultivable**, ***(Option e)*** only maintained in rabbit testes.
Serology (antibody detection)
• Non-treponemal or STS (standard tests for syphilis) reagin antibodies are detected by using cardiolipin antigen. ▪ Old methods: Wassermann test (CFT) and Kahn test. ▪ Newer methods (slide flocculation tests) ▪ VDRL ***(Option a)*** (veneral disease research laboratory) test-blood, plasma, serum, CSF can be tested ▪ RPR (Rapid plasma regain) test-blood, plasma, serum can be tested but not CSF ***(Option d)***. ▪ TRUST (toluidine red unheated serum test) ▪ USR (Unheated serum regain test)

Contd...

Contd...

- Specific/treponemal tests (specific antibodies are detected by using T.pallidum antigens).
  - TPI (Treponema pallidum immobilization test)
  - FTA-ABS (Fluorescent treponemal antibody absorption test)
  - TPA (T.pallidum agglutination test)
  - TPIA (T.pallidum immune adherence test)
  - TPHA (T.pallidum hemagglutination test)
  - TPPA (T.pallidium particle agglutination test)
- Group specific : RP CFT (Reiter protein Complement fixation test) uses Reiter strain.
- Polymerase chain reaction

❑ **Treatment:** Penicillin is **drug of choice for all stages of syphilis** ***(option c)***. In penicillin allergy-Tetracycline can be given.

❑ ***Option b:*** **Jarisch-Herxheimer reaction:** A dramatic yet mild reaction consisting of fever, chills, myalgias, headache, tachycardia, increased respiratory rate, increased circulating neutrophil count, and vasodilation with mild hypotension may follow the initiation of treatment for syphilis. This reaction is thought to be a **response to lipoproteins released by dying T. pallidum organisms.**

JIPMER Pattern Based

1. After eating seafood patient has explosive diarrhea. Which is the organism causing it?

a. Shigella species
b. Vibrio parahaemolyticus
c. Vibrio vulnificus
d. Salmonella typhimurium

Ans. b. Vibrio parahaemolyticus. *Ref: Mandell's Infectious Diseases p1419*

EXPLANATION

❑ Vibrio parahaemolyticus
- Is a cause of sea food poisoning with onset of signs and symptoms in 9–28 hrs after ingestion of inadequately cooked fish/shellfish.
- Most commonly seen in U.S and Japan.
- Diarrhea may be explosive/watery/full blown dysentery with blood, pus and superficial ulceration on proctoscopic examination.
- Self –limiting illness (3–4 days).

❑ Etiology of food borne diseases

Etiology	Foods
Bacterial	
Salmonella	Beef, poultry, eggs, dairy products
Staphylococcus aureus	Ham, poultry and egg salads, pastries
Campylobacter jejuni	Poultry, raw milk
Clostridium botulinum	Home-canned vegetables, preserved fish, honey (infants)
Clostridium perfringens	Beef, poultry, gravy
Shigella	Egg salad, lettuce

Contd...

Contd...

Etiology	Foods
Vibrio parahaemolyticus	Shellfish
Bacillus cereus	Fried rice, meats, vegetables
Yersinia enterocolitica	Milk, pork, chitterlings
Vibrio cholerae O1	Shellfish
Vibrio cholerae non-O1	Shellfish
Shiga toxin–producing *Escherichia coli*	Ground beef, raw milk
Viral	
Noroviruses	Salads, shellfish
Histamine fish poisoning	Tuna, bonito, mahi-mahi
Mushroom poisoning	Mushrooms
Heavy metals	Acidic beverages
Paralytic shellfish poisoning	Shellfish
Neurotic shellfish poisoning	Shellfish

2. Swollen belly syndrome is caused by:

a. Strongyloides fuellebroni
b. Giardia lamblia
c. Capillaria philippinensis
d. A. duodenale

Ans. a. Strongyloides fuellreboni *Ref: Parija Textbook of Parasitology*

Explanation

- It is a parasite of monkey/apes.
- Zoonosis affecting humans in Asia/Africa.
- Seen in infants in Western Papua New Guinea.
- This syndrome is a life-threatening condition characterized by diarrhea, respiratory distress, edema.
- Protein losing enteropathy leading to hypoalbuminemia.
- Infection spreads from mother to infants by breastfeeding.
- Eggs are present in stools not larvae.
- Treatment is by thiabendazole.

3. A patient developed hemorrhagic blisters at the bite site following dog bite. Which is the most likely causative organism?

a. Pseudomonas spp.
b. *Staphylococcus aureus*
c. *Capnocytophaga canimorsus*
d. Pasteurella spp.

Ans. b. *Staphylococcus aureus* *Ref: Mandell's Infectious Diseases p2939, 2992*

Explanation

- Among animal bites, dog bites are most common, followed by cat bites.
- Approximately 15 to 20% of dog bite wounds and more than 50% of cat bite wounds become infected.

- For dog bite infections, *Staphylococcus aureus* and streptococcal species are the most commonly isolated pathogens, with Pasteurella and other organisms next in frequency.
- For cat bite infections, Pasteurella spp. are the most common pathogens.
- The zoonotic species *Capnocytophaga canimorsus* and *C. cynodegmi* are normal inhabitants of the oral cavity of dogs and cats. Zoonotic-associated infections arise via exogenous introduction of bacteria into wounds from penetrating traumas (dog bite) or by inapparent inoculation of bacilli into abraded surfaces or tissues via intimate contact with pets.

4. Bacillary angiomatosis caused by:

a. *Bartonella henselae*
b. *Bartonella quintana*
c. *Bartonella bacilliformis*
d. *Coxiella burnetii*

Ans. a. *Bartonella henselae* and b. *Bartonella quintana*

Ref: Essentials of Medical Microbiolgy by Dr. Apurba Sankar Sastry p395

Explanation

- **Both can cause:**
  - *B. henselae* causes hepatosplenic lesions.
  - *B. quintana* cause subcutaneous and lytic bony lesions.
  - In case question do not specify answer B. henselae.
- **Features of Bartonella species are given in the table below:**

Bartonella	Diseases	Reservoir	Transmission
B. henselae	Cat scratch disease Bacillary angiomatosis Bacillary peliosis Bacteremia Endocarditis	Cats, other felines	Exposure to cat bite/scratch
B. quintana	Trench fever Chronic bacteremia Endocarditis Bacillary angiomatosis	Humans	Louse (Pediculus humanus corporis)
B. baciliformis	Bartonellosis (Carrion's disease) Oroya fever Verruga peruana	Humans	Sandfly (Lutzomyia verrucarum)

5. Sputum microscopy of a patient reveals the structure of a fungus as large yeast cells, broad based budding and a thick wall. Identify the fungus.

a. *Histoplasma capsulatum*
b. *Blastomyces dermatitidis*
c. *Basidiomycetes*
d. *Candida albicans*

Ans. b. *Blastomyces dermatitidis*

Ref: Essentials of Medical Microbiolgy by Dr. Apurba Sankar Sastry p564

Explanation

- *Blastomyces dermatitidis*: It is a dimorphic fungi, which causes blastomycosis/North American blastomycosis/Gilchrist's disease/Chicago disease.
  - Acute pulmonary blastomycosis is **most common form**.

- In the yeast form, is seen as thick-walled, round yeast cells of 8–15 um size with single broad based budding (figure of 8 appearance).

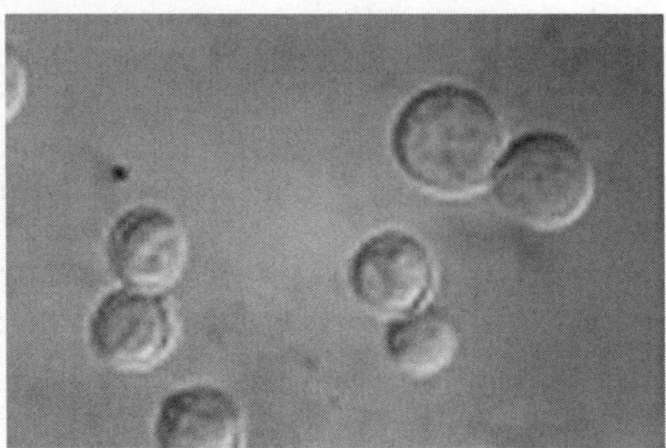

- *Histoplasma capsulatum*: It is a dimorphic fungus, which causes histoplasmosis.
  - Pulmonary histoplasmosis is most common form.
  - In the yeast form, it appears as oval yeast cells (2–4 um in size) with narrow based budding within the macrophages and underlying granulomatous response.

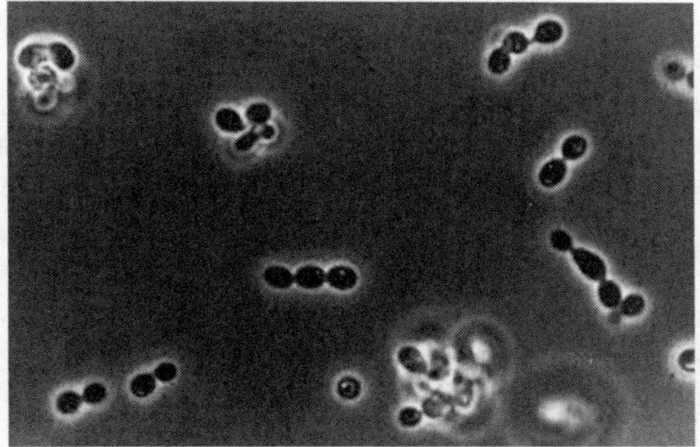

- *Candida albicans*: It is a yeast like fungus
  - It produces spectrum of infections ranging from skin and mucosal to invasive and allergic infections.
  - On gram stain they appear as oval budding yeast cells (4–6 um) with pseudohyphae.

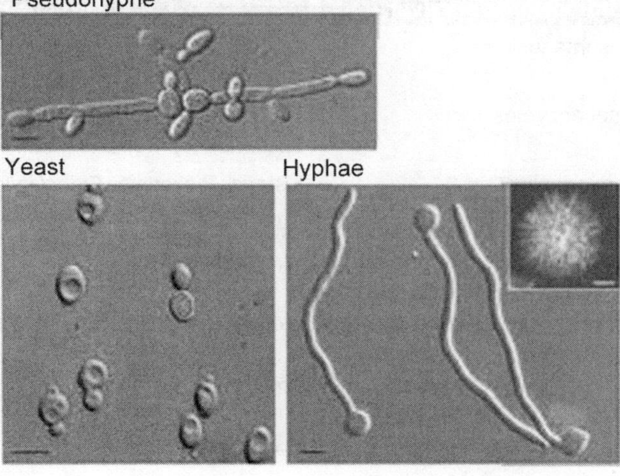

- **Basidiomycetes:** These includes members of phylum basidiomycota and they produce sexual spore—basidiospore.
  Cryptococcus sp e.g., which are detected by negative staining.

6. All the following organisms can cause arthritis *except*:

a. *Wuchereria bancrofti* b. *Echinococcus granulosus*
c. *Dracunculus medinensis* d. *Trichuris trichiura*

Ans. d. *Trichuris trichiura*

Ref: Paniker's Parasitology p210; Mandell's Infectious Diseases p3589; American College of Rheumatology, Arthritis and Rheumatism, Vol 38, September 1995, p1338-1339

EXPLANATION

- **Wuchereria bancrofti** causes lymphatic filariasis and occult filariasis.
  - Occult filariasis results due to hypersensitivity reaction to malarial antigen, classical features of lymphatic filariasis are absent.
  - C/F → Arthritis, massive eosinophilia, hepatosplenomegaly, cough, dyspnea, glomerulonephritis, thrombophlebitis, tenosynovitis (*Panikers Parasitology, p210*).
  - **Dracunculus medinensis** → It makes a painful papule that enlarges to form blister, local erythema, urticaria, fever, nausea, pruritius.
  - Complications: Sepsis, local abscess, pyogenic arthritis *(Mandell's infectious diseases p no. 3589).*
- Case study reveals a case of monoarthritis caused by **Echinococcus granulosus** (*American College of Rheumatology, Arthritis and Rheumatism, Vol 38, September 1995, p1338-1339*).

7. Mycobacterium tuberculosis escapes immunity by:

a. Inhibition of phagolysosome fusion b. Resistance to lysosomal enzymes
c. Adaptation to cytoplasmic replication
d. Prevents engulfment by macrophages through its capsule.

Ans. a. Inhibition of phagolysosome fusion

Ref: Essentials of Medical Microbiolgy by Dr. Apurba Sankar Sastry p92

EXPLANATION

- The following table gives mechanism used by various organisms for their intracellular survival

Mechanism of intracellular survival	Organism
Inhibition of phagolysosome fusion	Legionella species, *Mycobacterium tuberculosis*, Chlamydia species.
Resistance to lysosomal enzymes	*Salmonella typhimurium*, Coxiella species, *Mycobacterium leprae, Leishmania species.*
Adaptation to cytoplasmic replication	Listeria, Rickettsia, *Francisella tularensis.*

- Sequence of Pathogenic events of *M. tuberculosis*:
  Inhalation of infected droplet nuclei with *M. tuberculosis*

↓

Majority of bacteria are expelled out by mucosal ciliary cells

↓

<10% of small droplets reach alveoli

↓

Bacilli adheres to macrophages

↓

Internalization of bacilli

↓

Phagocytosis by macrophages

↓

Impairs phagosome lysosome fusion by inhibiting increase in intracellular calcium by phosphatidylinositol-3-phosphate

↓

Bacilli replicates inside macrophage

↓

Rupture of macrophage releasing bacillary contents infecting other phagocytes and cycle continues.

8. Plasmodium falciparum vaccine strain:

a. RTS, S/AS01

b. RTS, RS

c. Spf16

d. NYVAC-PF01

Ans. a. RTS, S/AS01 *Ref: Paniker Textbook of Parasitology p83*

EXPLANATION

Malarial vaccines

- Malarial vaccine is an area of intensive research.
- Several vaccines are under development, effective safe vaccine is still unavailable.
- **SpF66:** 1st vaccine developed that undergone field trial. It presents a combination of antigens from the sporozoite (using CS repeats) and merozoite parasites.
- **NYVAC-PF.7:** It blocks transmission of the parasite from vertebrate host to mosquitoes. Highly attenuated NYVAC vaccinia virus strain has been utilized to develop a multistage vaccine.
- **RTS, S/AS01:** Commercial name is mosquirix. It is most promising vaccine, engineered using genes from outer protein of P. falciparum and a portion of Hepatitis B virus, plus a chemical adjuvant to boost immune response.
  R → Circumsporozoite protein (repeats)
  T → T-cell epitopes
  S → HBsAg
  S → Genetically engineered transformed yeast strain.

9. Which contaminates disinfectants?

a. Staphylococcus species

b. Pseudomonas species

c. CONS

d. Shigella species

Ans. b. Pseudomonas species *Ref: Essentials of Medical Microbiolgy by Dr. Apurba Sankar Sastry p339*

EXPLANATION

- It is oxidase positive, pigment producing non-fermenting gram negative bacilli.
- A major pathogen among hospitalized patients and in patients with cystic fibrosis.
- Virulence factors:
  1. They colonize with the help of pili or fimbriae and polar flagellum.
  2. Toxin mediated immune evasion and tissue injury.
  3. Pigment production—Pyocyanin (blue green pigment of *P. aeruginosa*), fluorescein (or pyoverdin-greenish yellow color), pyorubin (red color), pyomelanin (brown-black color).

4. Alginate coat—Slimy layer that facilitates biofilm formation.
5. Capsule—Few strains have capsule which prevents phagocytosis.
6. Multidrug resistance to several antibiotics-leading to treatment failure.
7. Multi-disinfectant resistance-bacilli can grow in various disinfectants, thus spreading infection in hospitals.

Clinical manifestations: Ventilator-associated pneumonia, chronic respiratory tract infections, bacteremia, infective endocarditis, ear infections (swimmer's ear in children and malignant otitis externa in elderly diabetics), corneal ulcer, endophthalmitis, Shanghai fever (mild febrile illness resembling typhoid fever), skin infections in burns patient, ecthyma gangrenosum, dermatitis, green-nail syndrome, osteomyelitis, cellulitis, UTI, post-operative meningitis.

Lab diagnosis: (1) Sample-pus, urine, wound swab.

(2) Direct gram stain-gram negative bacilli with pus cells.

(3) Culture on bacterial media like nutrient agar, blood agar, MacConkey agar, selective media like Cetrimide agar.

(4) Biochemical reactions-catalase and oxidase positive,

ICUT: – + – K/K, gas (–), H_2S, OF test shows oxidative pattern (it's a non-fermenter).

Treatment: Piperacillin, mezlocillin, ticarcillin, ceftazidime, cefoperazone, cefepime, imipenem, aztreonam, tobramycin, amikacin, gentamicin, ciprofloxacin, polymyxin B, colistin.

10. Causative organism of Boggy swelling of hair:

a. Trichophyton mentagrophytes
b. E. flocosum
c. M. canis
d. T. concentricum

Ans. a. Trichophyton mentagrophytes

Ref: Essentials of Medical Microbiolgy by Dr. Apurba Sankar Sastry p555

Explanation

- DERMATOPHYTOSES (tinea or ringworm) is the most common superficial mycoses affecting skin, hair, nail caused by group of fungi called dermatophytes.
  - Trichophyton species: Infect skin, hair, nail.
  - Microsporum species: Infect skin and hair.
  - Epidermophyton species: Infect skin and nail.
- Depending on habitat, they are classified as follows:
  Anthropophilic: These fungal species exclusively affect humans.
  Zoophilic: They infect animals and birds.
  Geophilic: These fungal species are isolated from soil.
- Pathogenesis: Fungal spores are acquired by direct contact with soil, animals, humans infected
- In skin, they grow in centrifugal pattern in the stratum corneum forming characteristic annular or ring shaped pruritic lesions
- They invade hair shaft from within or from outside leading to alopecia:
- In nails, they invade through lateral or superficial nail plates.
- Clinical types of dermatophytoses:

Clinical types	Area involved
Tinea capitis (scalp infection): Scaly patches on scalp with broken hair. It is of following types:	
1. Kerion	Painful inflammatory reaction producing boggy lesions. Agent: Trichophyton verrucosum, Trichophyton mentagrophytes.
2. Favus	Cup like crust (scutula) around infected hair follicle. Agent: Trichophyton schoenleinii.

Contd...

Contd...

Clinical types	Area involved
3. Ectothrix	Arthrospores on the surface of hair shaft Agent: M. audouinii, M. canis, T. mentagrophytes.
4. Endothrix	Arthrospores formed within the hair, filling the hair shaft leading to alopecia. Agent: T. tonsurans and T. violaceum.
Tinea corporis	Infection of non-hairy skin of body (trunk and limbs)
Tinea pedis (athlete foot)	Infection of web space of foot later spreading to sole (moccasin pattern.)
Tinea cruris (jock itch)	Infection of groin area.
Tinea barbae	Infection of beard and moustache area of face.
Tinea faciei	Infection of non-bearded area of face.
Tinea imbricate	Concentric lesions of skin agent: T. concentricum
Tinea unguium	Infection of nail bed agent : T. mentagrophytes, E. floccosum
Tinea manuum	Infection of palmar aspect of hands.

- **Laboratory diagnosis:**
  1. Wood's lamp examination: Sample-skin scrapings, hair plucks, nail clippings.
  2. Direct examination: KOH mount using 10% from skin scrapings or 20–40% for nail clippings.
  3. Culture: on Sabouraud dextrose agar with cycloheximide. Macroscopic features like growth rate, texture, pigmentation- microscopic features appreciated by LPCB mount.
  4. Hair perforation test is positive for T. mentagrophytes and M. canis.
  5. Urease test positive for T. mentagrophytes.
  6. Molecular methods: PCR.
- **Treatment:** Oral terbinafine or itraconazole, whitfield ointment or tolnaftate.

11. Function of CRISPR is:

a. Bacterial genome editing mechanism to protect against virus infection
b. Phage infection protection by bacteria
c. Mechanism used by viruses to produce reassortants
d. Genotypic mixing seen in viruses for genetic reactivation

Ans. a. Bacterial genome editing mechanism to protect against virus infection

Ref: www.horizondiscovery.com

Explanation

- CRISPR is clustered regularly interspaced short palindromic repeats.
- It is one of the ancient naturally-occurring defence mechanism seen in wide range of bacteria.
- Scientists found out, that DNA sequence of bacterial genome has many repeated unique sequences, these unique sequences matched the DNA of viruses that attacked bacteria.
- CRISPR is part of bacteria's immune system, which keeps bits of dangerous viruses, so they recognize and defend against those viruses next time they attack.
- Cas (CRISPR-associated proteins) is second part of defense mechanism, which snips DNA and slice the DNA of invading viruses.
- Genes of Cas are always placed near CRISPR sequences.
- Number of Cas enzymes are present, best known is Cas9. Its from *Streptococcus pyogenes*.

12. Hepatitis C virus high efficacy testing in blood bank is by:

a. NS1
b. NS2
c. NS3
d. E1

Ans. c. NS3 *Ref: Essentials of Medical Microbiolgy by Dr. Apurba Sankar Sastry p536*

Explanation

- Hepatitis C virus: **Most common cause of Post-transfusion hepatitis in developing countries.**
- Morphology: +ve sense ssRNA and proteins (3 structural proteins like core protein, E1 and E2 glycoproteins; 6 non-structural proteins like NS1, NS2, NS3, NS4A, NS4B, NS5A, NS5B).
- **Genetic diversity**:
  - Higher rate of mutation seen in E2 envelope protein >NS5B.
  - E2 is target against most neutralizing antibodies, genetic diversity of E2 results in mutant strains escaping body's immunity.
  - HCV genotypes:
    - Genotype 1 is **most common type worldwide**
    - Genotype 4 seen in Egypt
    - Genotype 5 seen in South Africa
    - Genotype 6 seen in Hong Kong
    - Genotype 1 and 3 **common in India.**
- **Transmission:**
  - Parenteral (blood transfusion, blood products, organ transplantation, injection drug users, contaminated needles and sharps)
  - Vertical (from mother to fetus < lower rate (6%) than HBV (20%)
  - Sexual (rare)
  - **It doesn't spread by breast feeding/food/casual contacts of hugging, shaking hands.**

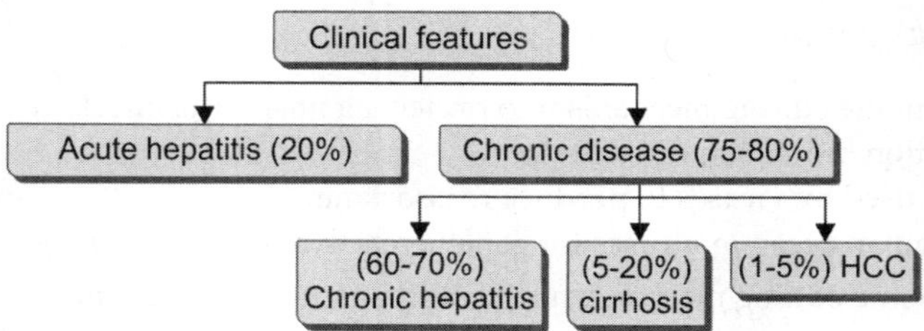

  - Extrahepatic: mixed cryoglobulinemia, arthritis, glomerulonephritis.
- **Epidemiology**:
  - Worldwide infections every year 3–4 million people, are infected with HCV with more than 3.5 lakhs deaths.
  - Prevalence rate: India (1%)
  - Africa (10%) > South America, Asia > World (3%).
- Laboratory diagnosis.

Serum antibody detection	Antigen detection
• Anti-HCV antibodies are detected by Third-generation ELISAs using Core antigens, NS3, NS4, NS5 to detect anti-HCV antibodies	• Hepatitis C virus RNA is most sensitive and **gold standard test.**

Contd...

Contd...

• **Acute diagnosis:** Anti-HCV (C33c, C22-3, NS5) are detected.	• Branched-chain DNA (bDNA) assay
• **Chronic diagnosis:** Anti-HCV (C100-3, C33c, C22-3, NS5) are elevated.	• Reverse transcriptase PCR
	• Real time RTPCR
	• Transcription mediated Amplification (TMA).

- **Treatment:**
  - Combined therapy with pegylated interferon plus ribavirin.
  - Start treatment within 2–3 months after onset of disease and continued till 24 weeks.

13. Resistance in bacteria is by:

a. Transposon
b. Plasmid
c. Transduction
d. All of the above

Ans. d. All of the above

Ref: Essentials of Medical Microbiolgy by Dr. Apurba Sankar Sastry p67

Explanation

- Plasmid
  - They are extrachromosomal ds circular DNA molecules that exist in free state in the cytoplasm of bacteria, and also found in some yeasts.
  - Plasmids are not essential for life.
  - They can be present singly or in multiple numbers up to 40 plasmids per cell.
  - They are capable of independent replication.
  - **Episome**: Plasmids integrating with chromosomal DNA of bacteria.
  - **Curing**: The process of eliminating the plasmids from bacteria. It can be spontaneous or induced by acridine, radiations, thymine starvations, growth at higher temperature.
  - **Classification of plasmids**:

1. **On ability to perform conjugation**
   - Conjugative plasmids
   - Non-conjugative plasmids.
2. **On compatibility between plasmids**
   - Compatible plasmids
   - Incompatible plasmids
3. **On function**
   - *Fertility or F-plasmids:* Help in bacterial conjugation by forming the conjugation tube.
   - *Resistance plasmids:* They code for resistance genes to various antibiotics.
   - *Col plasmids:* They code for bacteriocins.
   - *Virulence plasmids:* They code for virulence factors and toxins.
   - Metabolic plasmids.

- Plasmids are also vectors in genetic engineering.
  - Transposons
    - Also called as jumping genes or mobile genetic elements.

  - Transposons or transposable elements are bacterial genes that are capable of intracellular transfer between chromosome to chromosome, plasmid to plasmid, and chromosome to plasmid or vice versa.
  - Transposons were first discovered by Barbara McClintock during her maize studies in 1940s and she was awarded noble prize in 1983.
- Transduction
  - Transmission of bacteriophages from one bacterium to another, a part of host DNA may accidentally get incorporated into bacteriophage and then gets transferred to recipient bacterium.
  - Two types of life-cycle: (a) lytic or virulent cycle (b) lysogenic or temperate cycle.
  - Transduction transfers bacterial genes coding for drug resistance, e.g. plasmid coded penicillin resistance in staphylococci.

Forensic Medicine and Toxicology

Author: Bahram Gor, Co-author: Krishna Kumar Singh

AIIMS May 2017

1. Which of the following is correct regarding corporobasal index of sacrum?

a. Breadth of first sacral vertebra × 100/breadth of fifth lumbar vertebra
b. Breadth of fifth lumbar vertebra × 100/breadth of all sacral vertebra
c. Breadth of first sacral vertebra × 100/breadth of base of sacrum
d. Breadth of fifth lumbar vertebra × 100/breadth of base of sacrum

Ans. c. Breadth of first sacral vertebra × 100/breadth of base of sacrum

Ref: Biswas - Review of Forensic Medicine and Toxicology, 2nd/ed p54-55; The Essentials of Forensic Medicine and Toxicology, 33rd/ed p62-64; and Spitz and Fisher's, Medicolegal Investigation of Death, 4th/ed p245

EXPLANATION

Various indexes helpful in determining sex:

S. No.	Index	Formula	Values	
			Male	Female
1.	Ischiopubic index	**Pubic length in mm** × 100 Ischial length in mm	73–94	91–115
2.	Sciatic notch index	**Width of sciatic notch** × 100 Depth of sciatic notch	4–5	5–6
3.	Corporobasal index	**Breadth of first sacral vertebra** × 100 Breadth of base of sacrum ***(Answer)***	45	40.5
4.	Sternal index	**Length of manubrium** × 100 Length of body	46.2	54.3
5.	Sacral index	**Transverse diameter of base of sacrum** × 100 Anterior length of sacrum	<114	>114

- ❑ Out of these five, only corporobasal index is more in females compared to males, other index values are more in male.
- ❑ Sciatic notch index is most reliable criteria to determine sex within pelvis.
- ❑ Some more index with lesser importance:
  - Kimura's Base-wing index = $\frac{\text{Width of wing (ala of sacrum)}}{\text{Width of base (transverse diameter of body of S1)}} \times 100$
  - Chilotic line index = $\frac{\text{Sacral part of chilotic line}}{\text{Pelvic part of the chilotic line}} \times 100$

- "Chilotic line: It is an anthropometric line extending from the posterior aspect of the iliopectineal eminence to the closest point on the anterior auricular margin (the pelvic segment) and then to the iliac crest (the sacral portion). Since the pelvic segment is predominant in males, the chilotic index may be used to identify the sex of human skeletal remains."

2. Which of the following is false regarding teeth features and ethnicity?

a. In negroes the teeth are broad and extra cusps
b. Caucasians have Carabelli's cusp on labial surface of mandibular molar
c. Shovel shaped incisors in Mongoloids
d. Absent upper 3rd molar in Mongoloids

Ans. b. Caucasians have Carabelli's cusp on labial surface of mandibular molar

Ref: Biswas - Review of Forensic Medicine and Toxicology, 2nd/ed p58; and Spitz and Fisher's Medicolegal Investigation of Death, 4th/ed p261

Explanation

Teeth features typical to Mongoloids:

- **Bull tooth (Taurodontism):** Taurodontism is an abrasion of teeth that lacks the constriction at the level of the cementoenamel junction characterized by elongated pulp chambers and apical displacement of bifurcation or trifurcation of the roots, giving it a rectangular shape. The term means 'bull-like' teeth derived from similarity of these teeth to those of cud chewing animals.
- Congenital lack of upper third molars ***(option d)***
- Enamel pearls on premolars
- Pointed canines
- Shovel shaped incisors (classical feature) ***(option c)***.

Teeth features typical to Negroids:

- Teeth are broad ***(option a)***
- Presence of fourth molar
- Maxillary and mandibular diastemas.

Teeth features typical to Caucasians:

- ***Carabelli's tubercle (Option b)*** is an anomalous cusp on the mesial palatal surface of the upper first permanent molars, most commonly seen among Europeans (75–85%) (50% of American whites and 34% of Afro-Americans).

3. An adult came to casualty with complaints of palpitation, high pulse rate and angina like pain. On examination everything was normal except for episodic tachycardia with occasional extrasystole and amblyopia. Most likely cause is:

a. Chronic nicotine poisoning
b. Cannabis intoxication
c. Odynophagia
d. Cocainism

Ans. a. Chronic nicotine poisoning

Ref: Poisoning & Drug Overdose 5th/ed; and Biswas - Review of Forensic Medicine; and Toxicology, 2nd/ed p436,499,501,508

Explanation

Clinical Features of nicotine poisoning

- Nicotine binds to nicotinic cholinergic receptors, resulting initially, via actions on ganglia, in predominantly sympathetic nervous stimulation.

- With higher doses, parasympathetic stimulation and then ganglionic and neuromuscular blockage may occur. Direct effects on the brain may also result in vomiting and seizures.

Acute poisoning

- **CVS:** Tachycardia followed by bradycardia, hypotension, arrhythmia, tachypnea followed by respiratory depression and collapse.
- **GI:** Burning acid sensation, nausea, vomiting, abdominal pain, salivation.
- **CNS:** Headache, restlessness, confusion, vertigo, sweating, convulsions and coma.

Chronic poisoning

- **Respiratory:** Cough, wheeze, dyspnea, chronic bronchitis and lung cancer may develop.
- **CVS:** Anemia, **palpitations, irregularity of heart, angina pectoris** and Berger's disease.
- **GI:** Anorexia, vomiting and diarrhea.
- **CNS:** Impaired memory, **blindness**, tremors, insomnia, anxiety and headache.

Fatal dose

- Nicotine: 60–100 mg
- Tobacco: 15–30 g

  Fatal period: 5-15 min

***Option b:* Clinical features of cannabis poisoning**

Onset of symptoms occurs within a few minutes of smoking or within half hour of oral ingestion. The duration of action is usually 6–12 hours; symptoms are most marked in the first 1–2 h.

I. Stage of excitement

- Feeling of euphoria, detachment, well-being grandiosity, dreaminess, subjective sense of slowing of the passage of time, increased self-confidence, rapidly changing emotions, talkativeness and laughing.
- Impairment of thinking and short-term memory, decreased concentration, disorientation, illusions, visual hallucinations, altered sexual feelings, impaired judgment, and perceptual and psychomotor dysfunctions resulting in impaired driving and motor vehicle accidents.
- Increased appetite (the '*munchies*') and thirst, nausea, headache, conjunctival injection, dizziness, dry mouth, slurred speech, orthostatic hypotension, tachycardia and increased urinary frequency.

II. Stage of narcosis

- Giddiness, incoordination, confusion, ataxia and paresthesias.
- The person passes into deep sleep and wakes up without depression/nausea/hangover.
- Rarely, drowsiness may be followed by coma, collapse and death.
- **Fatal dose**
  - Bhang: 10 g/kg body wt
  - Charas: 2 g
  - Ganja: 8 g
- **Fatal period:** About 12 h

***Option c:* Clinical features of arsenic poisoning:**

Some people take arsenic daily as a tonic or as aphrodisiac and they acquire tolerance to 250–300 mg or more in one dose. Such people are known as ***arsenophagists.***

Chronic poisoning features:

- **GIT:** Nausea, vomiting, abdominal cramps, loss of appetite, diarrhea, salivation.
- **Ocular:** Congestion, watering of the eyes, photophobia.
- **RS:** Cough, hoarseness of voice, bronchial catarrh, hemoptysis, dyspnea.
- **Skin and nails:** There may be a rash resembling fading measles rash. Speckled brown pigmentation, mostly on the skin flexures, temples, shoulders, eyelids and neck (**raindrop appearances** with patches of leukoplakia). Hyperkeratosis of the palms and soles with irregular thickening of the nails and development of white bands of opacity in the nails of fingers and toes (called **Aldrich-Mees' lines**). Brittle nails and alopecia are also seen.

- **CNS:** Tingling, numbness of hands and feet, polyneuritis, anesthesia, paraesthesia with painful swelling *(erythromelalgia)*, encephalopathy. Neuritis resembles chronic alcoholism.
- **CVS:** Cardiac failure, dependent edema.
- **Renal:** Chronic nephritis.
- **Hepatic:** Hepatomegaly, jaundice, cirrhosis of the liver.
- **Hematologic:** Bone marrow suppression, hypoplasia, anemia, thrombocytopenia and leukemia.

Fatal dose: 120–200 mg of arsenic trioxide (adults), 2 mg/kg (children).

Fatal period: 1–2 days.

Option d: **Clinical features of cocaine poisoning:**

Signs and symptoms of acute poisoning include elevated pulse, blood pressure, respiration and temperature. Onset occurs within **7 s** after inhalation, **15 s** after taking iv, **3 mins** after nasal insufflation and **10 mins** after oral ingestion. **(Potential question zone: asked in SR July 2017 session)**

I. **Stage of excitement**
- **Local:** Feeling of numbness or tingling at the place of application.
- **Face:** Flushed.
- **Skin:** Pale.
- **GIT:** Bitter taste, dryness of mouth, vomiting, diarrhea, hyperactive bowel sounds
- **CNS:** Feeling of well-being, euphoria, restlessness, excitement, talkativeness, delirium, maniacal, hallucinations, tremors (e.g. twitching of small muscles, especially facial and finger) and tonic-clonic seizures. Reflexes are exaggerated.
- **RS:** Tachypnea, dyspnea, cyanosis.
- **CVS:** Tachycardia, hypertension, ventricular arrhythmias, hyperthermia.
- **Ocular:** Pupils are dilated resulting in blurred vision.

II. **Stage of depression**
- After an hour, respiration becomes slow, there is profuse sweating, and patient becomes calm and dull.
- **Fatal dose:** 20 mg IV; 500 mg to 1.4 g orally.
- **Fatal period:** Few minutes to 1–2 h.

4. A young adult visited casualty with H/O some substance abuse. His pulse was 130 bpm, respiratory rate 30/min, blood gas analysis revealed metabolic acidosis, hypocalcemia and electrolyte imbalance. Blood urea was 100 mg/dL, creatinine 3.4 mg/dL. Urine analysis showed calcium oxalate crystals. He improved on gastric lavage, ethanol, sodium bicarbonate, calcium gluconate and 4-methylpyrazole. What is the substance he consumed?

a. Ethylene glycol
b. Methyl alcohol
c. Formaldehyde
d. Paraldehyde

Ans. a. Ethylene glycol

Ref: Biswas - Review of Forensic Medicine and Toxicology, 2nd/ed p488,490; The Essentials of Forensic Medicine and Toxicology, 33rd/ed p582-583

EXPLANATION

Ethylene glycol poisoning

- **CNS:** Usually develop within half hour to 12 h after ingestion. The individual develops nausea, vomiting, slurred speech, tipsy sensation, severe headache, delusions, dizziness, feeling of breathlessness, convulsions and coma.
- **CVS:** Usually appear 12–24 h after ingestion. Tachycardia, tachypnea and congestive heart failure are present.

- **Renal:** Acute tubular necrosis. This usually is seen 24–72 h after ingestion. **Oxalate crystals** are seen in the urine.

  Oxalate crystals are the crux here in the question.

Methyl alcohol poisoning

- **GIT:** Nausea, vomiting, cramps in abdomen, spirit like odor in the nostrils and mouth, dehydration.
- **RS:** Dyspnea, cyanosis, respiratory depression.
- **CNS:** Headache, dizziness, vertigo, restlessness, muscular weakness, hypothermia, delirium, amnesia, convulsion (terminal event), coma.
- **Renal:** Strongly acidic urine, acidosis, scant urine.
- **Ocular:** Pupils—Fixed and dilated. Visual disturbances, like photophobia, blurred or misty vision *(snowfield vision)*, central or peripheral scotoma, decreased light perception, concentric diminution of visual fields causing temporary or complete blindness due to optic neuritis and atrophy from accumulation of formic acid within the optic nerve. Retinal edema and hyperemia may be seen.
- **Pancreas:** Pancreatitis may occur.

5. Death in Jack-knife position is due to:

a. Burking
b. Positional asphyxia
c. Traumatic asphyxia
d. Wedging

Ans. b. Positional asphyxia *Ref: Knight's Forensic Pathology 3rd/ed p365*

EXPLANATION

- **Positional asphyxia:** Persons who have been trapped upside down or even only in a 'jack-knife' position, with the upper half of their body bent acutely downwards from the waist, may have such impairment of their respiratory movements that they become hypoxic and suffer marked disturbance of their circulatory system, especially the venous return to the heart. Seen in drunkenness and other disability.

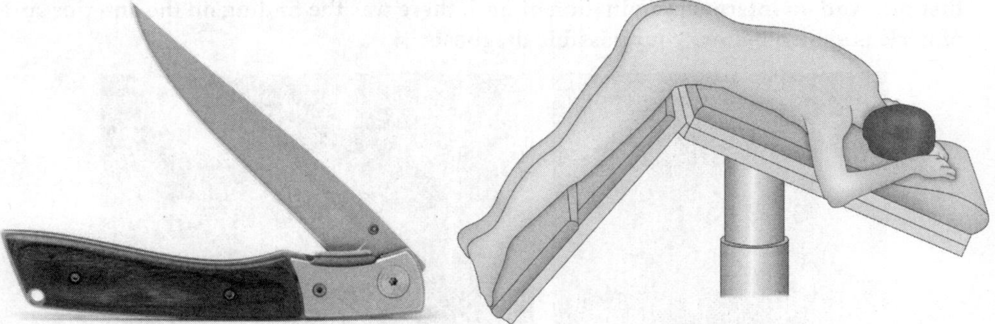

- **Suffocation**

  Definition: It is a form of asphyxia caused by mechanical obstruction to the passage of air into the respiratory tract *by means other than constriction of neck or drowning.*

Classification

i. Smothering	ii. Choking	iii. Gagging
iv. Overlying	v. Traumatic asphyxia	vi. Burking

- *(Option A)* **Burking:** A combination of homicidal smothering and traumatic asphyxia.
  Method: Usually done by two persons. One used to kneel or sit on the chest and close the nose and mouth of the victim with his hands, and other one used to pull him around the room by the feet.

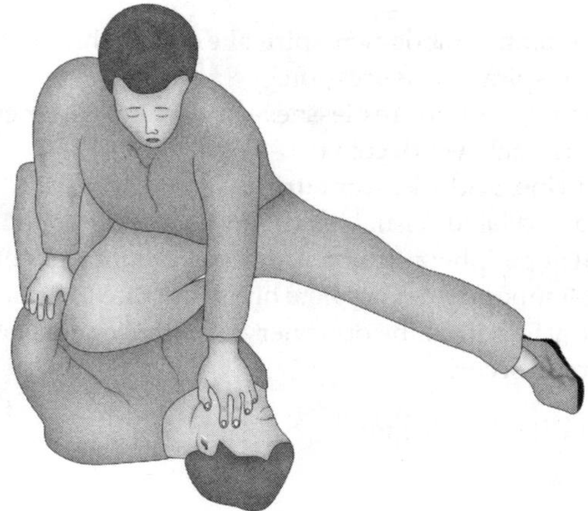

- *(Option d)* **Wedging:** It is a form of mechanical asphyxia in which the face, neck or thorax is compressed between two firm structures. It is common in 3–6 months old children when they start to move to the corners of beds and cribs, but they do not have the muscle development to free themselves out of a wedged position. They become wedged between the mattress and either the wall, bed frame, a piece of furniture, mesh or another mattress.
- *(Option c)* **Traumatic asphyxia:** Asphyxia resulting from respiratory arrest due to mechanical fixation of chest, so that the normal movements of chest wall are prevented. For instance, house collapse, accidentally or in wars/earthquake, stampede by crowd.

6. A person was brought to the casualty brought dead and autopsy was performed to find the cause of death. On external examination only finding found was a mark on the chin as in first pic. And on internal examination of neck there was the finding on the anterior surface of neck as shown below. Your possible diagnosis is:

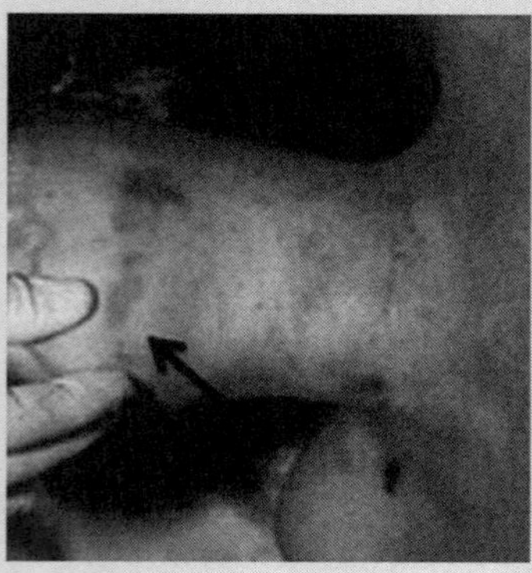

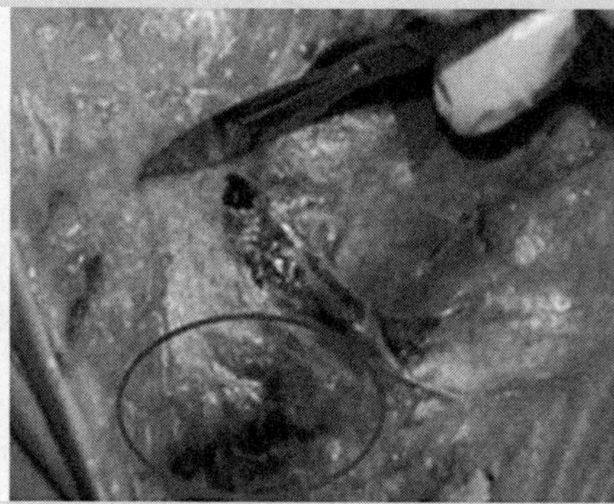

a. Throttling
b. Hanging
c. Smothering
d. Ligature strangulation

Ans. a. Throttling *Ref: Biswas - Review of Forensic Medicine and Toxicology, 2nd/ed p148-151; Knight's Forensic Pathology 3rd/ed p353*

Explanation

- As shown in first figure, there is extensive bruise over neck, especially below chin, left angle of mandible, lower part of anterior neck and shoulder. Fingernail abrasions are seen below chin (both suggestive of throttling as these are absent in smothering). These features may be present in ligature strangulation but will present with a ligature mark. Very rare in hanging (if victim itself tries to take out the noose as a fear of death after action of hanging).
- In second figure, neck muscle bruising (hematoma) suggest it to be either ligature strangulation or throttling but as external features are corroborative of throttling, it is a sure shot case of throttling.

External findings

- **Throttling** refers to strangulation, usually by hand, the word rarely being applied to ligature strangulation.
- Bruises made by tips of thumbs are more prominent than with other fingers.
- Multiple curvilinear abrasions on the neck may also result from use of victim's hands in an effort to dislodge the assailant's grip.
- If these are from the assailant, they are usually vertical.

Internal findings

- Extravasation of blood in subcutaneous tissues underneath the external marks of bruising and abrasions is the *most significant internal sign.*
- Tear/laceration of platysma or sternomastoid muscles may be seen.
- Hemorrhages, varying from pinpoint ecchymosis to extensive extravasation may be found in mucous membrane of larynx, epiglottis, pharynx, and peritonsillar region.
- Inward compression fracture of hyoid bone is the **most diagnostic finding of throttling (Potential question zone).**

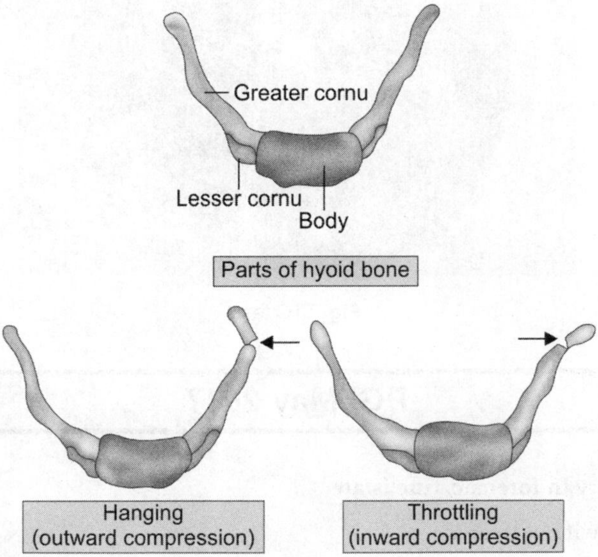

7. On staining with triphenyltetrazolium, while performing autopsy of a patient who died of 'Myocardial infarction', the color of normal viable part of heart will be:

a. White
b. Red
c. Blue
d. Dark brown

Ans. b. Red *Ref: The Essentials of Forensic Medicine and Toxicology, 33rd/ed p146; Knight's Forensic Pathology 4rd/ed p531*

EXPLANATION

- ❑ Immersion of tissue slices in a solution of triphenyl tetrazolium chloride (TTC) gives brick red color to intact areas (where dehydrogenase enzymes are preserved).
- ❑ Infarcted areas appear pale.
- ❑ This is seen in about 4 hours.
- ❑ Results are variable.

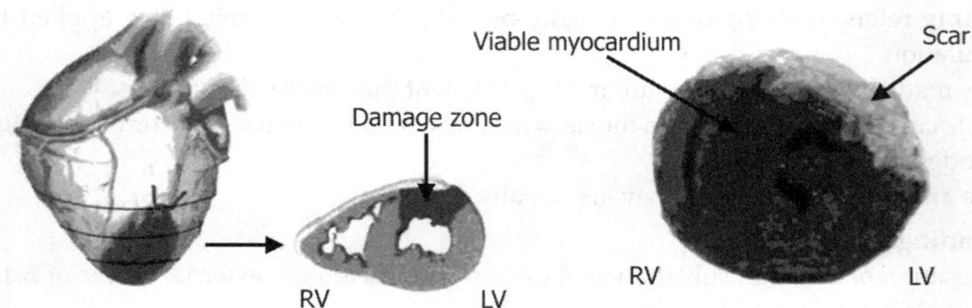

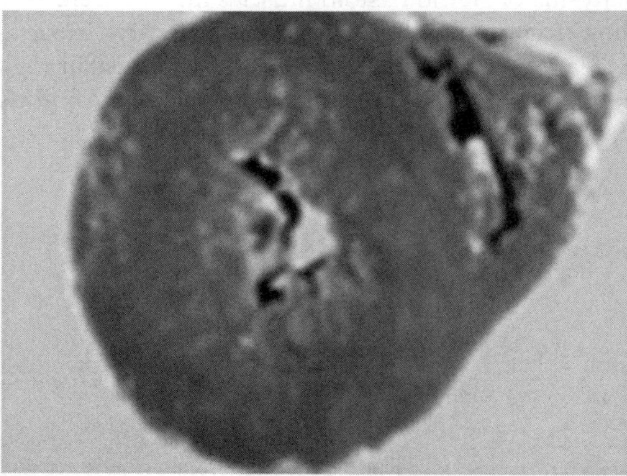

Fig. TTC test.

PGI May 2017

1. Dangerous injury in forensic, true is/are:

a. Endangers life if not treated
b. Grievous injury
c. Emasculation
d. Tooth loss/loosening

Ans. a. Endangers life if not treated

Ref: The Essentials of Forensic Medicine and Toxicology, 33rd/ed p293; and Biswas - Review of Forensic Medicine and Toxicology, 2nd/ed p265

EXPLANATION

Dangerous injuries are those which cause imminent danger to life by its direct or imminent effects because of being extensive in nature, involving important structures or organs of the body and also being likely to prove fatal in absence of medical/surgical aid.

Injuries sufficient to cause death in ordinary course of nature, examples of dangerous injury are:

i. Injuries to the brain (intracranial hemorrhages) and spinal cord.
ii. Injuries to heart or large blood vessels.
iii. Injuries to respiratory organs.
iv. Injuries involving GIT, e.g. rupture of liver, spleen, perforation of intestines, etc.
v. Injuries (wounds) to highly vascular organs, like liver/spleen.
vi. Extensive burns or scalds (affecting > 1/3rd of the body surface area).
vii. Combined effect of number of injuries, none of which by itself may be sufficient to cause death, but together may cause it.
viii. Squeezing of testes (Not emasculation **option c**).

- The term 'endangers life' is much broader term than the expression 'dangerous to life'. **All dangerous injuries can endanger life**, but not vice-versa.
- An injury caused on a vital part of the body cannot be called as grievous hurt, unless the nature and dimensions of the injury or its effects are such that the doctor is of the opinion that it actually endangers the life of the victim (**option b**).
- Mere looseness of teeth will not amount to dislocation by the injury. Fracture or dislocation of a bone or a tooth causes great pain and suffering to the injured person and is considered as grievous hurt but still not a dangerous injury (**option d**).

2. Dying declaration true is/are:

a. Doctor cannot record dying declaration, if police person is not present
b. Police or magistrate can record it
c. If incomplete then it is invalid
d. Given to magistrate only

Ans. b. Police or magistrate can record it

Ref: The Essentials of Forensic Medicine and Toxicology, 33rd/ed p10
Biswas - Review of Forensic Medicine and Toxicology, 2nd/ed p39

Definition of dying declaration: It is a written or oral statement of a person, who is dying as a result of some unlawful act, relating to the material facts of the cause of death or the circumstances surrounding it.

Procedure:

❑ The doctor should certify that the person is conscious and his mental faculties are normal **(Compos mentis)**.
❑ Oath is not administered because of the belief that a dying person tells the truth.
❑ *No leading questions* are asked.
❑ Who can record the 'dying declaration' ***(Clarifies option a, b and d)***?
  - Ideally, a **Magistrate** should be called to record the declaration.
  - When death is imminent, the statement may be recorded, in the presence of two witnesses, by the **doctor or the police officer** without losing time in waiting for the Magistrate ***(option a)***.
  - The declaration can be made to a **police officer, public servant, village headman or a private person,** but its evidential value will be less ***(Option b)***.

- While recording the statement, if the declarant becomes unconscious, the person recording it must record as much information as he has obtained and sign it himself. It will be still valid and admissible in court ***(option c)***.
- If the declarant survives, the declaration is not admitted, but has *corroborative value,* and the person is called to give oral evidence.

JIPMER Pattern Based

1. All of the following is true about kevorkian sign *except*:

a. Persist even after 3 years of death
b. Appear within minutes of death
c. Visualized using ophthalmoscope
d. Cattle tracking sign

Ans. a. Persist even after 3 years of death

Ref: The Essentials of Forensic Medicine and Toxicology, 33rd/ed p154; and Biswas - Review of Forensic Medicine and Toxicology, 2nd/ed p118

Explanations

Changes in eyes (molecular death)

- Loss of corneal and pupillary reflexes.
- Shape of the pupils of both the side may differ.
- Opacity of the cornea: The cornea becomes permanently hazy after about 10–12 h of death due to decomposition.
- **Tache noire:** If the eyelids remain open for 3-4 h after death, there is formation of two yellow triangles (base on the limbus, apex at the lateral or medial canthus and sides are formed by the margins of the upper and lower eyelids) on the sclera at each side of the iris, which become brown and then black.
- **Loss of intraocular tension:** Intraocular tension falls rapidly after death. It becomes zero in 4–8 h from 10–22 mm Hg during life **(Potential question zone)**.
- **Changes in the retina:** The blood in retinal vessels appears fragmented or segmented (cattle tracking or shunting) ***(option d)*** within seconds to minutes after death ***(option b)***, and persists for about an hour (Kevorkian sign).This occurs all over the body due to loss of blood pressure, but it can be seen only in retina by an ophthalmoscope ***(option c)***.

2. The brick red color of postmortem lividity is seen in poisoning due to:

a. Carbon monoxide
b. Hydrogen sulfide
c. Phosphorus
d. Cyanide

Ans. d. Cyanide

Ref: The Essentials of Forensic Medicine and Toxicology, 33rd/ed p159

Explanation

Cause	Color
CO	Cherry red
Cyanide/hydrocyanic acid	Bright red/brick red
Nitrites, Potassium chlorate, Potassium bicarbonate, Nitrobenzene	Chocolate/copper brown
Phosphorus	Yellow/dark brown
Hydrogen sulfide	Bluish green

3. Lichtenberg figures are seen in:

a. Heat stroke
b. Radiation injury
c. Lightning
d. Electrocution

Ans. c. Lightning *Ref: The Essentials of Forensic Medicine and Toxicology, 33rd/ed p334; and Knight's Forensic Pathology 3rd/ed p336*

EXPLANATION

Lightning stroke

- The physical damage in fatal cases can vary from virtually nil to gross burning, fractures and tissue destruction. Cutaneous marks may be present, the well-known **'fern-like' or 'arboresque' pattern**, also referred to as **'Lichtenberg' figures** (because of their similarity to the pattern described by a German physicist, Georg Christoph Lichtenberg, in 1777 AD) being much less common than the standard texts suggest.
- Also known as **Arborescent or Filigree burn.**
- It appears within minutes to one hour of accident.
- Irregular red marks, often linear first-degree burns, may follow skin creases, especially if damp from sweating.
- These marks may be many inches long and generally follow the long axis of the body toward the ground.
- Frank blistered or charred burns are also present in some cases.

4. A 22-year-old was brought after consuming herbicide containing paraquat, features include all *except*:

a. Diarrhea
b. Hyperreflexia
c. Fast heart rate
d. Confusion

Ans. b. Hyperreflexia *Ref: VV Pillay - Modern Medical Toxicology, 4th/ed p398; The Essentials of Forensic Medicine and Toxicology, 33rd/ed p526*

EXPLANATION

Paraquat

Paraquat and diquat are widely used herbicides which belong to the bipyridine group available under the trade name, 'Gramoxone' and 'Weedol'.

Action:

Paraquat undergoes a NADPH dependent reduction to form a free radical which acts with molecular oxygen to reform the cation to produce superoxide free radicals and hydroxyl radical (OH) which disrupt cellular function leading to cell death.

Systemic features:

- **Local:** Irritation and inflammation of skin, cornea, conjunctiva and nasal mucosa.
- **GIT:** Ulceration and corrosion of mouth, oropharynx, and esophagus; nausea, vomiting, hematemesis, **diarrhea**, dysphagia.
- **RS:** Cough, hemoptysis, dyspnea due to pulmonary edema, aphonia, aspiration.
- **Renal:** Oliguria, renal failure.
- **CVS:** Hypovolemia, shock, **arrhythmias**.
- **Hepatic:** Cholestasis.
- **CNS: Confusion**, convulsions, cerebral edema, coma.

Orthopedics

Author: Bahram Gor, Co-author: Naveen Kumar A

AIIMS May 2017

1. A patient presented with fracture of femur. On 3rd day of admission he developed sudden breathlessness. Which of the following is the most common cause?

a. Pulmonary hypertension
b. Post-trauma MI
c. Fat embolism
d. Hypovolemic shock

Ans. c. Fat embolism *Ref: Maheshwari 3rd/ed p34, Ebnezer 4th/ed p30*

EXPLANATION

Given history of fracture and presentation on 3rd day favor the diagnosis of fat embolism. This is most often tested topic—see details below.

- ❑ *"Fat embolism is a dreaded complication occurring* ***within 72 hours*** *of skeletal trauma".* –Ebnezer
- ❑ *"Fat embolism is one of the most serious complications, the essential feature being occlusion of small vessels by fat globules. Symptoms are evident a day or so after the injury".* –Maheshwari
- ❑ ***Option d:*** Shock- presents as early complication within hours after injury with features of sunken eyeballs, tongue—pale and dry, pale look, low BP, cold clammy skin, cold nose, peripheral pulses feeble or absent, drowsy or unconscious.
- ❑ ***Option b:*** Post-trauma MI—patient will have symptoms of MI like chest pain, sweating. Even though this can be kept as d/d in this case but not more common than fat embolism.

FAT EMBOLISM REVIEW

- ❑ It is a dreaded complication often associated with multiple fractures, major bone fractures (10–45%) occuring within 72 hours of trauma.
- ❑ Pathogenesis: Release of marrow fat into circulation causing:
  - ▪ Obstruction of vessels (obstructive theory) or
  - ▪ Induces a toxic vasculitis, followed by platelet-fibrin thrombosis (toxic theory)
- ❑ Clinical features (C/F):
  a. Cerebral
  b. Pulmonary
  c. Petechial rashes: [occurs in axilla, chest, and conjuctiva/fleeting type/fades rapidly/retinal rashes are pathognomic, diagnosed by fundoscopy]
- ❑ Diagnostic criteria—Gurd's criteria
  - ▪ 1 Major criteria:
    - Axillary and subconjunctival petechiae,
    - $PaO_2 < 60$ mm Hg
    - CNS depression.
  - ▪ 4 Minor criteria:
    - Pulse > 110/min
    - Pyrexia >38.5°C
    - Retinal embolism

- Fat in urine
- Reduced platelet count
- Increased erythrocyte sedimentation rate (ESR)
- Fat globules in sputum

❑ Chest X-ray:
  ▪ Snowstorm appearance (pathognomic)

❑ ECG—prominent S wave

❑ Treatment
  ▪ Respiratory support, steroids (anti-inflammatory), heparin (anti-platelet), low molecular wt dextran, intravenous alchohol, antibiotics.

2. In the given picture which movement of Hip is tested?

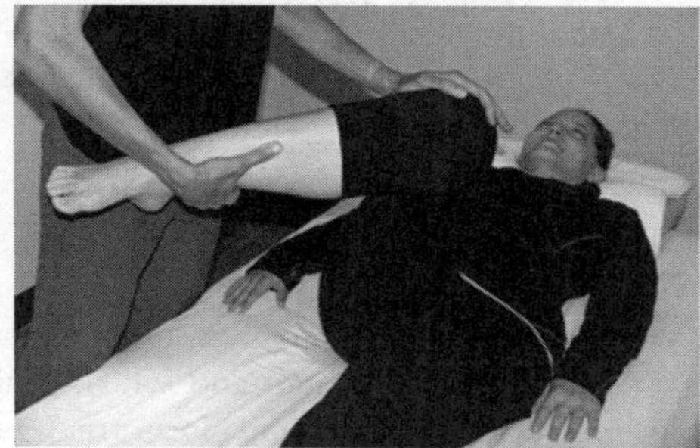

a. Abduction
b. Adduction
c. Internal rotation
d. External rotation

Ans. c. Internal rotation *Ref: 2nd edition Bruce Reider, AB, MD, p183*

EXPLANATION

In the given picture as the hip and knee are flexed and leg is moved from the body there will be internal rotation movement in the hip. This question is even though easy one but little tricky. So don't be in hurry to answer. Best way to answer such questions is to imagine yourself in patient position and imagine your hip position.

In this particular question, hip is tested in flexion, although foot moves laterally hip rotates internally.

Below picture shows rotation of hip in flexion and extension

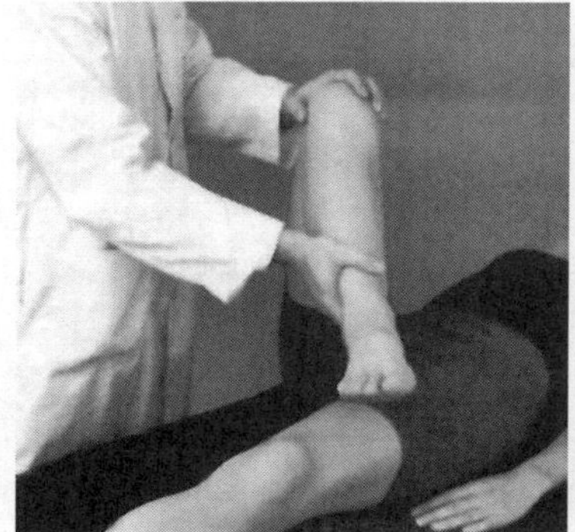

Hip external rotation in flexion

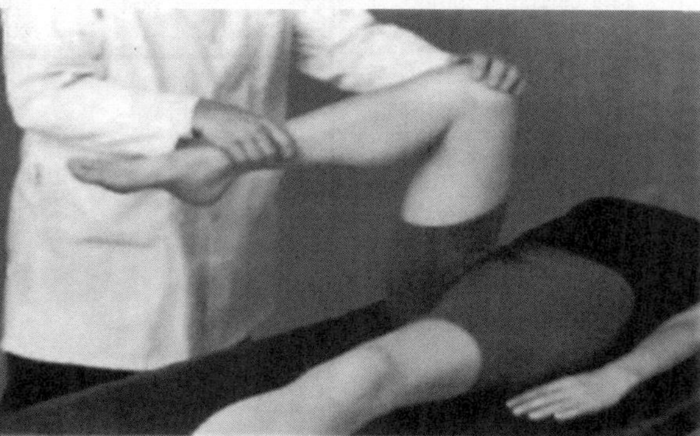

Hip internal rotation in flexion

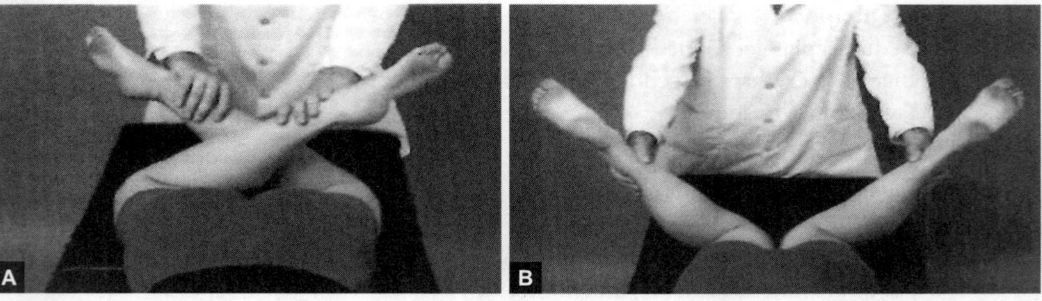

Hip rotation in extension, prone position: A, External rotation; B, Internal rotation

3. Hand to knee gait in polio is due to weakness of which muscle?

a. Gluteus maximus
b. Gluteus medius
c. Soleus and gastrocnemius
d. Quadriceps

Ans. d. Quadriceps *Ref: Tureks 6th/ed p74*

EXPLANATION

Quadriceps is made of four muscles (vastus medialis, vastus lateralis, vastus intermedialis, and rectus femoris) which forms anterior portion of thigh and whose major function is extension of thigh, paralysis of this muscle leads to hand knee gait. In normal gait, quadriceps functions to keep knee in extension during stance phase. When quadriceps is weak, patient uses his hand to push anterior thigh to prevent buckling of knee and also shifting center of gravity anteriorly along the axis of upper limb to leg through knee joint.

Pathological Gait

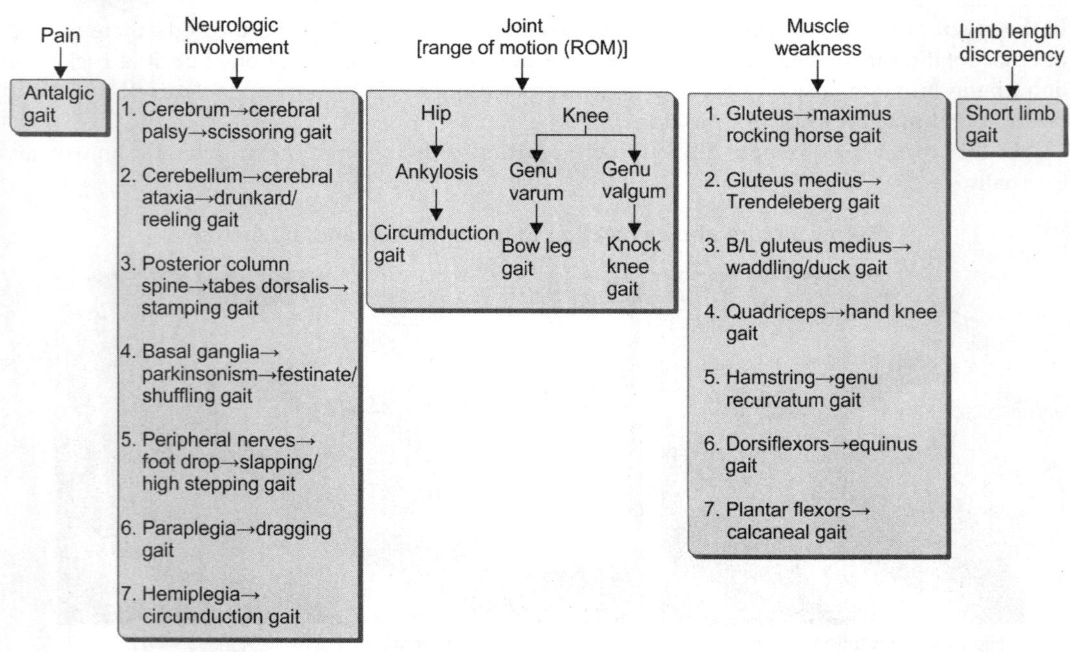

4. Haglund deformity is associated with:

a. Knee
b. Elbow
c. Ankle
d. Wrist

Ans. c. Ankle *Ref: Campbell 12th/ed Vol-4, p3643*

Explanation

Haglund deformity is name given to tender swelling over posterior aspect of ankle joint over the insertion of Achilles tendon. A Haglund deformity, or pump bump, is caused by chronic inflammation of the Achilles bursa that separates the Achilles tendon from the overlying skin.

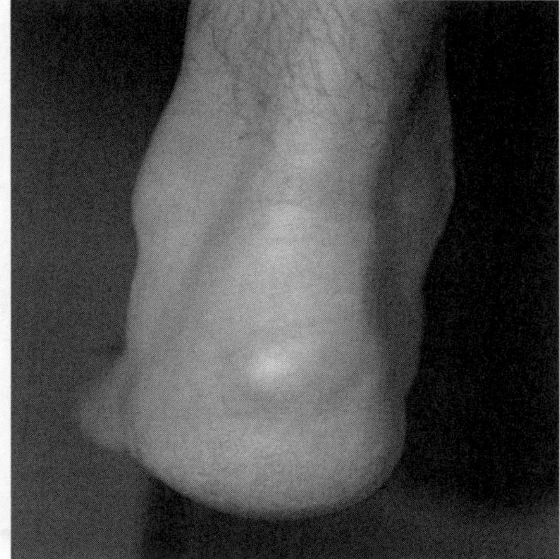

5. March fracture following stress is seen in which part of second metatarsal?

a. Shaft
b. Base
c. Neck
d. Head

Ans. c. Neck *Ref: Rockwood and Greens Adult Fractures, 6th/ed p676*

Explanation

March fracture is the *stress fracture* most commonly occurs at *neck* portion of the *second metatarsal* due to *overuse* especially in *militants and runners.*
This is direct and most often repeated question.

- The 'second metatarsal neck' is the most likely site for stress fracture.
- Other common sites—femur neck, posteromedial femur shaft,anterior aspect of tibial shaft, mid 3rd and lower 3rd tibia shaft and tarsal navicular bone.
  (for other named fractures refer explanation of Q4. of *JIPMER Orthopedics*).

6. A patient came with complaints of inability to move his 4th and 5th digit, cannot hold pen and he was not able to hold paper between fingers. Which of the following site given below is the probable cause of injury to the nerve in question?

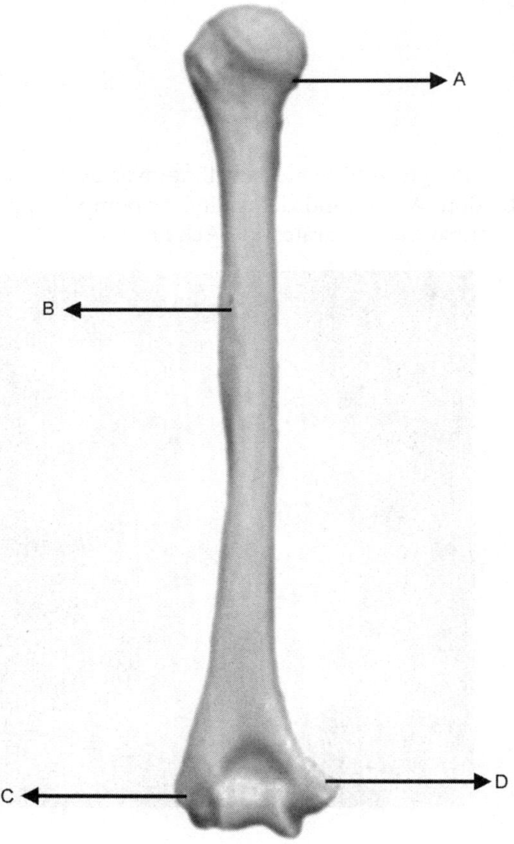

a. Point A
b. Point B
c. Point C
d. Point D

Ans. d. Point D *Ref: Netter's Clinical Anatomy p38/Turek's 6th/ed Ebnezer 4th/ed p319*

Explanation

Inability to move 4th and 5th finger [medial two lumbricals and medial half flexor digitorum profundus (FDP) paralysis] inability to hold paper (introssei paralysis) all suggests ulnar nerve injury. Anatomically ulnar nerve lies more superficial and also close to bone while it passes under the groove of **medial epicondyle** which is more likely to be the site of injury.

- Nerve injuries is one of the most commonly asked questions. Anatomy of nerve supply should be on your finger tips. Diagram and table given below are self-explanatory. Please memorize it before going to exam.
- Picture given below shows anatomy of nerves of upper limb and their sensory distribution.

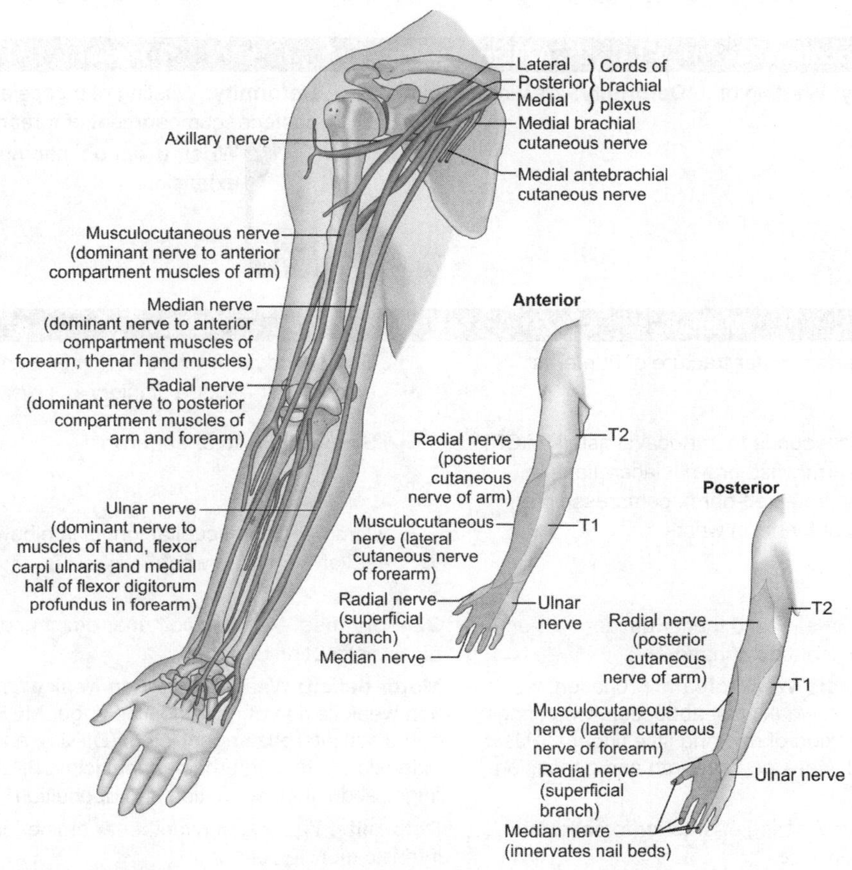

❑ Table below shows the clinical feature of nerve injuries.

Musculocutaneous	Axillary	Radial
NB/injuries are rare as protected by bulk of biceps muscle Stab wounds to upper arm	Fracture of surgical neck of humerus Stab wounds to posterior shoulder Compression by shoulder dislocation of pressure of crutches on armpits	Fracture of proximal humerus, humeral shaft or proximal radius Stab wounds to antecubital fossa (ACF)/forearm/wrist Compression by pressure of crutches on armpits, falling asleep/ lying on arm, tight plaster cast or prolonged tourniquet use
Sensory loss: Numb lateral forearm	**Sensory loss:** Numb sergeant's patch	**Sensory loss:** Numb posterior arm and forearm numb radial distribution of hand
Motor deficit: Weak elbow flexion weak forearm supination absent biceps reflex	**Motor deficit:** Very weak shoulder abduction from 15–90°, weak shoulder flexion, weak shoulder extension, weak shoulder external rotation	**Motor deficit:** Weak elbow extension, absent triceps reflex, weak wrist extension, weak finger metacarpophalangeal joint (MCPJ) extension, absent supinator reflex

Contd...

Contd...

Musculocutaneous	Axillary	Radial
Deformity: Wasting of biceps	**Deformity:** Wasting of deltoid	**Deformity:** Wasting of triceps and posterior compartment of forearm. 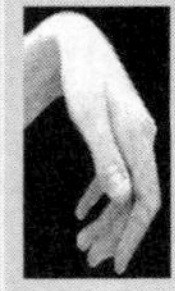 **Wrist drop** on attempted wrist extension

Median	Ulnar
Supracondylar fracture of humerus	Supracondylar fracture of humerus, medial epicondylar fracture of injury
Stab wounds to aortocaval fistula (ACF)/ forearm/wrist, or wrist lacerations in deliberate self-harm, compression at carpal tunnel in wrist	Stab wounds to forearm/wrist
	Compression at cubital tunnel in elbow or Guyon's canal in wrist
Sensory loss: Numb thenar eminence, numb median distribution of hand	**Sensory loss:** Numb hypothenar eminence, numb ulnar distribution of hand
Motor deficit: Weak forearm pronation, weak wrist flexion, weak wrist abduction, weak finger flexion—flexion of ring and little finger DIPJs preserved, weak grip strength and opposition	**Motor deficit:** Weak wrist flexion weak wrist adduction weak flexion of ring and little finger MCPJs and distal interphalangeal joints (DIPJs), and weak extension at their interphalangeal joints (IPJs) weak finger abduction, adduction and opposition
Deformity: Wasting of anterior forearm and thenar eminence 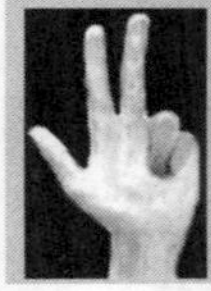 **Hand of benediction** on attempted finger flexion	**Deformity:** Wasting of hypothenar eminence and intrinsic muscles of hand 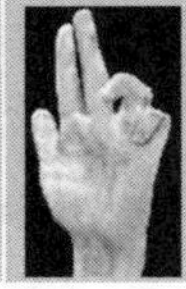 **Claw hand** on attempted finger extension

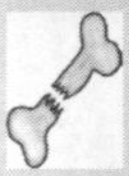

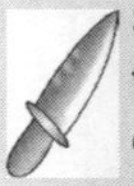

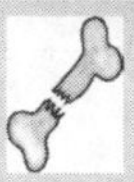

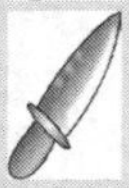

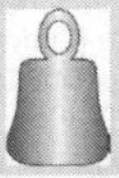

7. A patient sustained leg injury in an RTA, X-ray knee was done as given below. What will be the best management?

a. K wire
b. Patellectomy
c. Compression plate
d. Tension band wiring

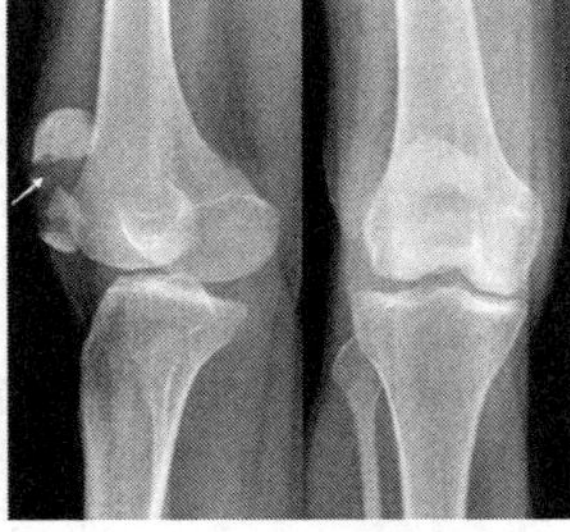

Ans. d. Tension band wiring *Ref: Maheshwari 3rd/ed, p12*

EXPLANATION

The given X-ray shows displaced fracture patella with two separate fragments. In such cases treatment of choice will be open reduction and fixation with tension band wiring.

- Treatment of fracture patella
  - Undisplaced → cylindrical cast
  - Clean break with separation of fragments → tension band wiring
  - Comminuted → patellectomy

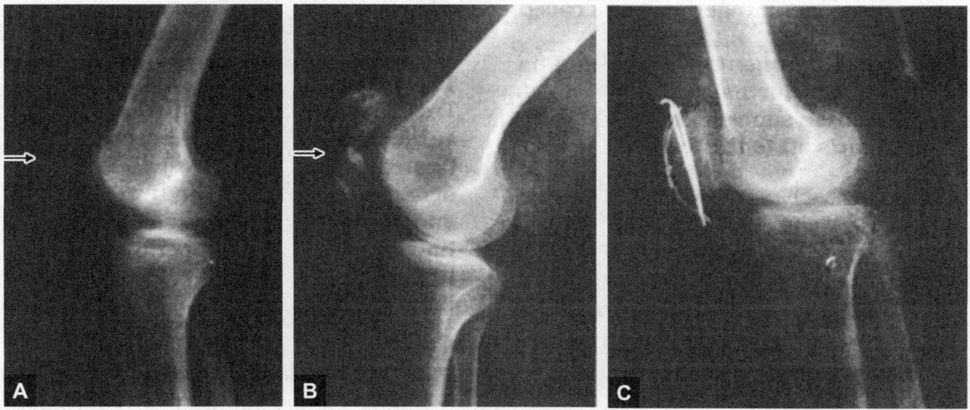

A and B: Preoperative X-ray showing fracture patella C. Postoperative X-ray after fixation with tension band wiring

8. A middle-aged-woman with history of back pain came to OPD. On examination she was positive for schober test. Her sclera, nose and ears were hyperpigmented. Most likely diagnosis is?

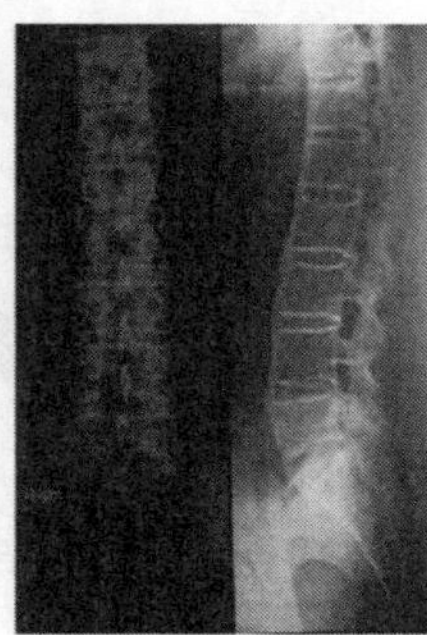

a. Hypoparathyroidism
b. Ochronosis
c. Fluorosis
d. Ankylosing spondylitis

Ans. d. Ankylosing spondylitis *Ref: Textbook of Basic Radiology p78/Robbins Pathology p361*

EXPLANATION

This is tricky question here. In the given question 3 hints have been given

1. **Positive schober test: Classically used to determine decrease in lumbar spine motion, most commonly as result of ankylosing spondylitis but may also be associated with other condition that decrease range of motion in lumbar spine like pain, segmental fusion (in other terms it is not pathognomic for ankylosing spondylitis (AS) but just signifies decrease in lumbar flexion).**

2. **Pigmentation of sclera, nose and ears even though are associated with onchronosis among given options but it is not pathognomic.**
3. **X-ray shown here clearly shows acute lymphoblastic leukemia (ALL) calcification, bamboo spine, end plate sclerosis, osteoporosis of rest of bone, squaring of vertebra → all features pointing to diagnosis of AS.**

Option a: Hypoparathyroidism: Clinical manifestations of chronic hypoparathyroidism include nonspecific mental symptoms such as lethargy, irritability, and depression, as well as cataracts, alopecia, and poor tooth formation. Bony changes are minimal.

Option b: Onchronosis: An inherited defect in enzyme system involved in metabolism of phenylalanine and tyrosine. The retained homogentisic acid selectively binds to collagen in connective tissues, tendons, and cartilage, imparting to these tissues a blue-black pigmentation **(ochronosis)** most evident in the ears, nose, and cheeks. The most serious consequences of ochronosis, however, stem from deposits of the pigment in the articular cartilages of the joints. The vertebral column, particularly the intervertebral disc, is the prime site of attack, but later the knees, shoulders, and hips may be affected. Typical feature of onchronosisis is ***disc space calcification*** which is not evident in given X-ray.

Option c: Fluorosis: Fluorine directly stimulates osteoblastic activity fluoroapatite crystals are laid down in bone and these are unusually resistant to osteoclastic resorption → generalized osteosclerosis which is not evident on given X-ray.

Option d: Ankylosing spondylitis- due to inflammatory granulation tissue. The outer annular fibers are eroded and eventually replaced by bone, forming the beginning of a **syndesmophyte**, which then grows by continued endochondral ossification, ultimately bridging the adjacent vertebral bodies visible on plain films as bony bridges connecting successive vertebral bodies anteriorly and laterally. Ascending progression of this process leads to the **"bamboo spine."** Other lesions in the spine include **diffuse osteoporosis** (loss of trabecular bone despite **accretion of periosteal bone**), erosion of vertebral bodies at the disc margin, "**squaring**" or "**barreling**" of vertebrae. X-ray given here and positive schober test goes much with AS even though pigmentation cannot be explained but definitely diagnosis will be AS based on X-ray.

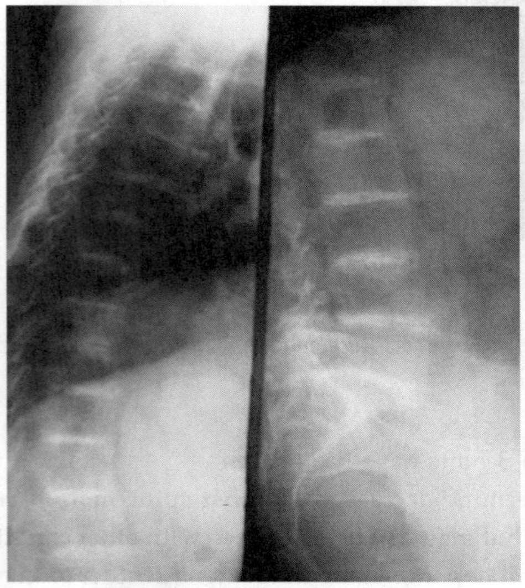

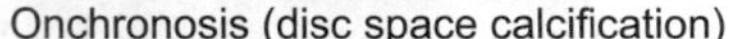

Onchronosis (disc space calcification)

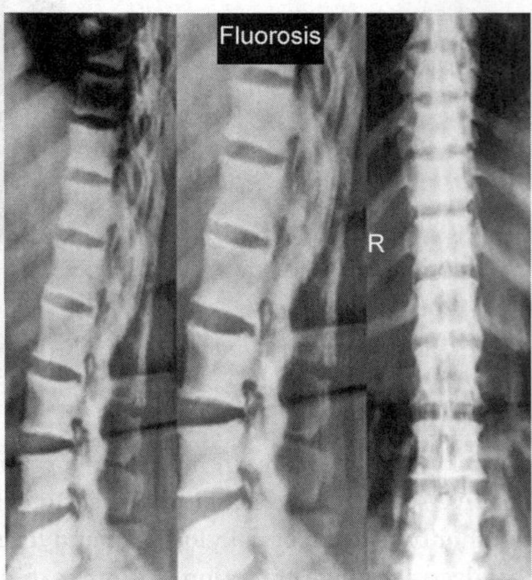

Fluorosis (genaralized osteosclerosis)

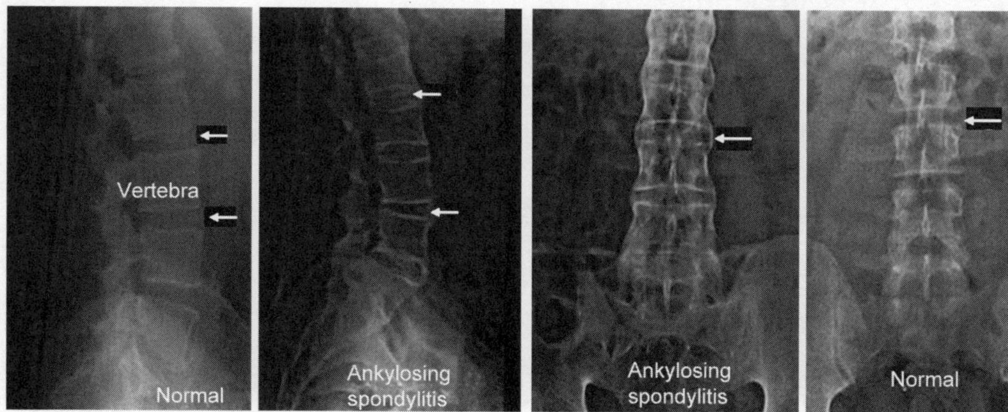

There is a ligament (arrows) in front of the vertebrae. It is flexible and not normally seen in a normal person. It gets calcified, thick in Ankylosing Spondylitis and is seen.

There is a ligament (arrows) on sides of the vertebrae. It is flexible and not normally seen in a normal person. It gets calcified and thick in Ankylosing Spondylitis and is seen.

For review of ankylosing spondylitis refer question number 12 of PGI

9. Which of the following is true regarding Gallezi fracture dislocation?

a. Interosseous membrane tear with triangular fibrocartilage complex (TFCC) tear and radial shaft fracture
b. Interosseous membrane tear + Radial shaft fracture
c. Radial collateral ligament tear with interosseous membrane tear with radial shaft fracture
d. Interosseous membrane tear with triangular fibrocartilage complex (TFCC) tear and ulnar shaft fracture

Ans. a. Interosseous membrane tear with triangular fibrocartilage complex (TFCC) tear and radial shaft fracture *Ref: Rockwood and Greens Fracture Adults Vol 1 p967*

Explanation

- A Galeazzi or Piedmont fracture refers to a fracture of the radial diaphysis at the junction of the middle and distal thirds with associated disruption of the distal radioulnar joint (DRUJ) [DRUJ includes TFCC and interosseous membrane]
- A Monteggia lesion denotes a fracture of the proximal ulna accompanied by radial head dislocation [monteggia-M for medial]

(For other named fracture refer explanation of Q4. of JIPMER Orthopedics)

10. Which of the following image is of bone holding forceps?

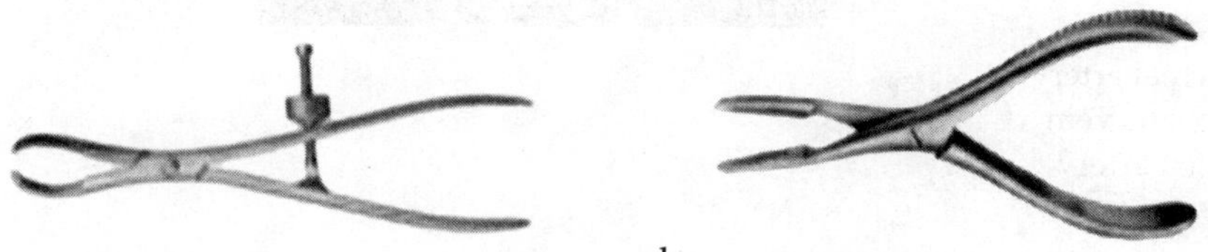

a.

b.

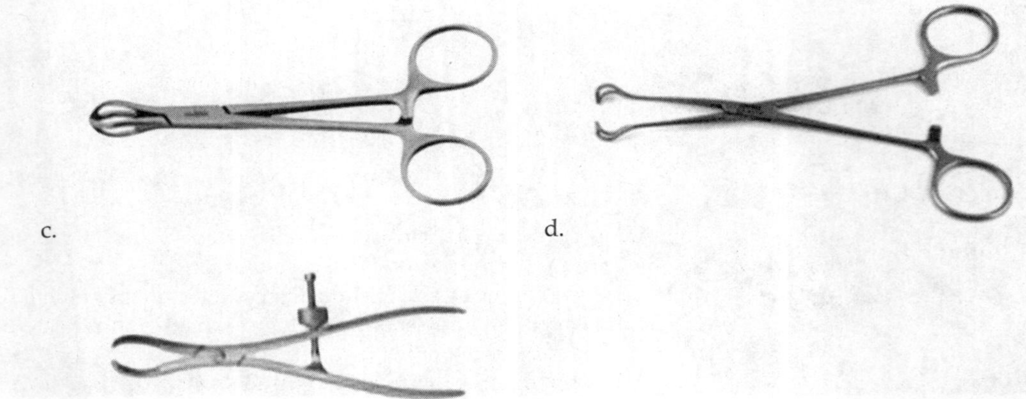

Ans. a.

Ref: Practical Orthopedics By John Ebnezar p339, Maheshwari 5th/ed p372, SRB's Surgical.

EXPLANATION

The given options are:

a. AO type bone holding forceps
b. Sequestrum holding forceps
c. Lane's tissue forceps
d. Babcock's forceps

11. A 14-year-old boy fell on outstretched hand, X-ray is as shown below. Which of the following vascular structure is most commonly injured?

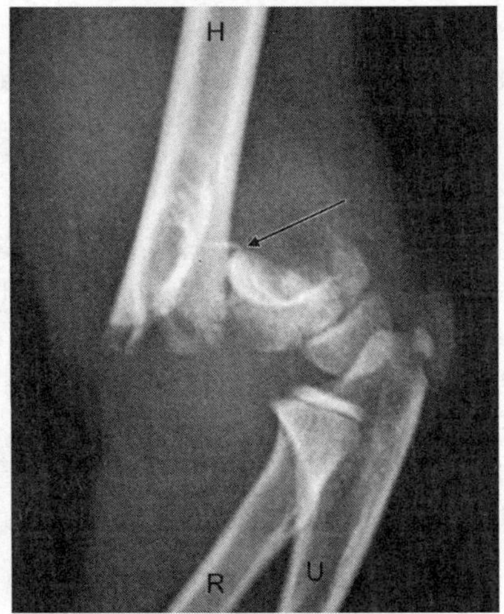

a. Brachial artery
b. Cephalic vein
c. Radial artery
d. Ulnar artery

Ans. a. Brachial artery *Ref: John Ebnezer 4th/ed p154*

Explanation

As brachial artery passes through cubital fossa it runs anteriorly in front of distal humerus in close proximity to bone. In extension type of supracondylar fracture proximal fragment is anteriorly displaced and more likely to injure brachial artery.

Neurovascular involvement in supracondylar fracture [extension type]

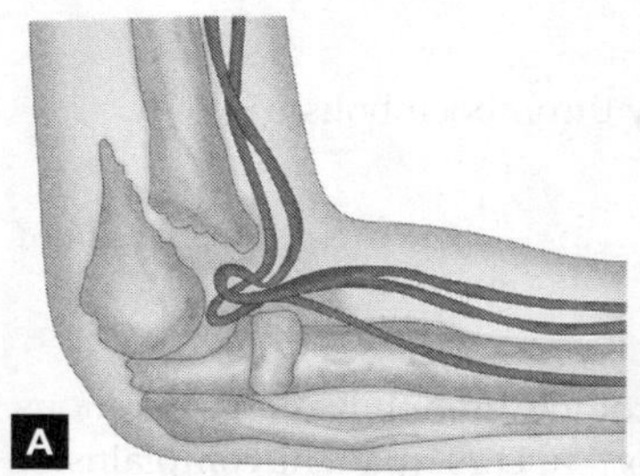

B

- Neurological involvement: Overall incidence is around 7%.
- Radial nerve: Most commonly affected and is usually injured in posteromedial displacement.
- Median nerve: Injured during posterior displacement.
- Anterior interosseous nerve: Injury is seen in posterolateral displacement of the distal fragment
- Ulnar nerve: Injured in overhead skeletal traction and in flexion type of supracondylar fracture.
- Vascular injury: The incidence is between 0.5% and 1%. Common with extension type and isusually due to direct injury of brachial artery by the fracture.

Picture A: showing injury to brachial artery in supracondylar fracture

Box B: Showing incidence of neurovascular involvement in supracondylar fracture humerus

12. An elderly patient slipped in bathroom and sustained injury over hip. X-ray is shown below. Attitude of her limb will be:

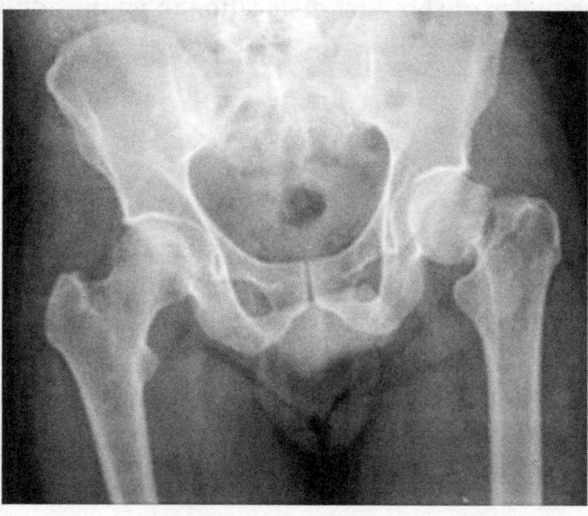

a. Shortened and externally rotated
b. Shortened, externally rotated and abducted
c. Shortened, internally rotated and adducted
d. Flexed and adducted and internally rotated

Ans. a. Shortened and externally rotated *Ref: Maheshwari, 4th/ed, p114*

Explanation

Picture shows fracture neck of femur associated with decreased neck shaft angle. In this case patient will be having shortening, external rotation and adduction so better to go with ***option a***.

Common Signs in Fracture Neck of Femur

- External rotation of the leg, the patella facing outwards.

- ❑ Shortening of the leg, usually slight.
- ❑ Tenderness in the groin.
- ❑ Attempted hip movements painful, and associated with severe spasm.
- ❑ Active straight-leg-raising not possible.

13. A 23-year-old boy badminton player sustained injury on left ankle, he was immobilized for 3 months, the cast was removed and patient was able to walk normally. Later, he complained of pain and swelling in the left calf, left ankle and foot. His mother massaged him for 30 min. After a while he developed acute onset of breathlessness and was brought to emergency and died. Most likely cause of death is?

a. Fat embolism
b. Pulmonary thromboembolism
c. Myocardial infarction (MI)
d. Stroke

Ans. b. Pulmonary thromboembolism *Ref: Ebnezer 4th ed*

EXPLANATION

In the given question patient is immobilized for 3 months → Prolong immobilzation → Venous stasis (Virchow's triad- vessel wall injury/stasis/hypercoagulability) → DVT (patient complains of pain in leg and calf) → clot dislodgement after massage → pulmonary embolism.

- ❑ **Option a:** Fat embolism common during first 48 hrs after major bone fracture.
- ❑ **Option c and d:** MI and stroke less common in 23 years young boy and also doesn't fit with history and presentation.

14. Most common sequelae of shoulder dislocation in young adult is:

a. Recurrent dislocation
b. Rotator cuff tear
c. Adhesive capsulitis
d. Subcapsular tendinitis

Ans. a. Recurrent dislocation *Ref: Ebenezer 4th ed*

EXPLANATION

Recurrent dislocation is the most common complication of shoulder dislocation.

- ❑ This is a very common complication of anterior dislocation of shoulder and accounts for greater than 80% of dislocations of the upper extremity.
- ❑ Age at the time of initial dislocation is an important prognostic factor,
  - Recurrence rate being 55% in patients 12 to 22 years old
  - 37% in 23 to 29 years old, and
  - 12% in 30 to 40 years old.

PGI May 2017

1. Which one of the following is true about fracture healing?

a. Primary healing doesn't involve woven bone
b. Primary healing has an intermediate cartilage stage formation
c. Secondary healing doesn't have intermediate cartilage
d. Micromovements at fracture site help in fracture healing
e. Secondary healing involve woven bone formation.

Ans. a. Primary healing doesn't involve woven bone; d. Micromovements at fracture site help in fracture healing and e. Secondary healing involve woven bone formation *Ref: Tureks 6th/ed*

Explanation

Option a and b: Primary healing occurs when bone is rigidly fixed with plate by direct growth of osteons hence doesn't involve stage of intermediate cartilage or woven bone formation.

Option c and e: Secondary healing occurs in non-rigidly fixed fracture (e.g. conservatively managed/intramedullary nailing) which involves intermediate cartilage formation and woven bone formation.

Option d: Micro movements at fracture site stimulates mesenchymal cells to become chondroblasts, osteoblasts and fibroblasts which helps in fracture union.

Flowchart shows stages of primary/secondary fracture healing

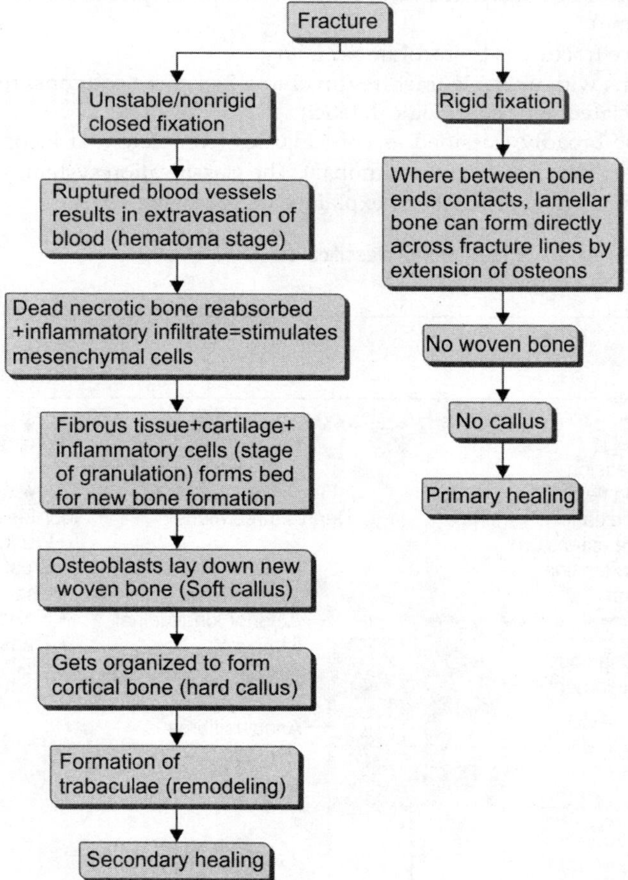

2. True about spinal trauma is/are:

a. 40% mortality rate
b. Spinal shock recovers completely
c. Brown sequard syndrome is the most common spinal cord injury

d. Chance fracture is the most common cervical spine injury
e. Patients with no neurological deficit requires no fixation

Ans. b. Spinal shock recovers completely

Ref: Campbell 13th/ed, Maheshwari, Ebnezer

EXPLANATION

- Spinal trauma
  - Incidence—6% of all trauma
  - Mortality—17 % **(Option a)**
  - Male: female = 4:1
- **Option b:** Spinal shock- complete loss of sensory, motor, reflexes following spinal cord injury but recovers completely
- **Option c:** Posterior cord syndrome is most common among spinal cord syndromes. (not brown sequard syndrome)
- **Option d:** Chance fracture is thoracolumbar injury.
- **Option e:** Patients with unstable fracture (involving 2 or more columns) requires fixation even though not associated with neurological deficits.

Spinal trauma can be broadly classified as cord injuries (complete and incomplete cord injuries) and vertebral fractures (cervical or thoracolumbar). The classification system, special named spinal fractures and their management has been explained in following charts.

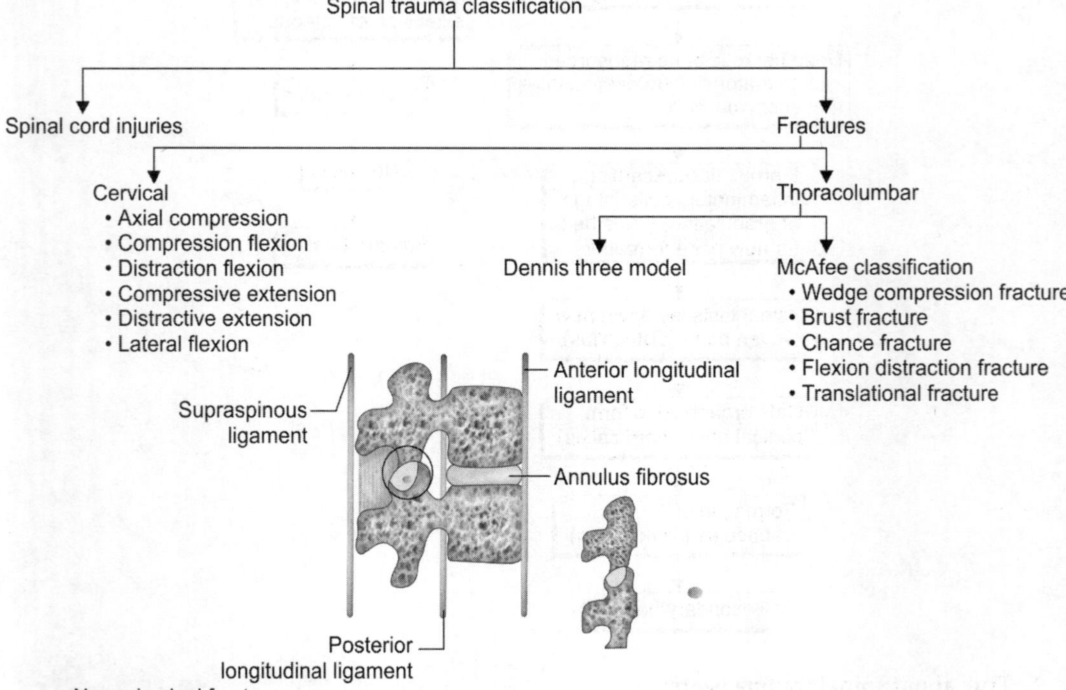

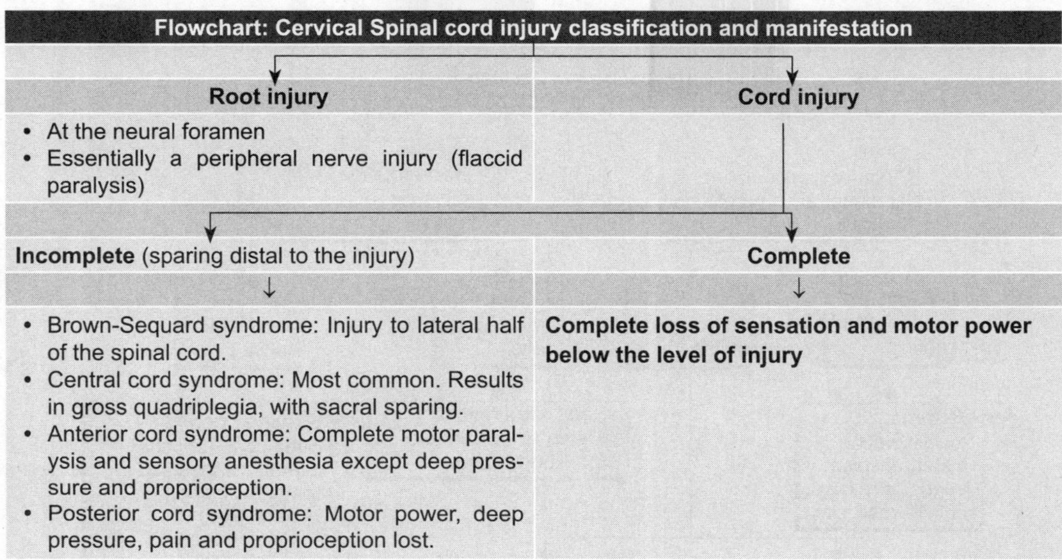

Flowchart: Cervical Spinal cord injury classification and manifestation

Root injury	Cord injury
• At the neural foramen • Essentially a peripheral nerve injury (flaccid paralysis)	
Incomplete (sparing distal to the injury) ↓	**Complete** ↓
• Brown-Sequard syndrome: Injury to lateral half of the spinal cord. • Central cord syndrome: Most common. Results in gross quadriplegia, with sacral sparing. • Anterior cord syndrome: Complete motor paralysis and sensory anesthesia except deep pressure and proprioception. • Posterior cord syndrome: Motor power, deep pressure, pain and proprioception lost.	**Complete loss of sensation and motor power below the level of injury**

Flowchart: Management of cervical spinal cord injury.

- Injury to cervical spine
  - No neurological deficit
    - Alignment maintained (A) → Cervical traction for 6 wks → Collar or SOMI brace for 6 wks
      - Spontanaeous bony fusion → Discard the collar
      - No bony fusion → Assess stability of the spine by cine-radiograph
        - Stable → Cont. conservative treatment
        - Unstable → Spinal fusion
    - Alignment not maintained → Reduction by traction
      - Successful → Same as (A)
      - Unsuccessful → ORIF
  - Neurological deficit
    - Alignment maintained → Same as (A)
    - Alignment not maintained → Rediction
      - Successful → Same as (A)
      - Unsuccessful → CT/MRI → Decompression + ORIF

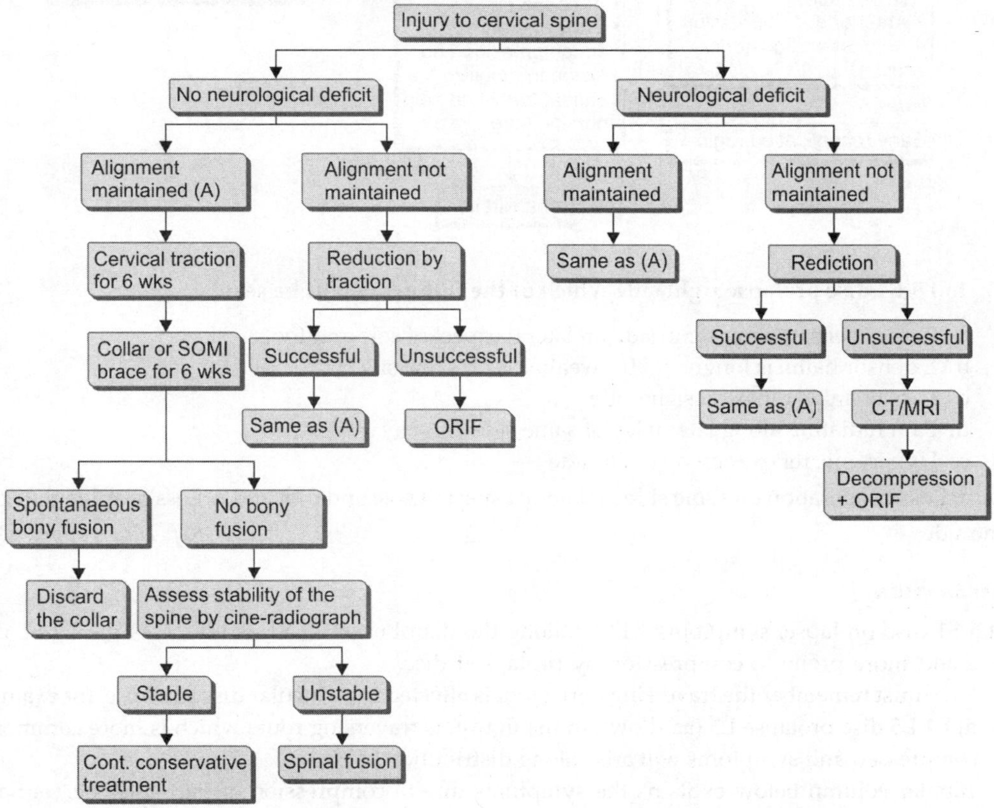

SOME: Sternal-occipital-mandibular-immobilization;
ORIF: Open reduction internal fixation.

Flowchart: Thoracolumbar injury manifestions and management

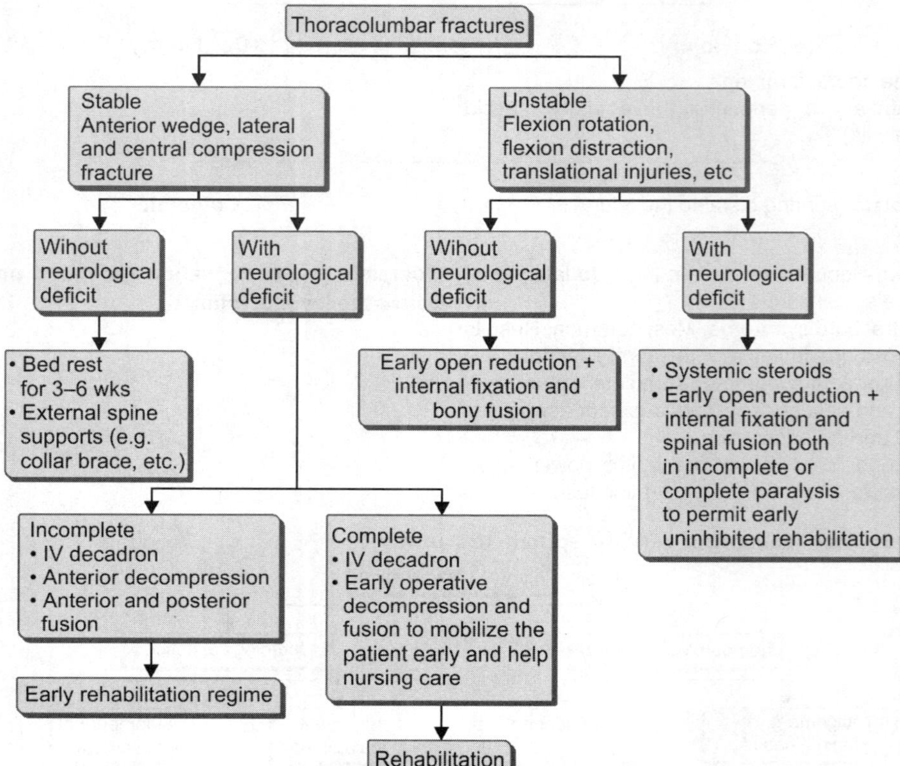

3. In L5-S1 disc prolapse right side which of the following will be seen?

a. Loss of sensation on same side on lateral aspect of sole and foot.
b. Extensor hallucis longus (EHL) weakness on same side
c. Loss of ankle reflex on same side
d. Pain radiating along lateral leg of same side
e. Hypertonic reflexes on opposite side

Ans. a. Loss of sensation on same side on lateral aspect of sole and foot and c. Loss of ankle reflex on same side *Ref: Tureks 6th/ed p389.*

Explanation

In L5 S1 disc prolapse, symptoms will be along the distribution of S1 as it crosses the L5 S1 disc space and more prone to compression by prolapsed disc.

- One must remember the traversing nerve root is affected in particular disc prolapse, for example in L4 L5 disc prolapse L5 (as shown in the figure) is traversing route which is more commonly compressed and symptoms will arise along distribution of L5.
- Tabular column below explains the symptoms due to compression of particular nerve. So in particular disc prolapse traversing nerve root will be compressed and symptoms will be along the distribution of that nerve.

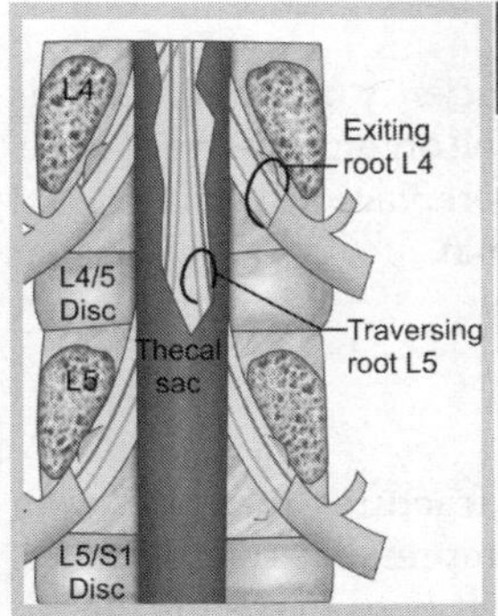

Nerve root	Pain referral	Motor	Sensory	Deep tendon reflex (DTR)
L4	Medial leg	Ankle dorsiflexion	Medial ankle	Knee
L5	Lateral leg, dorsal foot	Great toe dorsi-flexion	First web space between 1st and 2nd toe	No reliable reflex
S1	Posterior calf, lateral or sole of foot	Foot plantar flexion	Lateral aspect of the sole of foot	Ankle

4. Which of the following is true about ponseti regimen?

a. Adductus corrected first
b. Varus corrected last
c. Equinus corrected last
d. Cavus corrected first
e. All corrected simultaneously

Ans. c. Equinus corrected last and d. Cavus corrected first *Ref: Tachdjians Paediatric Othopaedics 4th/ed p856*

Explanation

Ponseti is conservative method of management of congenital talipes equinovarus (CTEV) using above elbow casts in which the deformity is corrected in sequential order. Mneumonic to remember order of correction will be **CAVE** (Cavus → Adductus + Varus → Equinus)

Ponseti Regimen

- ❑ Conservative management of CTEV with above knee casts
- ❑ Age-started as soon as diagnosed (within first week)
- ❑ Has two phases—1) correction 2) maintenance

1. *Correction steps* → *Cavus* (corrected by supination of foot)

↓

Adduction and varus (by abduction and external rotation with index finger on head of first metatarsal with thumb on head of talus used as fulcrum)

↓

Equinus (corrected last by Achilles tendon tenotomy)

2. Maintenance → DB splint (70 degree-abduction and 15 degree dorsiflexon) timing-should be wore 23 hrs till walking age then only in night till age of 5 years, CTEV shoes while walking)

5. True about osteomalacia is/are:

a. Decreased bone osteoid
b. Loosers zone
c. Normal serum calcium levels
d. Decreased vit D
e. Alkaline phosphatase increased

Ans. b. Loosers zone; c. Normal serum calcium levels; d. Decreased vit D and e. Alkaline phosphatase increased *Ref: Ebnezer 4th/ed, Maheshwari 3rd/ed and Mercer Textbook of Orthopaedics*

Explanation

- Osteomalacia—inadequate mineralization of bone primarily due to deficiency of vitamin D. This results in failure to replace the turnover of calcium and phosphorus in the organic matrix of bone. Hence, the bone content is de-mineralized and the bony substance is replaced by soft osteoid tissue. The osteoid is increased at the cost of mineralized bone **(option a)**.

Review of Osteomalacia

- C/F- bone pains, muscle weakness and fractures
- X-ray– Diffuse rarefaction of bones
  - Pseudofractures or loosers zone **(option b)** result from stress fractures that heal with unmineralized bone and are seen as radiolucent lines on the compression side of bones. Multiple pseudofractures may be seen bilaterally, with radiolucent lines perpendicular to the axis of long bones developing from healing stress fractures. This finding is referred to as "Milkman syndrome," named after the radiologist who described it; it is almost pathognomonic for osteomalacia.
  - Spine: The bodies of spine are biconcave and are called "codfish spine".
  - Hip show protrusioacetabuli and triradiate pelvis.
- Inv
  - Serum chemistries are similar in osteomalacia and rickets; patients have normal calcium levels, low vitamin D levels, elevated parathyroid hormone (PTH) levels, and elevated alkaline phosphatase levels. **(option c, d and e)**

[Decreased vit D → decrease Ca → elevated PTH → increases alkaline phosphatase (ALP) and normalizes Ca levels and decreases P levels]

  - Diagnostic-bone biopsy from iliac crest
- Causes:

Conditions that cause osteomalacia or rickets
• Vitamin D-deficient conditions
▪ Dietary lack of vitamin D
▪ Insufficient exposure to sunlight
▪ Vitamin D deficiency of prematurity
▪ Use of seizure medications
▪ Liver disease
▪ Intestinal disease or surgery
▪ Vitamin D-dependent rickets
▪ Renal osteodystrophy
• Hypophosphatemic rachitic syndromes
▪ X-linked dominant hypophosphatemic rickets
▪ Autosomal dominant hypophosphatemic rickets
▪ Fanconi syndrome
▪ Use of aluminum-containing antacids
• Impaired mineralization
▪ Hypophosphatasia
▪ Use of bisphosphonates

6. False about neurogenic claudication:

a. Shiny skin
b. Walking distance fixed
c. Normal back
d. Painless on walking uphill
e. Back pain

Ans. a. Shiny skin; b. Walking distance fixed; c. Normal back and e. Back pain

Ref: Macnab's Backache 4th/ed p256

EXPLANATION

This table is self-explanatory.

Evaluation	Vascular claudication	Neurogenic claudication
Walking distance	Fixed	Variable
Palliative factor	Standing	Sitting/bending
Provocative factor	Walking	Walking/standing
Walking uphill	Painful	Painless
Bicycle test	Positive (painful)	Negative
Pulse	Absent	Present
Skin	Loss of hair; shiny	
Weakness	Rarely	Occasionally
Back pain	Occasionally	Commonly
Back motion		Limited
Pain character	Cramping—distal to proximal	Numbness, aching—proximal to distal
Atrophy	Uncommon	Occasionally

7. True about sciatica is/are:

a. Associated L5-S1 prolapse
b. Radicular pain present
c. Incontinence suggest severity
d. Diabetes can cause sciatica
e. MRI is diagnostic

Ans. a. Associated L5-S1 prolapse; b. Radicular pain present; c. Incontinence suggest severity and d. Diabetes can cause sciatica

Ref: Macnab's Backache 4th/ed p232

EXPLANATION

Sciatica is a symptom and not a diagnosis. It means a radiating pain (***option b)*** along the distribution of sciatic nerve either due to inflammation of the sciatic nerve or because of compression of one of the roots" constituting the sciatic nerve.

- The sciatic nerve (L3, L4, L5, S1 and S2) is the largest nerve in the body and is composed of the tibial and common fibular (peroneal) nerves. The sciatic nerve innervates muscles of the posterior compartment of the thigh (tibial component), which are largely extensors of the thigh at the hip and flexors of the leg at the knee. It also innervates all muscles below the knee, via its tibial and common fibular components.
- Clinical features depends on the nerve root compressed site of pain, sensory and motor deficits changes which has been discussed in Question 4 of PGI.
- **Option c:** Cauda equine syndrome is severe form of sciatica characterized by dramatic increase in back pain and the occurrence of bilateral leg pain and perineal numbness with bowel and bladder incontinence and absence of bilateral ankle reflexes.
- **Option e:** The diagnosis of sciatica is a clinical diagnosis. It is made after a history and physical examination and before expensive testing such as MR imaging. Only when a patient fails to respond to conservative care or presents with severe neurologic compromise it is time to start investigating.

D/D of Sciatica

- ❑ Proximal to disc:
  - Conus and cauda equina lesions (e.g., neurofibroma, ependymoma)
- ❑ Disc level
  - Herniated nucleus pulposus **(option a)**
  - Stenosis (canal or recess)
  - Infection: Osteomyelitis or discitis (with nerve root pressure)
  - Inflammation: Arachnoiditis
  - Neoplasm: Benign or malignant with nerve root pressure
- ❑ Extraspinal causes
  - Pelvis
    - Cardiovascular conditions (e.g., peripheral vascular disease)
    - Gynecologic conditions
    - Orthopedic conditions (e.g., osteoarthritis of hip)
    - Sacroiliac joint disease
    - Neoplasms
  - Peripheral nerve lesions
    - Neuropathy (diabetic, tumor, alcohol) **(option d)**
    - Local sciatic nerve conditions (trauma, tumor)
    - Inflammation (herpes zoster)

8. Injury to dorsal surface of proximal interphalangeal joint of middle finger:

a. Swan neck deformity
b. Boutonniere deformity
c. Mallet finger
d. Central slip avulsion
e. Flexion at distal interphalangeal (DIP)

Ans. b. Boutonniere deformity and d. Central slip avulsion

Ref: Snells Anatomy 8th/ed, Campbell 13th/ed

EXPLANATION

Injury at proximal interphalangeal (PIP)→***central lip avulsion***→ hyperactivity of lateral band→Flexion at PIP and Hyperextension at DIP→***Boutonniere deformity***

Anatomy of dorsal digital expansion of finger

Figures 1 and 2: Posterior view of normal dorsal extensor expansion. The extensor expansion near the proximal interphalangeal joint splits into three parts: a central part, which is inserted into the base of the middle phalanx, and two lateral parts, which converge to be inserted into the base of the distal phalanx.

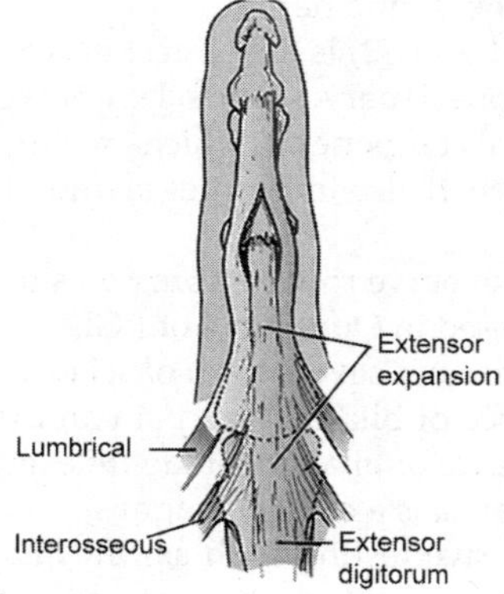

Fig. 1.

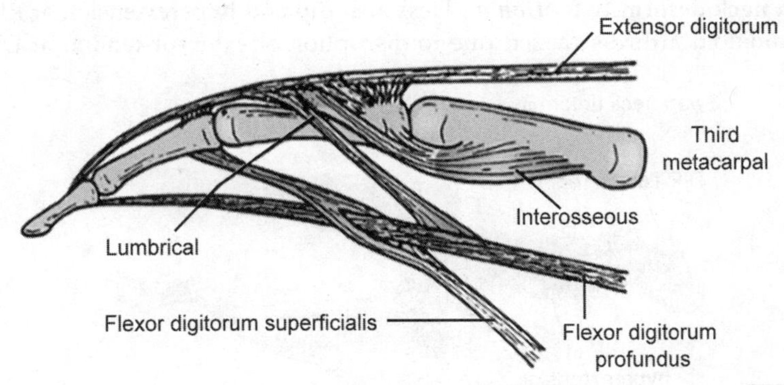

Fig. 2.

Figure 3 Mallet or baseball finger (*option c*): The insertion of the extensor expansion into the base of the distal phalanx ruptured; sometimes a flake of bone on the base of the phalanx is pulled off.

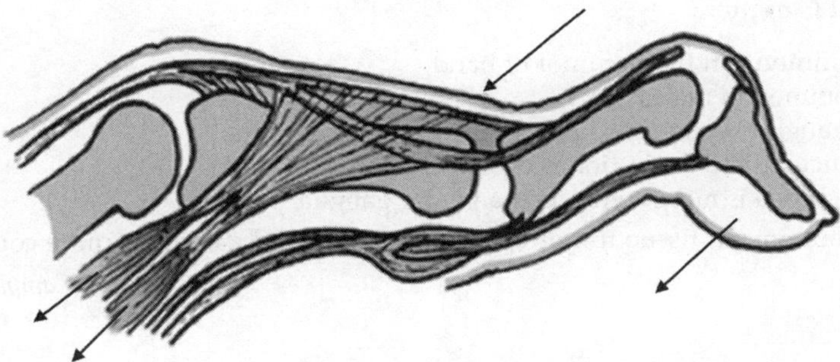

Fig. 3.

Figure 4 Boutonniere deformity (*option b*): The insertion of the extensor expansion into the base of the middle phalanx is ruptured. The arrows indicate the direction of the pull of the muscles and the deformity.

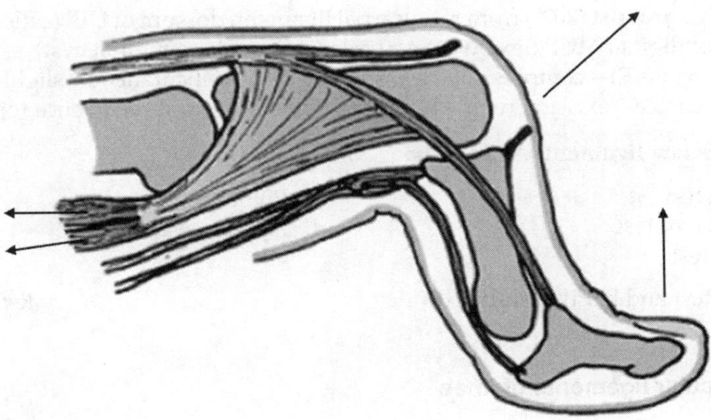

Fig. 4.

Figure 5 Swan neck deformity (*option a*): Flexion at dip and hyperextension at PIP usally associated with rheumatoid arthritis caused due to disruption of extensor tendon at DIP.

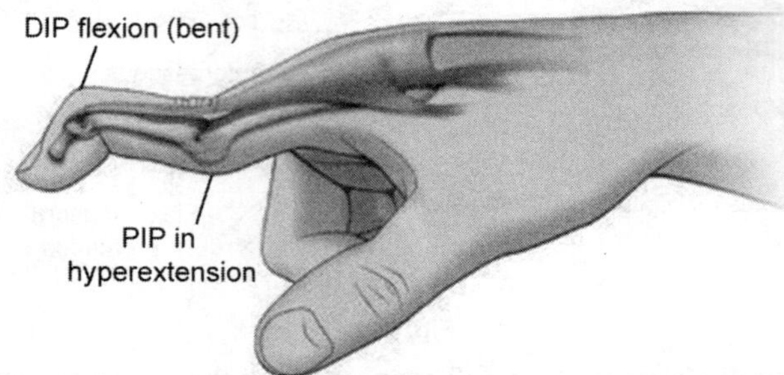

Fig. 5.

9. True about Ganglion:

a. Most common soft tissue tumor of hand
b. More common in males
c. Dorsal ganglion commonly arises from extensor tendons
d. Cyst puncture and aspiration is choice of treatment
e. Dorsal ganglia is more common than volar ganglia

Ans. a. Most common soft tissue tumor of hand and e. Dorsal ganglia is more common than volar ganglia *Ref: Campbell 13th/ed, p3506*

Explanation

- ❑ Ganglions are the most common cause of focal masses **(option a)** in the hand and characteristically arise from the synovium of joints or tendon sheaths or from tendons.
- ❑ Most common among females **(option b)** in 3rd to 4th decade
- ❑ Theories—benign tumors/ herniation of synovial fluid/ mucoid degeneration
- ❑ Most common (M/C) sites—dorsum (70%)—arises from scapholunate ligament **(option c and e)**, palpable between 2nd and 4th dorsal extensor compartment
- ❑ Other sites—volar wrist (20%) from radiocarpal ligament, dorsum of DIP (called as mucous cyst) volar aspect of digit at MCP flexion crease (volar retinacular ganglion cyst)
- ❑ On examination (O/E)—compressible, transilluminating, subcutaneous, slightly mobile
- ❑ Treatment of choice—excision with whole of capsule to prevent recurrence **(option d)**.

10. Anterior cruciate ligament (ACL) tests:

a. Lachman test
b. Pivot shift test
c. Reverse pivot test
d. Apley's test
e. Thessaly test

Ans. a. Lachman test and b. Pivot shift test *Ref: Campbell 13th/ed*

Explanation

Tests for intrarticular ligaments of knee

- ❑ ACL:
  - Anterior drawer test

- Lachman test
- Anterior rotatory drawer test
- Pivot shift test
- Jerk test

❑ Posterior cruciate ligament (PCL)
- Posterior drawer test
- Godfrey's sign

❑ Menesci
- McMurray test
- Apley's grinding test
- Thessaly test
- Squat test

❑ Collateral ligament
- Varus and valgus stress tests

❑ Posterolateral corner (PLC)
- Dial test
- External rotation recurvatum test
- Reverse pivot shift test

11. True about ankylosing spondylitis:

a. Associated with HLAB 27
b. Pain relieves on rest
c. Has associated post uveitis in 30% people
d. Chronic enthesitis
e. Causes atrioventricular defects

Ans. a. Associated with HLAB 27; c. Has associated post uveitis in 30% people and d. Chronic enthesitis *Ref: Turek's 6th/ed, p348*

EXPLANATION

Ankylosing spondylitis (AS) is seronegative [rheumatoid (RA) factor negative] spondyloarthropathy associated with HLA B27

Option b: AS is inflammatory arthropathy characterized by pain at rest and relieved on exercise

Option d: Enthesitis is characteristic feature of *AS* which involves inflammation at site of tendon and ligament insertion.

Option c and e: All extra-articular features are discussed in explanation part of this question.

Review of Ankylosing Spondylitis

❑ Important points
- Seronegative (absence of RA factor)
- Axial skeleton affected (sacroiliac joint and spine)
- HLA B27 positive (85%)

❑ Pathology:
- Enthisitis—involvement of ligament and tendon insertions

❑ C/F:
- 30–40 yrs male (10:1)
- Insidious onset low back
- > 3 minutes
- Morning stiffness
- Relieved on exercise

❑ O/E:
- Sacroiliac (SI) joint stiffness—Gaenslen's test, pump handle, pelvi compression (+ve)
- Spine-
  - ↓ Occiput-wall distance,

- ↓ Finger floor distance,
- ↓ Bimalleolar straddle,
- ↓ Thoracic chest wall expansion,
- ↓ Lumbar spine motion (shober test)

❑ Diagnostic criteria—modified New York criteria

❑ X-ray signs:
- Spine—syndesmetophyte, bamboo spine, squaring of vertebra, dragger sign, road rally sign, corner shine sign, romanus lesion
- Sacroiliac (SI) joint—star sign
- HP—whiskering sign

❑ Extra-articular—anterior uveitis (30%), atlantoaxial subluxation, 3rd degree heart block, prostatitis, aortatitis, apical lobe fibrosis, chrons/ulcerative

❑ Synonyms—Von Bechtrew's disease, Marie-Strumple syndrome, Poker's back

12. True about Perthes disease is/are:

a. May be asymptomatic
b. Progressive avascular necrosis of femoral head
c. Common in females
d. May involve other joints
e. Positive Trendelenburg test

Ans. a. May be asymptomatic and e. Positive Trendelenburg test

Perthes disease is self limiting (***option b***) avascular necrosis is femoral head most common in late born male child (***option c***) in 4 to 12 years age group usually involving unilateral hip joint (*option d*) may be asymptomatic (***option a***) or present with mild hip pain/ limp.
It involves destruction of femoral head affecting lever and fulcrum system of hip→positive Trendelenburg test (***option e).*** *Ref: Tachdjains 6th/ed p857*

Explanation

Perthes disease review

❑ Self limiting avascular necrosis of femoral epiphysis

❑ Etiology unknown: Two hypothesis
- Single arterial source of blood supply in 4–7 years (Trueata's)
- Venous obstruction increasing intraosseous pressure (Caffey's)

❑ Commonly affects:
- Age 4–12 years
- Males (4:1); late born male child (3rd or 4th)
- Low economic status

❑ C/F:
- Asymptomatic or painless limp
- Restricted abduction and internal rotation
- Positive Trendelenburg and shortening
- Other joints unaffected

❑ Pathology: Stages
- Avascular stage → stage of resorption and fragmentation → stage of reossification → healing stage

❑ Staging: Catterall, Salter-Thompson, lateral pillar, Elizabethtown

❑ X-ray signs:
- Waldenstorm's sign (increased medial joint space)
- Gage's sign (V shaped lucent defect on lateral side of epiphysis)
- Salter sign (subchondral fracture)

- Head at risk signs
  - Lateral subluxation of femoral head
  - Lateral calcification
  - Horizontal physis
  - Gage's sign
  - Metaphyseal cysts
- Complication: Healing results in abnormal femoral head shape leading to early degenerative changes
- Treatment: Containment of head within acetabulum
  - Conservative—abduction bracing
  - Surgical—Varus derotation osteotomy/Salter's osteotomy

13. Avascular necrosis of femoral head:

a. Weight bearing is indicated on affected side
b. Plain X-ray findings can be missed in early stages
c. CT is useful in early diagnosis
d. Corticosteroids are beneficial
e. May be asymptomatic

Ans. b. Plain X-ray findings can be missed in early stages and e. May be asymptomatic

Ref: Ebnezer and Maheshwari 3rd/ed

EXPLANATION

- Delay weight-bearing on the necrotic bone until it is revascularized, thereby preventing its collapse (***option a***). *Ref: Maheshwari 3rd/ed*
- Avascular necrosis of a bone is usually asymptomatic in the early stages. In the later stage, the patient may complain of pain, limp and slight loss of movements. In very advanced cases, the patient will show features of osteoarthritis ***(option e)***. *Ref: Ebnezer*
- In the early stages, avascular necrosis can be detected by bone scan, radioisotope study. In the later stages, radiograph shows dense changes in the bone, collapse and osteoarthritis features (***option b and c***).
- Common cause—*(Mnemonic-SCLERA)*
  - S—Steroids (**option d**—long-term steroid intake is one of the causative agent and not used for treatment)
  - C—Caisson's disease
  - LE—Lupus erythematosis
  - R—Radiation therapy
  - A—Alcoholism and fracture neck
- Common sites:
  - Head of femur
  - Body of the talus
  - Proximal pole of scaphoid.

14. True about hemophilic arthropathy

a. Deepening of intercondylar notch
b. Subarticular osteoporosis
c. Prolonged bleeding time
d. Subchondral cysts
e. Aspiration is contraindicated

Ans. b. Subarticular osteoporosis and d. Subchondral cysts *Ref: Tureks 6th/ed, p416*

EXPLANATION

Hemophilic arthropathy is chronic joint inflammatory disease affecting due to repeated intra-articular bleeding due to deficiency of coagulation factors.

X-ray and management have been summarized in explanation part.

Hemophilic Arthropathy Review

- Hemophilia
  - Hemophilia A: ↓ factor VIII (80%) [x linked]
  - Hemophilia B: ↓ factor IX (15%) [x linked]
  - Hemophilia C: (AD)
- Severity of factor VIII deficiency-
  - < 1% Severe,< 5% minor trauma, < 5–25% trauma or surgery.
- Pathogenesis
  - Bleeding → synovial irritation → inflammation → repeated attacks → synovial hyperplasia and pannus → articular cartilage distruction → fibrous ankylosis.
- Lab investigation:
  - The classical feature of this disease is bleeding time is normal, but the clotting time is prolonged **(option c)**.
- X-ray
  - Early-subarticular osteoporosis **(option b)**, subchondral cysts **(option d)** joint interval is normal, squaring of the patella, intercondylar notch of femur and trochlear notch of ulna widened **(option a)**
  - Late-joint destroyed and fibrous ankylosis.
- Treatment
  - Acute: Knee aspiration, **(option a)** splintage and immobilization, replacement of factor
  - Late: Deranged joint—synovectomy/contracture release/arthrodesis/replacement

JIPMER Pattern Based

1. All true about desert rheumatism except:

a. Caused by *Coccidioides immitis*
b. Associated with erythmanodosum
c. Migratory recurrent attacks of joint pains with symptom free period between attacks
d. Common in hot and dry areas

Ans. c. Migratory recurrent attacks of joint pains with symptom free period between attacks

Ref: Kelly's rheumatology

EXPLANATION

Desert rheumatism is **triad** of fever, joint pains and erythema nodosum (***option b***) caused by *Coccidioides immitis* (***option a***) or Coccidioides posadasii, common in hot deserts (***option d***) of California [also called California fever/San Joaquin Valley fever]. Infection is acquired by inhaling fungal spores.

- Presentation may be in three forms as
  - Acute self limiting respiratory infection
  - Chronic form
  - Disseminated form
- **Option c**: But not associated with migratory joint pains.

2. Interosseous skeletal tumor best detected by:

a. X-ray
b. CT
c. MRI
d. Bone scan

Ans. c. MRI *Ref: Campbell 13th/ed, p944*

EXPLANATION

Option b: **CT** is most helpful in assessing ossification and calcification and in evaluating the integrity of the cortex.

Option d: **Technetium bone scans** are used to determine the activity of a lesion and to determine the presence of multiple lesions or skeletal metastases.

Option c: **MRI** has replaced CT as the study of choice to determine the size, extent, and anatomical relationships of bone and soft-tissue tumors. It is the most accurate technique for determining the limits of disease within and outside bone.

3. Russels traction used for:

a. Femur shaft
b. Trochanteric fracture
c. Low backache
d. Fracture humerus

Ans. b. Trochanteric fracture

EXPLANATION

See Question Number 4 of JIPMER Orthopedics

4. Agnes hunt traction:

a. Flexion deformity of hip
b. Trochantric fracture
c. Fracture shaft of humerus
d. Low backache

Ans. a. Flexion deformity of hip *Ref: Campbell, Ebnezer and Maheshwari*

EXPLANATION

These are commonly asked memory based questions in orthopedics. These charts are must to memorize.

Commonly asked tractions, fractures, splints and cast

Name	Use
Gallow's traction	Fracture shaft of the femur in children below 2 years
Bryant's traction	Same
Russell's traction	Trochanteric fractures
Buck's traction	Conventional skin traction
Perkin's traction	Fracture shaft of femur in children
Agnes-Hunt traction	Correction of hip deformity
Well-leg traction	Correction of adduction or abduction deformity of hip
Dunlop traction	Supracondylar fracture of humerus
Smith's traction	Supracondylar fracture of humerus

Contd...

Contd...

Name	Use
Calcaneal traction	Open fractures of ankle or leg
Metacarpal traction	Open forearm fractures
Head-Halter traction	Cervical spine injuries
Crutchfield traction	Cervical spine injuries
Halo-pelvic traction	Scoliosis

Splints

Name	Use
Cramer-wire splint	Emergency immobilization
Thomas splint	Fracture femur—anywhere
Bohler-Braun splint	Fracture femur—anywhere
Aluminium splint	Immobilization of fingers
Denis Browne splint	Congenital talipes equinovarus (CTEV)
Cock-up splint	Radial nerve palsy
Knuckle-bender splint	Ulnar nerve palsy
Toe-raising splint	Foot drop
Volkmann's splint	Volkmann's ischemic contracture (VIC)
Four-post collar	Neck immobilization
Aeroplane splint	Brachial plexus injury
Sternal occipital mandibular immobilizer (SOMI) brace	Cervical spine injury
Anterior spinal hyperextension (ASHE)	Dorso-lumbar spinal injury brace
Taylor's brace	Dorso-lumbar immobilization
Milwaukee brace	Scoliosis
Boston brace	Scoliosis
Lumbar corset	Backache

Casts

Name of the cast	Use
Minerva cast	Cervical spine disease
Risser's cast	Scoliosis
Tum-buckle cast	Scoliosis
Shoulder spica	Shoulder immobilization
U-slab	Fracture of the humerus
Colles' cast	Colles' fracture
Hip spice	Fracture of the femur
Cylinder cast	Fracture of the patella
Patella tendon bearing (PTB) cast	Fracture of the tibia
A spica is a cast where a limb and a part of the trunk are included, e.g., hip spica, shoulder spica.	

Disease and location

Name	Site affected
Perthes' disease	Femoral head
Panner's disease	Caplitulum
Kienbock's disease	Lunate bone
Osgood-Schlatter's disease	Tibial tubercle
Sever's disease	Calcaneal tuberosity
Kohler's disease	Navicular bone
Freiberg's disease	Metatarsal head
Schuermann's disease	Ring epiphysis of vertebrae
Calve's disease	Central bony nucleus of vertebral body

Named Fractures

- Barton's: Distal radius, intra-articular fracture
- Chauffer's: Radial styloid fracture
- Colles': Distal radius, extra-articular fracture with dorsal tilt of the distal fragment
- Galleazzi: Fracture of distal V2 of the radius with dislocation of distal radio-ulnar joint
- Monteggia: Fracture of proximal V2 of the ulna with dislocation of head of the radius
- Night-stick: Isolated fracture shaft of the ulna
- Smith's: Distal radius fracture, extra-articular with volar tilt of the distal fragment
- Bennett's: Fracture of base of the 1st metacarpal, intra-articular
- Boxers': Fracture of neck of 5th metacarpal
- Mallet: Avulsion of attachment of extensor tendon from base of the distal phalanx
- Rolando: Fracture of base of 1st metacarpal, extraarticular
- Hangman's: Fracture pedicle-lamina of C2 vertebra
- Malgaigne's: Pelvic-ring disruption with both pubic rami and sacro-iliac injury on the same side
- Bumper: Comminuted fracture of lateral condyle of the tibia
- Cotton's: Trimalleolar ankle fracture
- Pott's: Bimalleolar ankle fracture
- March: Stress fracture of shaft of 2nd metatarsal
- Aviators: Fracture of the neck of the talus
- Jone's: Fracture of the base of the 5th metatarsal

Signs and Tests

- Adson's test: For thoracic outlet syndrome
- Allen's test: For testing patency of radial and ulnar arteries
- Alli's test: For CDH
- Anvil test: For testing tenderness of the spine
- Ape thumb: For median nerve injury
- Apley's grinding test: For meniscus injury
- Apprehension test: For recurrent dislocation of the shoulder
- Barlow's test: For CDH
- Blue sclera: Osteogenesis imperfect
- Bryant's test: For anterior dislocation of the shoulder
- Callaways' test: For anterior dislocation of the shoulder
- Chovstek's sign: For tetany
- Claw hand: For ulnar nerve injury

- ❑ Coin test: For dorso-lumbar tuberculosis of spine
- ❑ Cozen's test: For tennis elbow
- ❑ Drawer test: For ACL and PCL injuries
  - Anterior: For ACL injury.
  - Posterior: For PCL injury
- ❑ Finkelstein's test: For de Quervain's tenovaginitis
- ❑ Foot drop: For common peroneal nerve injury
- ❑ Froment's sign: For ulnar nerve injury
- ❑ Gaenslen's test: For SI joint involvement
- ❑ Galleazzi sign: For congenital dislocation of the hip (CDH)
- ❑ Gower's sign: For muscular dystrophy
- ❑ Hamilton-ruler test: For anterior dislocation of the shoulder
- ❑ Kanavel's sign: For infection in ulnar bursa
- ❑ Lasegue's test: For disc prolapsed
- ❑ Lachmann test: For ACL injury
- ❑ Ludloff s sign: For avulsion of lesser trochanter
- ❑ McMurray's test: For meniscus injury
- ❑ Nagffziger test: Disc prolapsed
- ❑ Ober's test: For tight ilio-tibial band (e.g., in polio)
- ❑ O'Donoghue triad: Triad of MCL, ACL and medial meniscus injuries occurring together
- ❑ Ortolani's test: For CDH
- ❑ Pivot-shift test: For ACL injury
- ❑ Policeman tip: For Erb's palsy
- ❑ Sulcus sign: For inferior dislocation of the shoulder
- ❑ Thomas' test: For hip flexion deformity
- ❑ Trendelenburg's test: For unstable hip due to any reason (e.g., CDH)
- ❑ Tinel's sign: For detecting improving nerve injury
- ❑ Volkmann's sign: For ischemic contracture of forearm muscles
- ❑ Wrist drop: For radial nerve injury
- ❑ Runner's knee: Patellar tendinitis.

5. Question on osteomalacia. All true *except*:

a. Characterized by a diffuse reduction in the bone density due to a decrease in the bone mass
b. Characerized by excess of osteoid
c. Loosers zone on X-ray is pathognomic
d. Bone biopsy is diagnostic

Ans. a. Characterized by a diffuse reduction in the bone density due to a decrease in the bone mass

EXPLANATION

Refer Question No. 6 of PGI orthopedics

Ophthalmology

Author: Jyotsana Priya, Co-author: Shivani Sinha

AIIMS May 2017

1. An infant had conjunctivitis, which later developed into respiratory distress and pneumonia. Chest X-ray showed bilateral lung infiltrates. WBC count 14,300/dL, differential counts were N: 40% L: 56%. Which of the following is the most likely organism?

a. *Chlamydia trachomatis*
b. *H. influenzae*
c. *N. gonorrhoeae*
d. *Streptococcus pneumoniae*

Ans. a. *Chlamydia trachomatis*

Ref: Parsons' Diseases of the Eye. 22nd/ed p177-78; Kanski Clinical Ophthalmology a Systemic Approach 7th/ed p141

Explanation

Time of onset after birth	Differential diagnosis	Features	Treatment	Associated systemic findings/history
Within first 48 hours	*Neisseria gonorrhoeae*	*Discharge*: Mucopurulent to purulent *Conjunctiva*: Intensely inflamed, bright red, swollen. ***Marked chemosis*** is distinguishing feature, dense infiltration of bulbar conjunctiva. Risk of corneal ulceration and perforation	Ceftriaxone injection IM, gentamicin drops, bacitracin eye ointment	Parental symptoms of sexually transmitted infections
Within first 48 hours	Chemical	Spontaneous resolution. ***Crede's*** method: prophylactic instillation of silver nitrate 1% if maternal infection was suspected leading to conjunctivitis	Wash eyes, erythromycin ointment, observe, usually improves in 24 hours	Instillation of prophylactic chemical preparations
48–72 hours	Other bacteria		Neomycin-bacitracin eye ointment, gentamicin or tobramycin drops	
5–7 days	Herpes simplex virus (HSV 2)		Acyclovir 3% eye ointment, systemic acyclovir if systemic involvement	Features of encephalitis

Contd…

Contd...

Time of onset after birth	Differential diagnosis	Features	Treatment	Associated systemic findings/history
>1 week	*Chlamydia trachomatis* (D-K)	Relatively common cause. Less severe than gonococcal *Discharge*: Purulent *Conjunctiva*: Swollen and edematous Complicating superficial keratitis occurs as a rule in smouldering cases	Erythromycin or chlortetracycline eye ointment, oral erythromycin for systemic infection.	Pneumonitis, rhinitis and otitis

2. "Silent choroid" on FFA is feature of:

a. Best's disease
b. Age related macular degeneration
c. Stargardt's disease
d. Cystoid macular edema

Ans. c. Stargardt's disease *Ref: Yanoff Ophthalmology 4th/ed p492;629*

Explanation

- ***Silent choroid or dark choroid*** refers to appearance of prominent retinal circulation against hyperfluorescent choroid.
- Helpful in making diagnosis of Stargardt disease but present only in one fourth of cases
- Despite the accumulation of lipofuscin like material in RPE like Stargardt disease, patients with best dystrophy do not exhibit silent choroid.

Cystoid macular edema (CME):

- On FA, CME often has a honeycomb pattern of dye accumulation at the perifoveal area. CME in the macular periphery has a honeycomb configuration because of the vertical nature of the external plexiform layer fibers.
- The cystoid spaces have a stellate configuration in the central portion of the macula because the external plexiform layer fibers are oblique in this area.
- Petalloid pattern also present.

3. Which of the following will not cause hypotonic maculopathy?

a. Suprachoroidal hemorrhage
b. Cyclodialysis of uvea
c. Corneal perforation
d. Filtration site leak

Ans. a. Suprachoroidal hemorrhage *Ref: Kanski Clinical Ophthalmology a Systemic Approach 7th/ed p288-89*

Explanation

- Maculopathy develops in eyes developing hypotony defined as IOP less than 5 mm of Hg

Causes

- The *most common cause* is excessive drainage following glaucoma filtration surgery (even more if antimetabolite used in surgery)
- Trauma resulting in cyclodialysis cleft, penetrating injury)

- ❑ Chronic uveitis (impaired ciliary body function and tractional ciliary body detachment due to cyclitic membrane)
- ❑ Retinal detachment.

Features:

Vision variably affected
Chorioretinal folds present
B scan: Choroidal effusion
A scan: Reduced axial length

Ref: Kanski Clinical Ophthalmology a Systemic Approach 7th/ed p644-45

Suprachoroidal hemorrhage:

- ❑ Involves bleed into suprachoroidal space from ruptured long or short posterior ciliary artery
- ❑ Can lead to expulsive hemorrhage (0.04%)
- ❑ Signs:
  - Progressive swallowing of anterior chamber, ***increased IOP*** and prolapse of iris
  - Vitreous extrusion, loss or partial obscuration of red reflex
  - Appearance of dark mound behind pupil

4. Visual pathway defect at the level of optic chiasma will result in:

a. Binasal hemianopia
b. Bitemporal hemianopia
c. Central scotoma
d. Bilateral hemianopia

Ans. b. Bitemporal hemianopia

Ref: Albert and Jakobiec's Principles and Practice of Ophthalmology 3rd/ed p393

Explanation

- ❑ The classic chiasmal visual-field defect is a bitemporal depression or scotoma more near fixation
- ❑ Chiasmal compression from below by a pituitary adenoma, the pattern most often observed is a bitemporal superior hemianopia (Fig. 1).
- ❑ Conversely, compression of the chiasm from above (craniopharyngioma or dysgerminoma)– typically produces an inferior bitemporal hemianopia (Fig. 2).

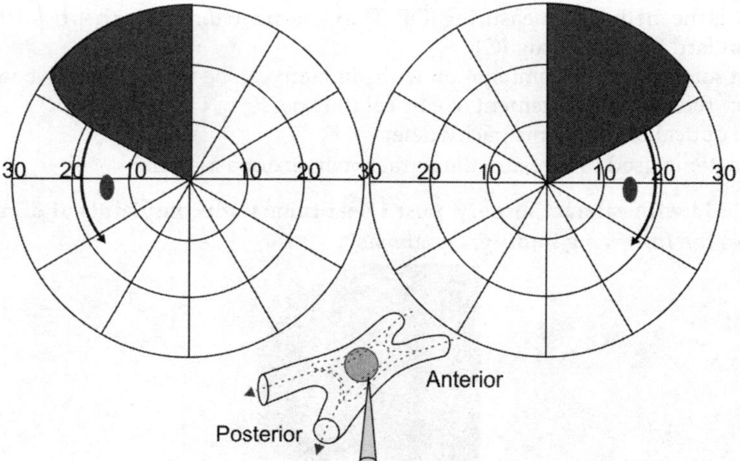

Fig. 1: Bitemporal superior partial hemianopia

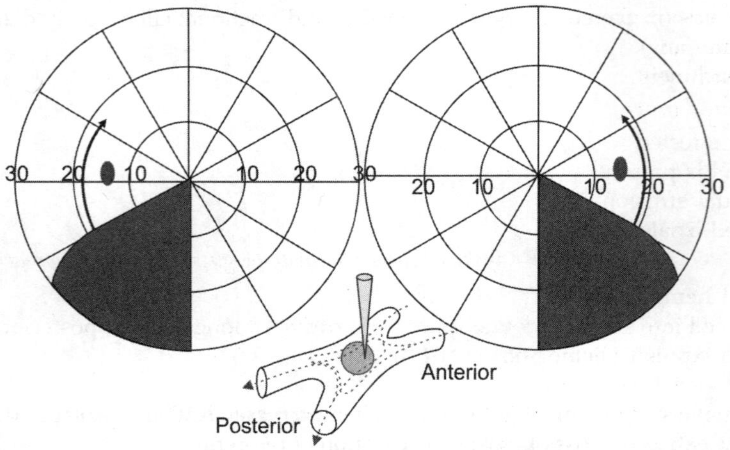

Fig. 2: Bitemporal inferior partial hemianopia

5. Identify the test shown below:

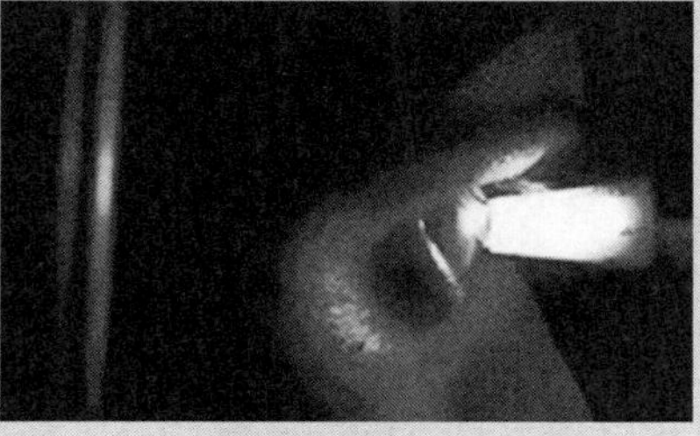

a. Tonometry
b. Laser interferometry
c. Pachymetry
d. Refractometer

Ans. a. Tonometry *Ref: AK Khurrana Theory and Practice of Refraction 3rd/ed p371*

Explanation

- Tonometry is the method of measuring IOP. The Goldmann tonometer has been the international clinical standard for measuring IOP
- LASER interoferometry in combination with slit lamp can be used to assess axial length
- Pachymetry refers to measurement of corneal thickness
  - Can be optical or ultrasonic pachymeter
- Refractrometer is used to measure the refractive index of a material

6. A 60-year-old with cataract surgery, post 1 year came with complaints of diminished vision and shows the following finding. Diagnosis?

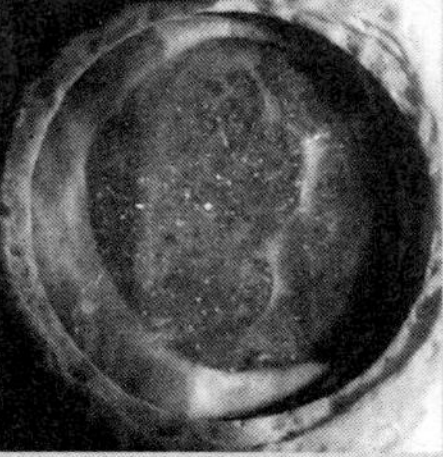

a. Irvine-Gass syndrome
b. After cataract
c. UGH syndrome
d. Endophthalmitis

Ans. b. After cataract *Ref: Yanoff Ophthalmology 4th/ed p629; Albert and Jakobiec's Principles and Practice of Ophthalmology 3rd/ed p1542-1553*

Irvine-Gass syndrome

- Pseudophakic CME is also known as Irvine-Gass syndrome is the most common cause of unexpected poor vision following cataract surgery
- Phacoemulsification cataract surgery has decreased the incidence of CME to ~9% of patients exhibiting angiographic CME, and 0–2% of patients exhibiting clinical CME.
- Complicated cataract surgery increases the risk of CME.
- There is a high incidence of CME in diabetic patients, more so in diabetic retinopathy.
- Inflammation is the most important factor associated with pseudophakic CME. The prostaglandins seem to have an important role in intraocular inflammation. The use of topical prostaglandin analogues (latanoprost) have been associated with postoperative CME after cataract surgery in glaucoma patients.

Diagnosis

- OCT may be more sensitive than angiography or clinical examination in detecting mild CME.

Treatment

- Corticosteroids: Topical, peribulbar and oral
- NSAIDs: Topical
- Carbonic anhydrase inhibitors: Oral

After cataract/secondary cataract/posterior capsule opacification

In adults, the time from surgery to visually significant opacification varies from months to years

- The rate of opacification declines with increasing age.
- In younger age groups, almost 100% opacification occurs within 2 years after surgery.
- **Incidence is lower if:**
  - Meticulous cortical cleanup is performed.
  - Hydrophobic acrylic lenses with square lens edge designs have also been found to decrease posterior capsule opacification by decreasing the migration of lens epithelial cells.

Pathogenesis

Posterior capsule opacification occurs as a result of the formation of opaque secondary membranes by active lens epithelial proliferation, transformation of lens epithelial cells into fibroblasts with contractile elements, and collagen deposition. The anterior lens epithelial cells proliferate onto the posterior capsule at the site of apposition of the anterior capsule flaps to the posterior capsule. The contraction caused by the myoblastic features of the lens epithelial cells produces wrinkling of the posterior capsule. Collagen deposition results in white fibrotic opacities.

Types

- Fibrosis that develops months to years postoperatively is caused by migration of anterior lens epithelium, fibroblastic metaplasia, and collagen production. Heavy fibrosis occurs frequently at the edge of a PC-IOL placed in the bag with apposition of anterior and posterior capsules.
- Formation of small Elschnig pearls and bladder cells (cells of Wedl), the second major form of opacity, occurs months to years after surgery. This type of opacity occurs from proliferating lens epithelial cells, which can form layers of several cells thick.

Treatment

Nd: YAG capsulotomy

UGH Syndrome

- Uveitis combined with glaucoma and hyphema results from an IOL implant rubbing against the iris.
- It was a more frequent problem with early versions of iris-fixated and AC-IOLs but is also reported with posterior chamber implants.
- Causes include imperfections in implant construction, improperly sized lenses, or imperfectly positioned lenses.
- Initially, patients are treated conservatively with ocular anti-inflammatory and antiglaucoma medications. Patients with persistent glaucoma, recurrent hemorrhage, or endothelial decompensation require removal of the implant.
- If the trabecular meshwork has not been irreversibly damaged, the glaucoma will subside.

Endophthalmitis

Can occur as acute or chronic.

Acute endophthalmitis:

- It occurs within 2–5 days of surgery and is usually fulminant
- Common organism are gram positive, coagulase negative micrococci, *Staphylococcus aureus*, streptococci and enterococcus.

Signs

- Ciliary injection
- Conjunctival chemosis
- Hypopyon
- Decreased visual acuity
- Ocular pain

Chronic endophthalmitis:

- Over several weeks
- Causative organism: *Propionibacterium acnes* and *Staphylococcus epidermidis*

Signs

- Decreased visual acuity
- Uveitis with or without hypopyon
- Sometimes plaque like material on posterior capsule

Treatment of Endophthalmitis

- Culture of aqueous or vitreous aspirate
- Intravitreal, topical or subconjunctival antibiotic

7. Identify the below finding:

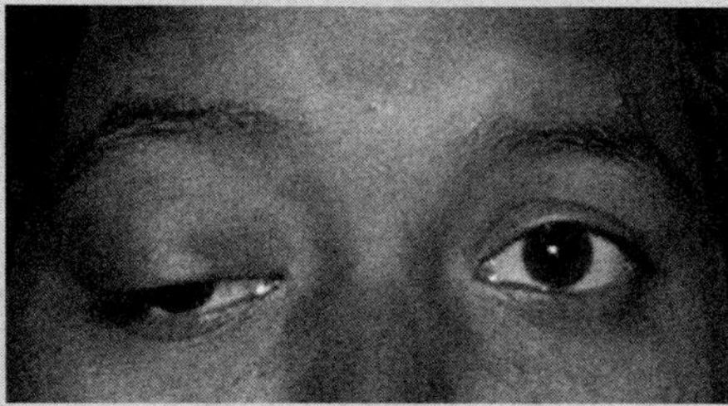

a. Ptosis of right eye
b. Entropion of right eye
c. Lagophthalmos right eye
d. Ectropion left eye

Ans. a. Ptosis of right eye

Explanation

- ❑ *Ptosis* refers to drooping of eyelids. The absence of lid crease in upper eyelids in this patient indicates that it is congenital ptosis
- ❑ Rolling inwards of the lid margin is called as ***entropion***
- ❑ ***Lagophthalmos*** refers to the inability to fully close their eyelids.
    - The symptoms are of dry and irritated eyes.
    - Common morbidities of lagophthalmos are corneal exposure and subsequent keratopathy, which may progress to corneal ulceration and infectious keratitis
- ❑ Eversion of the lid margin and the eyelashes away from the globe is called ***ectropion***.

PGI May 2017

1. True about CRAO:

a. Embolism of artery main cause
b. Painful loss of vision
c. Trucking of vessel is seen
d. Involvement of Ophthalmic Artery
e. Pale disc is a characteristic feature

Ans. c. Trucking of vessel is seen

Ref: Yanoff ophthalmology. 4th/ed p518-521; Parsons' Diseases of the Eye 22nd/ed p320-21

Explanation

- ❑ Central retinal artery obstruction (CRAO) is an abrupt diminution of blood flow through the central retinal artery severe enough to cause ischemia of inner retina.
- ❑ Mean age is 60 yrs
- ❑ Men affected more 2:1
- ❑ Majority of CRAO caused by thrombus formation at or just proximal to lamina cribrosa. 20–25% cases are due to emboli
- ❑ Atherosclerosis main cause, inflammation (vasculitis, mucormycosis)
- ❑ Manifestation:
    - Abrupt painless diminution of vision (DOV) but no light perception uncommon, can occur if associated with ophthalmic artery
    - Amaurosis fugax precedes visual loss in 10%
    - Ischemic whitening of retina more so at posterior pole
    - Cherry rod spot at macula
    - Cattle truck appearance: when obstruction is not complete, the flow may be partially restored in the course of few days in which case gentle pressure upon the globe may break up the column of venous blood into red beads separated by clear spaces
    - NVD (2%) and NVI (18%) may result
    - Inner retinal atrophies apart from outer retina which receives nourishment from choroid
    - If cilioretinal retinal artery is present macular sparing occurs.

Diagnosis:

- ❑ FA: Delayed arm to retina time
- ❑ OCT: Acute phase inner retinal thickening and later thinning
- ❑ ERG: Absent b wave with intact a wave

Pathology:

- ❑ Coagulative necrosis of inner retinal tissue

Treatment

- ❑ Breathing carbogen to increase retinal oxygenation
- ❑ Increase in retinal blood flow by lowering IOP: Ocular massage, paracentesis or ocular hypotensive drug
- ❑ Intravenous thrombolysis

2. Ocular features seen in diabetes:

a. Cataract
b. Papillopathy
c. Rhegmatogenous retinal detachment is characteristic of advanced diabetic retinopathy.
d. Papillitis
e. Removal causes cystoid macular edema

Ans. a. Cataract; b. Papillopathy and e. Removal causes cystoid macular edema

Ref: Parsons' Diseases of the Eye 22nd/ed p268; Yanoff Ophthalmology 4th/ed p518-521

EXPLANATION

- ❑ Senile cataract tends to develop at an earlier age and more rapidly in diabetic subjects
- ❑ Cataracts are dependent on duration of diabetes and progresses more rapidly
- ❑ Mechanism being glycation, carbamylation and increased oxidative damage
- ❑ True diabetic cataract occurs in young people. Manifests as fluid vacuoles under anterior and posterior part of capsule and later results in snowstorm snowflake cataract
- ❑ Diabetics are more susceptible to papilledema characterized by acute disc edema without the pale swelling of AION.
- ❑ Papillitis is not associated with diabetics
- ❑ Patients with diabetes more so with DR are at increased risk of developing CME post cataract surgery
- ❑ The retinal detachment common is tractional retina detachment.

3. True regarding congenital ptosis:

a. Lid lag
b. Lagophthalmos
c. Levator palpebrae resection surgery is done
d. Lid skin crease visible
e. Amblyopia

Ans. c. Levator palpebrae resection surgery is done and e. Amblyopia

Ref: Parsons' Diseases of the Eye 22nd/ed p461-62

EXPLANATION

- ❑ Lid lag is a feature of thyroid ophthalmopathy
- ❑ Usually bilateral
- ❑ Due to defective development of muscles
- ❑ Important feature is dystrophic levator muscle which leads to wider palpebral aperture in down gaze as dystrophic muscle can neither contract nor relax normally
- ❑ The second important distinguishing feature is absent lid crease

- Two types:
  - Simple congenital ptosis
  - Complicated congenital ptosis where there is associated maldevelopment of surrounding structure like defective Bell's phenomenon, jaw winking (Marcus Gunn ptosis)
- Blepharophimosis syndrome associated ptosis
- **Management:**

Ptosis surgery	Requisite levator action	Amount of ptosis that can be treated	Indication
Fasanella- Servat	Good	<2 mm	Horner syndrome
Levator resection-anterior approach	Moderate	Any	Large resection in ptosis (congenital acquired)
Levator resection-conjuctival approach	Moderate	Any	Moderate ptosis congenital or acquired
Levator resection with aponeurotic reinsertion	Moderate	Any	Acquired ptosis
Frontalis suspension	Poor	>2 mm	Congenital esp Marcus Gunn

4. Blue sclera is associated with:

a. Osteogenesis imperfecta
b. Thin sclera
c. Keratoconus
d. Scleritis
e. Keratoglobus

Ans. a. Osteogenesis imperfecta; b. Thin sclera; c. Keratoconus and e. Kertoglobus *Ref: Parsons' Diseases of the Eye 22nd/ed p230-31*

EXPLANATION

- Sclera is normally bluish in color but the effect decreases with age
- Osteogenesis imperfecta: Frequent bone fractures (fragilitas ossium), blue sclera and deafness. Affects both sexes
- Other systemic disease :
  - Ehler Danlos syndrome
  - Marfan syndrome
  - Pseudoxanthoma elasticum
- Local ocular disease associated are:
  - Keratoconus
  - Keratoglobus
- Histologically, sclera is thin so uveal pigment shines through thin sclera and produces blue color

5. Corneal ulcer is:

a. Loss of integrity in corneal endothelium
b. Loss of integrity in corneal epithelium
c. Loss of integrity in corneal epithelium and loss of sensation
d. Breach of epithelium with corneal thinning
e. Breach of epithelium with underlying inflammation

Ans. b. Loss of integrity in corneal epithelium and e. Breach of epithelium with underlying inflammation *Ref: Parsons' Diseases of the Eye 22nd/ed p193-94*

Explanation

- Loss of integrity of corneal epithelium alone is termed as epithelial abrasion/erosion
- Heals within 12–24 hrs by regeneration of the epithelial cells from periphery

Corneal ulcer:

- Loss of epithelium with inflammation is termed as corneal ulcer
- The inflammation is visible as a grayish haze or loss of clarity
- If it is accompanied by outpouring of leukocytes color is more off white or yellowish
- Corneal ulcer can be sterile or infective

6. In cataract surgery what can prevent endophthalmitis?

a. Preop antibiotics
b. Postop antibiotics
c. Intracameral antibiotics
d. Clean instruments and OT
e. Use of povidone iodine

Ans: All

Ref: Barry P, Cordovés L, Gardner S. ESCRS guidelines for prevention and treatment of endophthalmitis following cataract surgery: data, dilemmas and conclusions. European Society of Cataract and Refractive Surgeons, 2013.

Explanation

- The ESCRS study found that the risk for contracting postoperative endophthalmitis was significantly reduced, approximately 5-fold, by an intracameral injection of 1 mg cefuroxime at the close of surgery.

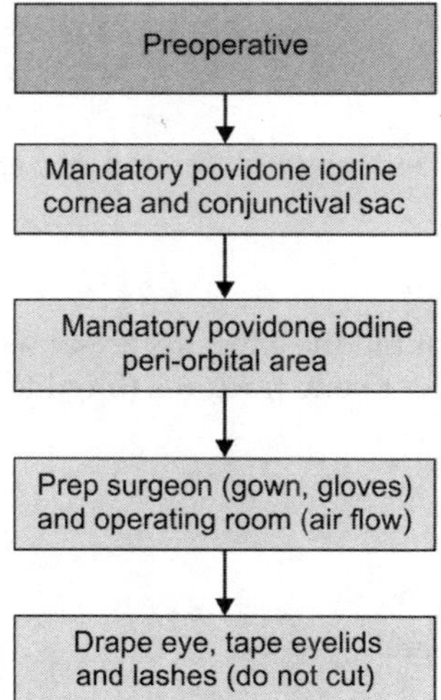

- All instruments for surgery should be sterile. Single use is even more robust.
- Preoperative topical antibiotics seems to reduce the no of bacteria in conjunctival sac
- Vancomycin and other reserve antibiotics should not be used for prophylaxis
- In order to reduce the risk of infection particularly after clear corneal incision until wound is secure use of preoperatively applied topical antibiotics is recommended for two weeks but not proven.

7. With regard to medial longitudinal fasciculus following is true:

a. MLF lesions affect the horizontal saccades
b. Left INO involves defective left adduction and ataxic nystagmus of the right eye on right gaze.

c. Convergence intact
d. In one and half syndrome, the only residual movement is abduction of the ipsilateral eye which also exhibits ataxic nystagmus
e. MLF lesion leads to loss of accomodation

Ans: a. MLF lesions affect the horizontal saccades; b. Left INO involves defective left adduction and ataxic nystagmus of the right eye on right gaze and c. Convergence intact

Ref: Kanski Clinical Ophthalmology a Systemic Approach 7th/ed p839-40.

EXPLANATION

Lesion affecting horizontal saccades:

- PPRF lesion gives rise to ipsilateral horizontal gaze palsy with inability to look in the direction of the lesion.
- MLF lesion is responsible for the clinical syndrome of internuclear ophthalmoplegia (INO). A left INO is characterized by
  - Straight eyes in the primary position.
  - Defective left adduction and ataxic nystagmus of the right eye on right gaze.
  - Left gaze is normal.
- *Convergence is intact* if the lesion is discrete; this may help to differentiate INO from myasthenia. Vertical nystagmus occurs on attempted upgaze.
- Bilateral INO is characterized by:
  - Limitation of left adduction and ataxic nystagmus of the right eye on right gaze.
  - Limitation of right adduction and ataxic nystagmus of the left eye on left gaze.
- Convergence is intact if the lesion is discrete but may be absent if the lesion is extensive.
- PPRF and MLF combined lesions on the same side give rise to the *'one-and-a-half syndrome'* which is characterized by a combination of ipsilateral gaze palsy and INO so that the only residual movement is abduction of the contralateral eye which also exhibits ataxic nystagmus.

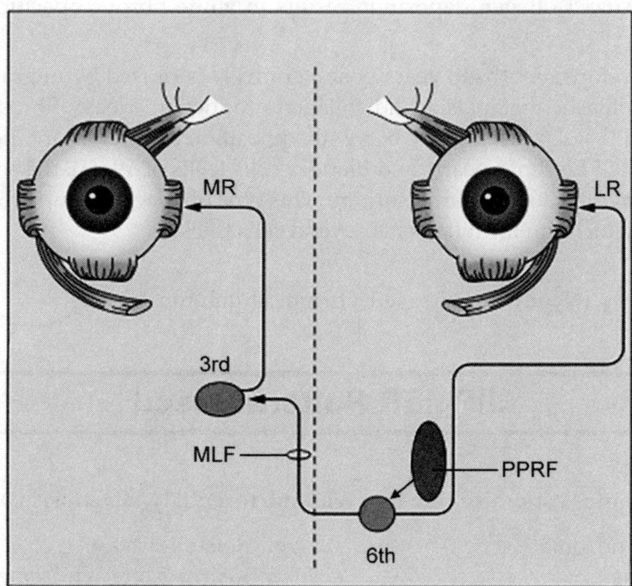

Fig. 3: Showing anatomical pathways for horizontal eye movements (PPRF = paramedian pontine reticular formation; MLF = medial longitudinal fasciculus; MR = medial rectus; LR = lateral rectus)

8. True about after cataract is/are:

a. Meticulous cortical cleanup prevents its formation
b. Best treated by Nd:YAG laser
c. More common in diabetic
d. Less with hydrophilic acrylic IOL
e. More in elderly compared to young secondary cataract

Ans. a. Meticulous cortical cleanup prevents its formation; b. Best treated by Nd:YAG laser; c. More common in diabetic and d. Less with hydrophilic acrylic IOL

Ref: Albert and Jakobiec's Principles and Practice of Ophthalmology. 3rd/ed p1542-1553

EXPLANATION

After cataract/secondary cataract/posterior capsule opacification

- In adults, the time from surgery to visually significant opacification varies from months to years
- The rate of opacification declines with increasing age.
- In younger age groups, almost 100% opacification occurs within 2 years after surgery.
- Incidence is lower if:
  - Meticulous cortical cleanup is performed.
  - Hydrophobic acrylic lenses with square lens edge designs have also been found to decrease posterior capsule opacification by decreasing the migration of lens epithelial cells.

Pathogenesis

Posterior capsule opacification occurs as a result of the formation of opaque secondary membranes by active lens epithelial proliferation, transformation of lens epithelial cells into fibroblasts with contractile elements, and collagen deposition. The anterior lens epithelial cells proliferate onto the posterior capsule at the site of apposition of the anterior capsule flaps to the posterior capsule. The contraction caused by the myoblastic features of the lens epithelial cells produces wrinkling of the posterior capsule. Collagen deposition results in white fibrotic opacities.

Types

- Fibrosis that develops months to years postoperatively is caused by migration of anterior lens epithelium, fibroblastic metaplasia, and collagen production. Heavy fibrosis occurs frequently at the edge of a PC-IOL placed in the bag with apposition of anterior and posterior capsules.
- Formation of small Elschnig pearls and bladder cells (cells of Wedl), the second major form of opacity, occurs months to years after surgery. This type of opacity occurs from proliferating lens epithelial cells, which can form layers of several cells thick.

Treatment

Nd: YAG capsulotomy (Neodymium-doped yttrium aluminum garnet)

JIPMER Pattern Based

1. Retinitis pigmentosa and bird like face with microcephaly, diagnosis is:

a. Cockayne syndrome
b. Refsum disease
c. Usher disease
d. Kearns Sayre syndrome

Ans. a. Cockayne syndrome

Ref: Kanski Clinical Ophthalmology a Systemic Approach 7th/ed p654-56;852-53

EXPLANATION

Cockayne syndrome is characterized by:

- ❑ Bird like face
- ❑ Microcephaly
- ❑ Premature aging
- ❑ Dwarfism
- ❑ Cachexia
- ❑ Sunken eyes
- ❑ Usually dies before 30
- ❑ Other ocular association: RP, pupillary unresponsiveness, hypermetropia, nystagmus, hypoplastic irides and cataract

Bardet–Biedl syndrome

- ❑ Inheritance is genetically heterogeneous.
- ❑ Systemic features include hypogonadism in males, polydactyly, truncal obesity, renal anomalies and mental handicap.
- ❑ Fundus typically shows a bull's eye maculopathy due to cone-rod dystrophy. Less frequently findings are typical RP, RP sine pigmentosa and retinitis punctata albescens.

Usher syndrome

- ❑ Usher syndrome accounts for about 5% of all cases of profound deafness in children, and is responsible for about half of all cases of combined deafness and blindness.
- ❑ There are three major types
- ❑ Inheritance is AR (genetically heterogeneous).
- ❑ Classification
  a. Type I (75% of patients): Congenital, profound deafness with vestibular dysfunction; visual loss due to RP with extinguished ERG occurs in the 1st decade.
  b. Type II (23%): Congenital, moderate to severe deafness with normal vestibular function; visual loss occurs in the 2nd decade.
  c. Type III (2%): Progressive hearing loss and progressive vestibular dysfunction and relatively late- onset pigmentary retinopathy.
- ❑ Systemic features include premature ageing beginning in infancy, dwarfism, skeletal anomalies, deafness, photosensitivity, mental handicap and early demise.
- ❑ Fundus shows salt and pepper pigmentation and optic atrophy.
- ❑ Other ocular features are miosis, cataract and orbital fat atrophy.

Refsum disease

- ❑ Inheritance is AR. The infantile and adult forms are genetically distinct
- ❑ Pathogenesis. Deficiency in phytanic acid alpha- hydrolase results in accumulation of phytanic acid throughout the body. Early detection and treatment with a diet low in phytanic acid can arrest disease progression.
- ❑ Systemic features
  - Infantile disease is characterized by dysmorphic facies, mental handicap, hepatomegaly and deafness
  - Adult disease is characterized by cerebellar ataxia, polyneuropathy, anosmia, deafness, cardiomyopathy and ichthyosis
- ❑ Fundus appearance may be similar to RP or merely show salt-and-pepper changes.
- ❑ Other ocular features include cataract, prominent corneal nerves, optic atrophy, nystagmus and poorly dilating pupils.

Kearns–Sayre syndrome

- Kearns–Sayre syndrome is characterized by chronic progressive external ophthalmoplegia
- Pathogenesis. Mitochondrial cytopathy associated with mitochondrial DNA deletions. Histology of extraocular muscles shows 'ragged red bres' due to intramuscular accumulation of abnormal mitochondria
- Presentation is in the first and second decades with an insidious onset progressive external ophthalmoplegia.
- Signs
  - Cerebellar ataxia and heart block.
  - Fatigue and proximal muscle weakness are common.
  - Deafness, diabetes, short stature, renal disease and dementia may be present.
- The fundus usually has a 'salt and pepper' appearance most striking at the macula; less frequently findings are typical RP or choroidal atrophy similar to choroideremia.

Other association with RP

- *Bassen–Kornzweig syndrome (abetalipoproteinaemia)*

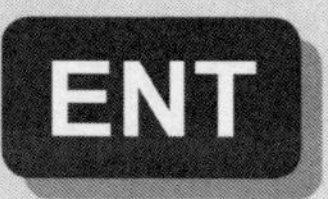

Author: Jyotsana Priya, Co-author: Vishakha Gupta

AIIMS MAY 2017

1. Audiogram of 30-year-old female is shown below. Most likely diagnosis is:

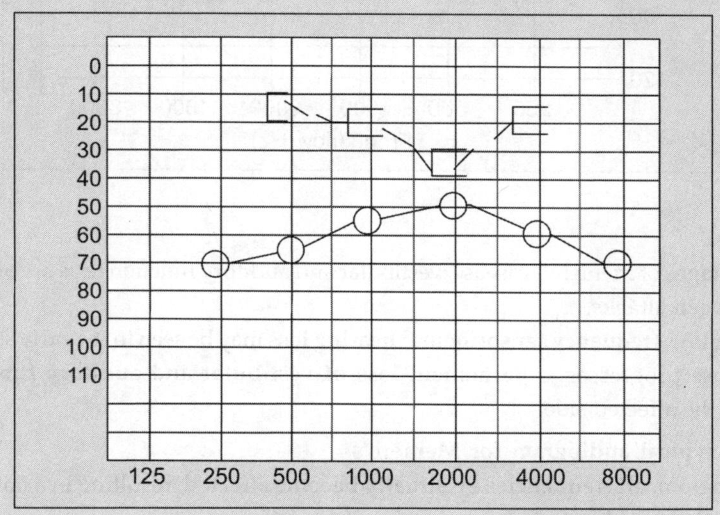

a. Otosclerosis
b. Meniere's
c. Ototoxicity
d. Otitis media

Ans. a. Otosclerosis

Ref. Scott-Brown's Otorhinolaryngology, Head and Neck Surgery 7th/ed p3462,3758

EXPLANATION

Otosclerosis:

- Pure tone audiometry shows **loss of air conduction,** more for lower frequencies.
- Bone conduction is normal. In some cases, there is a **dip in bone conduction curve.** It is different at different frequencies but **maximum at 2000 Hz** and is called the **Carhart's notch**.
- Carhart's notch disappears after successful stapedectomy

Shown below a typical audiogram for otosclerosis

- Audiogram showing classical appearance of a conductive impairment in clinical otosclerosis.
- The **air-bone gap is greater at the lower frequencies** and a Carhart notch is present at 2 kHz.

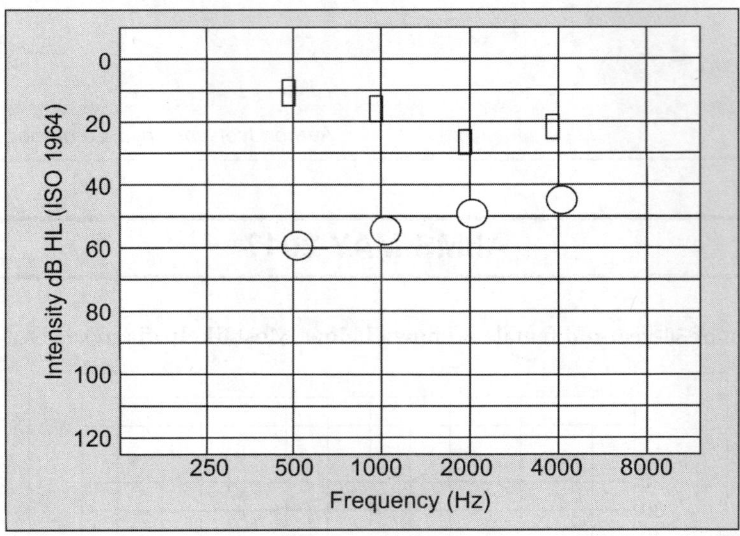

Meniere's disease

- In the **early stages** of Meniere's disease, vestibular and auditory function tests are often **completely normal between attacks.**
- A fluctuating **low-frequency sensorineural hearing loss** may be seen in the early stages of disease.
- As the disease progresses, a **permanent loss of vestibular and auditory function** becomes apparent on the affected side.

Shown below a typical audiogram for Meniere's

- On the audiogram, **all frequencies eventually become affected**, resulting in a **flat sensorineural hearing loss that is at least moderate in severity.**

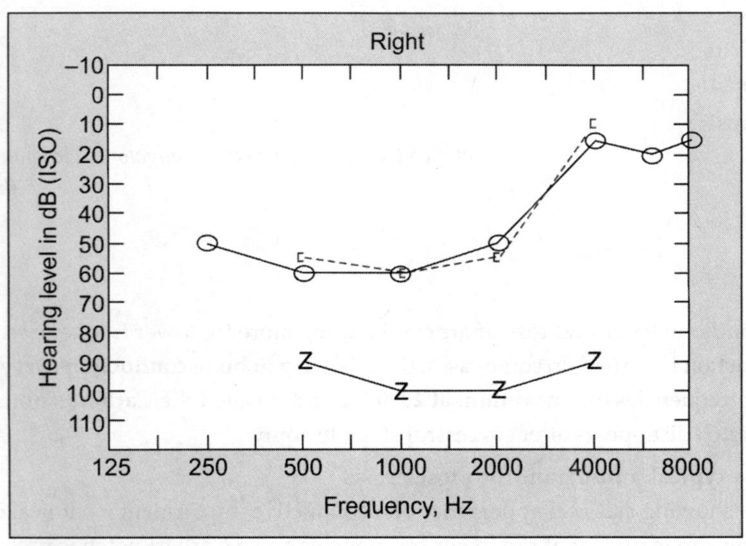

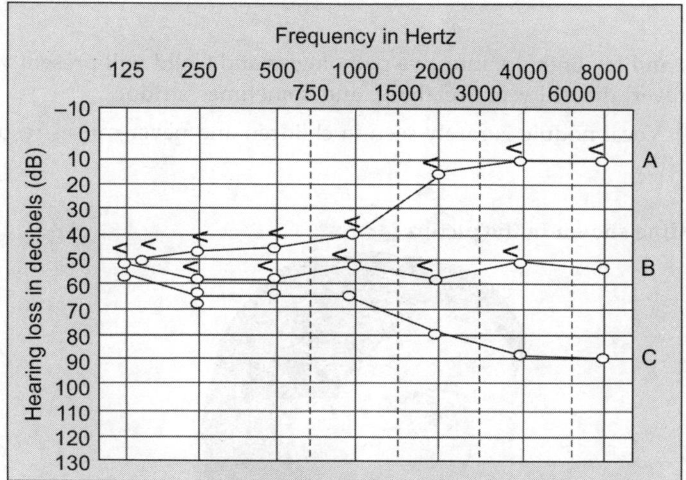

(A) Audiogram is early Meniere's disease. Note: Hearing loss is sensorineural and more in lower frequencies—the rising curve. As the disease progresses, middle and higher frequencies get involved and audiogram becomes flat or falling type (B&C).

2. Which of the following arteries is never ligated in epistaxis control?

a. Internal maxillary artery
b. External carotid artery
c. Internal carotid artery
d. Anterior ethmoidal artery

Ans. c. Internal carotid artery

Ref. Scott-Brown's Otorhinolaryngology, Head and Neck Surgery 7th/ed p1603

Explanation

Epistaxis control

- **Ligation is reserved for intractable bleeding** where the source cannot be located or controlled by the other techniques.
- Ligation should be performed as close as possible to the likely bleeding point; thus the **hierarchy of ligation** is:
  - Sphenopalatine artery;
  - Internal maxillary artery;
  - External carotid artery;
  - Anterior/posterior ethmoidal artery.

3. A 5-year-old child presents with gradually progressive hoarseness in voice for the last 3 months and difficulty in breathing for the last 2 weeks. Most likely diagnosis is:

a. Respiratory papillomatosis
b. Acute epiglottitis
c. Croup
d. Vocal cord nodule

Ans. a. Respiratory papillomatosis

Ref: Scott Brown 7th/ed Vol 1, p1176, Dhingra 6th/ed p305; Current Otolaryngology 2nd/ed, Chapter 32

Explanation

About Option (b) and (c): Both are infective pathologies and Child will present with toxic features like severe pain, fever, difficulty in breathing, and sometimes stridor

About Option (d): Vocal nodule is rarely seen in children and never causes respiratory difficulty.

4. Identify the line shown in the picture?

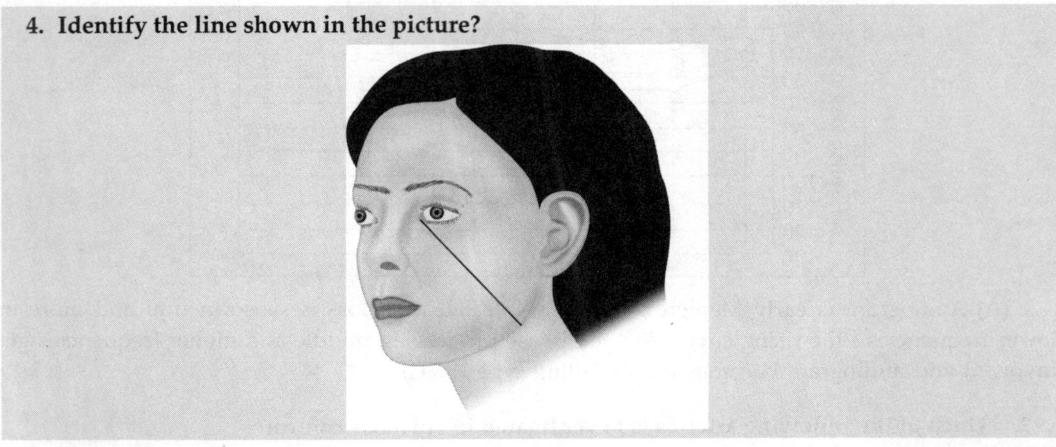

a. Sebileau line
b. Ohngren's line
c. Donaldson line
d. Frankfurt line

Ans. b. Ohngren's line

Ref. Diseases of Ear, Nose and Throat 5th/ed, Pl Dhingra p221

Explanation

Ohngren line:

The line extends an imaginary plane from the medial canthus to the angle of the mandible, which gives a rough estimate of the dividing line between tumors that may be resected with a good prognosis (below the line) and those with a poor prognosis (above the line).

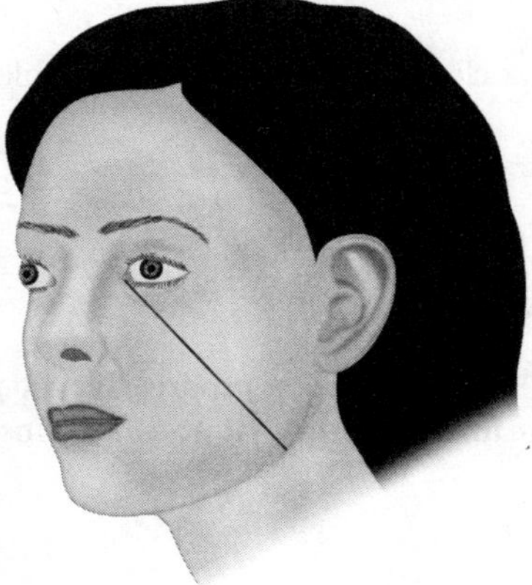

Ref. Cummings Otolaryngology–Head and Neck Surgery 6th/ed p1180

Donaldson's Line: Imaginary line from the lateral semicircular canal bisecting perpendicularly the posterior semicircular canal, marks the superior limit of where the endolymphatic sac is found.

Sebileau Line:

Lederman's classification (maxillary carcinoma) uses two horizontal lines of Sebileau; one passing through the floors of orbits and the other through floors of antra, thus dividing the area into:

a. Suprastructure: Ethmoid, sphenoid and frontal sinuses and the olfactory area of nose.
b. Mesostructure: Maxillary sinus and the respiratory part of nose.
c. Infrastructure: Containing alveolar process.

This classification further uses vertical lines, extending down the medial walls of orbit to separate ethmoid sinuses and nasal fossa from the maxillary sinuses.

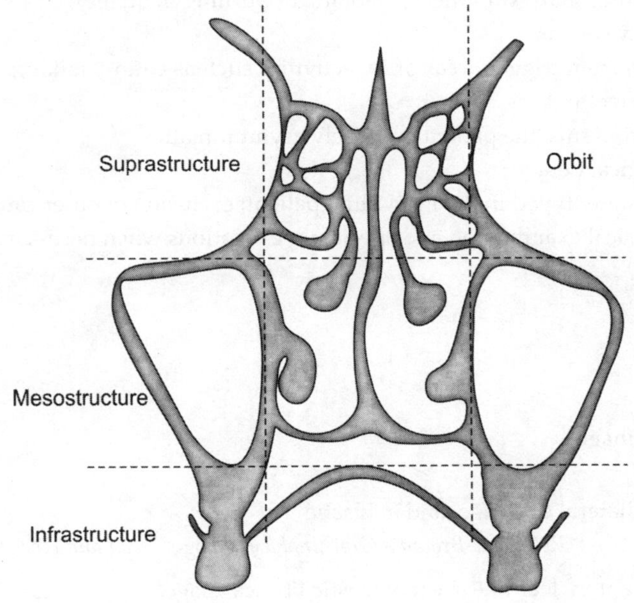

PGI MAY 2017

1. Criteria for trigeminal neuralgia is/are:

a. Bilateral
b. Stabbing pain
c. Associated with nerve deficit
d. Severe intensity of pain
e. Paroxysmal attacks of facial pain that lasts less than two minutes

Ans. b. Stabbing pain; d. Severe intensity of pain and e. Paroxysmal attacks of facial pain that lasts less than two minutes

Ref. Scott-Brown's Otorhinolaryngology, Head and Neck Surgery 7th/ed p1829,1830

- ❑ **Trigeminal neuralgia (idiopathic trigeminal neuralgia; benign paroxysmal trigeminal neuralgia; Tic Doloureux)**
- ❑ Trigeminal neuralgia (TN) causes episodes of unilateral intense, stabbing, electric shock-like pain in the jaw or the face.

- ❑ TN onset is mainly in the 50–70 year age group.
- ❑ The cause is unclear, but one hypothesis is that there may be compression around the trigeminal root in the posterior cranial fossa, possibly due to a cerebral blood vessel becoming atherosclerotic, and therefore less flexible with age, and then pressing on the roots of the trigeminal nerve causing neuronal discharge.

TN has the following main characteristics (International Headache Society):

- ❑ Paroxysmal attacks of facial or frontal pain which lasts a few seconds to less than two minutes.
- ❑ The pain also has the following features:
  - Distribution along one or more divisions of the trigeminal nerve;
  - Sudden intense, sharp superficial, stabbing or burning in quality;
  - Pain intensity severe;
  - Precipitation from trigger areas or by activities such as eating, talking, washing the face or cleaning the teeth;
  - Between paroxysms, the patient is entirely asymptomatic;
  - No neurological deficit;
  - Attacks are stereotyped in the individual patient; exclusion of other causes of facial pain by history, physical examination and special investigations when necessary.

2. Epiglottis:

a. Oval
b. Mucous
c. Serous
d. Bilateral drainage
e. Elastic

Ans. b. Mucous; d. Bilateral drainage, and e. Elastic

Ref. Scott-Brown's Otorhinolaryngology, Head and Neck Surgery 7th/ed p2133

- ❑ The epiglottis is a thin, leaf-like sheet of elastic fibrocartilage.
- ❑ The posterior surface of the cartilage is indented by numerous small pits into which mucus glands project.
- ❑ The anterior surface of the epiglottis is covered with mucous membrane superiorly and forms the posterior wall of the vallecula.
- ❑ The mucous membrane overlying the epiglottis is reflected on to the base of the tongue, forming the glossoepiglottic fold in the midline and laterally the lateral glossoepiglottic folds.

3. Cochlear implant absolutely contraindicated in:

a. Labyrinthine otosclerosis
b. Active middle ear disease
c. Agenesis of cochlea
d. Agenesis of auditory nerve
e. Uncontrolled epilepsy

Ans. c. Agenesis of cochlea and d. Agenesis of auditory nerve

Ref. Scott-Brown's Otorhinolaryngology, Head and Neck Surgery 7th/ed p3651
Cummings Otolaryngology–Head and Neck Surgery, 6th/ed p2431

Contraindications for the Cochlear Implantation:	
Absolute	**Relative**
• Agenesia of cochlea • Agenesia of cochlear nerve • Severe mental disease • Acute/chronic otitis media and mastoiditis Without eradication of the disease mental retardation to cooperate with speech training	• Inappropriate medical conditions (e.g. pulmonary, cardiac, hematologic) • Uncontrolled epilepsy • Not being available for postoperative rehabilitation • Active middle ear disease, either acute or chronic

4. Foreign bodies in child *except*:

a. Vegetable
b. Pebble
c. Button batteries
d. Coins
e. None

Ans. e. None *Ref. Scott-Brown's Otorhinolaryngology, Head and Neck Surgery 7th/ed p1184-1193*

5. Schwartz sign:

a. Indicate inactive otosclerosis
b. Red blush of tympanic membrane
c. Seen in area of round window
d. Seen in area of oval window
e. Indicate active otosclerosis

Ans. b. Red blush of tympanic membrane; c. Seen in area of round window and e. Indicate active otosclerosis *Ref. Diseases of Ear, Nose and Throat 5th/ed, PL Dhingra p461*

Schwartz sign is a pink reflex, seen through intact tympanic membrane, in the area of oval window. It indicates active otosclerosis usually during pregnancy.

JIPMER Pattern Based

1. Landmark of geniculate ganglion for facial nerve decompression:

a. Pyramid
b. Processus cochleariformis
c. Incus neck
d. Oval window

Ans. b. Processus cochleariformis *Ref. Diseases of Ear, Nose and Throat 5th/ed, PL Dhingra p103*

Explanation

- *Processus cochleariformis.* It demarcates the geniculate ganglion which lies just anterior to it. Tympanic segment of the nerve starts at this level.
- *Oval window and horizontal canal.* The tympanic segment of facial nerve runs above the oval window (stapes) and below the horizontal canal.
- *Short process of incus.* Facial nerve lies medial to the short process of incus at the level of aditus.
- *Pyramid.* Nerve runs behind the pyramid and the posterior tympanic sulcus.

2. A child with tubotympanic CSOM and suffering from meningitis. What is the congenital preformed route of spread of infection?

a. Hyrtl fissure
b. Foramen of Huschke
c. Fissure of Santorini
d. Petrosquamons septum

Ans. d. Petrosquamons septum *Ref. Diseases of Ear, Nose and Throat 5th/ed, PL Dhingra p4, 84*

Explanation

- Cartilaginous part of EAC has two deficiencies—the *"fissures of Santorini"* in this part of the cartilage and through them the parotid or superficial mastoid infections can appear in the canal, or vice versa.
- Antero-inferior part of the bony canal of EAC may present a deficiency (*foramen of Huschke*) in children up to the age of four or sometimes in adults, permitting infections to and from the parotid.
- *Infection* can easily travel beyond the middle ear cleft if preformed pathways exist.

Preformed Pathways

i. Congenital dehiscences, e.g. in bony facial canal, floor of middle ear over the jugular bulb.
ii. Patent sutures, e.g. petrosquamous suture.
iii. Previous skull fractures. The fracture sites heal only by fibrous scar which permits infection.
iv. Surgical defects, e.g. stapedectomy, fenestration and mastoidectomy with exposure of dura.
v. Oval and round windows.
vi. Infection from labyrinth can travel along internal acoustic meatus, aqueducts of the vestibule and that of the cochlea to the meninges.

3. All are true about otoacoustic emissions *except*:

a. OAEs are auditory evoked potentials
b. Measured in decibels (dBSPL)
c. Can be seen during sleep
d. Low intensity sounds

Ans. a. OAEs are auditory evoked potentials *Ref. 1. Shambaugh Surgery of the Ear 6th/ed p19; 2. Clinical Audio-Vestibulometry for Otologists and Neurologists: Anirban Biswas 5th/ed p244*

Explanation

- OAEs **are low-intensity sounds** that are generated by the cochlea either spontaneously or evoked by an auditory stimulus and propagate through the middle ear into the ear canal.
- OAEs are by-product of active processing by the outer-hair cell system. OAEs are present when outer-hair cells are healthy and absent when outer-hair cells are damaged. Thus, OAEs reveal, an incoming **the integrity of outer-hair cell function.**
- OAEs are biological phenomenon generated in normal cochlea when cochlea processes incoming auditory impulse. This is a mechanical activity taking place in outer hair cells before the inner hair cells transducer the mechanical activity into action potentials.
- It is a preneural activity and there are no action potentials generated. OAEs are not auditory evoked potentials.
- OAEs are sounds, they are measured in decibels (dBSPL).

There are two broad categories of OAEs: spontaneous and evoked.

A. Transient evoked OAEs (TEOAEs). Evoked by clicks. A series of click stimuli are presented at 80-85 dBSPL and response recorded.
B. Distortion product OAEs (DPOAEs). Two tones are simultaneously presented to the cochlea to produce distortion products. They have been used to test hearing in the range of 1000-8000 Hz.

Uses

- ❑ OAEs are used as a screening test of hearing in neonates and to test hearing in uncooperative or mentally challenged individuals after sedation. **Sedation does not interfere with OAEs.**
- ❑ They help to distinguish cochlear from retrocochlear hearing loss. OAEs are absent in cochlear lesions, e.g. ototoxic sensorineural hearing loss. They detect ototoxic effects earlier than pure-tone audiometry.
- ❑ OAEs are also useful to diagnose retrocochlear pathology, especially auditory neuropathy. Auditory neuropathy is a neurologic disorder of CN VIII. Audiometric tests, e.g. SNHL for pure tones, impaired speech discrimination score, absent or abnormal auditory brainstem response, show a retrocochlear type of lesion but OAEs are normal.

4. Cotton Myer's classification for subglottic stenosis grade 2:

a. <50%
b. 71–99%
c. 30%
d. 51–75%
e. 51–70%

Ans. e. 51–70% *Ref. Scott-Brown's Otorhinolaryngology, Head and Neck Surgery 7th/ed p2282*

EXPLANATION

Myer's and Cotton

- ❑ Devised a classification scheme for grading circumferential subglottic stenosis from I-IV.
- ❑ This grading system applies mainly to circumferential stenosis and does not apply to other types of SGS or combined stenoses.
- ❑ The scale describes stenosis as a percent of area that is obstructed.
- ❑ The system contains 4 grades, as follows:
  - **Grade I:** Obstruction of 0–50% of the lumen obstruction
  - **Grade II:** Obstruction of 51–70% of the lumen
  - **Grade III:** Obstruction of 71–99% of the lumen
  - **Grade IV:** Obstruction of 100% of the lumen (i.e. no detectable lumen)

5. A Singer who is unable to increase pitch of her voice after thyroid surgery is due to injury of:

a. Unilateral recurrent laryngeal nerve
b. Bilateral recurrent laryngeal nerve
c. Unilateral superior laryngeal nerve
d. Bilateral superior laryngeal nerve

Ans. c. Unilateral superior laryngeal nerve *Ref. Scott Brown's Otorhinolaryngology, Head and Neck Surgery 7th/ed p1426*

EXPLANATION

- ❑ **The pitch of the voice is defined as the "rate of vibration of the vocal folds".**
- ❑ **Pitch is the physiological property which permits placing of a note in the scale from low to high.**
- ❑ **Alteration in pitch is achieved by changes in length, tension, shape and size of vocal cord.**
- ❑ **Length and tension changes in vocal cord are controlled by thyroarytenoid muscle and cricothyroid. Cricothyroid muscle lengthen and tense the ipsilateral true vocal cord.**
- ❑ **Cricothyroid muscle is supplied by external branch of superior laryngeal nerve.**
- ❑ **Paralysis of superior laryngeal nerve causes paralysis of cricothyroid muscle and ipsilateral anesthesia of the larynx above the vocal cord. Paralysis of cricothyroid can also occur when external laryngeal nerve is involved in thyroid surgery, tumors, neuritis or diphtheria.**

Preventive and Social Medicine

Author: Bahram Gor, Co-author: Abhishek Pathania

AIIMS May 2017

1. A researcher said he has discovered a new drug which is effective in chronic hypertensive with a p-value of <0.10. Which of the following is true regarding the same?

a. The test is 90% reproducible
b. 90% of test results could have occurred by chance
c. Not more than 10% of the people benefitted by the drug could be due to chance
d. 90% of patients will be benefitted by giving the drug

Ans. c. Not more than 10% of the people benefitted by the drug could be due to chance

Ref: A Dictionary of Epidemiology, Porta M, 5th/ed p199, Park 24th, p126

Explanation

This question is based on the concept of p-value and if one knows the definition and utility of p-value such questions can never go wrong.

p-value

- The letter P stands for probability.
- The *p-value* is probability of null hypothesis being true.
- Null hypothesis states that there is 'no difference between two treatments' or the observed difference is due to chance alone
- In other words p-value is the probability that the difference observed could have occurred **by chance alone.**
- p-value < 0.05 means → < 5% probability of null hypothesis being true or in other words, probability of observing the difference due to chance alone is <5%
- To simplify p-value = 0.05 means, if a study is repeated 100 times, then 5 times null hypothesis will be accepted and 95 times the null hypothesis will be rejected.
- For the given question null hypothesis will be *'drug has no antihypertensive effect'* or *'the antihypertensive effect of the drug is due to chance alone'*.
- p-value of <0.10 means, the probability of *'the antihypertensive effect of the drug is due to chance alone'* is < 10%. Or in other words, ***"not more than 10% of the people benefitted by the drug could be due to chance". (Thus the answer)***

Hint: Whenever we talk about p-value, we talk about chance, i.e. probability that the event occurs by chance alone. In this example, event is control of hypertension.

2. Which point in the below natural history of disease marks the onset of symptoms?

D

A B C

Stage of susceptibility	Stage of subclinical disease	Stage of clinical disease	Stage of recovery, disability or death

a. A
b. B
c. C
d. D

Ans. c. C *Ref: Leon Gordis Epidemiology, 5th/ed p21*

EXPLANATION

The question is regarding the natural history of disease and the four stages are shown in the figure.

- Natural history of disease refers to the progression of a disease process in an individual over time, in the absence of treatment.
  In the given question,
- Point A is the onset of disease in the susceptible host.
- Point B has been correctly labeled (subclinical disease; pathologic changes)
- Point C is the onset of symptoms and
- Point D is the time when symptoms can be used to diagnose the disease clinically.

3. A child with Sputum negative and chest X-ray suggestive of tuberculosis. Next step to do according to revised RNTCP criteria?

a. NAAT
b. Culture
c. Line probe assay
d. Tuberculin test

Ans. a. NAAT *Ref: Technical and Operational Guidelines for TB Control in India 2016*

EXPLANATION

- The latest RNTCP guidelines suggest cartridge-based nucleic acid amplification test (CBNAAT) in such cases.
- *Option c:* Line probe assay and culture are the last resort when diagnosis is unclear.
- *Option d:* Tuberculin test is not used for diagnosis according to the new guidelines.

The new algorithm for pulmonary TB is as follows:

Diagnostic algorithm for pulmonary TB

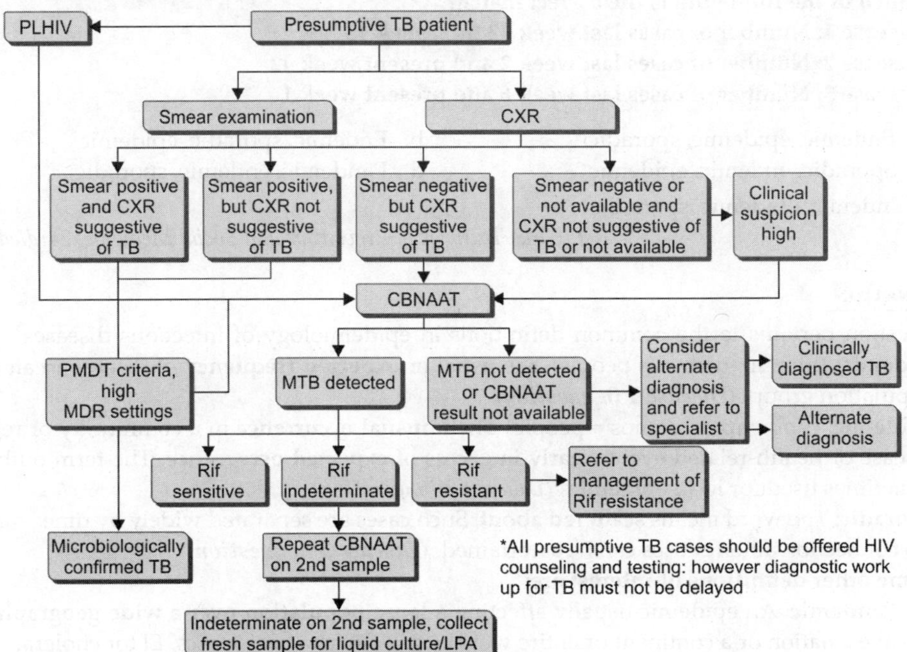

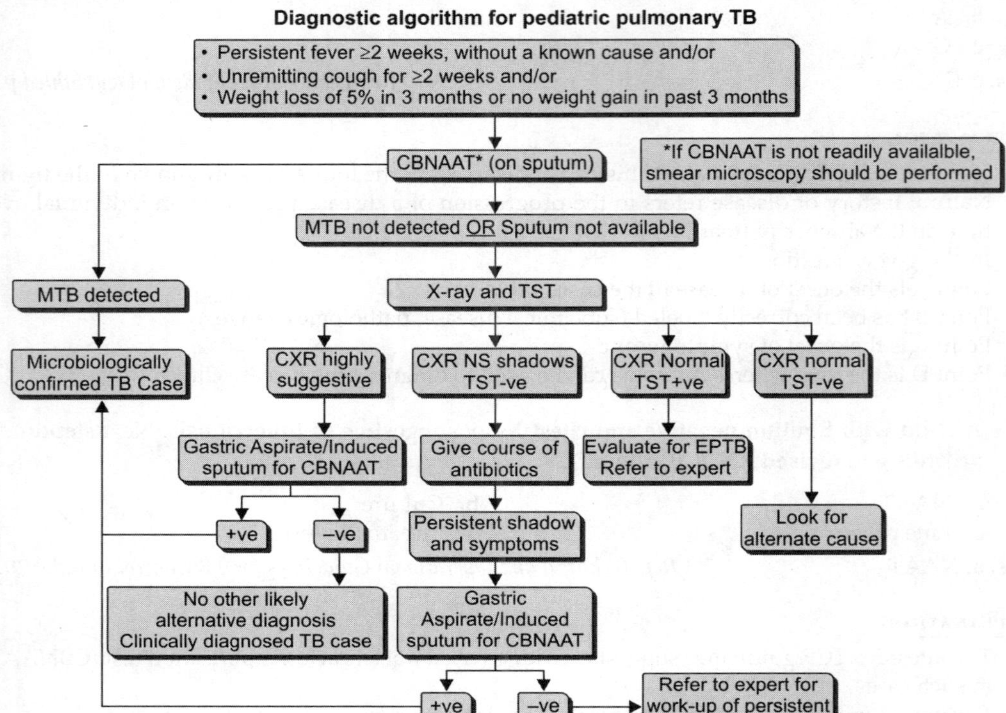

4. The following are the disease frequencies in a population. Based on the number of cases which of the following is the correct match?
Disease 1: Number of cases last week 42 this week 43
Disease 2: Number of cases last week 2 and present week 42
Disease 3: Number of cases last week 6 and present week 1

a. Endemic, epidemic, sporadic
b. Endemic, sporadic, epidemic
c. Sporadic, endemic, epidemic
d. Pandemic, endemic, sporadic

Ans. a. Endemic, epidemic, sporadic

Ref: Parks Textbook of Preventive and Social Medicine, 24rd/ed p98,99

EXPLANATION

The question pertains to the common definitions in epidemiology of infectious diseases.

- **Endemic:** (En = in; demos = people) The usual or **expected frequency** of disease in an area or population group. ***(Disease 1 in question)***
- **Epidemic:** (Epi = upon; demos = people) The **unusual occurrence** in a community or region of disease or health-related event clearly in excess of **expected occurrence**. The term outbreak is sometimes used for local epidemics ***(Disease 2 in question).***
- **Sporadic:** The word means **scattered about**. Such cases are separated widely by time and space. No connection among cases can be ascertained. ***(Disease 3 in question)***
- **Some other definitions of interest are:**
  - **Pandemic:** An epidemic usually affecting a **large population over a wide geographic area** like a nation or a continent or entire world e.g. influenza pandemics, El tor cholera.

- **Exotic:** Diseases which are imported into a country in which they do not occur, e.g. Rabies in UK, Yellow fever in India.
- **Infection:** The entry and development or multiplication of an infectious agent in the body of man or animals.
- **Contamination:** The presence of infectious agent on a body surface, clothes, instruments, food, milk or dressings.
- **Infestation:** The lodgment, development and reproduction of arthropods on surface of body or in clothing, e.g. lice, itch mite.

5. A radiotherapist prescribes a new drug combination of chemotherapy and immunotherapy for metastatic melanoma. It prolongs the survival. Which of the following is true in this situation?

a. Incidence reduces and prevalence increases
b. Incidence remains the same and prevalence increases
c. Incidence reduces and prevalence remains the same
d. Incidence increases and prevalence reduces

Ans. b. Incidence remains the same and prevalence increases

Ref: Parks Textbook of Preventive and Social Medicine, 24th/ed p65,66

EXPLANATION

The question tests your understanding of disease incidence and prevalence. Even if you just know that **incidence is the new cases** and **prevalence is the total number of cases** suffering from the disease, you can come to the conclusion that a curative or palliative treatment cannot change the number of new cases and therefore incidence remains the same no matter what type of treatment is available.

- **Incidence:** (new cases)
  - Incidence can be **decreased by primary prevention,** e.g. immunization can decrease incidence of measles (communicable diseases) likewise lifestyle modifications (e.g. adequate physical activity) decrease incidence of noncommunicable diseases.
  - Better diagnostic modalities might sometimes lead to **increase** in incidence as more cases are diagnosed.
- **Prevalence:** The total number of cases (old + new)
  - Prevalence on the other hand is given by formula
  - $P = I \times D$
  - I = incidence i.e. new cases
  - D = duration i.e. for how long cases suffer from the disease
  - The factors affecting incidence are discussed above, while things that affect duration is 'Treatment Modality': Two types of treatment modalities can be there:
    - **Curative:** As the patient is cured of disease, therefore will not be considered a case and thus a curative treatment will lead to decrease in prevalence.
    - **Palliative:** As in the present question, the new treatment combination does not cure the disease (melanoma) but prolongs survival. Thus, the overall period for which cases suffer from the disease and hence it will lead to increase in prevalence.
- An important thing to note is that diseases which are rapidly cured or are fatal usually have a low prevalence.

6. Which Biomedical waste is in the bag shown below?

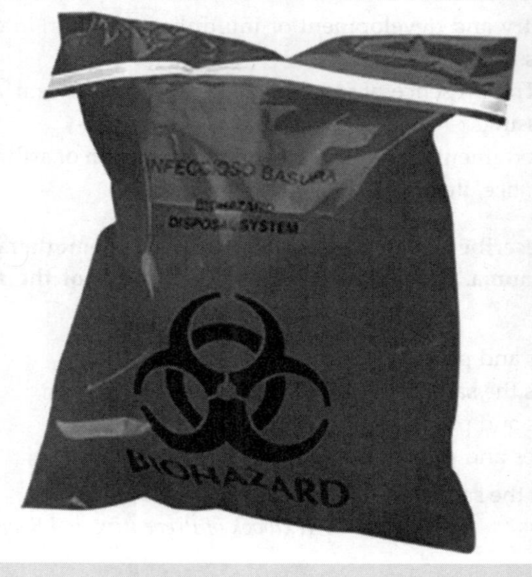

a. Laboratory wastes
b. Human anatomical waste
c. Sharp waste
d. Soiled plastic waste

Ans. d. Soiled plastic waste

Ref: The Bio-Medical Waste Management Rules, 2016. Available online at: http://cpcbenvis.nic.in/pdf/BMW_Rules_2016.pdf

EXPLANATION

Solid plastic waste (recyclable) is disposed in red bags as per the 2016 BMW handling and management rules.

- Most exams have at least one question from waste management rules. The 2016 rules are:

Category	Type of waste	Type of bag or container to be used	Treatment and disposal options
YELLOW	Human Anatomical Waste Animal Anatomical Waste	Yellow colored non-chlorinated plastic bags	Incineration or plasma pyrolysis or deep burial
	Soiled waste **Items** contaminated with blood, body fluids like dressings, plaster casts, cotton swabs **and *bags containing residual or discarded blood and blood components***		Incineration or plasma pyrolysis or deep burial In absence of above facilities, auto claving or microwaving hydroclaving followed by shredding or mutilation or combination of sterilization and shredding. Treated waste to be sent for energy recovery

Contd...

Contd...

Category	Type of waste	Type of bag or container to be used	Treatment and disposal options
	Expired or discarded medicines	Yellow colored non-chlorinated plastic bags **or containers**	Expired `cytotoxic drugs and items contaminated with cytotoxic drugs to be returned back to the manufacturer or supplier for incineration at temperature >1200°C or to common bio-medical waste treatment facility or hazardous waste treatment, storage and disposal facility for incineration at >1200°C Or Encapsulation or Plasma Pyrolysis at >1200°C. All other discarded medicines shall be either sent back to manufacturer or disposed by incineration
	Chemical waste	**Yellow colored containers** or non-chlorinated plastic bags	Disposed of by incineration or plasma pyrolysis or Encapsulation in hazardous waste treatment, storage and disposal facility
	Chemical liquid waste	Separate collection system leading to effluent treatment system	After resource recovery, the chemical liquid waste shall be pre-treated before mixing with other waste water.
	Discarded linen, mattresses, beddings contaminated with blood or body fluid	Non-chlorinated yellow plastic bags or suitable packing material	Non-chlorinated chemical disinfection followed by incineration or plasma pyrolysis or for energy recovery
	Microbiology, Biotechnology and other clinical laboratory waste	Autoclave safe plastic bags or containers	Pre-treat to sterilize with nonchlorinated chemicals on-site as per National AIDS Control Organisation or World Health Organisation guidelines thereafter for incineration
R E D	**Contaminated Waste (Recyclable)** Wastes generated from disposable items such as tubing, bottles, intravenous tubes and sets, catheters, urine bags, syringes (without needles and fixed needle syringes) and vaccutainers with their needles cut) and gloves	Red colored non-chlorinated plastic bags or container	Autoclaving or microwaving/ hydroclaving followed by shredding or mutilation or combination of Sterilization and shredding. Treated waste to be sent to registered or authorized recyclers or for energy recovery or plastics to diesel or fuel oil or for road making, whichever is possible. Plastic waste should not be sent to landfill sites

Contd...

Contd...

Category	Type of waste	Type of bag or container to be used	Treatment and disposal options
W H I T E Translucent	**Waste sharps including Metals:** Needles, syringes with fixed needles, needles from needle tip cutter or burner, scalpels, blades, or any other contaminated sharp object that may cause puncture and cuts. This includes both used, discarded and contaminated metal sharps	Puncture proof, Leak proof, tamper proof containers	Autoclaving or Dry Heat Sterilization followed by shredding or mutilation or encapsulation in metal container or cement concrete; combination of shredding cum autoclaving; and sent for final disposal to iron foundries (having consent to operate from the State Pollution Control Boards or Pollution Control Committees) or sanitary landfill or designated concrete waste sharp pit
B L U E	Glassware Broken or discarded and contaminated glass including medicine vials and ampoules except those contaminated with cytotoxic wastes	Cardboard boxes with blue colored marking	Disinfection (by soaking the washed glass waste after cleaning with detergent and Sodium Hypochlorite treatment) or through autoclaving or microwaving or hydroclaving and then sent for recycling
	Metallic body Implants		

- Vaccutainers are the vials (tubes) used for collection of blood samples.
- These are color coded according to type of blood sample that is collected.
  - *Red/yellow/grey:* Used for collecting blood for the tests that use Serum. e.g. RET/LFT, Serum electrolytes, blood sugar, Rapid tests for HIV, HBsAg etc.
  - *Purple:* Used for collecting blood samples for tests done on whole blood and contain anti-coagulant e.g. for complete hemogram, hematocrit.
  - *Light blue:* Usd for coagulation tests like Prothromin time (PT) and international Normalized Ratio (INR)
- A specialized needle is first inserted into the vein (after local anti-sepsis) and when this is attached to vaccutainer, blood automatically flows into the vaccutainer (negative pressure in the vaccutainer). This procedure does not involve syringe for sample collection.
- A Pictorial question with vaccutainer (of any color) is likely to be asked in coming exams.
- Remember Vaccutainer of any color is to be discarded in red colored bag according to new rules.

7. A study was conducted with the objective to compare the incidence of postpartum depression among mothers according to the sex of their child using a depression score (Edinburgh depression scale). One group with female babies and one with male babies. Which test should be used to compare?

a. Students t-test
b. Paired t-test
c. Chi square test
d. Pearson's coefficient

Ans. c. Chi square test

Ref: Interpretation and Uses of Medical Statistics, Leslie E. Daly, 5th/ed; Chapter 5 and Chapter 3.

EXPLANATION

- In the present question, as the prevalence of depression (a proportion) is used to compare two groups (male babies and female babies) therefore Chi square test is used.
- Chi square test is to be applied when we **compare proportions and percentages**. Fischer's exact test is used when sample size of any of the comparison groups is less than 30.
- As Fischer's test is not in option undoubtedly Chi-square test is the answer.
- ***Option a and b:*** Students t test (paired) is used for **comparing means** *in paired data* (e.g. Comparison of means of pretest and post test data of same individuals)
  - Unpaired students t test is used to compare means *in different group* of individuals.
  - Z test is a variant of Students t-test *for large sample size* usually above 30.
  - If there are *more than two groups then means* are compared using ANOVA, e.g. comparing mean Hb of adults, adolescents and elderly (three groups).
- ***Option d:*** Pearsons correlation coefficient (r): Used to **measure strength of association** between two quantitative (numerical) variables
  - Its value lies from –1 to 0 to +1
  - A scatter plot is used to represent correlation
  - R = +1 means perfect positive association
  - R = 0 means no correlation
  - R = –1 means perfect negative association
  - Association is said to be strong if value of $r > 0.8$
  - Moderate if value of r is between 0.3 to 0.7
  - Weak if value of r is less than 0.3
- In the present question, as the prevalence of depression (a proportion) is used to compare two groups (male babies and female babies) therefore Chi square test is used. If the mean score of the depression scale was to be compared among the two groups, then we would have used students paired t-test.

9. Below is the graph of CD4 count in HIV patients. From the graph below identify the mean CD4 count:

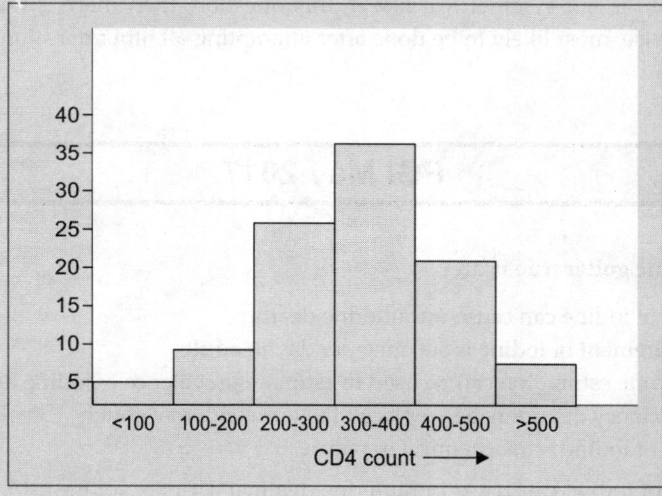

a. Mean will be 300
b. Mean more than 350
c. Mean anywhere between 300 and 400
d. Mean less than 300

Ans. c. Mean anywhere between 300 and 400 *Ref: Interpretation and Uses of Medical Statistics, Leslie e. Daly, 5th/ed, Chapter 5 and Chapter 3*

EXPLANATION

The question tests your mathematical skills of bar diagram from the sixth standard textbook of mathematics. Studying medicine we tend to forget such basic calculations. To solve such questions following steps are to be followed:

1. Calculate mid-points of each column of histogram
2. Multiply the histogram column height with the mid-point - total values
3. Calculate total population from the vertical axis - total population
4. Calculate mean = total values/total population

For the sake of simplicity, let us assume that the last bar saying >500 is 500–600 as no upper limit is given and meanwhile we should remember that mean is affected by outliers. (e.g. even if one patient has CD4 count of 5000, it will lead to a big rise in overall mean)

- There are six bars in the diagram. The mid-points of each are 50, 150, 250, 350, 450 and 550.
- **Now bar 1 has 5 patients:** 5 × 50 = 250
- **Bar 2 has 10 patients:** 10 × 150 = 1500
- **Bar 3 has 25 patients:** 25 × 250 = 6250
- **Bar 4 has 35 patients:** 35 × 350 = 12250
- **Bar 5 has 20 patients:** 20 × 450 = 9000
- **Bar 6 has 8 patients:** 8 × 550 = 4400

Therefore the answer is 250 + 1500 + 6250 + 12250 + 9000 + 4400/5 + 10 + 25 + 35 + 20 + 8 = 33650/103 = **327** ***(Answer)***

As time is short in the exam and calculation is going to take time, observe few important things

- **The shape of histogram:** As we can see the shape is somewhat like a symmetrical bell, therefore, the center represents the mean and can safely be marked as the answer.
- If the histogram is not symmetrical like in this question, then there is no other way but to calculate stepwise, most likely to be done after attempting all other questions, towards the end of examination.

PGI May 2017

1. About endemic goiter true is/are:

a. Deficiency of iodine can cause intrauterine death
b. Daily requirement of iodine is 500 mcg per day in adults
c. Urinary iodine estimation can be used to estimate prevalence of iodine deficiency
d. Iodine deficiency disorders has replaced the term endemic goiter
e. Deficiency of iodine is geochemical in nature

Ans. a. Deficiency of iodine can cause intrauterine death; c. Urinary iodine estimation can be used to estimate prevalence of iodine deficiency; d. Iodine deficiency disorders has replaced the term endemic goiter and e. Deficiency of iodine is geochemical in nature *Ref: Parks 23rd p624*

EXPLANATION

- Endemic goiter was the term used previously, which has been replaced by iodine deficiency disorders as it encompasses several other conditions like hypothyroidism, cretinism, dwarfism, IUD, etc. which are also caused by iodine deficiency ***(Option d)***.
- Deficiency of iodine has been known to cause intrauterine death and growth retardation ***(Option a).***
- Daily requirement of Iodine is 150 mcg per day in adults and 250 mcg in pregnant women. ***(Option b which is wrong)***
- Prevalence of Iodine deficiency disorders can be estimated by
  - Prevalence of goiter
  - Prevalence of cretinism
  - Urinary excretion of iodine ***(Option c)***
  - Prevalence of neonatal hypothyroidism.
- The last option has been directly taken from park, and means that deficiency of iodine in soil results in deficiency in human beings. ***(Option e).***

2. Correct combination of diseases and their incubation periods is/are:

a. Leptospirosis — 5 to 20 days
b. Hepatitis A — 10 to 50 days
c. Measles — 10 to 15 days
d. Chickenpox — 7 to 10 days
e. Cholera — 7 to 10 days

Ans. a. Leptospirosis – 5 to 20 days; b. Hepatitis A - 10 to 50 days and c. Measles – 10 to 15 days

Ref: Parks 24th/Chapter 5, Epidemiology of Communicable Diseases

EXPLANATION

Incubation of communicable diseases mentioned are correct except for **chickenpox which is 14 to 16 days**

Disease	Incubation period
Chicken pox *(Option d)*	14 to 16 days
Measles *(Option c)*	10 to 14 days
Rubella	18 days (14 to 21 days)
Mumps	18 days (14 to 21 days)
Influenza	18 to 72 hours
Diphtheria	2 to 6 days
Pertusis	7 to 14 days
Tuberculosis	3 to 6 weeks (variable from weeks to months)
Poliomyelitis	7 to 14 days
Hepatitis A *(Option b)*	10 to 50 days
Hepatitis B	30 to 180 days
Hepatitis C	40 to120 days
Hepatitis E	2 to 9 weeks
Hepatitis D	2 to 12 weeks

Contd...

Contd...

Disease	Incubation period
Cholera ***(option e)***	Few hours to 5 days
Typhoid fever	10 to 14 days
Food poisoning Salmonella Staph. aureus Botulism Cl perfringens Bacillus cereus – emetic Bacillus cereus – diarrheal	 12 to 24 hours 1 to 6 hours 12 to 36 hours 6 to 24 hours 1 to 6 hours 12 to 24 hours
Amoebiasis	2 to 4 weeks
Ascariasis	2 months
N. americanus	7 weeks
A.duodenale	5 weeks to 9 months
Dengue fever	3 to 10 days
Malaria • Falciparum • Vivax • Malarie • Ovale	 12 days 14 days 28 days 17 days
Filariasis	8 to 16 months
Rabies	3 to 8 weeks
Yellow fever	3 to 6 days
Japanese encephalitis	5 to 15 days
KFD	3 to 8 days
Brucellosis	1 to 3 weeks
Leptospirosis *(Option a)*	10 days (4 to 20 days)
Plague Bubonic Septicemic Pneumonic	 2 to 7 days 2 to 7 days 1 to 3 days
Scrub typhus	10 to 12 days
Murine typhus	1 to 2 weeks
Indian tick typhus	3 to 7 days
Q fever	2 to 3 weeks
Taeniasis	8 to 14 weeks
Hydatid disease	Months to years
Leishmaniasis	1 to 4 months
Trachoma	5 to 12 days
Tetanus	6 to 10 days

Contd...

Contd...

Disease	Incubation period
Leprosy	3 to 5 years
Syphilis	Variable
Yaws	3 to 5 weeks
Pinta	7 to 21 days

3. True about measles is/are:

a. Period of communicability is approx. 3 days before and 5 days after appearance of rash
b. Period of communicability is approx. 4 days before and 4 days after appearance of rash
c. Period of communicability is approx. 5 days before and 3 days after appearance of rash
d. Caused by DNA paramyxovirus
e Incubation period is 10–14 days following infection

Ans. b. Period of communicability is approx. 4 days before and 4 days after appearance of rash and e. Incubation period is 10–14 days following infection *Ref: Parks 24th, p156*

EXPLANATION

Measles is also known as rubeola meaning red spots. Measles is amenable to elimination.

Epidemiological determinants of measles:

- **Agent:** RNA paramyxovirus ***(Option d which is wrong)***
- **Source of infection:** Case of measles, No carriers.
- **Infective material:** Secretions of nose, throat, respiratory tract.
- **Communicability:** 4 days before and after the appearance of rash ***(Option b)***
- One infection provides lifelong immunity.
- **Most susceptible age:** 6 months to 3 years
- Severe in malnourished children
- In India epidemics are common in winters and early spring
- **Transmission:** Through droplets.
- Portal of entry is respiratory tract
- **Incubation period:** 10 days for fever and 14 days for rash (average) ***(Option e)***
- **Three phases after infection:** Prodromal stage, eruptive phase and post measles stage.
- **Rash:** Dusky red macular or maculopapular rash. Begins behind the ears and spreads to face and necks and then to whole of body in 2 to 3 days. Disappears in the order of onset after 3–4 days.
- **Kopliks spot:** Appear a day or two before onset of rash. Look like table salt crystals and appear on buccal mucosa opposite to first and second lower molars. They are pathognomonic of measles.
- **Complications:** Diarrhea, pneumonia, otitis media.
- **Most common life-threatening complication:** Pneumonia (20–80% cases in developing countries)
- Subacute sclerosing pan encephalitis **SSPE** and febrile convulsions are serious complications. Frequency of SSPE 1:300,000 cases.
- All cases of severe measles or in areas of high fatality rates should be treated with Vitamin A.

Measles vaccine:

- Only live attenuated vaccine are recommended for use
- Freeze dried product (lyophilized)
- **Dose:** 0.5 mL, >1000 viral infective units
- Reconstituted vaccine is very heat labile and should be used within 6 hours and stored in dark after reconstitution

- Administered at 9 months, can be given at 6 months in outbreaks.
- **Route of administration:** Subcutaneous
- Immunity develops in 10–12 days and remains lifelong
- **Contraindications:** High fever, pregnant women, H/O anaphylaxis to neomycin, gelatin, sorbitol (vaccine contains these) and severe immunocompromised states.
- Can be given to asymptomatic HIV positive children (after the age of 6 months) and adults.
- Second dose of vaccine is recommended in countries where coverage of first dose is above 80%
- **WHO defines measles elimination as** the absence of endemic measles for a period of >12 months in the presence of adequate surveillance. Indicator used is less than 1 case per million population
- **Elimination strategy:** Catch up, keep up and follow-up.

4. Revised RNTCP:

a. There are five National Reference Laboratories (NRLs)
b. A DMC serves a population of 1,00,000
c. Daily regimen for pediatric TB
d. Daily regimen for TB + HIV patients
e. Bedaquilline in Drug resistant TB patients

Ans. b. A DMC serves a population of 1,00,000; c. Daily regimen for pediatric TB; d. Daily regimen for TB + HIV patients and e. Bedaquilline in Drug resistant TB patients

Ref: Parks 24th, p447-48

Explanation

- **Laboratory network under RNTCP:**
    - **Designated microscopy centre (DMC):** Most peripheral laboratory and serves a population of about one lac (50,000 in tribal and hilly areas). Sputum microscopy is done at DMCs. ***(Option b)***
    - **Intermediate reference laboratory (IRLs):** At-least one for each state. Drug sensitivity testing, culture and monitoring and supervision of quality assurance in state.
    - **National reference laboratories (NRLs):** Total **six in number**. Work closely with NRLs and performs trainings for staff in quality assurance and various tests like CBNAAT, DST and culture. In the present question, ***option a*** is wrong as there are Six NRLs and not five.
- **Newer initiatives in RNTCP:**
    1. Daily regimen for pediatric TB.
    2. Daily regimen for all forms of TB in five states.
    3. Daily regimen for all TB/HIV co-infected patients across the country.
    4. Pilots for universal access to TB cases.
    5. Bedaquilline conditional access programme.

5. Disease/s caused by ticks is/are:

a. Trench fever
b. Tularemia
c. Tick typhus
d. Epidemic typhus
e. Oriental sore

Ans. b. Tularemia and c. Tick typhus *Ref: Parks 24th, p817*

Explanation

Out of the given options, tularemia and tick typhus (rocky mountain spotted fever) are caused by ticks. Trench fever and epidemic typhus are transmitted by lice. Oriental sore is transmitted by sand fly.

❑ **Diseases transmitted by hard ticks are:**
- Tick typhus
- Viral encephalitis (Russian spring-summer encephalitis)
- Viral fevers (Colorado tick fever)
- Viral hemorrhagic fevers (KFD in INDIA)
- **Tularemia**
- Tick paralysis
- Human babesiosis

❑ **Diseases transmitted by soft ticks are:**
- Q fever
- Relapsing fever
- KFD

6. True about malaria is/are:

a. Gametocytes are found in mosquitoes
b. Relapses occur
c. Choroquine resistant malaria occurs in India
d. Vector is female Culex mosquito
e. *Plasmodium malariae* has widest geographic distribution in the world

Ans. a. Gametocytes are found in mosquitoes; b. Relapses occur and c. Choroquine resistant malaria occurs in India *Ref: Parks 24th, p274,282*

❑ Both microgametes and macrogametes are found in mosquitoes and then zygote is formed in mosquito ***(Option a)***.

❑ Infective stage
- For mosquito → gametes
- For man → sporozoites from saliva of mosquito.

❑ **Option b:** Relapses are usual in → vivax and ovale malaria.
- Chloroquine resistant malaria was first reported in the year 1973 from Assam.

❑ Life cycle of malarial parasite is commonly asked in PG entrance exams. A simple diagram which should be remembered is:

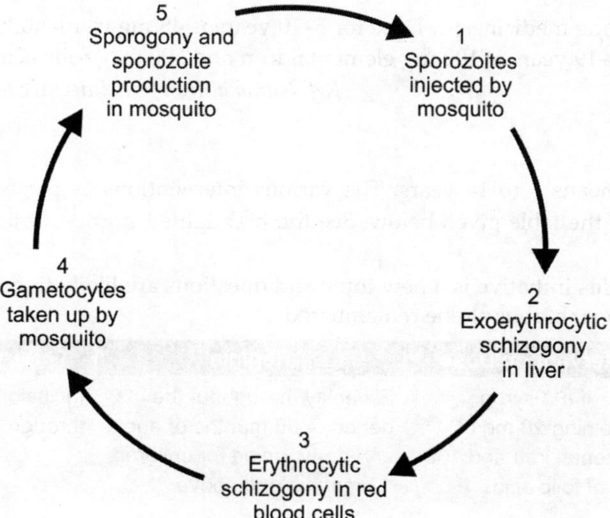

About Option d:

- ❑ Vector for malaria are female mosquitoes of the genus Anopheles.
- ❑ Remember, Aedes mosquito is vector for Dengue, Chikungunya and Yellow fever (not found in India).
- ❑ Anopheles mosquito is vector for Malaria
- ❑ Culex mosquito is vector for Japanese encephalitis (found in India)

Option e: *P. vivax* has widest distribution in the world.

7. Which of the following drugs can be used in case of Rifampicin resistance Leprosy?

a. Clofazimine
b. Rifapentine
c. Moxifloxacine
d. Clindamycin
e. Minocycline

Ans. a. Clofazimine; b. Rifapentine; c. Moxifloxacine and e. Minocycline

Ref: Rao PN, Jain S. Newer Management Options in Leprosy. Indian J Dermatol 2013;58:6-11

Explanation

All medicines except clindamycin can be used to manage rifampin resistant cases of Leprosy.

Medicines used in drug resistant leprosy are Rifapentin, moxifloxacin, clarithromycin, clofazimine, minocycline, ofloxacin.

No guidelines for rifampicin resistance leprosy are there in India.

It is a Pharmacology, dermatology and medicine question.

8. Iron folic acid supplementation in school going children. True statements are:

a. Deworming done once a year
b. Teachers to provide medicines
c. Dose for 5–10 years is 45 mg elemental iron and 400 mcg folic acid
d. Dose for 10–19 years is 100 mg elemental iron and 500 mcg folic acid
e. IFA to be given weekly

Ans. b. Teachers to provide medicines; c. Dose for 5–10 years is 45 mg elemental iron and 400 mcg folic acid; d. Dose for 10–19 years is 100 mg elemental iron and 500 mcg folic acid and e. IFA to be given weekly *Ref: National Iron Plus Initiative for Anaemia Control*

Explanation

School going children means 5 to 14 years. The various interventions as per National Iron plus initiative is described in the table given below. See the highlighted portion of table, you will find answers.

- ❑ The National iron plus initiative is a new topic and questions are likely to come in most of the exams. The following table should be remembered.

Age group	Intervention/Dose	Regime	Service delivery
6–60 months.	1 mL of IFA syrup containing 20 mg of elemental iron and 100 mcg of folic acid	Biweekly throughout the period 6–60 months of age and de-worming for children 12 months and above	Inclusion in MCP card through ASHA/ANM

Contd...

Contd...

Age group	Intervention/Dose	Regime	Service delivery
5–10 years	Tablets of **45 mg elemental iron** and **400 mcg** of folic acid	**Weekly** throughout the period 5–10 years of age and biannual de-worming	In school through **teachers** and for out of school children through Anganwadi Centre (AWC)
10–19 years	**100 mg elemental iron** and **500 mcg** of folic acid	**Weekly** throughout the period 10–19 years of age and **biannual de-worming**	In school through **teachers** and for those out of school through AWC
Pregnant and lactating women	100 mg elemental iron and 500 mcg of folic acid	1 tablet daily for 100 days, starting after the first trimester, at 14–16 weeks of gestation. To be repeated for 100 days post-partum.	ANC/ANM/ASHA Inclusion in MCP card
Women in reproductive age (WRA) group	100 mg elemental iron and 500 mcg of folic acid	Weekly throughout the reproductive period	Through FHW during house visit for contraceptive distribution

MCP – mother and child protection card. Contains all details for antenatal care, postnatal care and immunization; ANM – Auxiliary nursing midwife, FHW – Female Health Worker, IFA – Iron Folic Acid

- ❑ From the table it is clear that ***Option a*** is wrong as deworming (400 mg albendazole) is to be done twice a year. All other options are correct.

9. Vaccine/s contraindicated in HIV:

a. MMR
b. Varicella
c. Hepatitis A
d. Hib
e. DPT

Ans. a. MMR and b. Varicella

Ref: Parks 23rd p103; Harrison Principles of Internal Medicine 19th/ed p788.

Explanation

- ❑ Live vaccines should not be administered to persons with pregnancy and immunocompromised states.
- ❑ Killed or inactivated vaccines are contraindicated only when there is specific allergy (H/O severe reaction) on prior dosage.
- ❑ ***Option a and b:*** **MMR and Varicella** are the live vaccine among the given options.
- ❑ ***Option e:*** **DPT** is a toxoid.
- ❑ ***Option d:*** **Hib** is either a polysaccharide or glycoconjugate.
- ❑ ***Option c:*** Hepatitis A is an inactivated vaccine
- ❑ See table for vaccines

Live attenuated	Killed whole organism	Toxoid/ Protein	Polysaccharide	Glycoconjugate	Recombinant
Tuberculosis (BCG)	Typhoid	Diphtheria	Pneumococcus	Hib	HBV
Yellow fever	Cholera	Tetanus	Meningococcus	Pneumococcus	Lyme disease
Polio (OPV)	Plague	Acellular Pertussis	Hib	MenACWY	Cholera toxin B
Measles	Pertussis	Anthrax	Typhoid (Vi)		HPV
Mumps	Influenza	Influenza subunit			
Rubella	Typhus				
Typhoid	Polio (IPV)				
Varicella	Rabies				
Rotavirus	JE				
Cholera	TBE				
Cold-adapted influenza	HAV				
Rotavirus reassortants					
Zoster					

BCG: Bacille Calmette-Guerin; HAV: Hepatitis A virus; HBV: Hepatitis B virus; Hib: Haemophilus influenzae type b; IPV: Inactivated polio vaccine; JE: Japanese encephalitis; Men: Meningococcus, OPV: Oral polio vaccine; TBE: Tick-borne encephalitis.

- What Harrison says
  - MMR and varicella are contraindicated if CD4 <200 and can be given if CD4 >200
  - Zoster is contraindicated if CD4 <200 and there is no recommendation for CD4 >200

10. True about sandflies:

a. Do not fly by choice
b. Breeding in overhead water tanks
c. Smaller than mosquitos
d. Cause chikungunya
e. Cannot fly normally

Ans. a. Do not fly by choice and c. Smaller than mosquitos *Ref: Parks 24th, p812*

Explanation

Sandflies

- Small light to dark brown insects.
- They are **smaller than mosquitoes** ***(Option c)***
- Lay eggs (breed) in damp and dark places in vicinity of cattle shed and poultry ***(Option b)***
- They can fly over small distances but usually hop about and **do not fly by choice** ***(Option a)***
- Only female bites and more so at night.
- Diseases transmitted by Sandflies are:

Species	Diseases carried
Phlebotomusargentipes	Kala-azar
Phlebotomuspapatasii	Sandfly fever Oriental sore
Phlebotomussergenti	Oriental sore
S. punjabensis	Sandfly fever

11. Which of the following are true regarding IPV?

a. Intradermal
b. 0.1 mL is intradermal dose
c. 0.5 mL is intramuscular dose
d. Intramuscular
e. Given at 14 weeks

Ans. All are true *Ref: WHO; http://www.who.int/immunization/diseases/poliomyelitis/endgame_objective2/inactivated_polio_vaccine/en/*

Explanation

IPV can be given as both intramuscular (0.5 mL) and intradermal (0.1 mL); intramuscular is given at week 14 and intradermal at week 6 and 14.

The photograph will help in remembering about IPV.

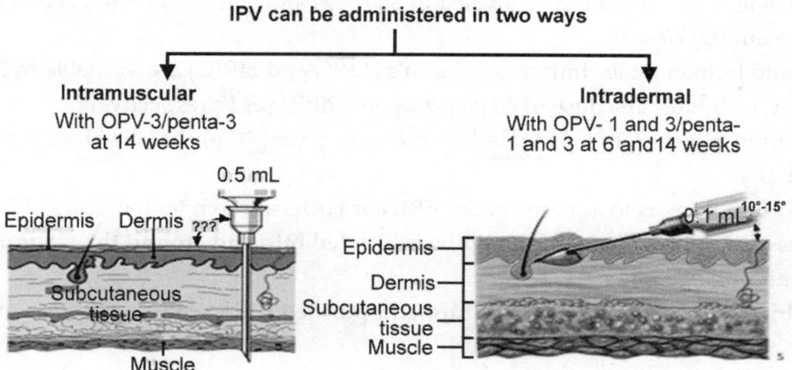

12. True about rabies post exposure prophylaxis:

a. If a person with complete pre-exposure prophylaxis gets a dog bite then there is no need of anti-rabies Ig
b. Local treatment of wound is necessary in all dog bites
c. Vaccine is not given if more than 3 days have passed since dog bite
d. Category 2 bites are treated by ARV
e. Category 3 bites are treated by ARV and Ig

Ans. a. If a person with complete pre-exposure prophylaxis gets a dog bite then there is no need of anti-rabies Ig; b. Local treatment of wound is necessary in all dog bites; d. Category 2 bites are treated by ARV and e. Category 3 bites are treated by ARV and Ig

Ref: National Guidelines on Rabies Prophylaxis, GOI, 2015

Explanation

National Guidelines on Rabies Prophylaxis have come up in the year 2015.

Salient features of the guidelines are:

- According to these there are three categories as: ***(Option d and e** in Table below)*

Category	Types of contact	Recommended PEP
I	• Touching or feeding of animals • Licks on intact skin • Contact of intact skin with secretions/excretions of rabid animal/ human case	None, if reliable case history is available
II	• Nibbling of uncovered skin • Minor scratches or abrasions without bleeding	Wound management Anti-rabies vaccine
III	• Single or multiple transdermal bites or scratches, licks on broken skin • Contamination of mucous membrane with saliva (i.e. licks)	Wound management Rabies immunoglobulin Anti-rabies vaccine

- Local management of wound is advised in all cases and consists of wound toilet and wound management ***(Option b).***
- Equine and human **r**abies **i**mmuno**g**lobulin's (ERIG and HRIG) are available in India and are given in Cat III bites at a dose of 40 *IU per kg* and 20 *IU per kg* respectively.
- If the bitten persons is vaccinated previously (complete), he/she does not require Ig. ***(Option a)***
- An important thing is to administer the ERIG or HRIG at room temperature (25°C to 30°C).
- RIG as is anatomically feasible should be **infiltrated into and around the wound/s**.
- Should never be given IV.
- **Anti-rabies Vaccine (ARV):** Cell culture and purified duck embryo vaccines are used with potency above >2.5 IU per IM dose.
- All Category II and III are given the same dose and regimen irrespective of age and weight.
- **IM regimen**: Days 0, 3, 7, 14 and 28. Dose 0.5 mL in deltoid.
- **ID regimen**: Days 0, 3, 7 and 28. Dose 0.1 mL at each site, one inch above insertion of deltoid. Also known as Updated Thai Red Cross Schedule.

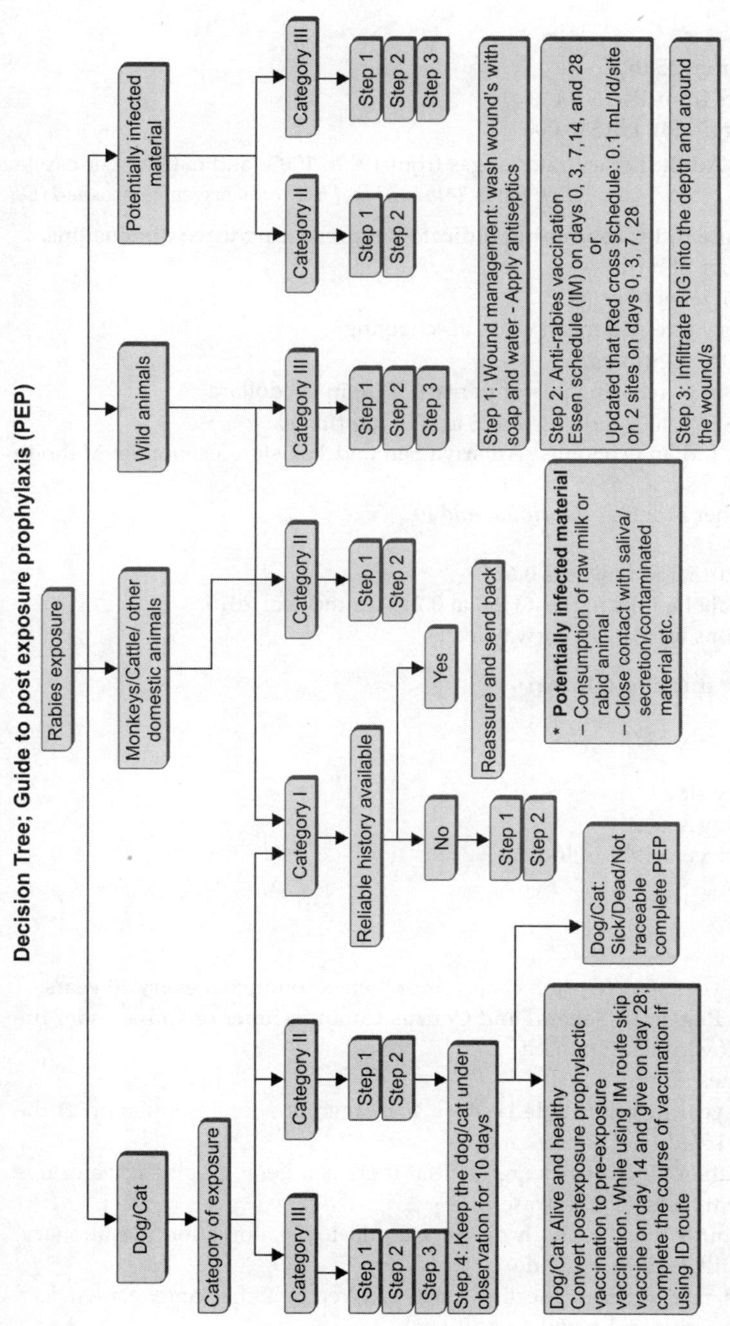
Decision Tree; Guide to post exposure prophylaxis (PEP)
Rabies exposure
Dog/Cat
Monkeys/Cattle/ other domestic animals
Wild animals
Potentially infected material
Category of exposure
Category III
Category II
Category I
Category II
Category III
Category II
Category III
Step 1
Step 2
Step 3
Step 4: Keep the dog/cat under observation for 10 days
Reliable history available
No
Yes
Reassure and send back
Dog/Cat: Alive and healthy
Convert postexposure prophylactic vaccination to pre-exposure vaccination. While using IM route skip vaccine on day 14 and give on day 28; complete the course of vaccination if using ID route
Dog/Cat: Sick/Dead/Not traceable complete PEP
* Potentially infected material
– Consumption of raw milk or rabid animal
– Close contact with saliva/ secretion/contaminated material etc.
Step 1: Wound management: wash wound's with soap and water - Apply antiseptics
Step 2: Anti-rabies vaccination
Essen schedule (IM) on days 0, 3, 7,14, and 28
or
Updated that Red cross schedule: 0.1 mL/Id/site on 2 sites on days 0, 3, 7, 28
Step 3: Infiltrate RIG into the depth and around the wound/s

13. Which of the following about human development index (HDI) are not true?

a. Ranges from 0 to 1
b. Ranges from 0 to 100
c. Life expectancy ranges from 25 to 85
d. Adult literacy rate ranges from 1% to 100%
e. GDP per capita ranges from $100 to $40,000

Ans. b. Ranges from 0 to 100; d. Adult literacy rate ranges from 1% to 100% and e. GDP per capita ranges from $100 to $40,000 *Ref: Parks 24th, p17 and hdr.undp.org/en/composite/HDI*

- **HDI is defined as a composite index combining indicators representing three dimensions:**
  - **Longevity**: Life expectancy at birth
    - Ranges **from 25 to 85 years** ***(Option c)***
  - **Knowledge**: Adult literacy rate and mean years of schooling
    - Ranges **from 0 to 100%** ***(Option d)***
  - **Income**: GDP per capita in purchasing power parity (PPP$) in US dollars
    - Ranges **from $100 to $ 75,000** (earlier it was $40,000) ***(Option e)***
- The HDI was developed by Indian economist Amartya Sen and Pakistani economist Mahbub ul Haq.
- HDI ranges from 0 to 1. Higher is better. ***(Option a and b)***
- **Norway** has highest at 0.949.
- HDI for **India was 0.609** in 2015 and now it **is 0.624**.
  - In India, the state of Kerala had the highest HDI at 0.712 for the year 2015.
- India ranks 131st in the nations list which Norway leads.

14. Which of the following are true about India?

a. Year of big divide-1881
b. Year of big divide-1921
c. India is in Low stationary stage
d. India is in Early expanding stage
e. Census was started in the year 1921 in India

Ans. b. Year of big divide-1921 *Ref: Parks 24th, Chapter 9, p513*

EXPLANATION

- First census was done in the year **1881** ***(Option e)*** and since then is conducted **every 10 years**.
- Census is conducted by the **Registrar General and Census Commissioner of India** under the Ministry of Home Affairs, Government of India
- It has been conducted **15 times** till now.
- The year **1921 is called the year of big divide** because since then, the total population of the country has been increasing steadily. ***(Option a and b)***
- The history of world population **since 1650** suggests that there is a demographic cycle of five stages through which a country passes. These are:
  1. **High stationary**: **High** birth rate and **high** death rate and total population is stationary. India was in this stage till 1920 (big divide)
  2. **Early expanding**: Death rate begins to decline, birth rate remains the same, e.g. African nations (possibly due to improved health conditions)
  3. **Late expanding**: **India** is in this phase. Death rate declines further, birth rate begins to fall. ***(Option c and d are wrong)***

4. **Low stationary**: Low death and birth rates and again population is stationary, e.g. Developed countries
5. **Declining**: Birth rate falls below death rate and population starts declining, e.g. Germany, Hungary

Therefore, only ***option b*** is correct.

JIPMER Pattern Based

1. True about correlation coefficient:

a. Denoted by r^2
b. Its value can never be Zero
c. Can be used to calculate value of one variable if other is known
d. Value lies between –1 to +1

Ans. d. Value lies between –1 to +1 *Ref: Park 23rd, p889.90*

- **Correlation:** Often we wish to know if there is linear relation between two variables, e.g. height and weight. To find out the strength of association between the two variables we calculate the coefficient of correlation and it is denoted by 'r'.
- The value of r can lie between –1 to +1
- If r = 0 then there is no association between the two variables.
- **Regression:** Used when we wish to calculate unknown value of a variable, when we know value of another variable.
- The known variable is called independent variable and denoted by x and the unknown variable is called dependent variable denoted by y.
- Equation for linear regression is given by

$$y = a + bx$$

Where y is dependent variable, a is constant, **b is the regression coefficient** and x is independent variable.

Coming to the present question

- ***Option a*** is wrong as correlation coefficient is denoted by r and not r^2.
- ***Option b*** has to be false if option d is correct. In such questions, where there are two mutually exclusive options, i.e. of the two statement one explains the other and only one can be true, you easily rule out the other two even if you do not know about them. Thus, in this question even if you do not know a thing about correlation (which by now you do pretty well) you can conclude answer has to be either option c or d.
- ***Option d*** is the only true statement among all four.
- ***Option c*** is the definition of regression.

2. Two tests are applied in series. Effect on sensitivity and specificity:

a. Both increase
b. Sensitivity increases, specificity decreases
c. Sensitivity decreases, specificity increases
d. Both decrease

Ans. c. Sensitivity decreases, specificity increases *Ref: Parks 24th/ed p149 and Daly's 5th, p413,414*

Explanation

- **Sensitivity:** Ability of a test to identify correctly all those **who have** the disease or true positives.
- **Specificity:** Ability of test to identify all those **who do not have** the disease or true negatives.

- **Testing in series**: Means application of tests one after the other, e.g. RPR is used in screening of Syphilis which is followed by FTA-ABS. Using tests in **series increases specificity only** and decreases sensitivity ***(Answer)***
- **Testing in parallel:** Two test are applied simultaneously. Done in HIV testing. Using two tests in **parallel increases sensitivity only** and decreases specificity.

Remember, **Sensitivity and specificity are inversely related.**

3. Randomization is done in clinical trials to:

a. Avoid selection bias inside the study group
b. To avoid bias from general population
c. To eliminate comparability
d. Option not recalled

Ans. a. Avoid selection bias inside the study group *Ref: Parks 24th, p86*

EXPLANATION

- **Randomization** is a statistical procedure by which participants are allocated to study and control groups in a Randomized control trail.
- **Randomization is the heart of a control trial**. It ensures investigator has no control over allocation process and thus **eliminates selection bias** and thus every individual gets equal chance of being allocated to either of the groups.
- **By definition distortions that result from procedures used to select subjects and from factors that influence participation in the study is called selection bias.**
- The estimated effect of cigarette smoking on heart disease will be biased if study participants are volunteers and the decision to volunteer is affected by smoking status.

4. If the same individual participates in both study and experimental group (patient serves as his or her own control), it is called:

a. Cross over study
b. Case control study
c. Cohort study
d. Experimental study

Ans. a. Cross over study *Ref: Parks 24th, p88*

EXPLANATION

- Cross over type of study designs are the randomized controlled trials, in which each patient serves as his own control. A better understanding can be taken from the diagram.
- Here the patient is initially either enrolled into intervention group or control group, after a specified duration the person is crossed over alternate group (e.g. patient initially enrolled in intervention arm, later after a period (say 3 months) he is crossed to control arm, i.e. he now receives control treatment, e.g. placebo).

Cross over trial

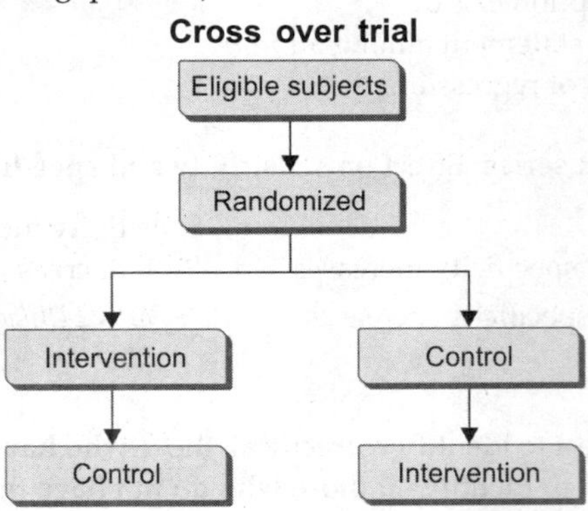

- They have added advantage that all the participants receive the intervention at some time. The number of patients and time are also reduced.
- **Cannot be used when:**
  - Drug cures the disease
  - Drug is effective only in certain stage of disease
  - Disease changes radically during the period of time required for the study.

5. The evaluation of a particular program or intervention is better known as its:

a. Efficacy
b. Effectiveness
c. Efficiency
d. Benefit

Ans. b. Effectiveness *Ref: A Dictionary of Epidemiology, Porta M. 5th/ed, p76*

EXPLANATION

Effectiveness: It is a measure of the extent to which a specific intervention, procedure, regimen, or service, when deployed in the field in the **usual circumstances**, does what it is intended to do.

Efficacy: The extent to which a specific intervention, procedure, regimen, or service produces a beneficial result **under ideal conditions**.

Efficiency: The effects or end results achieved in relation to the effort expended in terms of **money, resources, and time**.

Benefit: Advantage or improvement resulting from an intervention.

Unless it is specified that ideal conditions are present, effectiveness is the answer of choice.

Author: Bahram Gor

AIIMS May 2017

1. A 40-year-old male with hisotry of (H/O) one episode of vomiting and fall near an alcohol shop. When he was brought to casualty, pulse was fast and feeble and had slurred speech. On awakening, patient had unrelieved retrograde amnesia. Which of the following is the most likely cause?

a. Concussion
b. Drunkenness
c. Diffuse axonal injury
d. Cerebral venous thrombosis

Ans. b. Drunkenness *Ref: Harrison Principles of Internal Medicine 19th/ed p457e-1,2724,2194*

Explanation

Cerebral venous thrombosis is easily ruled out. Fall near alcoholic shop, with feeble pulse and retrograde amnesia all favor in the diagnosis of drunkenness. Concussion may also present with all the features but slurred speech and rapid pulse is not seen in it, and moreover to produce concussion there should be H/O blow/jolt to head that lead to fall. Diffuse axonal injury occurs with severe head trauma.

The retrograde amnesia involves an inability to recall experiences that occurred before the onset of the amnestic state. Relatively recent events are more vulnerable to retrograde amnesia than are more remote and more extensively consolidated events.

Option (a) A brief period of both retrograde and anterograde amnesia is characteristic of concussion and it recedes rapidly in alert patients. Memory loss spans the moments before impact, but may encompass the previous days or weeks (rarely months). With severe injuries, the extent of retrograde amnesia roughly correlates with the severity of injury.

Option (b) Standing near an alcohol shop is a clue to alcoholism. *"Approximately 35% of drinkers (and a much higher proportion of alcoholics) experience a blackout, an episode of temporary anterograde amnesia, in which the person forgets all or part of what occurred during a drinking evening." .... Harrison's 2724.*

Option (c) Diffuse axonal injury (DAI) is associated with severe head trauma and may be seen on CT as multiple areas of punctate hemorrhage in deep white matter and corpus callosum. DAI is associated with poor prognosis.

Option (d) Cerebral venous thrombosis is most frequently observed in the superior sagittal and transverse sinuses and is associated with headache and increased intracranial pressure.

2. A 56-year-old man came to casualty with history of massive hemoptysis. His routine investigation chest X-ray was normal. Which of the following is not done to prevent hemoptysis?

a. Bronchial artery embolization
b. Pulmonary artery embolization
c. Bronchoscopic ligation
d. Resection of affected lung lobe

Ans. c. Bronchoscopic ligation *Ref: Harrison 19th/ed p246; Schwartz 9th/ed Chap 19*

EXPLANATION

Bronchoscopic interventions are done in massive hemoptysis but does not includes ligation. Ligation is not possible by bronchoscopy.

For the most part, the treatment of hemoptysis will vary based on its etiology Flowchart 1. However, large-volume, life-threatening hemoptysis generally requires immediate intervention regardless of the cause. The ***first step is to establish a patent airway*** usually by endotracheal intubation and subsequent mechanical ventilation. The volume of the hemoptysis is also important not only in determining the cause, but in gauging the urgency for further diagnostic and therapeutic maneuvers. ***Massive hemoptysis is defined as hemoptysis of greater than 200–600 cc in 24 hours***. Massive hemoptysis should be considered a medical emergency.

Option (a) It is generally employed when there is persistent brisk hemoptysis despite correction of coagulopathy and after bronchoscopy. The bronchial arteries should be the first vessels studied in most patients with massive hemoptysis because they are the most common source of bleeding. Severe hemoptysis from bronchial arteries can be treated with angiographic embolization of the culprit bronchial artery. This intervention should only be entertained in the most severe and life-threatening cases of hemoptysis because there is a risk of unintentional spinal-artery embolization and consequent paraplegia with this procedure.

Option (b) The pulmonary arteries are generally studied only if bronchial arteriography does not identify a bleeding source or if there is a high suspicion for arteriovenous malformation (AVMs) or pulmonary embolism. Overall, the pulmonary arteries are the bleeding source in fewer than 10% of patients with massive hemoptysis.

Option (c) As large-volume hemoptysis usually arises from an airway lesion, it is ideal to identify the site of bleeding by either chest imaging or bronchoscopy (more commonly rigid rather than flexible). Endobronchial lesions can be treated with a variety of bronchoscopically directed interventions, including cauterization and laser therapy. ***There are a variety of bronchoscopic techniques that may control pulmonary hemorrhage, but none have been indisputably proven to be of benefit. They include balloon tamponade, iced saline lavage, topical medications, laser therapy, and electrocautery.***

Option (d) In extreme conditions, surgical resection of the affected region of lung is considered.

Note: ***Blood products in massive hemoptysis:*** Patients with massive hemoptysis should be suspected for coagulation abnormalities. Those who are receiving an anticoagulant or have an elevated prothrombin time, partial thromboplastin time, or international normalized ratio should receive fresh frozen plasma. Those who are thrombocytopenic should receive a platelet transfusion. Patients who are uremic or taking an antiplatelet agent (e.g. aspirin, clopidogrel) or transfused platelets. Finally, the administration of recombinant factor VIIa should be considered.

3. A 20-year-old female came with complaints of headache, vomiting and decrease in movement of right leg. In the past she had episodes of violent and aggressive behavior and abdominal pain. Which of the following is the most probable diagnosis?

a. Conversion disorder
b. AIDP with migraine
c. Right side paralysis
d. Acute intermittent porphyria

Ans. d. Acute intermittent porphyria *Ref: Harrison's Principles of Internal Medicine 19th/ed p2527*

EXPLANATION

The given history is characteristic of acute intermittent porphyria (AIP), see below for features of AIP.

Acute Intermittent Porphyria

- ❑ Autosomal dominant condition resulting from the half-normal level of hydroxymethylbilane (HMB) synthase activity

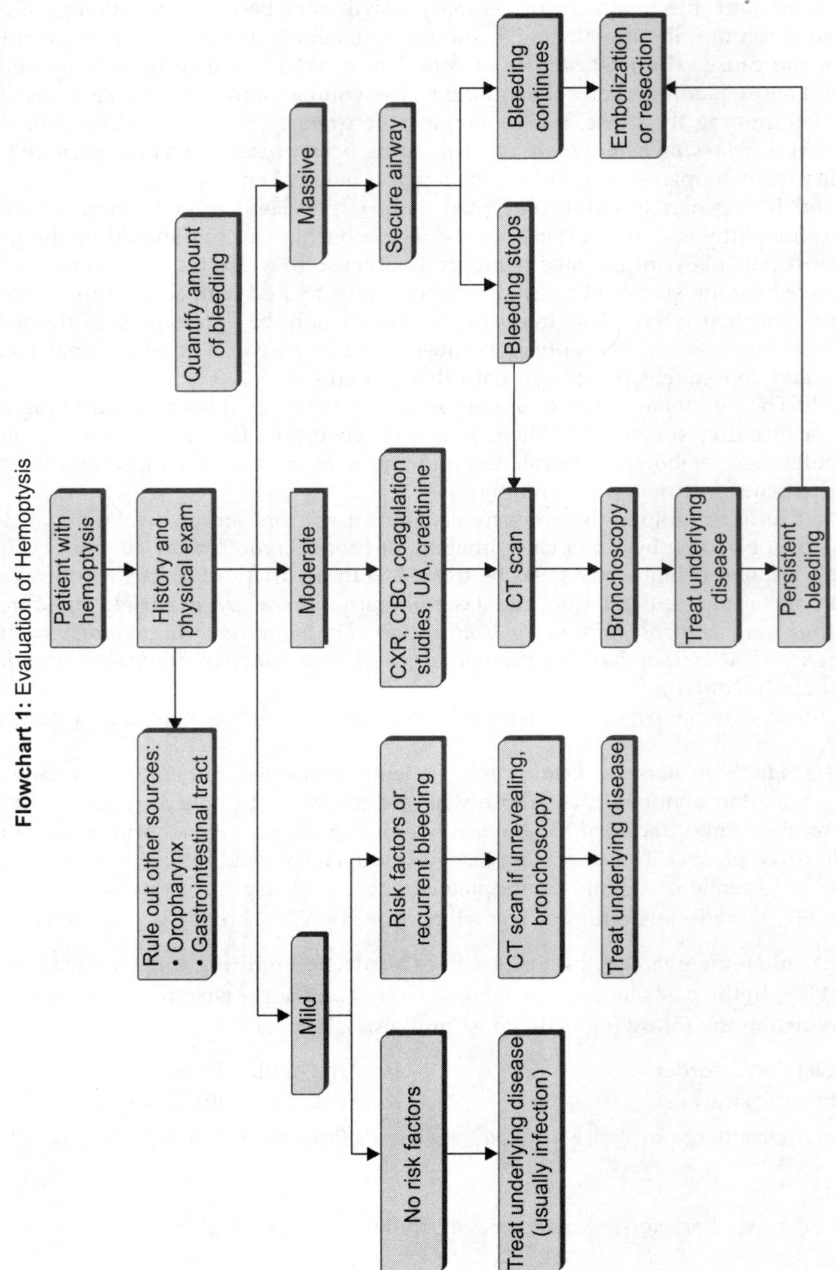

Flowchart 1: Evaluation of Hemoptysis

- Symptoms are **more common in women**, suggesting a role for estrogens or progestins.
- Sometimes exacerbated by exogenous steroids, including oral contraceptive preparations containing progestins. Surprisingly, pregnancy is usually well tolerated, suggesting that beneficial metabolic changes may ameliorate the effects of high levels of progesterone.
- Clinical features (C/F):
  - Abdominal pain (most common symptom), is usually steady and poorly localized but may be cramping.
  - Abdominal tenderness, fever, and leukocytosis are usually absent or mild because the symptoms are neurologic rather than inflammatory.
  - **Nausea; vomiting**; constipation; tachycardia; hypertension; mental symptoms; pain in the limbs, head, neck, or chest; muscle weakness; sensory loss; dysuria; and urinary retention are characteristic. Tachycardia, hypertension, restlessness, tremors, and excess sweating are due to sympathetic overactivity.
  - The peripheral neuropathy is due to axonal degeneration (rather than demyelinization) and primarily affects motor neurons.
  - Deep tendon reflexes initially may be normal or hyperactive but become decreased or absent as the neuropathy advances.
  - Progression to respiratory and bulbar paralysis and death occurs especially when the diagnosis and treatment are delayed. Sudden death may result from sympathetic overactivity and cardiac arrhythmia.
  - **Mental symptoms such as anxiety, insomnia, depression, disorientation, hallucinations, and paranoia can occur** in acute attacks. Seizures can be due to neurologic effects or to hyponatremia.

For various porphyria refer Question 2 of Biochemistry in AIIMS May 2017

4. A female comes with elevated TSH with subnormal level of free T4:

a. Primary hyperthyroidism
b. Secondary hypothyroidism
c. Primary hypothyroidism
d. Subclinical hypothyroidism

Ans. c. Primary hypothyroidism *Ref: Harrison's Principles of Internal Medicine 19th/ed p2292*

Explanation

A relatively straight question, see below.

Thyroid function tests: Assessment and diagnosis			
Assessment	**Serum TSH**	**Serum free T4**	**Serum T3**
Primary hypothyroidism ***(Option c)***	↑	↓	(N) or ↓
Secondary hypothyroidism ***(Option b)***	↓ (usually) or (N) or ↑ (rare)	↓	↓
Subclinical hypothyroidism ***(Option d)***	↑	(N)	(N)
Euthyroid hypothyroxinema	(N)	(N) or ↓	(N) or ↓
Euthyroid	(N)	(N)	(N)
Euthyroid hyperthyroxinemia	(N)	(N) or ↑	(N) or ↑
Euthyroid: T3 therapy	(N)	↓	(N) or ↑
Euthyroid: Thyroid extract therapy	(N)	Low-(N) or ↓	(N) or ↑

Contd...

Flowchart 2: Evaluation of Hypothyroidism

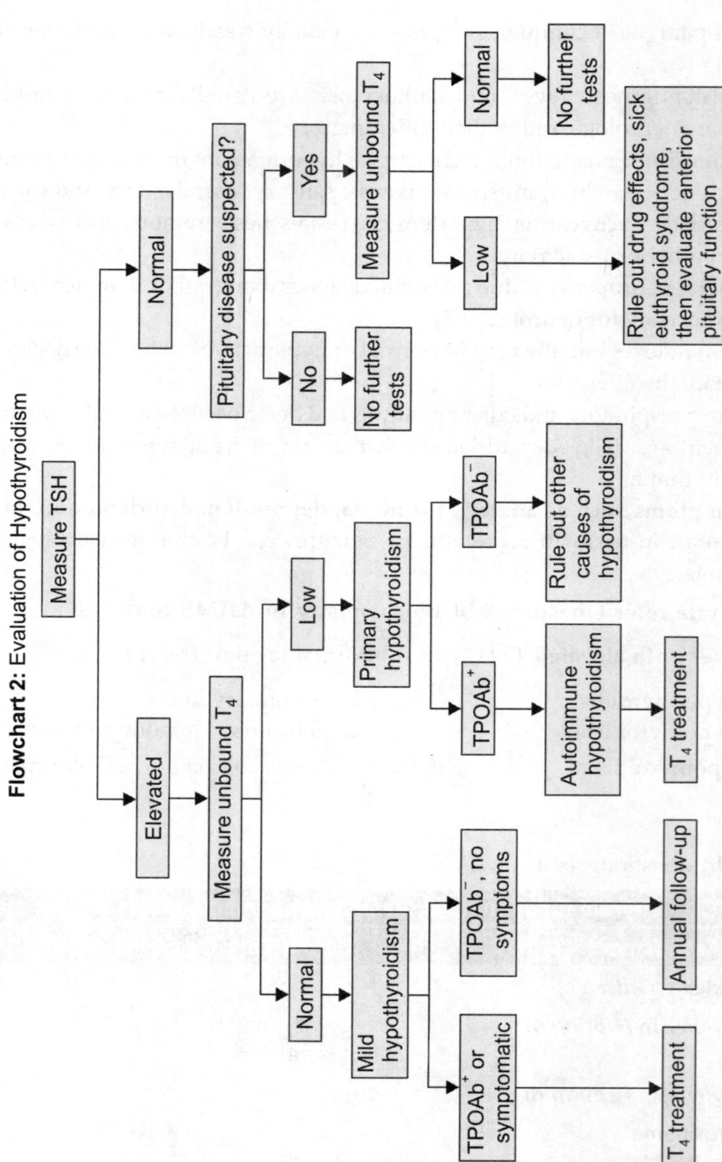

TSH: Thyroid-stimulating hormone; TPOAb: Thyroid peroxidase antibodies.

Contd...

Assessment	Serum TSH	Serum free T4	Serum T3
Hyperthyroidism	↓	↑ or (N)	↑
Subclinical hyperthyroidism	↓	(N)	(N)
TSH-mediated hyperthyroidism	(N) or ↑	↑	↑

5. A lady delivered a normal vaginal delivery and was discharged. On third day she came back with fever, tachycardia and seizures. Fundus showed papilledema with no focal deficits. Diagnosis is:

a. Meningitis
b. Acute migraine
c. Cerebral vein thrombosis
d. Subarachnoid hemorrhage

Ans. c. Cerebral vein thrombosis *Ref: Williams Obstetrics 24th/ed p1193*

EXPLANATION

Raised intracranial pressure (ICP) in puerperal period and absent focal neurological signs favor the diagnosis of cerebral vein thrombosis.

Option (a) Meningitis: Would be associated with fever, neck rigidity/photophobia and presence of early papilledema usually goes against acute bacterial/viral meningitis.

Option (b) Acute migraine: The history of fever and seizures does not go with the diagnosis of migraine.

Option (c) Cerebral vein thrombosis: Points in favor are predisposing factor in the form of prothrombotic state, H/O headache, papilledema, seizures.

In postpartum period if patient presents with headache and seizure, following DD should be considered.

a. Eclampsia
b. Cerebral venous thrombosis
c. Pituitary hemorrhage/Sheehan's syndrome

Cerebral venous thrombosis

- Thrombosis of the lateral or superior sagittal venous sinus usually occurs in the puerperium and often in association with preeclampsia, sepsis, or thrombophilia.
- It is more common in patients with inherited thrombophilias, lupus anticoagulant, or antiphospholipid antibodies.
- Headache is the most common presenting symptom, neurological deficits are common, and up to a third of patients have convulsions.
- Diagnosis is with MR venography.
- Management includes anticonvulsants for seizures, and although heparinization is recommended by most, its efficacy is controversial.
- Antimicrobials are given if there is septic thrombophlebitis, and fibrinolytic therapy is reserved for those women failing systemic anticoagulation.
- The prognosis for venous thrombosis in pregnancy is better than in non-pregnant subjects, and mortality rates are less than 10%.
- The recurrence rate is 1 to 2% during a subsequent pregnancy.

6. A middle-aged man presented with frontal bossing and large tongue and he had spade shaped hands. Which of the following tests will you do for diagnosis?

a. Thyroid hormone assay
b. Serum prolactin
c. Insulin like growth factor
d. Serum testosterone

Ans. c. Insulin like growth factor *Ref: Harrison Principles of Internal Medicine 19th/ed p2269*

EXPLANATION

The given clinical features (frontal bossing, large tongue and spade shaped hands) are suggestive of acromegaly in this middle aged patient. Among the given options IGF-1 (Insulin like growth factor) is used as a screening test in diagnosis of acromegaly.

ACROMEGALY

- **Clinical features**
  - It follows a indolent course, usually takes 10 years to become clinically diagnosable.
  - The overall survival in untreated patients with acromegaly is 10 years less than the age matched control population
  - Features are due to excess of growth hormone (GH) and insulin-like growth factor 1 (IGF1), leading to acral bony overgrowth, soft tissue swelling, visceromegaly and other features as follows:

Acral bony overgrowth	Soft tissue swelling	Visceromegaly	Other features
• ***Frontal bossing*** • ***Increased hand and foot size*** • Mandibular enlargement with prognathism • Widened space between the lower incisor teeth	• Increased heel pad thickness • Increased shoe or glove size • Ring tightening • Characteristic coarse facial features • A large fleshy nose	• Cardiomegaly • ***Macroglossia*** • Thyroid gland enlargement	• Hyperhidrosis • A deep and hollow-sounding voice • Oily skin • Arthropathy, kyphosis, carpal tunnel syndrome • Proximal muscle weakness and fatigue • Acanthosis nigricans, and skin tags

  - The most significant clinical impact of GH excess occurs with respect to the cardiovascular system.
  - Other important manifestations
    - 25% of patients develop diabetes mellitus
    - Increased risk of colonic polyps
- **Diagnosis:** It is based on clinical finding described above and investigations described below:
  - Single random GH level → is **not useful** because of pulsatile nature of GH secretion
  - IGF-1 levels → used as a **screening test** ***(Answer Option c)***
  - GH suppression test → **confirmatory test** [GH suppression to < 0.4 μg/L within 1–2 h of an oral glucose load (75 g)]
  - PRL is elevated in 25% of cases ***(Option b)***
  - Thyroid function ***(Option a)***, gonadotropins, and sex steroids may be attenuated because of tumor mass effects
  - MRI preferred over CT for demonstrating tumor
- Preferred primary treatment for both microadenoma and macroadenoma is transsphenoidal surgical resection.

7. A 12-year-old patient comes with history of bilateral ascending muscle weakness, along with areflexia. There is no history of trauma. Which of the following should be evaluated first?

a. Serum potassium
b. Serum calcium
c. Serum magnesium
d. Serum sodium

Ans. a. Serum potassium *Ref: Harrisons Principles of Internal Medicine 19th/ed p462-e 16*

EXPLANATION

History is similar to that of Guillain-Barré syndrome (GBS). Now among the given options hypokalemia can cause flaccid ascending paralysis, which is one of the differential diagnosis of GBS and it also causes hypokalemic periodic paralysis. Young age and no history of trauma mentioned in question it can be considered a case of hypokalemic periodic paralysis (PP).

- Hypocalcemia and hypomagnesemia cause tetany
- Hypercalcemia does not cause ascending paralysis

For GBS refer Question 21 of JIPMER.

HYPOKALEMIC PERIODIC PARALYSIS

- Due to a defect in muscle ion channels, and manifests as episodes of painless muscle weakness that may be triggered by rest after vigorous exercise, stress, or a high-carbohydrate meal.
- As the name suggests paralytic attacks occur periodically
  - Attacks begin in late childhood or teenage years.
  - **Frequency:** Disease free intervals of weeks to months are common, some patients experience several attacks per week.
  - **Duration:** Attack typically last several hours, but the duration can range from minutes to days.
  - **Trigger factors**: Attacks may be triggered by rest after vigorous exercise, stress, or a high-carbohydrate meal, often after a delay of several hours.
  - **Pathogenesis**: Often associated with an increased release of epinephrine or insulin, both of which cause movement of potassium into cells and low potassium blood levels.
- **Neurologic examination** during an attack:
  - Weakness, usually affecting proximal more than distal muscles, and the legs more than the arms.
  - Hyporeflexia or areflexia is typical.
  - Between attacks, the neurologic examination is usually normal; the myotonia typical of hyperkalemic PP is not a feature of hypokalemic PP.
- **Diagnosis:** Established family history = episodes of periodic paralysis or
  - Documentation of hypokalemia during a typical attack of weakness + other tests to rule out alternative diagnoses.

8. A young girl with the diagnosis of acute promyelocytic leukemia (APML) was treated medically. She developed fever and tachypnea and chest X-ray shows pulmonary infiltrates. Which is the drug she should be given next?

a. Doxorubicin
b. Methotrexate
c. Dexamethasone
d. Cytarabine

Ans. c. Dexamethasone

Ref: Harrisons Principles of Internal Medicine 19th/ed p686; Miguel A. Sanz and Pau Montesinos, How we Prevent and Treat Differentiation Syndrome in Patients with Acute Promyelocytic Leukemia; Blood 2014 123:2777-2782; doi: https://doi.org/10.1182/blood-2013-10-512640

EXPLANATION

The patient here presents with fever, tachypnea and pulmonary infiltrates, that developed after treatment. Acute promyelocytic leukemia (APML) is treated with oral tretinoin (DOC for APML). Frequent complication tretinoin is development of 'APML differentiation syndrome', this is treated by dexamethasone.

Review of Acute Promyelocytic Leukemia (APML)

- **APML:** A highly curable subtype of acute myeloid leukemia (AML), and approximately 85% of these patients achieve long-term survival with current approaches.

- Before tretinoin use earlier APML was responsive to cytarabine and daunorubicin, but previously patients treated with these drugs alone frequently died from disseminated intravascular coagulation (DIC) induced by the release of granule components by the chemotherapy-treated leukemia cells.
- With the introduction of tretinoin (oral drug) prognosis of APML has changed dramatically from adverse to favorable.
- Tretinoin decreases the frequency of DIC but produces another complication called the APML differentiation syndrome.
- **APML differentiation syndrome:**
  - Occurs **within the first 3 weeks** of treatment.
  - It is characterized by **fever**, fluid retention, dyspnea, chest pain, **pulmonary infiltrates**, pleural and pericardial effusions, and hypoxemia ***(Question)***
  - The syndrome is related to adhesion of differentiated neoplastic cells to the pulmonary vasculature endothelium.
  - Treatment:
    - **Dexamethasone:** Most commonly used drug to treat this syndrome ***(Answer)***
    - Other supportive measures like furosemide is used to treat fluid overload
    - If the syndrome is severe → temporary discontinuation of tretinoin
  - Severe APML differentiation syndrome = if patient develops renal failure or requires admission to the ICU due to respiratory distress
  - The mortality rate of this syndrome is about 10%.
- Mechanism of tretinoin: In APML t(15;17) leads to disruption of retinoic acid receptor alpha *(RARA)* gene that codes for retinoid acid receptor. Tretinoin acts through inducing differentiation of these leukemia cells bearing t(15;17).

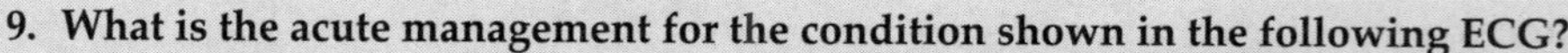

9. What is the acute management for the condition shown in the following ECG?

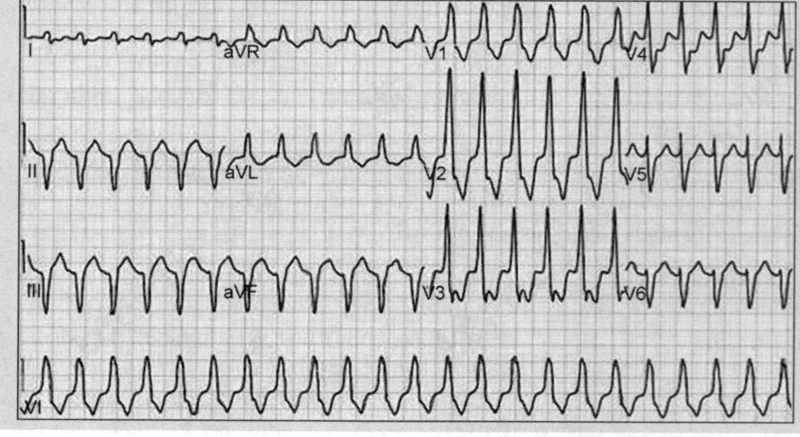

a. $MgSO_4$ b. DC cardioversion
c. Lignocaine d. Diltiazem

Ans. b. DC cardioversion *Ref: Harrison's Principles of Internal Medicine 19th/ed p1494*

Explanation

The given ECG shows wide QRS and tachycardia, which points towards diagnosis of wide complex tachycardia.

Option a: $MgSO_4$ is used in TDP.

Option c: Lignocaine is not indicated unless it is post myocardial infraction (MI) or ischemic ventricular tachycardia (VT).

A wide complex tachycardia (WCT) represents a unique clinical challenge for two reasons:

1. Diagnosing the arrhythmia is difficult: Although most WCTs are due to VT, the differential diagnosis includes a variety of supraventricular tachycardia (SVTs). Diagnostic algorithms to differentiate these two etiologies are complex and imperfect.
2. Urgent therapy is often required: Patients may be unstable at the onset of the arrhythmia or deteriorate rapidly at any time, particularly if the WCT is VT.

Acute management of sustained VT:

- Initial management follows advanced cardiac life support (ACLS) guidelines.
- If hypotension, impaired consciousness, or pulmonary edema is present → QRS synchronous electrical **cardioversion**
- For stable tachycardia → **trial of adenosine** is reasonable, as this may clarify a supraventricular tachycardia with aberrancy
- Intravenous **amiodarone is the drug of choice** if heart disease is present.
- Subsequent management is determined by the underlying heart disease and frequency of VT.
  - If VT recurs frequently or is incessant, → antiarrhythmic medications or catheter ablation may be required to restore stability.
  - ICDs are usually considered for VT associated with structural heart disease.

10. Definition of fever of unknown origin (FUO) includes all of the following *except*:

a. Fever persisting for more than 3 weeks
b. Two fever spikes more than 38.3°C
c. Undiagnosed after one week of investigation
d. No history of immunocompromised state

Ans. c. Undiagnosed after one week of investigation

Ref: Harrison's Principles of Internal Medicine 19th/ed p135

EXPLANATION

Undiagnosed after 1 week of investigation was included in old definition, now it is changed to set of investigations to be done.

Original definition of fever of unknown origin (FUO) by Petersdorf and Beeson in 1961
• An illness of >3 weeks' duration • With fever of ≥38.3°C (101°F) on 2 occasions • An uncertain diagnosis despite 1 week of inpatient evaluation ***(Option c)***.
Need for revised definition:
• As patient may not be admitted just for diagnostic evaluation and evaluation for 1 week is quantitative measure and it is changed to qualitative measure like specific set of investigations to be completed. • Also the immunocompromised individuals need separate evaluation and are excluded from the definition.
Now the definition of FUO is
1. Fever >38.3°C (101°F) on at least two occasions ***(Option b)*** 2. Illness duration of ≥3 weeks ***(Option a)*** 3. No known immunocompromised state ***(Option d)*** 4. Diagnosis that remains uncertain after a thorough ▪ History-taking ▪ Physical examination, and

Contd...

Contd...

- Following obligatory investigations:
  - Erythrocyte sedimentation rate (ESR) and C-reactive protein (CRP) level;
  - Platelet count; total leukocyte count (TLC) and differential leukocyte count (DLC)
  - Measurement of levels of (Hb), electrolytes, creatinine, total protein, alkaline phosphatase (ALP), alanine aminotransferase (ALT), aspartate aminotransferase (AST), lactic dehydrogenase (LDH), creatine kinase (CK), ferritin, antinuclear antibody (ANA) and rheumatoid arthritis (RA) factor;
  - Protein electrophoresis;
  - Urinalysis;
  - Blood cultures (*n* = 3); urine culture;
  - Chest X-ray; abdominal ultrasonography (USG); and tuberculin skin test (TST)

11. Window period for thrombolytic therapy in case of stroke is:

a. 1.5 hour
b. 2.5 hours
c. 3.5 hours
d. 4.5 hours

Ans. d. 4.5 hours *Ref: Harrison's Principles of Internal Medicine 19th/ed p2562*

Explanation

- ❑ The time of stroke onset is defined as the time the patient's symptoms were witnessed to begin or the time the patient was last seen as normal
- ❑ Patients who awaken with stroke have the onset defined as when they went to bed
- ❑ Efficacy of rtPA is confirmed in the < 3 h time window, and efficacy likely extended to 4.5 h and possibly to 6 h.
- ❑ In Europe and Canada, recombinant tissue plasminogen activator (rtPA) is approved in the 3–4.5 h window but in US and Canada, it is still only approved for 0–3 hour.

Administration of intravenous recombinant tissue plasminogen activator (rtPA) for acute ischemic stroke	
Indication	**Contraindication**
• Clinical diagnosis of stroke • Onset of symptoms to time of drug administration ≤4.5 hour • CT scan showing no hemorrhage or edema of >1/3 of the MCA territory • Age 18 ≥ years • Consent by patient or surrogate	• Sustained BP >185/110 mm Hg despite treatment • Platelets <100,000; HCT <25%; glucose <50 or >400 mg/dL • Use of heparin within 48 h and prolonged PTT, or elevated INR • Rapidly improving symptoms • Prior stroke or head injury within 3 months; prior intracranial hemorrhage • Major surgery in preceding 14 days • Minor stroke symptoms • Gastrointestinal bleeding in preceding 21 days • Recent myocardial infarction • Coma or stupor
Administration of rtPA	
• IV access with two peripheral IV lines (avoid arterial or central line placement) • Review eligibility for rtPA • Administer 0.9 mg/kg IV (maximum 90 mg) IV as 10% of total dose by bolus, followed by remainder of total dose over 1 hour • Frequent cuff blood pressure monitoring • No other antithrombotic treatment for 24 hour • For decline in neurologic status or uncontrolled blood pressure, stop infusion, give cryoprecipitate, and reimage brain emergently • Avoid urethral catheterization for ≥2 hour	

12. A 40-year-old female currently on a drug for psychiatric illness and hypertension presents with NYHA class III heart failure with dyspnea, pedal edema and K levels of 5.5 mEq/L and creatinine 2.5 mg%. Which of the following drug is best avoided?

a. Spironolactone
b. Amitriptyline
c. Enalapril
d. Digoxin

Ans. a. Spironolactone *Ref: KDT 7th/ed p523*

Explanation

The patient in the question is having hypertension and some psychiatric illness and now presents with heart failure, hyperkalemia and increased serum creatinine.

- Among the given options
- *Option d:* Digoxin is not a preferred drug in heart failure. But as it causes hypokalemia, it may be beneficial in this patient.
- *Option a*: Amitryptiline is a tricyclic antidepressants (TCA), it can potentially cause fatal arrhythmias and it is contraindicated during acute recovery phase following myocardial infarction. But the patient is having some psychiatric illness; use may depend on the risk benefit ratio. As the psychiatric illness, its severity, controlled or not, is not mentioned nothing can be commented on it.
- *Option a and c:* Both these drugs cause hyperkalemia. Hyperkalemia is a contraindication for use of spironolactone, for angiotensin-converting enzyme (ACE) inhibitors it is not a contraindication.
  - All drugs affecting rennin angiotensin aldosterone path can cause hyperkalemia.
  - Aldosterone action causes Na^+ reabsorption and K^+ and H^+ excretion, therefore when this action is inhibited **hyperkalemia** and **metabolic acidosis** may be seen. Thus renin inhibitors (Aliskerin) ACE inhibitors (enalapril) angiotensin receptor blocker (ARB) (sartans) and aldosterone antagonists (spironolactone, eplerenone); all cause hyperkalemia.
  - Lower the path inhibited by a drug more chances of hyperkalemia, thus Aldosterone antagonist cause more hyperkalemia than ACE inhibitors.
- Contraindications of ACE inhibitors (enalapril), aldosterone antagonist spironolactone and amitriptyline are as follows:

Contraindication (C/I) of enalapril	C/I of spironolactone	C/I of amitryptiline
• H/O angioedema on use of any ACE inhibitor • Patients with hereditary or idiopathic angioedema • Drugs that act directly on the renin-angiotensin system can cause injury and death to the developing fetus (avoid in pregnancy)	• Patients with anuria, acute renal insufficiency, significant impairment of renal excretory function • Hyperkalemia	• Hypersensitvity to drug • **Not recommended for use during the acute recovery phase following myocardial infarction.** • Not be given concomitantly with monoamine oxidase (MAO) inhibitors or cisapride

- Thus either amitriptyline or spironolactone can be answer, moreover spironolactone also causes CNS depression that may worsen the condition of given patient's psychiatric illness, therefore best answer among both will be spironolactone.

13. Which of the following is not a feature of myasthenia gravis?

a. Normal pupillary reflex
b. Ptosis
c. Absent deep tendon reflexes
d. Muscle fatigue

Ans. c. Absent deep tendon reflex *Ref: Harrison's Principles of Internal Medicine 19th/ed p2702*

Explanation

Absent deep tendon reflexes and autonomic features are present in Lambert-Eaton myasthenic syndrome (LEMS). These two features make LEMS easily distinguishable from myasthenia gravis (MG = normal reflexes and no autonomic symptoms).

- Myasthenia gravis is suspected on the basis of
  - Weakness and fatigability in the typical distribution ***(Option b and d)***
  - No loss of → tendon reflexes ***(Option c)***
  - No loss of → sensation or other neurologic function ***(Option a)***
- Once suspected the diagnosis should be confirmed:
  Diagnosis of myasthenia gravis = History + Physical examination + Lab testing.

Diagnosis of myasthenia gravis	
History of	Diplopia, ptosis, dysarthria, dysphagia, dyspnea
	Weakness in characteristic distribution: Proximal limbs, neck extensors, generalized
	Fluctuation and fatigue: worse with repeated activity, improved by rest
	Effects of previous treatments
Physical examination	Ptosis, diplopia
	Motor power survey: Quantitative testing of muscle strength
	Forward arm abduction time (5 min)
	Vital capacity measurement
	Absence of other neurologic signs
Laboratory testing	Anti-acetylcholine receptor (anti-AChR) radioimmunoassay 85% positive in generalized MG; 50% in ocular MG; If positive → **Diagnostic of MG** If negative → does not exclude MG. 40% of AChR antibody–negative patients with generalized MG have anti-MuSK antibodies.
	Repetitive nerve stimulation: Decrement of >15% at 3 Hz: highly probable
	Single-fiber electromyography: Blocking and jitter, with normal fiber density; **confirmatory, but not specific**
	Edrophonium chloride (Tensilon) 2 mg + 8 mg IV; highly probable diagnosis if unequivocally positive
	For ocular or cranial MG: Exclude intracranial lesions by CT or MRI

14. A 70-year-old smoker with brain metastasis with BP - 150/100 mm Hg, was admitted and started on antihypertensive drug thiazide. There are no neurological signs or pedal edema. Serum electrolytes were normal at admission, after starting of treatment, patient becomes confused and drowsy, his Se. Sodium was 123 mEq/L, urine-Na 110 mg/dL, Sr osmolarity –285 and Urine osmolarity 350. Most likely cause of hyponatremia is?

a. SIADH
b. Cerebral salt wasting
c. Diuretic induced hyponatremia
d. Pseudohypoaldosteronism

Ans. a. SIADH *Ref: Harrison's Principles of Internal Medicine 19th/ed p299*

Explanation

In this given history, patient is having hyponatremia with increased urinary sodium and normal serum osmolality. This history in the setting of lung malignancy (Smoker with brain metastasis) points towards diagnosis of SIADH.

Thiazide can cause hyponatremia but less likely based on much of the history.

SIADH: Euvolemic hyponatremia with increased urinary osmolality and increased urinary excretion of sodium.

For diagnostic approach of hyponatremia *see* Flowchart 3:

15. What complication of stroke does not require any treatment?

a. Spasticity
b. Neglect
c. Dysphagia
d. Fever

Ans: b. Neglect *Ref: Harrison's Principles of Internal Medicine 19th/ed p2573; Medical Complications after Stroke, Lancet Neurol 2010;9:105-18, Sandeep Kumar et al.*

Explanation

See below

- *Option d:* Fever
  - It can exacerbate neuronal injury by increasing metabolic demands on injured brain tissues.
  - Prompt treatment of hyperthermia might be effective in improving neurological outcomes
- *Option c:* Dysphagia
  - Patients with dysphagia are at particularly high risk for developing pneumonia, and severe dysphagia is estimated to lead to an 11-fold increase in this risk
  - A formal evaluation of swallowing function, appropriate dietary modifications and use of local anesthetics are crucial for preventing chest infections
- *Option a:* Spasticity
  - It cause pain, disability cosmetic disfigurement and psychosocial impact and hence should be treated with baclofen and tizanidine
- *Option b:* Neglect
  - It most often recovers spontaneously without treatment in 1 to 6 months
  - Active treatment may cause trouble to patient if recovery is partial
  - If persists > 6 months, neglect should be treated
  - Also note that neglect is one of the major precipitating event for falls which leads to hip fracture, thus treatment may be a necessary.

Based on above discussion most probably the answer appears to be neglect, but still not sure because their is no direct reference for such question.

16. Following parameters of CURB 65 score are true *except*:

a. Respiratory rate of > 30 /min
b. Confusion and blood urea greater than 7 mmol/L
c. Systolic blood pressure (SBP) less than or equal to 100 mm Hg, diastolic blood pressure (DBP) less than or equal to 60 mm Hg
d. Age > 65

Ans. c. Systolic blood pressure (SBP) less than or equal to 100 mm Hg, Diastolic blood pressure (DBP) less than or equal to 60 mm Hg *Ref: Harrison's Principles of Internal Medicine 19th/ed p806-807*

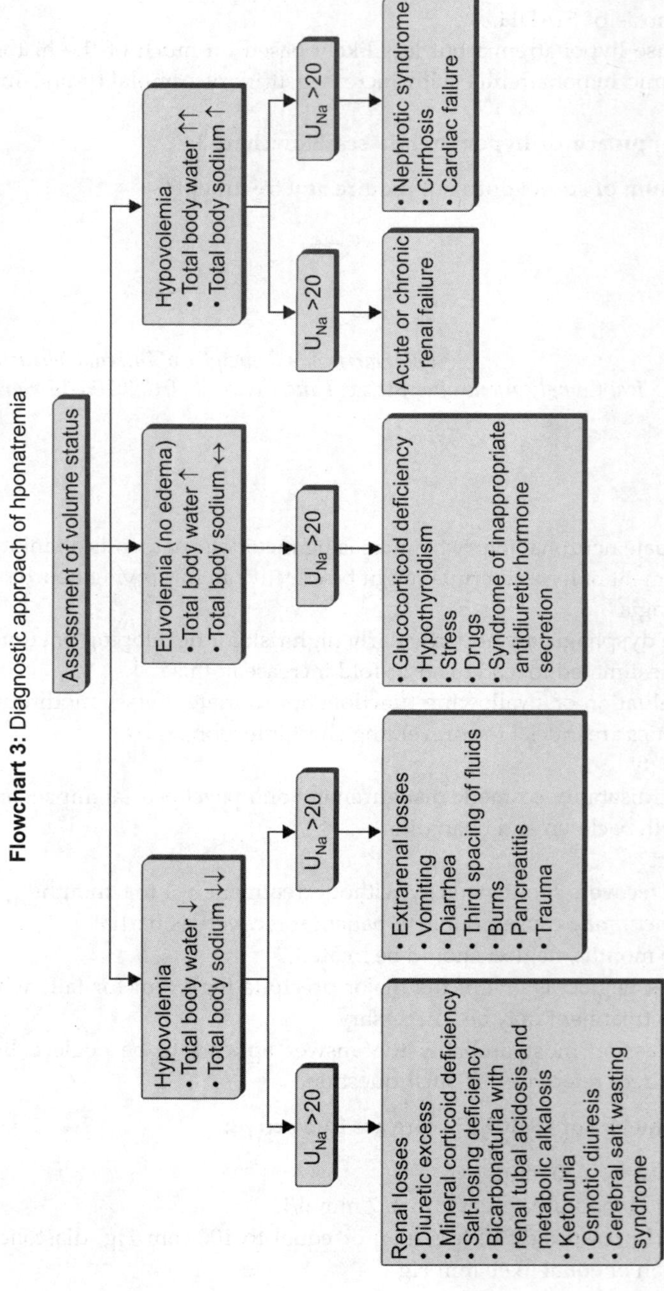

Flowchart 3: Diagnostic approach of hponatremia

Explanation

- In pneumonia treatment, it is often difficult to predict which patients require admission.
- Two currently used scoring systems used are PSI and CURB-65
- Pneumonia severity index (PSI): A prognostic model used to identify patients at low risk of dying
  - Points are given for 20 variables, including age, coexisting illness, and abnormal physical and laboratory findings.
  - Based on scores obtained patients are assigned to one of five classes with the following mortality rates: class 1, 0.1%; class 2, 0.6%; class 3, 2.8%; class 4, 8.2%; and class 5, 29.2%.

Class	1	2	3	4	5
Mortality	0.1%	0.6%	2.8%	8.2%	29.2%

  - PSI is often impractical in a busy emergency department setting because of the number of variables that must be assessed.
- CURB-65: *See below*

	CURB-65 Score
C	Confusion (disorientation to time, place and person)
U	Urea > 7 mmol/L (20 mg/dL)
R	Respiratory rate ≥30 breaths/minute
B	Blood pressure (SBP <90 mm Hg or DBP <60 mm Hg)
65	Age ≥65 years
	• 1 point is assigned for each criterion that is met. • Score = 0 → can be treated outside hospital (30 day mortality rate 1.5%) • Score = 1 → favors hospital admission, but a score 1 due to age alone ≥65 years without other comorbidities, not necessarily require hospital admission • Score = 2 → Patient should be admitted (30 day mortality rate 9.2%) • Score ≥ 3 → Patient may require ICU admission (overall mortality rate is 22%)

PGI May 2017

1. Splenomegaly seen in:

a. Hodgkins lymphoma
b. CML
c. Ovalocytosis
d. Autoimmune hemolytic anemia
e. Iron deficiency anemia

Ans. All *Ref: Harrison's Principles of Internal Medicine 19th/ed p410-412*

Explanation

- Spleen has various functions and splenomegaly may result in due to excess demand of function in various conditions as discussed below:

Functions of spleen	Cause of splenomegaly	Examples
Removes senescent and defective red blood cells	Reticuloendothelial hyperplasia	Spherocytosis, early sickle cell anemia, **ovalocytosis *(option c)*,** Thalassemia major, hemoglobinopathies, Paroxysmal nocturnal hemoglobinuria, pernicious anemia

Contd...

Contd...

Functions of spleen	Cause of splenomegaly	Examples
Generates immune response to certain pathogens	Immune hyperplasia; response to infection (viral, bacterial, fungal, parasitic)	Infectious mononucleosis, AIDS, viral hepatitis, cytomegalovirus, Subacute bacterial endocarditis, bacterial septicaemia, congenital syphilis, splenic abscess, tuberculosis, histoplasmosis, malaria
Synthesizes antibodies in the white pulp	Disordered immunoregulation	Rheumatoid arthritis (Felty's syndrome) SLE, collagen vascular diseases, serum sickness, **immune hemolytic anemias *(option d)*,** immune thrombocytopenias, immune neutropenias, drug reactions, angioimmunoblastic lymphadenopathy, Sarcoidosis, thyrotoxicosis (benign lymphoid hypertrophy), interleukin 2 therapy
Generates cellular components of blood under specific conditions where the bone marrow cannot meet the needs	Extramedullary hematopoiesis	Myelofibrosis, marrow damage by toxins, radiation, strontium, marrow infiltration by tumors, leukemias, Gaucher's disease

Apart from hyperfunction discussed above other causes that can lead to splenomegaly are as below:

Outflow obstruction (splenic vein or portal vein)		Cirrhosis, hepatic vein obstruction, intrahepatic or extrahepatic portal vein obstruction, cavernous transformation of the portal vein, splenic vein obstruction, splenic artery aneurysm, hepatic schistosomiasis, hepatic echinococcosis, congestive heart failure, portal hypertension (due to any cause)
Infiltration of spleen	Intracellular or extracellular depositions	Amyloidosis, Gaucher's disease, Niemann-Pick disease, Tangier disease, Hurler's syndrome and other mucopolysaccharidoses, hyperlipidemias
	Benign and malignant cellular infiltrations	**Leukemias (acute, chronic, lymphoid, myeloid, monocytic), lymphomas, Hodgkin's disease**, ***(option a and b),*** myeloproliferative syndromes (e.g., polycythemia vera, essential, thrombocytosis), angiosarcomas, metastatic tumors (melanoma is most common), eosinophilic granuloma, histiocytosis X, hamartomas, hemangiomas, fibromas, lymphangiomas, splenic cysts
Unknown cause		Idiopathic splenomegaly, **iron-deficiency anemia *(option e)*,** berylliosis

- Causes of massive splenomegaly (>8 cm below costal margin and/or weight >1kg) are:

1. Chronic myeloid leukemia (CML), chronic lymphocytic leukemia (CLL), hairy cell leukemia, lymphomas
2. Polycythemia vera, myelofibrosis with myeloid metaplasia, Gaucher's disease
3. Autoimmune hemolytic anemia, sarcoidosis
4. Diffuse splenic hemangiomatosis

2. Myasthenia gravis with MuSK antibodies—true is/are:

a. Thymic hyperplasia
b. Prominent proximal muscle weakness
c. More facial weakness
d. MuSK is more severe
e. Resistant to usual treatment of myasthenia

Ans. b. Prominent proximal muscle weakness; c. More facial weakness; d. MuSK is more severe and e. Resistant to usual treatment of myasthenia

Ref: CMDT 2017 page 1045 and Harrison's Principles of Internal Medicine 19th/ed p2702-2704

EXPLANATION

- Antibodies identified in myasthenia gravis (MG)
  1. Antibodies against AChR (acetylcholine receptor):
     - Found in 85% of patients with generalized MG and 50% of ocular MG
     - Presence is confirmatory but absence does not rule out MG
     - Used in diagnosis of MG
  2. Antibodies against MuSK (muscle-specific kinase):
     - Found in 40% of patients with AChR antibody negative
     - MuSK is a protein involved in clustering of ACh receptors at neuromuscular junctions
     - Used in diagnosis of MG
     - Typical features of MuSK antibodies positive patients compared to AChR antibody positive patients
     - Bulbar weakness is prominent (facial features) ***(option c)***
     - Response to anticholinesterase therapy is poor (which is standard therapy in MG) ***(option e)***
     - Response to thymectomy is poor *('**option a**' can be considered false)*
     - Responds well to rituximab
     - More likely to have facial, respiratory, and **proximal muscle weakness *(option b)*** than those with AChR antibodies. *(CMDT 2017)*
  3. Other antibodies: These are not available for commercial testing
     - Patients who are negative for both AChR and MuSK antibodies show positivity for these antibodies against
     - Low-density lipoprotein receptor related protein 4 (lrp4)
     - Agrin
     - lrp4 and agrin too play a role in clustering of AChR clustering.
- **About option a and d**
  - MG with anti-MuSK antibodies is often severe and requires aggressive treatment ***(option d)***
  - Usually does not respond to thymectomy
  - Thymic changes are much less in anti-MuSK MG compared to anti- AChR MG, though some changes are seen. For the purpose of this question because other options are about comparing anti-MuSK with anti-AChR antibodies this option can be taken as wrong.

3. Dubin Johnson syndrome—true is/are:

a. Autosomal dominant
b. Defect in udp glucoronsyl transferase
c. Reduced secretion of conjugated bilirubin in bile
d. Elevated AST/ALT
e. Kernicterus

Ans. c. Reduced secretion of conjugated bilirubin in bile

Ref: Harrison's Principles of Internal Medicine 19th/ed p281-282

EXPLANATION

- Dubin-Johson syndrome, an autosomal recessive condition is one of the cause of isolated hyperbilirubinemia
- Isolated hyperbilirubinemia means only serum bilirubin is raised and remaining liver function tests are normal ***(option d)***

- ❑ Isolated hyperbilirubinemia can be conjugated or unconjugated.
- ❑ Inherited causes of isolated unconjugated/indirect hyperbilirubinemia include Crigler-Najjar S and Gilberts syndrome
- ❑ Inherited causes of isolated conjugated/direct hyperbilirubinemia include Dubin-Johnson S and Rotor S
- ❑ *Option a:* Only Crigler-Najjar type 2 is autosomal dominant (AD), remaining inherited isolated hyperbilirubinemia are autosomal recessive (AR).
- ❑ *Option b:* UDPGT is defective in Crigler-Najjar S and Gilberts syndrome
- ❑ *Option e:* Kernicetrus is feature of Crigler-Najjar S.

Inherited causes of isolated hyperbilirubinemia				
Unconjugated or indirect hyperbilirubinemia			Conjugated or direct hyperbilirubinemia	
Crigler-Najjar type 1	Crigler-Najjar type 2	Gilbert's syndrome	Dubin-Johnson syndrome	Rotor syndrome
• **AR** • Mutations in the critical 3′ domain of the *UDPGT* gene; complete absence of **UDPGT** activity totally unable to conjugate bilirubin; and hence cannot excrete it. • Exceptionally rare found in neonates death in infancy or childhood. • Severe jaundice (Bl>20 mg/dL) neurologic impairment due to **kernicterus**	• **AD** • Mutations in gene causes reduction, but not complete absence of **UDPGT** activity. • Phenobarbital can be used to induce UDPGT activity. Common than type I. • Patients survive into adulthood • Se Bl 6–25 mg/dL. • Susceptible to **kernicterus** under the stress (illness or surgery)	• **AR** • Mutations in the promoter and, rarely, in the coding region; reduction in transcription **UDPGT** gene; activity is 1/3rd of the normal. Very common 3–7% of the population, males> females by a ratio of 2–7:1. • Se Bl <6 mg/dL. • Jaundice is often identified only during periods of fasting	• **AR** • Common than Rotor S. • Asymptomatic jaundice. • Mutations in the gene (ABCCA) that codes for MRP2 (protein) • MRP2 (Multidrug resistance protein) is a canalicular transporter that has role in excretion of conjugated bilirubin. • **Reduced excretion of bilirubin into the bile ducts *(Option c)***	• **AR** • Less common. • Asymptomatic jaundice. • Deficiency of the major hepatic drug uptake transporter proteins OATP1B1 and OATP1B3 • This results in **reduced reuptake of bilirubin that has been pumped into portal circulation** by MRP3

4. Diagnosis of Wilson's disease is by:

a. Se ceruloplasmin <20 mg/dL
b. Liver copper >250 μg/g dry weight of liver:
c. Kayser-Fleischer ring
d. Characteristic histology
e. 24 hour urine copper <40 μg

Ans. b. Liver copper >250 μg/g dry weight of liver and c. Kayser-Fleischer ring

Ref: Harrison's Principles of Internal Medicine 19th/ed p2521 and Robbins and Cotran Pathological Basis of Disease 8th/ed p1647

EXPLANATION

Robbins and Cotran Pathological basis of disease 8th/ed p1647:

This question is a direct statement from Robbins as follows *"The biochemical diagnosis of Wilson disease is based on a decrease in serum ceruloplasmin, an increase in hepatic copper content* ***(the most sensitive and accurate test)****, and increased urinary excretion of copper* ***(the most specific screening test)****. Serum copper levels are of no diagnostic value, since they may be low, normal, or elevated, depending on the stage of evolution of the disease. Demonstration of Kayser-Fleischer rings further favors the diagnosis."*

- ***Option a*** is considered false based on statement of Harrisons as follows *"Serum ceruloplasmin levels should not be used for definitive diagnosis, because they are normal in up to 10% of affected patients and are reduced in 20% of carriers."*
- ***Option b:*** The gold standard for diagnosis remains liver biopsy with quantitative copper assays.
- ***Option d:*** Histology of Wilson's disease is similar to that of viral- and drug-induced hepatitis, therefore histology cannot reliably diagnose Wilson's disease. Excess copper deposition can be demonstrated by special stains. But copper also accumulates in chronic obstructive cholestasis, therefore just demonstration of copper will not be diagnostic. Demonstration of hepatic copper content in excess of 250 μg per gram dry weight is most helpful for making a diagnosis.
- ***Option e:*** With increase in free serum copper urinary copper levels also increase.
- Other important features are as follows
  - Wilson's disease is due to mutation in ATP7B gene (chromosome 13) which leads to defective copper transport → leads to *decrease in copper transport into bile resulting in copper accumulation in liver.*
  - Defective copper incorporation into apoceruloplasmin leads to excess catabolism resulting in low blood levels of ceruloplasmin → leads to increase in free serum copper, which accumulates in CNS and cornea leading to neuropsychiatrical symptoms and Kayser-Fleischer ring respectively.
  - **The most common presentation is** *acute or chronic liver disease.*

Ref: Harrison's Principles of Internal Medicine 19th/ed p2521

- Diagnosis of Wilson's disease and usefulness of each test is as follows:

Test	Usefulness	Normal value	Wilson's disease	Carrier state
Serum ceruloplasmin	+	18–35 mg/dL	Low in 90%	Low in 20%
Kayser-Fleischer rings	++	Absent	Present in • >99% if neurologic or psychiatric involvement • 30–50% in hepatic presentation and presymptomatic state	Absent
Urine copper (24 h)	+++	20–50 μg	• >100 μg in symptomatic patients; • 60 to >100 μg in presymptomatic patients	Normal to 80 μg
Liver copper	++++	20–50 μg/g of tissue	>200 μg/g	Normal to 125 μg/g
Haplotype analysis	++++ (siblings only)	0 matches	2 matches	1 match

5. Features of pituitary apoplexy:

a. Ophthalmoplegia
b. Headache
c. Fever
d. Derailed consciousness
e. Seizure

Ans. a. Ophthalmoplegia; b. Headache and d. Derailed consciousness

Ref: Harrison's Principles of Internal Medicine 19th/ed p2257

EXPLANATION

See the table below:

Pituitary apoplexy	Sudden hemorrhage into the pituitary gland, often occurring into a pituitary adenoma
Causes	• May occur spontaneously in preexisting adenoma; postpartum (Sheehan's syndrome) • Or it may occur in association with diabetes, hypertension, sickle cell anemia, or acute shock
Clinical features	• Is an endocrine emergency that may result in severe hypoglycemia, hypotension • Acute symptoms: ▪ Severe headache with signs of meningeal irritation ***(option b)*** ▪ Bilateral visual changes, ophthalmoplegia ***(option a)*** • In severe cases pituitary apoplexy can cause cardiovascular collapse, loss of consciousness ***(option d)***, and even sudden death. • Hypopituitarism.
Diagnosis	CT or MRI
Treatment	• Patients with no evident visual loss or impaired consciousness → observed and managed conservatively with high-dose glucocorticoids • Patients with significant or progressive visual loss, cranial nerve palsy, or loss of consciousness → urgent surgical decompression • Severe ophthalmoplegia or visual deficits are indications for early surgery (earlier the surgery more will be visual recovery)

6. Hypothalmic pituitary axis controls all the following endocrine glands *except*:

a. Thyroid
b. Parathyroid
c. Pancreas
d. Adrenal
e. Testes

Ans. b. Parathyroid and c. Pancreas *Ref: Guyton 11th/ed p907*

EXPLANATION

Thyroid (TRH → TSH → T3, T4), adrenal (CRH → ACTH → cortisol) and testes (GnRH → FSH → see below) are under control of hypothalamo-pituitary axis.

Parathyroid and pancreatic hormones are not under control of hypothalamic or pituitary glands.

Hypothalamic and pituitary hormones and their major function is summarized further:

Hormones	Major functions
Hypothalamus	
TRH: Thyrotropin-releasing hormone	Stimulates secretion of TSH and prolactin
CRH: Corticotropin-releasing H	Causes release of ACTH
GHRH: Growth hormone–releasing H	Causes release of growth hormone
GHIH: Growth hormone inhibitory H (somatostatin)	Inhibits release of growth hormone
GnRH: Gonadotropin-releasing H	Causes release of LH and FSH
PIF: Dopamine or prolactin-inhibiting factor	Inhibits release of prolactin
Anterior pituitary	
Growth hormone	Stimulates protein synthesis and overall growth of most cells and tissues
Thyroid-stimulating hormone (TSH)	Stimulates synthesis and secretion of thyroid hormones (thyroxine and triiodothyronine)
Adrenocorticotropic hormone (ACTH)	Stimulates synthesis and secretion of adrenocortical hormones (cortisol, androgens, and aldosterone)
Prolactin	Promotes development of the female breasts and secretion of milk
Follicle-stimulating hormone (FSH)	Causes growth of follicles in the ovaries and sperm maturation in sertoli cells of testes
Luteinizing hormone (LH)	Stimulates testosterone synthesis in Leydig cells of testes; stimulates ovulation, formation of corpus luteum, and estrogen and progesterone synthesis in ovaries
Posterior pituitary	
Antidiuretic hormone (ADH) (also called vasopressin)	Increases water reabsorption by the kidneys and causes vasoconstriction and increased blood pressure
Oxytocin	Stimulates milk ejection from breasts and uterine contractions

7. Membranoproliferative GN type 1—true is /are:

a. Low C4 level
b. Double basement membrane appearance on light microscopy
c. Dense deposit along basement membrane on electron microscopy
d. Mesangial hypocellularity
e. Ig G and C3 deposition on

Ans. a. Low C4 level; b. Double basement membrane appearance on light microscopy and e. Ig G and C3 deposition on *Ref: Robbins Basic Pathology 9th/ed p527; Harrison's Principles of Internal Medicine 19th/ed p1840*

Explanation

Hypocomplementemia (low C4), double basement membrane and mesangial hypercellularity (not hypo) is seen in both MPGN1 and 2 *[Thus option a, b are true and option d is false]*. IgG and C3 deposition is seen in MPGN1 *[Option e is true]*. Dense deposit along basement membrane is a feature of MPGN 2 (dense deposit disease) *[Option c is false]*.

Membranoproliferative GN (MPGN) Review

- **MPGN** is manifested histologically by alterations in the
  - Glomerular basement membrane (thickening and deposits)
  - Mesangium (proliferation)
  - Proliferation of glomerular cells.
- **Presentation**:
  - Only with hematuria or proteinuria in the non-nephrotic range or
  - Combined nephrotic–nephritic picture.
- **Types**: On the basis of distinct ultrastructural, immunofluorescence, microscopic, and pathogenic findings
  - MPGN 1 (80%)
  - MPGN 2 (20%)
  - But these are now recognized to be separate entities, and MPGN 2 is now called as dense deposit disease
- **Pathogenesis of MPGN 1**
  - Circulating or in situ **immune complexes,**
  - Inciting antigen is not known, but it occurs in association with:
    - Hepatitis B and C antigenemia,
    - Systemic lupus erythematosus
    - Infected atrioventricular shunts, and
    - Extrarenal infections with persistent or episodic antigenemia.
- **Pathogenesis of dense deposit disease (MPGN 2)**
  - **The fundamental abnormality is excessive complement activation.** It can be due to:
    - Autoantibody against C3 convertase, called **C3 nephritic factor** (stabilize the enzyme) → uncontrolled cleavage of C3 → activation of the alternative complement pathway. OR
    - Complement regulatory protein **factor H** (Mutation or autoantibodies against it)
  - Excessive complement activation → Hypocomplementemia. Hypocomplementemia occurs in both MPGN 1 and 2, but it is marked in MPGN 2

Features	MPGN 1	Dense deposit disease (MPGN 2)
Fundamental pathogenic mechanism	• Circulating immune complexes • *In situ* immune complex formation	Excessive complement activation
Complement activated	Both classical and alternative pathway activated	Alternate pathway
Hypocomple-mentemia (70% cases of MPGN) ***(Option a)***	Not usual or less marked	Marked hypocomplementemia
Associated with	Associated with • HBV, HCV • SLE • Infected AV shunts, • Mixed cryoglobulinemia and • Extrarenal infections.	• C3 nephritic factor • Mutation or Ab against **factor H**
Light microscopy (similar in both)	• Glomeruli - **lobular appearance** (large) • **Mesangial and endothelial –proliferation *(Option d)*** and infiltrating leukocytes • **GBM - thickened,** double contour, or "tram track," appearance (evident with silver or PAS stains). ("**splitting" of the GBM** is due to extension of processes of mesangial and inflammatory cells into the peripheral capillary loops and deposition of mesangial matrix ***(Option b)***	

Contd...

Contd...

Features	MPGN 1	Dense deposit disease (MPGN 2)
Electron microscopy	• Subendothelial electron-dense deposits	• Lamina densa and the subendothelial space of the GBM are transformed into an irregular, **ribbon-like, extremely electron-dense structure**, resulting from the deposition of material of unknown composition. ***(Option C)***
	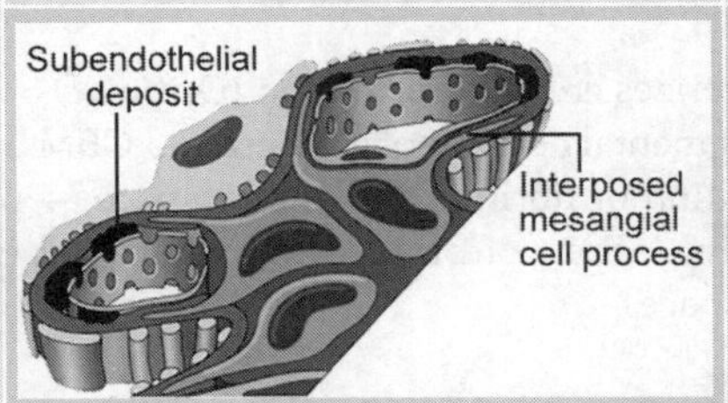 Subendothelial deposit Interposed mesangial cell process	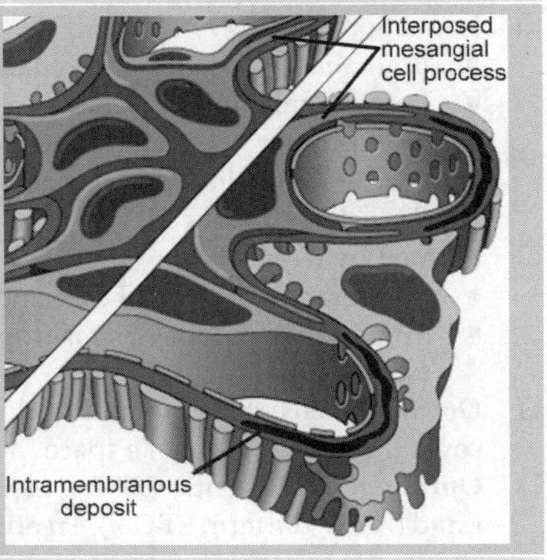 Interposed mesangial cell process Intramembranous deposit
Immunofluorescence microscopy	• C3- deposited in an irregular granular pattern, and • IgG and early complement components (C1q and C4) often **present**, indicative of an immune complex pathogenesis. ***(Option e)***	• C3 is present in irregular chunky and segmental linear foci in the basement membranes and in the mesangium. • IgG and the early components of the classical complement pathway (C1q and C4) are usually **absent**

8. True about crescents in kidney is/are:

a. Always respond to corticosteroids
b. Cover more than 10% of glomerulus
c. Presence of epithelial cells is characteristic of crescent
d. Made up of parietal epithelial cells and monocytes
e. More than 2 cell layer

Ans. c. Presence of epithelial cells is characteristic of crescent and d. Made up of parietal epithelial cells and monocytes *Ref: Robbins Basic Pathology 9th/ed p532; Harrison's Principles of Internal Medicine 19th/ed p1836*

EXPLANATION

Presence of epithelial cells is characteristic feature of crescent. It is made up of parietal epithelial cells and infiltrating leukocytes.

"The characteristic histologic finding associated with RPGN is the presence of crescents" .... Robbin's (532)

"Crescentic glomerulonephritis is the pathologic equivalent of the clinical presentation of RPGN" ...... Harrison's 1836

Crescentic GN Review:

- **Causes:** Many systemic and kidney diseases can cause crescents in kidney.
  - It may be associated with a known disorder or it may be idiopathic.
  - When the cause is identifiable
    - About 12% → anti-GBM antibody–mediated crescentic GN [**RPGN-1** (GP synd)]
    - 44% → immune complex GN with crescents [**RPGN-2** (SLE, HSP, MPGN, PSGN, IgA nephropathy, cryoglobulinemia)]
    - 44% have pauci-immune crescentic GN [**RPGN- 3** (Wegner's, Microscopic polyangitis)]
- Formation of crescent:
  - Epithelial cell proliferation characterizes crescent formation ***(Option c)***
  - Immune/inflammatory injury → segmental necrosis of glomeruli → GBM breaks → exudation of plasma proteins and the deposition of fibrin in Bowman's space → proliferation of the parietal epithelial cells → distinctive lesions of proliferation are called **crescents** owing to their shape as they fill Bowman's space.
- **Formed by *(Option d)***
  - Proliferation of parietal cells and
  - Migration of monocytes/macrophages into Bowman's space; Other types of leukocytes also may be present.
- ***Option b:*** Percentage glomerulus involvement is checked in FSGS not here in crescents it may cover the entire Bowman's space.
- ***Option a:*** In crescentic GN the glomerular injury is severe and progression of disease is very rapid (hence the term RPGN). Treatment here is treatment of cause (which are many as described above). Now in most of the cases steroids are useful, but the term 'always' and 'respond to' in given option "always respond to corticosteroids" make it a false statement.

9. Features of neurofibromatosis type 1 is/are:

a. Axillary freckling
b. Dysplasia of mandible
c. Optic glioma
d. Facial nerve palsy
e. Cafe-au-lait

Ans. a. Axillary freckling; b. Dysplasia of mandible; c. Optic glioma and e. Cafe-au-laut

Ref: Harrison's Principles of Internal Medicine 19th/ed p2343

EXPLANATION

- Basic pathology in NF1 is mutation in neurofibromin gene, on chromosome 17q.
- Normal function of neurofibromin: It is a tumor suppressor protein that maintains inactive state of oncoprotein Ras.
- When mutated, over activity of Ras leads to occurrence of cardinal tumors of NF1.
- Clinical features of NF1 are as follows:

System	Examples of manifestation	Relevant comments
Neurologic	Peripheral and spinal neurofibromas	Learning disabilities and seizures are also features
Ophthalmologic	Optic gliomas and iris hamartomas such as Lisch nodules	
Dermatologic	Cafe au lait macules, axillary freckling	
Skeletal	Scoliosis, macrocephaly, short stature, and pseudoarthrosis	Short stature is frequent in the absence of growth hormone deficiency in patients with NF1

Contd...

Contd...

System	Examples of manifestation	Relevant comments
Vascular	Stenoses of renal and intracranial arteries	
Endocrine	Pheochromocytoma, carcinoid tumors, and precocious puberty (due to extension of optic glioma into the hypothalamus → early activation of GnRH), growth hormone deficiency also reported	Endocrine abnormalities are not found in NF2 and are associated solely with NF1

- ❑ *Option b:* There is a exhaustive list of skeletal manifestations, though 'mandibular dysplasia' was not directly found in most literature but 'dysplasia of bone' has been mentioned and typically dysplasia of tibia has been mentioned.
- ❑ *Option d:* NF1 presents with peripheral and spinal neurofibromas. Cranial nerve involvement is a feature of NF2. There are case reports of facial nerve palsy in NF 1 hence not sure of this option. Hence this is true but very rare.

10. True about HIV-1 infection in pregnancy is/are:

a. Early detection during pregnancy reduces fetal morbidity
b. Zidovudine causes anemia
c. HAART is C/I in pregnancy
d. Cesarean section preferred
e. Chance of transmission to breastfed infant 10–20%

Ans. a. Early detection during pregnancy reduces fetal morbidity; b. Zidovudine causes anemia; d. Cesarean section preferred and e. Chance of transmission to breastfed infant 10–20%.

Ref: Harrison's Principles of Internal Medicine 19th/ed p1223, 50 and William's Obstetrics 24th/ed p1281

Explanation

- ❑ Mother to child transmission can occur any time during pregnancy (23–30%), delivery (50–65%) and/or breastfeeding (12–20%) ***(Option e)***.

Questions	Answers
Most commonly transmission occurs during	Perinatal period
Probability of transmission in absence of prophylaxis to the mother and to the infant	• 15–25% in industrialized countries • 25–35% in developing countries
Rate of MTCT in pregnant women receiving HAART	1% or less
Well documented risk factors associated with increased risk of transmission include	• High maternal plasma viremia levels. • Closer HLA match between mother and child • Prolonged interval between membrane rupture and delivery
Other potential risk factors (but not well documented) include	Presence of chorioamnionitis at delivery; STIs during pregnancy; illicit drug use during pregnancy; cigarette smoking; preterm delivery; and obstetric procedures such as amniocentesis, amnioscopy, fetal scalp electrodes, and episiotomy.

Contd...

Contd...

Questions	Answers
Recommendation for starting antiretroviral therapy in pregnancy	All pregnant HIV-infected women should receive HAART (highly active antiretroviral therapy), regardless of plasma HIV RNA copy, number or CD4+ T cell counts ***(option c)***.
Role of breastfeeding in transmission	
Estimated additional risk of transmission from breast milk, above that occurring during pregnancy and delivery	7 to 22% (approximately 15%) ***(option e)***
Risk factors that increase likelihood of transmission via breast feeding include	Detectable levels of HIV in breast milk; presence of mastitis; low maternal CD4+ T cell counts, and maternal vitamin A deficiency
Risk of HIV infection via breastfeeding is highest in	The early months of breastfeeding
Is breastfeeding a contraindication in HIV infected mothers?	• In developed countries, it is contraindicated since alternative forms of adequate nutrition, are available. • In developing countries, should be continued along with HAART therapy
Which has lower risk of transmission: Exclusive breastfeeding or mixed feeding?	Exclusive breastfeeding has lower risk of transmission

Harrison's Principles of Internal Medicine 19th/ed p50

- ❑ Most well documented risk for transmission is maternal HIV RNA levels.

Maternal HIV RNA levels	Risk of transmission and preferred intervention
<50 copies/mL	• Extremely rare that transmission may occur; but there are case reports of transmission with this level
<1000 copies/mL	• Transmission is very unlikely • Risk is approximately 1% regardless of mode of delivery or duration of membrane rupture (in patients receiving HAART) • Women may elect to attempt a vaginal birth following the spontaneous onset of labor
≥1000 copies/mL	• Risk of transmission is high • Scheduled prelabor cesarean at 38 weeks is recommended ***(option d)***

William's Obstetrics 24th/ed p1281

Other important points in mother to child transmission:

- ❑ Efavirenz is teratogenic to fetus if administered in first trimester
- ❑ Preferred agents for combination antiretroviral therapy in pregnancy
  - ▪ Nucleoside reverse transcriptase inhibitor (NRTI): Zidovudine, lamivudine
  - ▪ Non-nucleoside reverse transcriptase inhibitor (NNRTI): Nevirapine
  - ▪ Protease inhibitor (PI): Ritonavir/atazanavir, lopinavir/ritonavir
- ❑ Intervention apart from HAART during pregnancy includes: IV zidovudine infusion during delivery
- ❑ Perinatal complications to maternal HAART therapy:
  - ▪ Increased risk of preterm birth
  - ▪ Risk of neonatal neutropenia and anemia (due to zidovudine) ***(option b)***
  - ▪ No long-term sequelae in children to maternal HAART therapy has been reported
- ❑ Prophylaxis of neonate is by Nevirapine

About *option a:* Transmission can occur any time during pregnancy. Early the diagnosis earlier the HAART therapy can be initiated and thus maximum fetal benefit.

About *option e:* Relative proportion of transmission due to breastfeeding among all mother-to-child transmissions of HIV is 12 to 20%. And estimated risk of transmission due to breastfeeding above that occurring during pregnancy and delivery, in absence of treatment is 7 to 22%. However 'option e' seems to be correct in both scenarios.

11. Seen in leprosy is/are:

a. Saddle nose
b. Leonine facies
c. Small ear lobe
d. Lagophthalmos
e. Ptosis

Ans. a. Saddle nose; b. Leonine facies and d. Lagophthalmos

Ref: Harrison's Principles of Internal Medicine 19th/ed p1124,1125

EXPLANATION

In leprosy ear lobe is enlarged and pendulous not small. Could not find any evidence regarding ptosis as a feature leprosy, even in research articles. Moreover there is no evidence of oculomotor nerve involvement (most common cranial nerve involved are facial and trigeminal).

- Facial features of leprosy
  - Skin nodules, raised plaques, or diffuse dermal infiltration, when on the face, results in ***leonine facies. (Option b)***
  - Late manifestations include:
    - Loss of eyebrows (initially the lateral margins only) and eyelashes,
    - Pendulous earlobes, ***(Option c)*** and

Complications of leprosy

- **The extremities**
  - Primarily a consequence of neuropathy → insensitivity and myopathy.
  - *Most commonly affected nerve* is the ulnar nerve; results in
    - Clawing of the 4th and 5th fingers,
    - Loss of dorsal interosseous musculature in the affected hand
    - Loss of sensation in its distributions.
  - Median nerve involvement → impairs thumb opposition and grasp
  - Radial nerve dysfunction (rare) → wrist drop.
  - Plantar ulceration most common complication of leprous neuropathy.
  - Peroneal nerve palsy → Foot drop
  - Charcot's joints (uncommon)
  - Loss of distal digits (a consequence of insensitivity, trauma, secondary infection, and—in lepromatous disease—a poorly understood and sometimes profound osteolytic process.)
- **Nose**
  - Chronic nasal congestion and epistaxis (In lepromatous leprosy (LL), due to bacillary invasion of nasal mucosa)
  - **Saddle-nose deformity** ***(Option a)*** or anosmia (Long-untreated LL due to destruction of nasal cartilage)
- **Eye**
  - Lagophthalmos ***(Option d)*** and corneal insensitivity (due to cranial nerve palsies) → trauma, secondary infection, corneal ulcerations and opacities.
  - Uveitis in erythema nodosum leprosum (ENL) and LL (invasion by bacilli); → cataracts and glaucoma. Thus leprosy is a *major cause of blindness in the developing world.*
  - Slit-lamp evaluation in LL patients "corneal beading," (globi of *M. leprae*).

- **Testes**
  - *M. leprae* invades the testes, while ENL may cause orchitis.
  - Mild to severe testicular dysfunction: ↑ LH and ↑ FSH, ↓testosterone, and aspermia or hypospermia in 85% of LL patients but in only 25% of BL patients. → Impotence and infertility.
- **Amyloidosis**
  - Secondary amyloidosis is a complication of LL and ENL → abnormalities of hepatic and particularly renal function.
- **Nerve abscesses**
  - Can be seen in various forms, but is particularly seen in borderline tuberculoid (BT) form
  - *Most commonly occurs in* ulnar nerve
  - Affected nerve is swollen and exquisitely tender, with features of cellulitis in adjacent skin

12. Factitious fever:

a. More than 41°C
b. Looks very sick
c. Presence of diurnal variation
d. No change in pulse rate according to temperature
e. Absence of sweating during defeverscence

Ans. a. More than 41°C; d. No change in pulse rate according to temperature and e. Absence of sweating during defeverscence *Ref: Davidson's Principles and Practice of Medicine 22nd ed p297 and Harrison's Principles of Internal Medicine 19th/ed p138*

Explanation

- Factitious fever is one of the causes of pyrexia of unknown origin, which requires high clinician suspicion for diagnosis. Here the fever is engineered by the patient, for example, by IV injection of contaminated water.
- Common among young women in health care professions.

Clues for diagnosing factitious fever *(Davidson's)*

- Patient looks well ***(Option b)***
- Bizarre temperature chart with absence of diurnal variation ((***Option c***)
- Absence of temperature-related changes in pulse rate ***a (Option d)***
- Temperature > 41°C ***(Option a)***
- Absence of sweating during abatement of fever (defervescence) ***(Option e)***
- ESR and CRP will be normal despite high fever
- Evidence of self-injection or self-harm
- Normal temperature during observation period

Fraudulent fever *(Harrison's)*

- Patient is normothermic but manipulates the thermometer
- Simultaneous measurements at different body sites (rectum, ear, mouth) should rapidly identify this diagnosis.
- Here also dissociation between pulse rate and temperature.

13. Following matched pair/s is/are correct:

a. Pulsus parvus et tardus — Aortic stenosis
b. Bisferiens pulse—Aortic regurgitation
c. Pulsus paradoxus—Cardiac tamponade
d. Bisferiens pulse—Hypertrophic obstructive cardiomyopathy
e. Pulsus alternans—Hypertrophic obstructive cardiomyopathy

Ans. a. Pulsus parvus et tardus—Aortic stenosis; b. Bisferiens pulse—Aortic regurgitation; c. Pulsus paradoxus—Cardiac tamponade and d. Bisferiens pulse—Hypertrophic obstructive cardiomyopathy *Ref: Harrison's Principles of Internal Medicine 19th/ed, p1445*

Explanation

Pulse	Character	Associated condition
Pulsus parvus et tardus parvus 'small' + tardus 'slow'	A weak and delayed upstroke	Severe AS (aortic stenosis)
Anacrotic pulse	Slow, notched, or interrupted upstroke with a thrill or shudder.	Some patients with AS
Corrigan's or water-hammer pulse	Upstroke has a sharp rise and rapid fall-off	Chronic severe AR (aortic regurgitation)
Bifid or **bisferiens pulse**: pulsus 'stroke' + bis 'twice' + feriens 'striking'	Two upstrokes (systolic peaks) can be appreciated.	• Some patients with advanced AR • HOCM (hypertrophic obstructive cardiomyopathy)
Seen by sphygmomanometer		
Pulsus paradoxus	Refers to a fall in systolic pressure >10 mm Hg with inspiration	Pericardial tamponade also seen in massive pulmonary embolism, hemorrhagic shock, severe obstructive lung disease, and tension pneumothorax.
Pulsus alternans	Beat-to-beat variability of pulse amplitude	Severe left ventricular systolic dysfunction

14. Secondary hypertriglyceridemia seen in

a. Diabetes mellitus
b. Nephrotic syndrome
c. Hypothyroidism
d. Cholestatic jaundice
e. Alcohol consumption

Ans. a. Diabetes mellitus and e. Alcohol consumption

Ref: Davidson's Principles and Practice of Medicine 22nd/ed p453

	Predominant hypercholesterolemia	Predominant hypertriglyceridemia	Mixed hyperlipidemia
Elevated lipid results	TC ± TG	TG only or TG >> TC	TC + TG
Elevated lipoprotein	LDL > VLDL	VLDL ± LDL or chylo	VLDL + LDL
Risk of	↑ Coronary heart disease risk	↑ Pancreatitis	Both risk ↑
Primary causes	Polygenic (majority) Familial hypercholesterolemia (LDL receptor defect, defective Apo B100, increased function of PCSK-9) Hyperalphalipoproteinemia	Polygenic (majority) Lipoprotein lipase deficiency Familial hypertriglyceridemia	Polygenic (majority) Familial combined hyperlipidemia Dysbetalipoproteinemia

Contd…

Contd...

	Predominant hypercholesterolemia	Predominant hypertriglyceridemia	Mixed hyperlipidemia
Secondary causes ***(Question)***	Moderately common causes • Hypothyroidism ***(Option c)*** • Pregnancy • Cholestatic liver disease ***(Option d)*** • Drugs (diuretics, ciclosporin, corticosteroids, androgens, antiretroviral agents) Less common causes • Nephrotic syndrome ***(Option b)*** • Anorexia nervosa • Porphyria • Hyperparathyroidism	Common causes • Diabetes mellitus (type 2) ***(Option a)*** • Chronic renal disease • Abdominal obesity • Excess alcohol (***Option e***) • Hepatocellular disease • Drugs (β-blockers, retinoids, corticosteroids, antiretroviral agents)	From both mentioned previously

TC = Total cholesterol; TG = Triglycerides; chylo = chylomicrons; LDL = Low density lipoprotein; VLDL = Very low density lipoprotein

About option e: In question it is not mentioning whether it is excess consumption or regular consumption, however this line from Harrison would help in further clarification: *"Regular alcohol consumption inhibits hepatic oxidation of free fatty acids, thus promoting hepatic TG synthesis and VLDL secretion. Regular alcohol use also raises plasma levels of HDL-C and should be considered in patients with the unusual combination of elevated TGs and elevated HDL-C."* In both, regular consumption and excess consumption, it raises TG levels.

15. Which of the following can cause pulmonary embolism:

a. Oral contraceptives
b. Pregnancy
c. Mitral regurgitation
d. Excessive unaccustomed excersise

Ans. a. Oral contraceptives and b. Pregnancy *Ref: CMDT 2017 p314*

EXPLANATION

- ❑ Pulmonary embolism (PE) is leading preventable cause of death in hospitalized patients
- ❑ Identifying risk factors becomes important here since the condition is highly fatal and simultaneous highly preventable by appropriate prophylaxis.
- ❑ Many substances can embolize to pulmonary circulation like:

Substance	Examples
Air	During neurosurgery, central venous catheter
Amniotic fluid	During labor
Fat	Long bone fractures
Foreign bodies	Talc in injection drug users
Parasite eggs	Schistosomiasis
Septic emboli	Infectious endocarditis
Tumor cells	Renal cell carcinoma
Thrombus	MC embolus Most often originates from deep veins of lower limbs

- PE and DVT are two manifestations of the same disease.
- Risk factors for PE are risk factors for thrombus formation
- You all know risk factors for thrombus formation: 1. Venous stasis, 2. Injury to vessel wall and 3. Hypercoagulability (Virchow's triad!!)
- Risk factors for PE can be summarized as below:

Venous stasis	Injury to the vessel wall	Hypercoagulability
Immobility • Bed rest (esp. postoperative) • Obesity • Stroke Hyperviscosity • Polycythemia • Increased central venous pressure • Low cardiac output states • Pregnancy ***(option b)*** • COPD • Mitral stenosis	• Prior episode of thrombosis • Orthopedic surgery • Trauma	Medications • Oral contraceptives ***(option a)*** • Hormonal replacement therapy Disease • Malignancy • Surgery Inherited gene defects • Factor V Leiden (resistance to activated protein C) • Deficiency or dysfunction of protein C, protein S and antithrombin • Hyperhomocysteinemia • Antiphospholipid antibodies (lups anticoagulant >> anticardiolipin antibody)

About ***option c*** Mitral stenosis is associated with recurrent pulmonary emboli and not mitral regurgitation.

16. True about pectus excavatum is/are:

a. Compromise breathing
b. Worsens with puberty
c. Cardiac compromise
d. More common in females
e. Seen in Marfan's

Ans. b. Worsens with puberty and e. Seen in Marfan's

Ref: Davidson's Principles and Practice of Medicine 22nd/ed p731; Bailey and Love 26th edition 895

Explanation

- Pectus excavatum (funnel chest)
  - Idiopathic condition
  - Most common type of congenital chest wall abnormality
  - Typically noticed at birth, and within the first year of life.
  - Male predominance (M:F = 3:1) ***(Option d)***
  - Associated with Marfan syndrome and Poland syndrome ***(Option e)***
  - Worsening reported during rapid bone growth in the early teenage years. ***(Option b)***
  - Body of the sternum, usually only the lower end, is curved inwards.
  - ***Option a and c:***
    - The heart is displaced to the left and may be compressed between the sternum and the vertebral column but only rarely is there associated disturbance of cardiac function.
    - *"May restrict chest expansion and reduce vital capacity." .... Davidson's*
    - *It is never a cause of respiratory problems." .... Bailey and Love*

- Many patients are asymptomatic from a functional standpoint
- Operative correction is rarely performed, and only for cosmetic reasons.

❑ Pectus carinatum (pigeon chest)
- Frequently caused by severe asthma during childhood. Very occasionally, this deformity can be produced by rickets or be idiopathic
- Worsening in growth spurt (early teenage)
- Most patients are asymptomatic and the only justification for treatment is on cosmetic grounds.

17. About silicosis—true is/are:

a. More in basal part of lung
b. Concentrically arranged collagen fibers
c. Calcification more pronounced than hyaline
d. Lobar pneumonia
e. Diffuse calcification of lymph nodes

Ans. b. Concentrically arranged collagen fbers *Ref: Robbins Basic Pathology 9th/ed p476; Harrison's Principles of Internal Medicine 19th/ed p1690*

EXPLANATION

Option a: Silicosis is seen in upper part of lung, whereas asbestosis starts in lower part of lung.

Option b: Lymph node calcification is not diffuse (egg shell calcification—only outer rim of lymph node is calcified)

Option d: Silicosis patients are at increased risk of tuberculosis, atypical mycobacterial infections and fungal infections.

Silicosis Review

❑ Most prevalent chronic occupational disease in the world.

❑ **Cause**:
- Inhalation of crystalline silica, mostly in occupational settings.
- Sandblasting and hard-rock mining are at particular risk.

❑ **Silica**
- Crystalline form (most toxic and fibrogenic)
  - Quartz (most commonly implicated in silicosis)
  - Cristobalite, and tridymite.
- Amorphous forms,

❑ **Pathogenesis**:
- Inhaled silica → interacts with epithelial cells and macrophages.
- *Ingested silica particles → activation and release of mediators by pulmonary macrophages* (IL-1, TNF, fibronectin, lipid mediators, oxygen-derived free radicals, and fibrogenic cytokines)

❑ **Pathology:** Silicotic nodules
- Grossly:
  - Early stages—tiny, barely palpable, discrete, pale-to-blackened nodules in the **upper zones** of the lungs
  - With disease progression:
    - ~ Nodules may coalesce into hard, collagenous scars, → Progressive massive fibrosis (PMF).
    - ~ Intervening lung parenchyma may be compressed or overexpanded → honeycomb pattern.

~ Fibrotic lesions may also occur in the hilar lymph nodes and pleura. Sometimes, thin sheets of calcification occur in the lymph nodes and are appreciated radiographically as "eggshell" calcification (e.g., calcium surrounding a zone lacking calcification). (***Option e,*** not diffuse calcification)

- Microscopically
  - **Concentrically arranged hyalinized collagen fibers** surrounding an amorphous center. "Whorled" appearance of the collagen fibers ***(Option b)***
  - **Polarized microscopy—weakly birefringent silica** particles (in the center of the nodules)

❑ C/F

- Pulmonary fibrosis occurs in a dose-response fashion after many years of exposure.
- **Acute silicosis:**
  - Heavy exposure, e.g. sandblasting in confined spaces, tunneling through rock with a high quartz content (15–25%), or the manufacture of abrasive soaps → acute silicosis (even with 10 months of exposure).
  - C/F and pathological features - similar to pulmonary alveolar proteinosis
  - CXR - profuse miliary infiltration or consolidation
  - HRCT - characteristic pattern → "crazy paving".
  - Severe and progressive despite the discontinuation of exposure.
  - Whole-lung lavage may provide symptomatic relief and slow the progression.
- **Chronic exposure:** Long-term, less intense exposure
  - Small rounded opacities in the upper lobes may appear on the chest radiograph after 15–20 years of exposure,
  - Calcification of hilar nodes may occur in as many as 20% of cases and produces a characteristic "eggshell" pattern.
  - HRCT readily identifies silicotic nodules
  - **Simple silicosis:** Usually without associated impairment of lung function.
  - **Complicated silicosis:** The nodular fibrosis may be progressive in the absence of further exposure, with coalescence and formation of nonsegmental conglomerates of irregular masses >1 cm in diameter.
  - **Progressive massive fibrosis (PMF)**: Fibrotic masses become quite large. Significant functional impairment with both restrictive and obstructive components.

❑ Complications

- Infections that occur due to cytotoxicty to alveolar macrophages by silica (*Mycobacterium tuberculosis*, atypical mycobacteria and fungi) ***(Option d)***
- Autoimmune CTD (e.g. rheumatoid arthritis and scleroderma)
- Probable lung carcinogen.
- Some silicates, like *talc* and *vermiculite*, may be contaminated with asbestos. (Fibrosis of lung or pleura, lung cancer, and mesothelioma have been associated with chronic exposure to talc and vermiculite dusts).

18. In asbestosis, all are seen in CT *except*:

a. Causes pleural calcification
b. Fibrosis
c. Pleural effusion
d. Bilateral hilar lymphadenopathy
e. Option not recalled

Ans. d. Bilateral hilar lymphadenopathy *Ref: Robbins Basic Pathology 9th/ed p476; Thoracic imaging Richard Webb. p538- 544*

EXPLANATION

Lung disease associated with asbestos fiber inhalation is known as asbestosis, which usually develops 20–30 years after exposure to asbestos (specially amphibole fibers). Associated pleural disease is known as asbestosis-related disease.

RADIOLOGICAL FEATURES OF ASBESTOSIS

Chest Radiograph

- Irregular reticular opacities due to interstitial fibrosis. In early stages changes are noted as fine reticulation in lung bases posteriorly in subpleural location. Later reticulation progresses, becomes coarser and obscures heart border ('shaggy heart sign') along with honeycombing in mid lung zones.
- Calcified pleural plaques **(option a)** in 10 - 15% cases, usually bilateral. Appears round or irregular and geographic in shape when seen en face.
- Pleural effusion.

HRCT

- Parietal and visceral pleural thickening (focal or diffuse) with or without formation of parietal pleural plaques are the characteristic features. Plaques tend to spare costophrenic angles and appear 'mesa' shaped in cross-section. Diffuse pleural thickening involves more than quarter of chest wall.
- Benign exudative pleural effusion is an early finding **(option c).**
- Interstitial fibrosis **(option b)** in form of intra and interlobular septal thickening, traction bronchiectasis, architectural distortion, honeycombing (similar to idiopathic pulmonary fibrosis).
- Parenchymal bands (2-5 cm) in length are noted extending to pleural surface, giving crow- foot appearance when several bands seen in same location.
- Round atelectasis is focal lung collapse typically associated with pleural disease and hence seen in asbestosis. It is associated with curving of pulmonary vessels or bronchi into edge of lesion, so called 'comet-tail sign'.
- **Option d.** Hilar lymphadenopathy is not a feature of asbestosis and is seen mostly in silicosis and coal worker's pneumoconiosis.

Asbestosis Review

- Asbestos—crystalline hydrated silicates with a fibrous geometry.
- Occupational exposure to asbestos is linked to:
  - Parenchymal interstitial fibrosis (*asbestosis*)
  - Localized fibrous plaques or, rarely, diffuse fibrosis in the pleura
  - Pleural effusions
  - Lung carcinomas
  - Malignant pleural and peritoneal mesotheliomas
  - Laryngeal carcinoma.
- Pathogenesis:
  - Two distinct forms of asbestos:
    - **Serpentine** fiber—most of the asbestos used in industry
    - This is curly and flexible, therefore gets struck in upper respiratory tract and removed by mucociliary clearance
    - **Amphibole** fiber—less prevalent and more pathogenic
    - Straight, stiff, and brittle; may reach deeper in lungs and not very soluble as serpentine form.

- Both asbestos forms are ***fibrogenic***, and increasing exposure to either is associated with a higher incidence of all asbestos-related diseases.
- Oncogenecity: Functions as both a tumor initiator and a promoter.
  - Oncogenecity on the mesothelium is due to reactive free radicals generated by asbestos fibers
  - Potentially toxic chemicals (e.g., tobacco smoke) adsorbed onto the asbestos fibers contribute to the pathogenicity of the fibers

❑ Morphology

- Marked by diffuse pulmonary interstitial fibrosis, changes are similar to usual interstitial pneumonia except for asbestos bodies
- **Asbestos bodies**
  - Golden brown, fusiform or beaded rods with a translucent center.
  - Consist of asbestos fibers coated with an iron-containing proteinaceous material
  - Formed when macrophages attempt to phagocytose asbestos fibers; the iron is derived from phagocyte ferritin.
- **Begins in** the lower lobes and subpleurally, → middle and upper lobes of the lungs become affected as fibrosis progresses. *(Coal workers pneumoconiosis and silicosis begin in upper lobe)*[Q]
- **Lung architecture:** Contraction of fibrosed tissue → distorts the normal architecture → enlarged air spaces enclosed within thick fibrous walls → honeycombed.
- **Pleura:**
  - Visceral pleural fibrosis → adhesions between the lungs and the chest wall. Scarring may trap and narrow pulmonary arteries and arterioles, → pulm. HTN and cor pulmonale.
  - **Pleural plaques** (most common manifestation of asbestos exposure)
  - Well-circumscribed plaques of dense collagen, often containing calcium.
  - *Location:* Anterior and posterolateral aspects of the **parietal pleura** and over the domes of the diaphragm.
  - Do not contain asbestos bodies,
  - Rarely seen in persons with no history asbestos exposure (asbestos bodies are commonly seen in unexposed person, but the number is very less).
- Pleural effusion or diffuse pleural fibrosis is rare.

19. Exudative pleural effusion:

a. Cirrhosis of liver
b. Malignant subpleural metastasis
c. Pulmonary embolism
d. Congestive heart failure
e. Myxedema

Ans. b. Malignant subpleural metastasis and c. Pulmonary embolism

Ref: Harrison's Principles of Internal Medicine 19th/ed p1718

EXPLANATION

See table below:

Exudative pleural effusion	Transudative pleural effusion
Due to local factors that influence the formation and absorption of pleural fluid are altered.	Due to *systemic factors* that influence the formation and absorption of pleural fluid are altered.
General cause is local disease of pleura or lung that results in exudation of fluids	Also known as hydrothorax. General cause being systemic disease that results in transudation of fluids

Contd...

Contd...

Exudative pleural effusion	Transudative pleural effusion
Causes 1. Infection: Bacterial, fungal, parasitic, viral 2. Neoplastic diseases: Metastatic disease, mesothelioma ***(Option b)*** 3. Pulmonary embolization ***(Option c)*** 4. Surrounding structures pathology: Esophageal perforation, pancreatic disease, intraabdominal abscesses, diaphragmatic hernia 5. After surgical procedures or injury: Abdominal surgery, endoscopic variceal sclerotherapy, liver transplant, CABG, post-cardiac injury syndrome, Iatrogenic injury 6. Collagen vascular diseases: Rheumatoid pleuritis, SLE, drug-induced lupus, immunoblastic lymphadenopathy, sjogren syndrome, granulomatosis with polyangiitis (Wegener), Churg-Strauss syndrome 7. Asbestos exposure 8. Sarcoidosis 9. Uremia 10. Meigs' syndrome	**Causes** 1. Congestive heart failure ***(Option d)*** 2. Cirrhosis ***(Option a)*** 3. Nephrotic syndrome 4. Peritoneal dialysis 5. Superior vena cava obstruction 6. Myxedema ***(Option e)*** 7. Urinothorax
11. Yellow nail syndrome 12. Drug-induced pleural disease: Nitrofurantoin, dantrolene, methysergide, bromocriptine, procarbazine, amiodarone, dasatinib 13. Trapped lung 14. Radiation therapy 15. Hemothorax 16. Ovarian hyperstimulation syndrome 17. Pericardial disease 18. Chylothorax	
Exudative pleural effusions meet at least one of the following criteria: 1. Pleural fluid protein/serum protein >0.5 2. Pleural fluid LDH/serum LDH >0.6 3. Pleural fluid LDH > 2/3rd the normal upper limit for serum	Meet none

20. Indications of surgery in tuberculosis:

a. Tuberculous empyema
b. Streaky hemoptysis
c. Sputum +ve after 6 months of effective therapy
d. Bronchiectasis of lower lobe
e. Option not recalled

Ans. a. Tubercular empyma; c. Sputum +ve after 6 months of effective therapy and d. Bronchiectasis of lower lobe *Ref: RNTCP guidelines on PMDT in India 2012; p69*

EXPLANATION

- ❑ In MDR-TB patients with localized disease, surgery, as an adjunct to chemotherapy, can improve outcomes provided skilled thoracic surgeons and excellent postoperative care are available.
- ❑ When unilateral resectable disease is present, surgery should be considered for the following cases:
  - Absence of clinical or bacteriological response to chemotherapy **despite 6 to 9 months of treatment with effective anti-tuberculosis drugs *(Option c)***
  - High risk of failure or relapse due to high degree of resistance or extensive parenchymal involvement
  - Morbid complications of parenchymal disease e.g. **hemoptysis, bronchiectasis *(Option d)***, bronchopleural fistula, or **empyema *(Option a)***
  - Recurrence of positive culture status during course of treatment; and
  - Relapse after completion of anti-tuberculosis treatment.
  - If surgical option is under consideration at least six to nine months of chemotherapy is recommended prior to surgery.

Option b: Massive hemoptysis is a complication that is indication for surgery not streaky hemoptysis, which is often seen in later stages of tuberculosis.

21. Common infection/s in cystic fibrosis is/are:

a. *Staphylococcus aureus*
b. *Pseudomonas aeruginosa*
c. *Burkholderia pseudomallei*
d. *Burkholderia cepacia*
e. Option not recalled

Ans. a. *Staphylococcus aureus;* b. *Pseudomonas aeruginosa* and d. *Burkholderia cepacia*

Ref: Davidson's Principles and Practice of Medicine 22nd/ed p681

EXPLANATION

- ❑ Most common infection in cystic fibrosis **in childhood** period is *Staphylococcus aureus* ***(option a)***;
- ❑ **In adulthood**, many patients become colonized with *Pseudomonas aeruginosa* ***(option b)***.
- ❑ Most patients are eventually colonised with resistant strains, main culprits are; resistant strains of *P. aeruginosa, Stenotrophomonas maltophilia* and *Burkholderia cepacia* ***(option d)***.
- ❑ Frequently found, but benign colonisers that do not require specific treatment are: *Aspergillus* and non-tuberculous mycobacteria.

22. Neuroexitatory toxin:

a. Scorpion
b. Octopus
c. Wasp
d. Jelly fish
e. Cobra

Ans. a. Scorpion and d. Jelly fish

Ref: Davidson's Principles and Practice of Medicine 22nd/ed p224-228

EXPLANATION

- ❑ Among the given options scorpions (Indian scorpion and Brazilian scorpion) and Jelly fish produce neuroexcitatory symptoms
- ❑ ***Option b:*** Produces rapidly progressive paralysis
- ❑ ***Option c:*** Wasp stings allergic manifestations and may cause renal failure
- ❑ ***Option e:*** Cobra bite manifests with flaccid paralysis, local necrosis/blistering, shock
- ❑ **Neurotoxicity** in envenoming can be excitatory or paralytic
- ❑ **Excitatory neurotoxin or neuroexcitatory toxin**:

- Causes an 'autonomic storm', with profuse sweating, variable cardiac effects and cardiac failure, sometimes with pulmonary edema (notably Australian funnel web spider bite, Indian red scorpion).
- This can be rapidly fatal (many scorpions, funnel web spiders), or
- May cause distressing symptoms but constitute a lesser risk of death (widow spiders, banana spiders).

❑ **Neurotoxic flaccid paralysis**:
- Can develop very rapidly, progressing from mild weakness to full respiratory paralysis in less than 30 minutes (blue-ringed octopus bite, cone shell sting), or
- May develop far more slowly, over hours (some snakes) to days (paralysis tick).
- For neurotoxic snakes, the cranial nerves are usually involved first, with ptosis a common initial sign. From this, paralysis may extend to the limbs, with weakness and loss of deep tendon reflexes, then respiratory paralysis.

Type of venom	Clinical effects	Examples of venomous species
Neurotoxin		
Paralytic	Flaccid paralysis	• Some snakes (Kraits, Cobras, King **cobra**) • Paralysis ticks • Cone shells • Blue-ringed octopus
Excitatory	Neuroexcitation: Autonomic storm, cardiotoxicity, pulmonary edema	• **Some scorpions** (Indian scorpions, Brazilian scorpion) • Spiders • Jellyfish
Myotoxins	Systemic or local myolysis	**Some snakes:** • All sea snake (flaccid paralysis and/or myolysis) • Russel's viper (hemotoxic, myotoxic, nephrotoxic and local necrosis) • Few kraits like *Bangarus candidus* and *B. Multicinctus* (flaccid paralysis and myolysis)
Cardiotoxins	Direct or indirect cardiotoxicity; cardiac collapse, shock	• Some snakes (Puff adders) • Scorpions • Spiders • Jellyfish
Hemostasis system Toxins	Vary from rapid coagulopathy and bleeding to thrombosis, deep venous thrombosis and pulmonary emboli	• Many snakes (vipers) • Few scorpions • Brazilian caterpillars
Nephrotoxins	Renal damage	• Some snakes (Russel's viper) • Multiple bee • Wasp stings
Necrotoxins	Local tissue injury/necrosis, shock	• Some snakes (**Cobra** and most vipers) • Few scorpions • Spiders • Jellyfish • Stingrays
Allergic toxins	Induce acute allergic response (direct and indirect)	Almost all venoms but particularly those of social insects (bees, **wasps**, ants)

23. Following features is/are seen in hypomagnesemia but not in hypermagnesemia

a. Weakness
b. Seizures
c. Confusions
d. Tetany
e. Diminished deep tendon reflexes
f. Corrected by intravenous calcium

Ans. b. Seizures and d. Tetany *Ref: Harrison's Principles of Internal Medicine 19th/ed p2463*

EXPLANATION

Features of hypo and hypermagnesemia are as below:

Hypomagnesemia	Hypermagnesemia
Relatively common	Less common
Features are of neuromuscular excitation	Features are of neuromuscular depression and vasodilation
• **Tetany**, tremor, **seizures**, **muscle weakness**, ataxia, nystagmus, vertigo, apathy, depression, irritability, delirium, and psychosis. • Severe hypomagnesemia may present with **intractable seizures**, that will resolve only on administering magnesium	• Hypotension that is refractory to vasopressors or volume expansion may be an early sign • Nausea, lethargy, and **weakness** may progress to respiratory failure, paralysis, **confusion** and coma • Hypoactive tendon reflexes • Gastrointestinal hypomotility or ileus; facial flushing; pupillary dilation; paradoxical bradycardia; prolongation of PR, QRS, and QT intervals; heart block

Option a: Muscle weakness can be seen in both

Option c and e: Confusion and diminished tendon reflexes is a feature of hypermagnesemia

Option f: Hypomagnesemia is frequently associated with other electrolyte abnormalities like hypocalcemia, hypokalemia, hypophosphatemia, therefore calcium or potassium or phosphate supplementation may be needed. In severe hypermagnesemia IV calcium provides temporary improvement in signs and symptoms.

24. APACHE-2 scoring system uses:

a. Age
b. Glasgow coma scale
c. FiO_2
d. Chronic condition
e. Within first hour of admission to ICU

Ans. a. Age; b. Glasgow coma scale; c. FiO_2; and d. Chronic condition
Ref: Harrison's Principles of Internal Medicine 19th/ed p1730

EXPLANATION

- ❑ Severity of illness scoring systems are used in tool to assess severity in critically ill patients.
- ❑ Most commonly used scoring systems are APACHE-2 and SAPS (Simplified Acute Physiology Score)
- ❑ APACHE-2: **A**cute **P**hysiology **a**nd **C**hronic **H**ealth **E**valuation assigns numerical values to multiple variables (in the first 24 h after ICU admission). It is calculated as follows:

APACHE-2 score = APS + GCS + Age + Chronic condition

1. **APS:** Acute Physiology Score–This takes into account various physiological variables (more the score worse is the variable) and includes the following:
   - Rectal temperature
   - Mean blood pressure
   - Heart rate

- Respiratory rate
- Arterial pH
- Oxygenation: If $FiO_2 > 0.5$, use alveolar-arterial oxygen difference

If $FiO_2 \leq 0.5$, use PaO_2 partial pressure of oxygen
- Serum sodium
- Serum potassium
- Serum creatinine
- Hematocrit
- WBC count

2. **GCS:** Glasgow Coma scale
   - It is based on 1. Eye opening 2. Verbal activity and 3. Motor activity
   - In APACHE-2 scoring: Worse the condition more is the value of variable, hence "15 *minus* GCS-score" is used (In GCS score of 15 means the patient is healthy and 3 means worst condition)
3. Age (<45 years to >75 years → score 0 to 6)
4. Chronic condition- History of chronic condition
   - None = 0
   - If patient admitted after elective surgery = 2
   - If patient admitted after emergency surgery or for any reason other than elective surgery = 5

- ❑ APACHE- 2 score: For details of score for each variable (which is not necessary) refer to text given above. Minimum value = 0 Maximum value = 71
- ❑ If score is >35 then predicted mortality is more than 80%.
- ❑ ***Option e***: SAPS-3 (Simplified Acute Physiology Score - 3), utilizes a 1-hour rather than a 24-hour window for measuring physiologic derangement scores.

25. Ventilator associated pneumonia following is/are true except:

a. Maximum chance of occurring is within 5 days of admission
b. Most common in ICU patients
c. Due to aspiration of gastric contents
d. High volume low pressure cuff preferred
e. Disposable tube made of PVC is preferred

Ans. d. High volume low pressure cuff preferred and e. Disposable tube made of PVC is preferred

Ref: CMDT 2017 p273; Harrison's Principles of Internal Medicine 19th/ed p810; Zolfaghari PS, Wyncoll DL. The Tracheal Tube: Gateway to Ventilator-associated Pneumonia. Critical Care. 2011;15(5):310. doi:10.1186/cc10352.

EXPLANATION

Nosocomial pneumonia can be of following types:

- ❑ Hospital acquired pneumonia (**HAP**): Pneumonia developing after 48 hours of admission.
- ❑ Ventilator associated pneumonia (**VAP**): Pneumonia developing after 48 hours of endotracheal intubation.
- ❑ Health care associated pneumonia (**HCAP**): Pneumonia that occurs in a non-hospitalised patient with extensive healthcare contact. Some community members have extensive contact with the healthcare system and carry flora that more closely resemble hospitalised patients than healthy community residents. When pneumonia develops in these persons, the infection is referred as HCAP

VAP: epidemiology

- ❑ VAP is a common complication among patients requiring mechanical ventilation, which is common in ICUs ***(Option b)*** (Did not get any reference that directly quotes like given in option, but it seems true)

- ❑ Prevalence: 6 to 52 per 100 ventilated patients
- ❑ Risk for VAP depends on duration of ventilation
  - By definition it develops after 48 hours of intubation
  - Maximum chance of diagnosing VAP is in first 5 days ***(Option a)***, after that chance of diagnosing reaches a plateau.
  - However, cumulative rate of VAP in patients who remain ventilated for 30 days is 70%.
  - Please note that 'chance of diagnosing' and 'cumulative rate' are 2 different entities.
- ❑ Once the ventilated patient is transferred to chronic care facility or home care, the incidence of pneumonia drops significantly

VAP etio-pathogenesis and prevention

- ❑ Three factors are critical in the pathogenesis of VAP:
  - Colonization of the oropharynx with pathogenic microorganisms
  - Aspiration of these organisms from the oropharynx into the lower respiratory tract, and compromise of the normal host defense mechanisms
- ❑ ***Option c:*** Risk of aspiration is increased in intubated patient, role of gastric aspiration is as follows:
  - GERD patients are at increased risk of VAP
  - If gastric pH is increased (i.e. more towards alkaline) then it is a risk factor for VAP. Therefore acid suppressive therapies (PPI and H2 antagoists) should be given only to those hospitalized patients who are at high risk for stress gastritis
  - Thus ***option c*** is true
- ❑ The most obvious risk factor is the presence of endotracheal tube, its role is as follows:
  - Increases chances of aspiration by altering the normal mechanical factors preventing aspiration.
    - Endotracheal tube itself prevents large volume aspirations
    - Pooling of secretions above the cuff leads to microaspiration
  - The ET tube and repeated suctioning damages the tracheal mucosa, thereby facilitating tracheal colonization
  - Formation of glycocalyx biofilm by the bacteria
  - Repeated suctioning may also lead to dislodging of bacteria or fragments of glycocalyx; embolizing it to lower airways
  - **Factors related to cuff** of ET tube make and parts
    - Normal function of cuff is to produce a seal between the tube and the tracheal mucosa
    - Pooling of secretions and leakage around the ETT cuff leads to aspiration
    - The pressure delivered by cuff on trachea should be high enough to ensure delivery of mechanical ventilation and prevention of marked aspiration, but low enough to ensure perfusion to the tracheal capillaries. A cuff can be
      - ~ High volume (also known as high volume low pressure) → seal is not very good, but chances of tracheal ischemia are less ***(Option d)***
      - ~ Low volume (also known as Low volume high pressure) → seal is very good, but high chance of tracheal ischemia, these are abandoned nowadays due to tracheal ischemia
  - High volume cuffs tend to have large surface area and with low pressure, the material folds and forms microchannels through which aspiration may occur and thus high chance of VAP ***(Option d)***
  - **Chances of VAP is less with following features in ETT cuff:**
- ❑ Low volume low pressure
- ❑ Cylindrical shape of cuff
- ❑ Use of thinner material e.g. polyurethane, as it may go perfectly into tracheal mucosal folds and seal it completely (PVC is thicker), but these are costly ***(Option e)***.

JIPMER Pattern Based

1. Apheresis platelet donation—true is all except:

a. A person with below normal platelet count can donate
b. Person can donate again after 2 days
c. Person can donate 2 times maximum in a week
d. Not more than 24 donations can be done in 1 year

Ans. a. A person with below normal platelet count can donate

Ref: Hand book of Transfusion Medicine by Derek 5th/ed p20; Harrison's Principles of Internal Medicine 19th/ed p138 e-2

Explanation

- Specific Eligibility Criteria for Apheresis Platelet Donors
  - Age: 18–60 years and Weight- 50 kg (This is not just for platelet donation but also for all blood and blood product donations in India)
  - Donor platelet count must be > 1,50,000/dL ***(Option a)***
  - If taking anti-platelet medication:
    - Aspirin- defer for at least 2 full medication-free days
    - Clopidogrel or ticlopidine - defer for at least 14 full medication-free days
    - Frequency of donations:
      - Can donate up to 2 times in a week ***(Option c)***
      - 24 times in a year ***(Option d)***
    - Minimum interval between donations
      - Minimum of a 48 hour-interval needed after donating single unit ***(Option b)***
      - 7 days after donating double or triple units.

Other important points about platelet transfusion

- Threshold for prophylactic platelet transfusion is 10,000/μL.
  - In patients without fever or infections, a threshold of 5000/μL may be sufficient to prevent spontaneous hemorrhage.
  - For invasive procedures, the usual target level is 50,000/μL platelets.
- Platelets are produced in two ways:
  - **Random donor (RD) platelets:** Whole blood donations are centrifuged and the buffy coats (between the red cell and plasma layers) from four donations are pooled in the plasma of one of the donors.
  - **Single donor apheresis platelets (SDAP)**: Platelets are obtained from a single donor by apheresis. SDAP contain the equivalent of at least 6 units of RD platelets and have fewer contaminating leukocytes than pooled RD platelets.
  - Time required in collecting SDAP is 2 to 3 hours (in RD its 30 mins).
- Storage—20–24°C with agitation
- Shelf life—5 days (7 days if bacterial screening)

2. Ventilator associated pneumonia can be prevented by all *except*:

a. Elevation of head end of bed
b. Daily waking the patient from sedation
c. Oral hygiene with chlorhexidine
d. Change tube once in 2 weeks

Ans. d. Change tube once in 2 weeks *Ref: Harrison's Principles of Internal Medicine 19th/ed p823*

EXPLANATION:

- Option c: Oral hygiene with chlorhexidine is not a established strategy in preventing VAP, but yes it can prevent VAP
- Option d: Changing tube should be avoided, and if patient with VAP requires continuation of ventilatory support, then tracheostomy will be done.
- Prevention protocol in 'ventilator associated pneumonia' can be understood based on underlying pathogenic mechanism, see table below:

Pathogenic mechanism	Preventive strategy
Oropharyngeal colonization with pathogenic bacteria	
• Elimination of normal flora	• Avoidance of prolonged antibiotic Courses
• Large-volume oropharyngeal aspiration around time of intubation	• Short course of prophylactic antibiotics for comatose patients
• Gastroesophageal reflux	• Avoidance of high gastric residuals, prokinetic agents
Cross-infection from other colonized Patients	• Hand washing, especially with alcohol-based hand rub; • Intensive infection control education; • Isolation; • Proper cleaning of reusable equipment
Large-volume aspiration	• Endotracheal intubation; • Rapid-sequence intubation technique; • Avoidance of sedation; • Decompression of small-bowel obstruction
Microaspiration around endotracheal tube	
• Endotracheal intubation	• Noninvasive ventilation
• Prolonged duration of ventilation	• Daily awakening from sedation, ***(Option b)*** • Weaning protocols
• Abnormal swallowing function	• Early percutaneous tracheostomy
• Secretions pooled above endotracheal tube	• Head of bed elevated; ***(Option a)*** • Continuous aspiration of subglottic secretions with specialized ETT; • Avoidance of reintubation ***(Option d related)***; • Minimization of sedation and patient transport
Altered lower respiratory host defenses	• Lowering of hemoglobin transfusion threshold

3. A patient presented with pH of 7.32, bicarbonate 28 mEq/L and a pCO_2 of 50 mm Hg. The acid base abnormality here is:

a. Metabolic acidosis
b. Metabolic alkalosis
c. Respiratory acidosis
d. Respiratory alkalosis

Ans. c. Respiratory acidosis *Ref: Davidson's Principles and Practice of Medicine 22nd/ed 445*

EXPLANATION

See table on next page

Normal range	**pH** (7.35 to 7.45)// **HCO_3^-** (22 to 30 mEq/L)// **pCO_2** (35 to 45 mm Hg)		
Disturbance	pH	Primary change	Compensatory response
Metabolic acidosis	↓	HCO_3^- ↓	pCO_2 ↓
Metabolic alkalosis	↑	HCO_3^- ↑	pCO_2 ↑
Respiratory acidosis	↓	pCO_2 ↑	HCO_3^- ↑
Respiratory alkalosis	↑	pCO_2 ↓	HCO_3^- ↓

4. Vitamin A overdose leads to:

a. Lung cancer
b. Glaucoma
c. Hypothyroidism
d. Pseudotumor cerebri

Ans. d. Pseudotumor cerebri *Ref: See Question Number 5 of JIPMER Pattern Medicine*

EXPLANATION

Correct answer here is pseudotumor cerebri. All features are listed in explanation for next question (**question number 5 of JIPMER pattern medicine**).

Option b Hypothyroidism: Hypothyroid patients are prone to develop carotenemia, but vitamin A overdose does not cause hypothyroidism.

Option a (Lung cancer) high doses of carotenoids do not result in any toxic symptoms but should be avoided in smokers due to an increased risk of lung cancer. Thus it is partly correct.

5. Toxicity of which vitamin leads to acute fulminant hepatitis?

a. Vitamin B1
b. Vitamin B3
c. Vitamin B2
d. Vitamin B6

Ans. b. Vitamin B3 *Ref: Harrison's Principles of Internal Medicine 19th/ed p96 e-1 to 5*

EXPLANATION

Among given options only vit B3 and B6 overdose are associated with toxicity. Hepatic toxicity is the most serious toxicity of B3 (Niacin), hence the answer.

- Any vitamin deficiency can lead to disease state, but only few vitamins in excess can lead to disease state.
- Vitamin toxicity is manifested in
  - Vitamin B1–Thiamine (only high IV doses not by food source nor by supplements)
  - Vitamin B3 – Niacin
  - Vitamin B6 – Pyridoxine
  - Vitamin C
  - Vitamin A
  - Vitamin D, E, K (very rare)
- Vitamin toxicity from dietary sources has been mentioned only with vitamin A (in those who consumed polar bear liver)
- Life threatening toxicity is seen with vitamin B3 (hepatic and flushing) and vitamin A (raised ICP and skin). See table below to understand.

Two questions were asked in this same paper about vitamin intoxication, hence features of intoxication by various vitamin is summarized further:

Vitamin	Toxicity
Thiamine (vit-B1)	• Anaphylaxis after high IV doses. • No adverse effects either from food or supplements at high doses.
Niacin (vit-B3) (nicotinic acid and nicotinamide)	• Prostaglandin-mediated flushing (nicotinic acid supplements) ▪ Flushing *always starts in face* and may be accompanied by skin dryness, itching, paresthesia, and headache. ▪ Pharmaceutical preparations of nicotinic acid combined with laropiprant, a selective prostaglandin D2 receptor 1 antagonist, or premedication with aspirin may alleviate these symptoms ▪ Flushing is subject to tachyphylaxis and often improves with time. • Nausea, vomiting, and abdominal pain. • Hepatic toxicity (jaundice, ↑AST, ↑ALT) is the *most serious toxic reaction* caused by sustained-release niacin • Fulminant hepatitis requiring liver transplantation has been reported at doses 3–9 g/d of niacin ***(Answer).*** • Other toxic reactions include glucose intolerance, hyperuricemia, macular edema, and macular cysts • The combination of nicotinic acid + HMG-CoA reductase inhibitors → increases risk of rhabdomyolysis • Upper limit for daily niacin intake has been set at 35 mg
Pyridoxine (vit-B6)	• Severe sensory neuropathy, leaving patients unable to walk. • Photosensitivity and dermatitis • Upper limit for vitamin B6 has been set at 100 mg/d
Vitamin C	• Taking >2 g of vitamin C in a single dose may result in abdominal pain, diarrhea, and nausea • Chronic high-dose is assoscaited with increase risk of following: ▪ Kidney stones (because vit C is metabolized to oxalate) ▪ Promotes iron overload and iron toxicity ▪ Hemolysis in G6PD def. ▪ High doses may interfere with activity of certain drugs (e.g., bortezomib in myeloma patients). • Doses >1 g/d can cause false-negative guaiac reactions and interfere with tests for urinary glucose.
	• **Acute intoxication** ▪ 1st noted in Arctic explorers who ate polar bear liver (also seen after administration of 150 mg to adults or 100 mg to children. ▪ ↑ intracranial pressure, vertigo, diplopia, bulging fontanels (in children), seizures, and exfoliative dermatitis; may result in death. ▪ Transient bulging of fontanels occurs in 2% of infants, and transient nausea, vomiting, and headache occur in 5% of preschoolers. (Among children being treated for vitamin A deficiency)
Vitamin A	• **Chronic intoxication**: (industrialized countries) ▪ Seen in otherwise healthy adults who ingest 15 mg/d and children who ingest 6 mg/d over a period of several months. ▪ Manifestations include dry skin, cheilosis, glossitis, vomiting, alopecia, bone demineralization and pain, hypercalcemia, lymph node enlargement, hyperlipidemia, amenorrhea, and features of pseudotumor cerebri ***(Answer for Q4)*** with increased intracranial pressure and papilledema. Liver fibrosis with portal hypertension.

Contd...

Contd...

Vitamin	Toxicity
	• **In pregnancy:** ▪ Spontaneous abortion and congenital malformations, including craniofacial abnormalities and valvular heart disease. ▪ Daily dose of vit-A should not exceed 3 mg. ▪ Retinoid derivatives are also toxic, thus contraception should be continued for at least 1 year and possibly longer in women who have taken 13-*cis*-retinoic acid. • **In malnourished children:** ▪ Vitamin-A supplements are considered to amplify nonspecific effects of vaccines. • **Carotenoids:** ▪ High doses do not result in toxic symptoms but should be avoided in smokers due to an increased risk of lung cancer ▪ Carotenemia: Yellowing of the skin (creases of the palms and soles) *but not the sclerae.* ▪ Hypothyroid patients are particularly susceptible to the development of carotenemia due to impaired breakdown of carotene to vitamin A. ▪ Reduction of carotenes in the diet results in the disappearance of skin yellowing and carotenemia over a period of 30–60 days.
Vitamin D	• Intoxication is rare, may lead to hypercalcemia and associated symptoms
Vitamin E	• Toxicity is very rare as long as the liver functions normally • High doses reduce platelet aggregation and interfere with vitamin K metabolism and are therefore **contraindicated in** patients taking warfarin and antiplatelet agents
Vitamin K	• High doses of vitamin K can impair the action of oral anticoagulants

6. In Wernicke's encephalopathy which recovers early?

a. Ataxia
b. Ophthalmoplegia
c. Confusion
d. Psychosis

Ans. b. Ophthalmoplegia

Ref: Harrison's Principles of Internal Medicine 19th/ed p96 e-3

EXPLANATION

This statement from Harrison's gives the answer *"Cardiovascular and ophthalmoplegic improvement occurs within 24 h. Other manifestations gradually clear, although psychosis in Wernicke-Korsakoff syndrome may be permanent or may persist for several months."*

❑ **Treatment of thiamine deficiency**
  - In acute thiamine deficiency with either cardiovascular or neurologic signs,
    - 200 mg of thiamine three times daily should be given intravenously until there is no further improvement in acute symptoms;
  - Oral thiamine (10 mg/d) given until recovery is complete.
  - Other nutrient deficiencies should be corrected concomitantly.

❑ Cardiovascular and ophthalmoplegic improvement occurs within 24 h. ***(Answer)***
  - Other manifestations gradually clear,
  - Psychosis in Wernicke-Korsakoff syndrome may be permanent or may persist for several months.

7. Pickering syndrome:

a. Flash pulmonary edema
b. Obesity paradox
c. Flash pulmonary edema with renal artery stenosis
d. Metabolic syndrome

Ans. c. Flash pulmonary edema with renal artery stenosis *Ref: Flash Pulmonary Oedema and Bilateral Renal Artery Stenosis: The Pickering Syndrome; Eur Heart J. 2011;32(18):2231-2235. doi:10.1093/eurheartj/ehr056*

EXPLANATION

Please don't suppose this as an important topic, it is less likely to be repeated again.

- **Pickering syndrome** = Flash pulmonary edema seen in association with bilateral renal artery stenosis.
- There were many case reports of finding this association and was first reported by Pickering et al. In 1988, hence the proposed terminology of Pickering syndrome.
- Flash pulmonary edema is a general term used to describe a particularly dramatic form of acute decompensated heart failure. Term 'flash' is used because flooding of the alveolar space can occur within minutes resulting in an acute life-threatening emergency.
- Proposed pathogenesis is as follows:

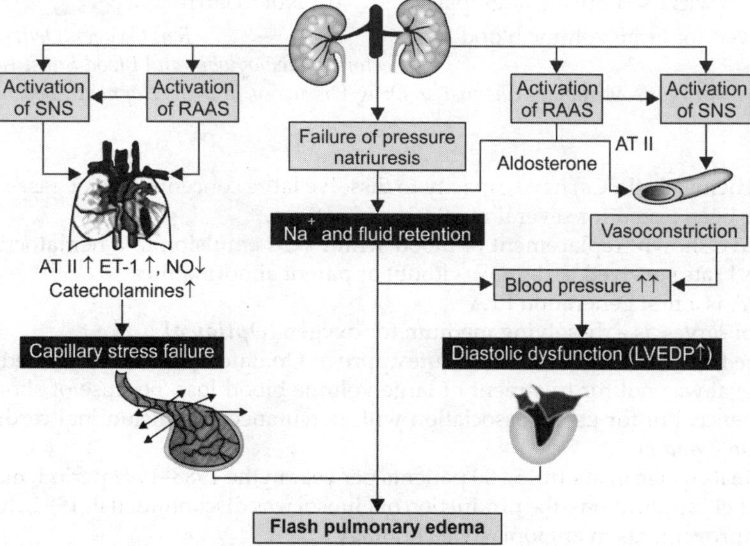

RAAS = Renin-angiotensin-aldosterone system;
SNS = Sympathitic nervous system;
ET-1 = Endothelin-1;
NO = Nitric oxide;
AT II = Angiotensin II;
LVEDP = Left ventricular end-diastolic pressure

8. Atypical pneumonia:

a. Pulmonary edema
b. Tuberculosis
c. Bronchiectasis
d. Option not recalled

Ans. See explanation *Ref: Davidson's Principles and Practice of Medicine 22nd/ed p682; Harrison's Principles of Internal Medicine 19th/ed p804*

EXPLANATION

Mostly options were not recalled correctly see below to know.
The classification as typical and atypical pneumonia based on clinical and radiological features is outdated and no longer recommended. A 'best guess' as to the likely organism may be made from the context in which pneumonia develops, but not from the clinical and radiological picture, which does not differ sufficiently from one organism to another; the term 'atypical pneumonia' has therefore been dropped.

Pathogens causing Community acquired pneumonia (CAP) are divided into typical and atypical.

Typical pathogens for CAP (bacterial)	Atypical organisms
• *S. pneumoniae*, • *Haemophilus influenzae* • In selected patients ▪ *S. aureus* ▪ *Klebsiella pneumoniae* ▪ *Pseudomonas aeruginosa*.	• *Mycoplasma pneumoniae* • *Chlamydia pneumoniae* • *Legionella* species (in inpatients) • Respiratory viruses (influenza viruses, adenoviruses, human metapneumovirus, and respiratory syncytial viruses)

9. Fluosol-DA—true is all *except*:

a. Serves as a dissolving medium for oxygen
b. Approved for large volume blood loss
c. Earlier it was used during angioplasty
d. Not in current use

Ans. b. Approved for large volume blood loss *Ref: Oxygen Delivery Via Allosteric Effectors of Hemoglobin and Blood Substitutes. Bruno et al. Burger's Medicinal Chemistry, Drug Discovery, and Development, Seventh Edition, 2010*

EXPLANATION

- ❑ Perfluorochemicals (PFCs) have capacity to dissolve large concentration of gases, linear or cyclic PFCs have been tested for several medical applications.
- ❑ Studies have shown 'replacement of blood with PFC's emulsion to a hematocrit less than 1%, "bloodless" rats survived and grew without apparent abnormalities
- ❑ Fluosol-DA is a first generation PFA
  - Fluosol serves as a dissolving medium for oxygen ***(Option a)***
  - It is the first and only blood substitute approved to date by the FDA for medical use
  - Approval was not for treatment of large volume blood loss, because of short intravascular persistence, but for use in association with percutaneous transluminal cardiac angioplasty ***(Option b and c)***
  - Despite its usage in about 15,000 patients per year in the 1988–1992 period, many of which in "off-label" applications, the production of Fluosol was discontinued in 1994, due to ***(Option d)***
    - Improvements in angioplasty technology
    - Storage difficulties, due to low stability at room temperature, the product had to be stored frozen.
    - And side effects: Ventricular arrhythmias, pruritus, bradycardia, chest pain, dyspnea, and increased respiratory rate.

10. All are involved in familial Mediterranean fever *except*:

a. CNS
b. Eye
c. Pericardium
d. Skin

Ans. b. Eye *Ref: Harrison's Principles of Internal Medicine 19th/ed p2212*

Explanation

Question is about differentiating features of hereditary recurrent fever syndromes summarised in the table below:

The Hereditary Recurrent Fever Syndromes						
	FMF	**TRAPS**	**HIDS**	**MWS**	**FCAS**	**NOMID**
Serosa	Y	Y	Y	Y	R	R
Skin	Y	Y	Y	Y	Y	Y
Joints	R	Y	Y	Y	Y	Y
Muscle	R	Y	-	Y	Y	Y
Eyes, ears	-	Y	-	Y	Y	Y
CNS	R	Y	y	Y	Y	Y
Amyloidosis	Y	15%	-	25%	-	Late comp

Abbreviations: **Y** = yes; **R** = rare; **FMF**, familial Mediterranean fever **TRAPS**, TNF receptor-associated periodic syndrome; **HIDS**, hyperimmunoglobulinemia D with periodic fever syndrome; **MWS**, Muckle-Wells syndrome; **FCAS**, familial cold autoinflammatory syndrome; **NOMID**, neonatal-onset multisystem inflammatory disease;

- ❑ Manifestation for organ involvement can be: (**Note:** *this is just to give idea of symptoms due to organ involvement, to know exact symptom associated with each condition refer table 392-1 page 2213 of Harrison's*):
  - **Serosa:** Pleurisy, peritonitis; pericardial effusions; pericarditis
  - **Skin:** Erysipeloid erythema (FMF), Centrifugally migrating erythema (TRAPS), Diffuse maculopapular rash and oral ulcers (HIDS) Diffuse urticaria-like rash (MWS and NOMID) Cold-induced urticaria-like rash (FCAS)
  - **Joint:** Arthralgia, acute/chronic mono/oligo/polyarthritis;, Epiphyseal, patellar overgrowth, clubbing
  - **Muscle:** Myalgia
  - **Eye:** Conjunctivitis, uveitis, episcleritis, disc edema or periorbital edema
  - **Ear:** Sensorineural hearing loss
  - **CNS:** Headache, aseptic meningitis, seizures

11. Pollutant released by combustion of fossil fuels causes exacerbation of asthma is:

a. Option not recalled
b. Nitrogen dioxide
c. Ammonia
d. Sulfur dioxide

Ans. d. Sulfur dioxide *Ref: Harrison's Principles of Internal Medicine 19th/ed p1691-1692*

Explanation

Among the given options sulfur dioxide and nitrogen dioxide are released by combustion of fossil fuels and sulfur dioxide is known to cause exacerbation in asthma patients (causes bronchospasm in asthma)

- ❑ Water-soluble gases such as ammonia and sulfur dioxide are absorbed in the lining fluid of the upper and proximal airways and thus tend to produce irritative and bronchoconstrictive responses.
- ❑ Particle size of air contaminants also
  - Particles >10–15 μm in diameter do not penetrate beyond the nose and throat
  - Particles <10 μm in size are deposited below the larynx
    - **Particles - 2.5–10 μm** (coarse-mode fraction):

- Contain crustal elements such as silica, aluminum, and iron
- Deposit relatively high in the tracheobronchial tree

- Particles < 2.5 μm (fine-mode fraction):
  - Created primarily by the **burning of fossil fuels**
  - Carried to the lower airways
- Particles < 0.1 μm in size, (ultrafine fraction)
  - May penetrate into the circulation and be carried to extrapulmonary sites.

Agent	Exposures	Accidental or high acute exposure	Chronic exposure
Sulfur dioxide	• Manufacture of sulfuric acid • Bleaches • Coating of nonferrous metals	• Mucous membrane irritant • Epistaxis • Bronchospasm (especially in people with asthma)	Chronic bronchitis
	• Food processing • Refrigerant • Burning of fossil fuels • Wood pulp industry		
Nitrogen dioxide	• Silage • Metal etching • Explosives • Rocket fuels • Welding • By-product **of burning fossil fuels**	• Cough, dyspnea • Pulmonary edema may be delayed 4–12 h • Possible result from acute exposure: Bronchiolitis obliterans in 2–6 weeks	• Emphysema in animals, • ? Chronic bronchitis, associated with reduced lung function in children with lifelong residential exposure
Ammonia	• Refrigeration • Petroleum refining • Manufacture of fertilizers • Explosives • Plastics and other chemicals	• Mucous membrane irritation, followed by chemical pneumonitis 2–3 days later • Bronchiectasis	• Upper respiratory tract irritation • Chronic bronchitis

12. Not a complication of cardioversion:

a. Myocardial septal perforation
b. ST elevation
c. Ventricular fibrillation
d. Hypokalemia

Ans. a. Myocardial septal perforation *Ref: Brawnwald's Cardiology 9th/ed p730*

EXPLANATION

This line from Brawnwald would answer this question *"Although direct-current shock has been demonstrated in animals to cause myocardial injury, studies in humans have indicated that elevations of myocardial enzymes after cardioversion are not common."*

Shock here does not result in myocardial injury (perforation = injury)

Complications of cardioversion:

❑ Postshock arrhythmias
- Caused by inadequate synchronization = shock occurring during the ST segment or T wave.
- Properly synchronized shock can produce ventricular fibrillation ***(Option c)***
- Postshock arrhythmias are usually transient and do not require therapy.

- ❑ Embolic episodes are reported to occur in 1 to 3% of patients converted from atrial fibrillation to sinus rhythm.
- ❑ Elevations of myocardial enzymes after cardioversion (rare).
- ❑ ST-segment elevation, sometimes dramatic, can occur immediately after elective direct-current cardioversion and last for 1 to 2 minutes, (If lasting more than 2 minutes then indicates myocardial injury other than shock) ***(Option b)***
- ❑ A decrease in serum K^+ and Mg^{2+} levels can occur after cardioversion of VT. ***(Option d)***

13. Brockenbrough effect is seen in:

a. Aortic stenosis
b. Right ventricular conduction abnormality
c. Hypertrophic obstructive cardiomyopathy
d. Restrictive cardiomyopathy

Ans. c. Hypertrophic obstructive cardiomyopathy *Ref: Harrisons 1462*

EXPLANATION

- ❑ Hypertrophic obstructive cardiomyopathy is confirmed by the Brockenbrough-Braunwald sign
- ❑ Brockenbrough-Braunwald sign: Following a premature ventricular contraction, there is an increase in the left ventricular–aorta pressure gradient with a simultaneous decrease in the aortic pulse pressure.

14. Contrast induced nephropathy defined as rise in serum creatinine by:

a. 0.5 mg/dL after 48 hours of contrast administration
b. 1 mg/dL after 48 hours of contrast administration
c. 1.5 mg/dL after 48 hours of contrast administration
d. 2 mg/dL after 48 hours of contrast administration

Ans. a. 0.5 mg/dL after 48 hours of contrast administration

Ref: Harrison's Principles of Internal Medicine 19th/ed p1461

EXPLANATION

See definition below

Contrast-induced acute kidney injury

- ❑ **Definition:** Increase in creatinine **> 0.5 mg/dL** or **25% above baseline** that occurs **48–72 hours after** contrast administration
- ❑ **Incidence:**
  - Occurs in approximately 2–7% of patients
  - Rates of 20–30% reported in high-risk patients
- ❑ High risk patients:
  - Diabetes mellitus
  - Congestive heart failure
  - Chronic kidney disease
  - Anemia
  - Older age
  - Dialysis is required in 0.3–0.7% of patients and is associated with a 5X ↑ in in-hospital mortality.
- ❑ **Preventive strategy:**
  - For all patients: Volume expansion with IV 0.9% saline for 3–12 hours before and continued 6–24 hours after the procedure
  - Diabetic patients on metformin *should stop metformin 48 hours* prior to the procedure to limit the associated risk of lactic acidosis.

- Other strategies include:
  - Administration of sodium bicarbonate 1 hour before and 6 hours after the procedure
  - Use of low- or iso-osmolar contrast agents
  - Limiting the volume of contrast to <100 mL per procedure.
- Pretreatment with N-acetylcysteine has not reduced the risk of contrast-induced acute kidney injury consistently and, therefore, is no longer recommended routinely. *(Potential all except type question)*

15. Criteria used for diagnosis of myocarditis is:

a. Agatston score
b. Dallas criteria
c. CHADS- VAS score
d. Option not recalled

Ans. b. Dallas criteria *Ref: Harrison's Principles of Internal Medicine 19th/ed p1559*

Explanation

Dallas criteria:

- ❑ The Dallas Criteria is for endomyocardial biopsy diagnosis of myocarditis
- ❑ On biopsy if following features are met then it is diagnostic of myocarditis:
  - Lymphocytic infiltrate
  - Evidence of myocyte necrosis
- ❑ Dallas Criteria is negative in 80–90% of patients with clinical myocarditis.
- ❑ Negative Dallas Criteria can reflect
  - Sampling error or
  - Early resolution of lymphocytic infiltrates
  - Also the test is insensitive when inflammation results from cytokines and antibody mediated injury.
- ❑ Other important scores that can be asked

  Voltage criteria → used for LVH

  (Option a) **Agatston score:** Most commonly used method to quantify coronary calcium after imaging (CT, EBCT or MDCT) .... page 1585 Harrison's

  (Option c) **CHA_2DS_2-VASc Score:** Used for predicting risk of stroke in atrial fibrillation and also to determine which patients need anticoagulant prophylaxis .... page 1485 Harrison's

  - CHA_2DS_2-VASc Score

Risk factors	Points	CHA_2DS_2-VASc score	Estimated annual stroke rate
C – congestive heart failure	1	0	0
H – hypertension	1	1	1.3%
A – age ≥75 y	2	2	2.2%
D – diabetes mellitus	1	3	3.2%
S – stroke or TIA, embolus	2	4	4.0%
V – vascular disease	1	5	6.7%
A – age 65–75 y	1	6–9	> 9%
Sex – female	1		

- Anticoagulation in AF patients is warranted for:
  - For patients who have had more than 48 h of AF and are undergoing cardioversion,
  - For patients who have a prior history of stroke, or
  - For patients with a CHA_2DS_2-VASc score of ≥2
  - May be considered in patients with a risk score of 1.

16. Best investigation for diagnosis of myasthenia gravis:

a. Tensilon test
b. Single fiber electromyography
c. Acetylcholinesterase antibody
d. Edrophonium test

Ans. b. Single fiber electromyography *Ref. Harrison's 19th/ed p/2702*

EXPLANATION

- Most sensitive electrophysiological assay in My sathenia gravis is 'single fiber electromyography
  - Sensitivity of SFEMG is >95% when tested in affected muscle
  - 95% sensitivity means: when 100 myasthenic patients are tested then this test will diagnose 95 patients as true positive, the remaining 5% patients are labelled falsely as not having MG
- Most specific test in Myasthenia gravis is → Anti AChR antibodies
  - Means Anti ACh R antibody if positive it is diagnostic of MG and if negative does not exclude the disease
- As AntiAChR antibody is not given in the options SFEMG is the answer

17. A 50-year-old man presents with ptosis and easy fatigability and weakness that improved after exercise. On examination he has proximal muscle weakness and depressed tendon reflexes. Which antibody can be detected in this person?

a. Anti-voltage-gated calcium channel antibody
b. Anti-Acetylcholine receptor antibody
c. Antinuclear antibody
d. Anti-muscle-specific kinase antibody

Ans. a. Anti-voltage-gated calcium channel antibody

Ref: Harrison's Principles of Internal Medicine 19th/ed p2703

EXPLANATION

The given case history is classically of Lambert-Eaton myasthenic syndrome (LEMS). ***Option c*** ANA seen in SLE, though moysitis can present with similar findings, no other features suggestive of SLE are given and more over weakness that improves on exercise is classical H/O of LEMS. ***Option b and d*** (anti-AChR and anti-MUSK) are seen in myasthenia gravis.

Lambert-Eaton myasthenic syndrome (LEMS)

- Features of LEMS that are similar to MG (myasthenia gravis) are:
  - Muscle weakness
    Most commonly affected muscles in LEMS → Proximal muscles of the lower limbs
  - Cranial nerve findings, like ptosis of the eyelids and diplopia, occur in up to 70% of patients
  - Nerve stimulation produces an initial low-amplitude response and, at low rates of repetitive stimulation (2–3 Hz), decremental responses like those of MG
- Features that are present in LEMS but not in MG are:
  - LEMS have *depressed or absent reflexes* and
  - Experience *autonomic changes* such as dry mouth and impotence.

- At high rates (50 Hz) of repetitive nerve stimulation, or following exercise, *incremental responses* occur.

- Etiopathogenesis:
  - LEMS is a *presynaptic* disorder of the NMJ (neuromuscular junction)
  - Autoantibodies directed against *P/Q-type calcium channels* at the motor nerve terminals (85% of patients)
  - These autoantibodies result in impaired release of ACh from nerve terminals
  - Usually associated with malignancy, most commonly *small-cell carcinoma of the lung* (SCCL)
  - SCCL may express calcium channels that stimulate the autoimmune response. The diagnosis of LEMS may signal the presence of a tumor long before it would be detected.
- Treatment of LEMS involves
  - Plasmapheresis and immunosuppression
  - 3,4-Diaminopyridine (3,4-DAP) and pyridostigmine for symptomatic relief.
    - 3,4-DAP acts by blocking potassium channels → prolonged depolarization of the motor nerve terminals → enhances ACh release.
    - Pyridostigmine prolongs the action of ACh.

18. Lorenzo oil therapy is used for:

a. Multiple slerosis
b. Amyotrophic lateral sclerosis
c. Adrenoleukodystrophy
d. Option not recalled

Ans. c. Adrenoleukodystrophy *Ref: Harrison's 2681*

EXPLANATION

Lorenzo's oil reduces levels of very long chain fatty acids which have a role in pathogenesis of adrenoleukodystrophy, but trials have failed to demonstrate it efficacy.

Adrenoleukodystrophy/Adrenomyeloneuropathy

- *X-linked dominant* disorder
- Adrenal insufficiency and neuropathy are the prime features
- Mild to moderate peripheral, progressive spastic paraplegia, spinocerebellar ataxia
- **Electrodiagnostic study:** 1° axonopathy with 2^{dry} demyelination.
- **Nerve biopsy:** Loss of myelinated and unmyelinated nerve fibers with lamellar inclusions in the cytoplasm of Schwann cells.
- **Urine:** Very long chain fatty acid (VLCFA) levels (C24, C25, and C26) are increased
- Laboratory evidence of adrenal insufficiency
- **Treatment**
  - Adrenal insufficiency → replacement therapy;
  - Neurologic manifestations → no proven effective therapy
    - Diets low in VLCFAs
    - **Lorenzo's oil** (erucic and oleic acids) reduce the levels of VLCFAs and increase the levels of C22 in serum, fibroblasts, and liver; however, several large, open-label trials of Lorenzo's oil failed to demonstrate efficacy. ***(Answer)***

19. Lennox-Gastaut syndrome is not seen with:

a. Trauma
b. Cryptogenic
c. Tumors
d. Option not recalled

Ans. None (among available options) *Ref: Harrison's Principles of Internal Medicine 19th/ed p2544*

EXPLANATION

All the given options can cause Lennox-Gastaut syndrome, the missing options might be the answer.

Lennox-Gastaut syndrome

- ❑ Occurs in children
- ❑ Defined by the ***triad of***
  1. *Multiple seizure types* (usually including generalized tonic-clonic, atonic, and atypical absence seizures);
  2. *EEG showing slow (<3 Hz) spike-and-wave discharges* and a variety of other abnormalities; and
  3. *Impaired cognitive function* in most but not all cases.
- ❑ Causes: Associated with CNS disease or dysfunction from a variety of causes, including
  1. *De novo* mutations (In cryptogenic cases- where cause is unknown) ***(Option b)***
  2. Developmental abnormalities
  3. Perinatal hypoxia/ischemia
  4. Trauma ***(Option a)***
  5. Infection and
  6. Other acquired lesions (includes tumors) ***(Option c)***
- ❑ Pathogenesis: It is a nonspecific response of the brain to diffuse neural injury.
- ❑ Prognosis: Poor due to the underlying CNS disease and the physical and psychosocial consequences of severe, poorly controlled epilepsy.

20. A patient with acute glomerulonephritis was treated with steroids, later the patient came with c/o hematuria, next step is:

a. Renal biopsy
b. Conservative
c. Azathioprine (steroid sparer)
d. Option not recalled

Ans. a. Renal biopsy *Ref: Harrison's Principles of Internal Medicine 19th/ed p1836*

EXPLANATION

Once the patient is diagnosed to be having acute glomerulonephritis, the next best step in management is to establish the cause which is best done by renal biopsy. This is done only in selected patient who are clinically stable, adequate clotting function and are willing to take the treatment. See the following lines from Harrison's:

"Once this initial information is collected, selected patients who are clinically stable, have adequate blood clotting parameters, and are willing and able to receive treatment are encouraged to have a renal biopsy."

"A renal biopsy in the setting of glomerulonephritis quickly identifies the type of glomerular injury and often suggests a course of treatment."

21. All involved in ascending paralysis, with areflexia *except*:

a. Olfactory nerve
b. Optic nerve
c. Facial nerve
d. Glossopharyngeal nerve

Ans. a. Olfactory nerve *Ref: Harrison's Principles of Internal Medicine 19th/ed p2694*

Explanation

Ascending paralysis with areflexia is suggestive of *Guillain-Barré syndrome*. Lower cranial nerves are frequently affected leading to bulbar paralysis, thus facial nerve and glossopharyngeal nerve are easily ruled out. Only Miller Fisher variant is associated with optic nerve involvement, that too very few case reports are available. Therefore the answer is Olfactory nerve.

Guillain-Barre Syndrome:

- ***"Rapidly evolving areflexic, ascending motor paralysis with or without sensory disturbance"*** remember each word of this line, this line itself is very high yield.
- Weakness or paralysis
  - First noticed as rubbery legs.
  - Evolves over hours to a few days and is frequently accompanied by tingling dysesthesias in the extremities.
  - Legs more affected than the arms
- Cranial nerve involvement
  - Facial diparesis is present in 50% of affected individuals. (**MC involved cranial nerve** is facial nerve)
  - The *lower cranial nerves* are frequently involved ➔ bulbar weakness with difficulty handling secretions and maintaining an airway;
- Pain in the neck, shoulder, back, or diffusely over the spine is also common in the early stages of GBS, occurring in ~50% of patients.
- Upto 30% require ventilator assistance at some time during the illness.
- **Fever and constitutional symptoms are absent** at the onset and, if present, diagnosis of GBS is doubtful.
- Cutaneous sensory deficits (e.g., loss of pain and temperature sensation) are usually relatively mild, but functions subserved by large sensory fibers, such as deep tendon reflexes and proprioception, are more severely affected.
- Bladder dysfunction may occur in severe cases but is usually transient.
- After reaching a plateau (within 4 weeks of onset), further progression is unlikely.
- Autonomic involvement is common
  - Loss of vasomotor control with wide fluctuation in BP, postural hypotension, and cardiac dysrhythmias.
- Subtypes of GBS
  - Most common variant → AIDP (acute inflammatory demyelinating polyneuropathy)
  - Two axonal variants, (clinically severe)
    - AMAN (acute motor axonal neuropathy) and
    - AMSAN (and acute motor sensory axonal neuropathy)
  - Limited or regional GBS
    - Miller Fisher syndrome (MFS), (ataxia and areflexia of limbs without weakness, and ophthalmoplegia, often with pupillary paralysis. (5% of all cases, ganglioside GQ1b antibodies) ***(Answer)***
    - Pure sensory forms;
    - Ophthalmoplegia with anti-GQ1b antibodies as part of severe motor-sensory GBS;
    - GBS with severe bulbar and facial paralysis, sometimes ass. with antecedent CMV infection and anti-GM2 antibodies
    - Acute pandysautonomia

22. Allgrove syndrome all true *except*:

a. Achalasia	b. Cushing syndrome
c. Neurologic impairment	d. Alacrima

Ans. b. Cushing syndrome *Ref: Harrison's Principle of Internal Medicine 19th/ed p2324*

EXPLANATION

Question is about causes of primary adrenal insufficiency, one of the cause is Allgrove syndrome also known as 'Triple A syndrome' is characterized by adrenal insufficiency, alacrima, achlasia and neurologic impairment. Not Cushing syndrome which is due to glucocorticoid excess.

- Causes of primary adrenal insufficiency along with other associated features are:

Condition	Gene	Adrenal insufficiency + associated feature
Triple A syndrome **(Allgrove syndrome)**	AAAS	**Alacrima, achalasia, neurologic impairment**
Smith-Lemli-Opitz syndrome	SLOS	Cholesterol synthesis disorder associated with mental retardation, craniofacial malformations, growth failure
Kearns-Sayre syndrome	Mitochondrial DNA deletions	Progressive external ophthalmoplegia, pigmentary retinal degeneration, cardiac conduction defects, gonadal failure, hypoparathyroidism, type 1 diabetes
IMAGe syndrome	CDKN1C	Intrauterine growth retardation, metaphyseal dysplasia, genital anomalies
Autoimmune polyglandular syndrome 1 (APS1)	AIRE	Hypoparathyroidism, chronic mucocutaneous candidiasis, other autoimmune disorders, rarely lymphomas
Autoimmune polyglandular syndrome 2 (APS2)	Associations with HLA-DR3, CTLA-4	Hypothyroidism, hyperthyroidism, premature ovarian failure, vitiligo, type 1 diabetes mellitus, pernicious anemia

- Causes other than those mentioned above for primary adrenal insufficiency are:
  - Isolated autoimmune adrenalitis
  - Congenital adrenal hyperplasia (CAH)
  - Congenital lipoid adrenal hyperplasia (CLAH) (*STAR, CYP11A1)*
  - Adrenal hypoplasia congenita (AHC) [*NR0B1 (DAX-1), NR5A1 (SF-1)]*
  - Adrenoleukodystrophy (ALD), adrenomyeloneuropathy (AMN) (*X-ALD)*
  - Familial glucocorticoid deficiency *MC2R MRAP STAR NNT MCM4*
  - Adrenal infections, adrenal infiltration, adrenal hemorrhage, drug-induced and bilateral adrenalectomy

23. Imerslund Grasbeck syndrome is:

a. Vitamin B12 deficiency with proteinuria
b. Selective proteinuria with nephrotic syndrome
c. Demyelination associated with vitamin deficiency
d. A renopulmonary syndrome

Ans. a. Vitamin B12 deficiency with proteinuria

Ref: Harrison's Principles of Internal Medicine 19th/ed p645

EXPLANATION

Selective malabsorption of cobalamin with proteinuria = **Imerslund's syndrome** or **Imerslund-grasbeck syndrome** or congenital cobalamin malabsorption; autosomal recessive megaloblastic anemia; MGA1)

- Autosomal recessive disease
- Most common cause of megaloblastic anemia due to cobalamin deficiency in infancy in Western countries.
- **B12 deficiency:** The patients secrete normal amounts of IF and gastric acid but are unable to absorb cobalamin. Other tests of intestinal absorption are normal
- **Proteinuria:** Over 90% of these patients show nonspecific proteinuria, but renal function is otherwise normal and renal biopsy has not shown any consistent renal defect
- A few have shown aminoaciduria and congenital renal abnormalities, such as duplication of the renal pelvis
- **Genetic defect:** In Finland, impaired synthesis, processing, or ligand binding of *cubilin* due to inherited mutations is found. In Norway, mutation of the gene for *AMN* has been reported.

24. Gertsmann syndrome not a feature:

a. Alexia,
b. Acalculia
c. Finger anomia
d. Option not recalled

Ans. a. Alexia *Ref: Harrison's Principles of Internal Medicine 19th/ed p179*

EXPLANATION

- The combination of the following is known as Gerstmann's syndrome:
  - *Acalculia* (impairment of simple arithmetic) ***(Option a)***
  - *Dysgraphia* (impaired writing)
  - *Finger anomia* (an inability to name individual fingers such as the index and thumb), ***(Option c)*** and
  - *Right-left confusion* (an inability to tell whether a hand, foot, or arm of the patient or examiner is on the right or left side of the body).
- In making this diagnosis, it is important to establish that the finger and left-right naming deficits are not part of a more generalized anomia and that the patient is not otherwise aphasic.
- When Gerstmann's syndrome arises acutely and in isolation, it is commonly associated with damage to the inferior parietal lobule (especially the angular gyrus) in the left hemisphere.

25. A 25-year-old lady on oral contraceptives developed severe headache, vomiting, papilledema and a CSF pressure of 28 cm of water. Diagnosis is:

a. Idiopathic cranial hypertension
b. Idiopathic cranial hypotension
c. Migraine
d. Cluster headache

Ans. a. Idiopathic cranial hypertension

Ref: Harrison's Principles of Internal Medicine 19th/ed p110, 2590,

EXPLANATION

In given history patient is having severe headache, elevated CSF pressure (Normal range- 10 to 18 cm of water when patient lying by side and 20 to 30 cm- sitting up) and papilledema, by this history ***option b*** (hypotension) and ***option d*** (cluster headache) are ruled out. Among the remaining options migraine seems unlikely because none of the classic features of migraine have been mentioned (Repeated attacks is must for diagnosing migraine). But OCP use is associated with migraine headache. However based on available options and given history best answer seems to be idiopathic intracranial hypertension (Pseudotumor cerebri).

Diagnostic Criteria for Migraine

Repeated attacks of headache lasting 4–72 h in patients with a normal physical examination, no other reasonable cause for the headache, and:	
At least 2 of the following features:	Plus at Least 1 of the following features:
Unilateral pain Throbbing pain Aggravation by movement Moderate or severe intensity	Nausea/vomiting Photophobia and phonophobia

Raised CSF Pressure Headache

NDPH due to raised CSF pressure can be the presenting symptom for patients with idiopathic intracranial hypertension (pseudotumor cerebri) **without visual problems, particularly when the fundi are normal**.

Persistently raised intracranial pressure can trigger chronic migraine. These patients typically present with a history of generalized headache that is present on waking and improves as the day goes on. It is generally worse with recumbency. Visual obscurations are frequent. **The diagnosis is relatively straightforward when papilledema is present,** but the possibility must be considered even in patients without funduscopic changes. Formal visual field testing should be performed even in the absence of overt ophthalmic involvement. Headache on rising in the morning or nocturnal headache is also characteristic of obstructive sleep apnea or poorly controlled hypertension.

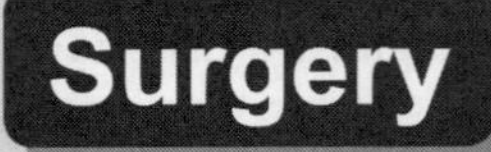

Author: Jyotsana Priya

AIIMS MAY 2017

1. A 27-year-old young male visited the emergency department with severe pain abdomen, vomiting and fever. On examination pain increased on doing maneuver shown below. What is this maneuver known as:

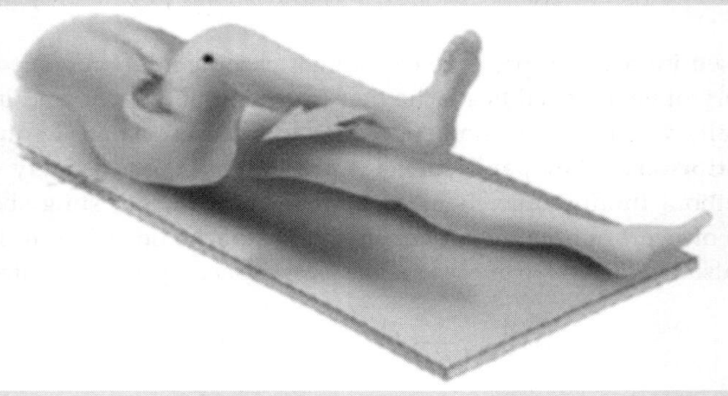

a. Rovsing's sign
b. Psoas sign
c. Obturator sign
d. Grey Turner sign

Ans. c. Obturator sign

Ref: Bailey and Love 26th/ed p1203

Explanation

Signs of acute appendicitis

Rovsing's sign

Deep palpation of the left iliac fossa may cause pain in the right iliac fossa, which is helpful in supporting a clinical diagnosis of appendicitis.

Psoas sign

Occasionally an inflamed appendix lies on the psoas muscle, and the patient, often a young adult, will lie with the right hip flexed for pain relief.

Obturator test; (Zachary Cope)

Spasm of the obturator internus is sometimes demonstrable when the hip is flexed and internally rotated. If an inflamed appendix is in contact with the obturator internus, this maneuvre will cause pain in the hypogastrium.

Grey Turner's sign is a sign of retroperitoneal hemorrhage.

The same topic is repeated in PGI paper also.

2. A 45-year-old female presented with 1.5 cm mass in upper quadrant of breast. On further investigation it was diagnosed as carcinoma breast. No axillary or systemic involvement was observed. Which of the following is preferred management?

a. Adjuvant chemoradiation
b. Adjuvant chemotherapy
c. Adjuvant radiotherapy
d. No adjuvant therapy

Ans. b. Adjuvant chemotherapy *Ref Sabiston 20th/ed p879*

EXPLANATION

Based on history provided the stage of Ca. Breast is Stage 1 (T1 N0 M0). It is reasonable to consider postmastectomy radiation therapy only for

- Selected patients with **stage II disease,**
  - Patients with extracapsular extension,
  - **Lymphovascular invasion,**
  - **Age 40 years or younger,**
  - Close surgical margins,
  - Or **a nodal positivity** ratio (ratio of positive nodes to total nodes examined) of 20% or greater and
  - Patients who have undergone **less than a standard level I or II axillary dissection.**
- And patients with **stage III breast cancer,** since they have high rates of locoregional recurrence after treatment with a modified radical mastectomy and adjuvant or neoadjuvant chemotherapy.

Decision making for systemic therapy in carcinoma breast cases.

Stage	Systemic therapy
I (<1 cm)	
HR +ve	Hormone and chemotherapy (H and C)
HR –ve	Chemotherapy (C)
HER 2 +VE	Transtuzumab and chemotherapy (T and C)
I (>1 cm)	
HR +ve	H and C
HR –ve	C
HER +ve	T and C
II lymph node –ve	
HR +ve	H and C
HR –ve	C
HER +ve	T and C
II lymph node +ve	
HR +ve	C and H
HR –ve	C
HER +ve	T and C

3. Most common site of post-ischemic stricture is:

a. Ascending colon
b. Hepatic flexure
c. Splenic flexure
d. Sigmoid colon

Ans. c. Splenic flexure *Ref: Sabiston 20th/ed p1356*

EXPLANATION

Splenic flexure is supplied by both inferior and superior mesenteric arteries, and there is a point where these two circulations meet, leading to formation of watershed area.

Ischemic colitis is a condition in which inflammation and injury of large intestine result from inadequate blood supply.

There are three categories of ischemic colitis—gangrenous, sricturing and transient.

Arterial Supply

- The colon is supplied by three major arterial sources: the superior mesenteric artery (SMA), the inferior mesenteric artery (IMA), and the bilateral iliac arteries.
- The **SMA** supplies the cecum, right colon, and proximal transverse colon through its ileocolic, right colic, and middle colic branches.
- The **IMA** supplies the distal transverse colon and left colon through its left colic branch.
- There is a variable branch, originating either from the left colic or the IMA itself, that supplies the distal left colon and sigmoid colon.
- Finally, the terminal IMA forms the superior hemorrhoidal artery that supplies blood to the rectum.
- The **iliac arteries** also supply the rectum through the inferior and middle hemorrhoidal branches.
- The colon has multiple vascular collaterals connecting the major arterial vessels that are important in understanding ischemic colitis.
- The **marginal artery of Drummond** runs parallel to the colon, connecting the SMA and IMA circulation.
- In patients with vascular disease who experience gradual occlusion of the IMA, this marginal artery can provide the majority of blood flow to the left and sigmoid colon.
- The **arc of Riolan** is a variable collateral vessel that connects the SMA, through the middle colic vessel, to the IMA, through the left colic.
- **Watershed areas** describe regions of the colon at the border of territory supplied by the two main arteries, the SMA and the IMA
  - **Griffith point** is the region of the splenic flexure where the circulations of the IMA and SMA meet.
  - **Sudeck point** describes an area in the sigmoid colon at the junction of the sigmoid and superior hemorrhoidal vessels.
  - These watershed areas are particularly susceptible to ischemia during periods of low blood flow.
- **The rectum**, on the other hand, has a robust **dual blood supply**, from both the IMA and the iliac circulation,and is rarely the victim of ischemic injury.
- **Management algorithm for ischemic colitis**

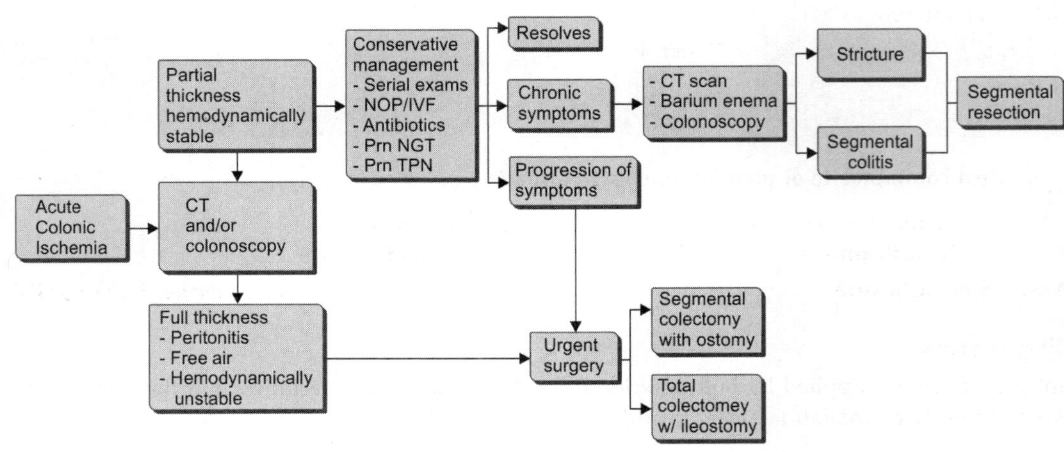

4. A 45-year-old female patient presents with bleeding per rectum and having frequency of stool refractory to treatment, upon colonoscopy geographical ulcer seen, histology from lesion given. Most likely diagnosis is?

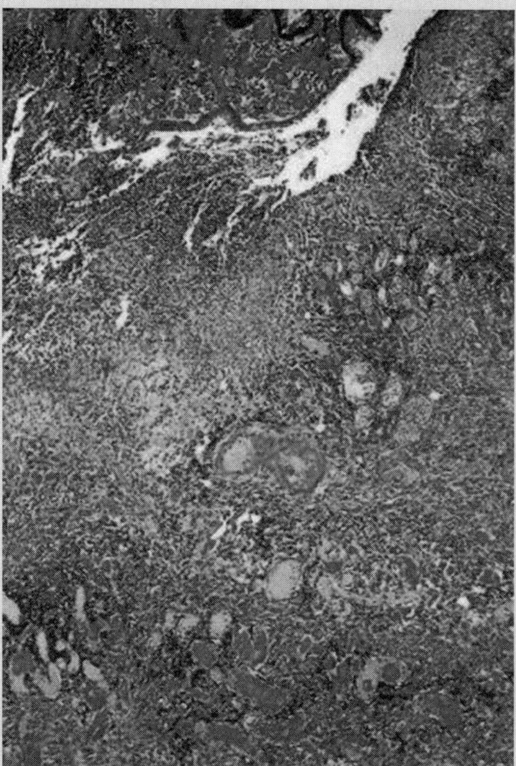

a. Pseudomembranous colitis
b. Crohn's disease
c. Ca colon
d. Visceral leishmaniasis

Ans b. Crohn's disease *Ref: http://crohnsandcolitis.org.nz/uploads/files/chapter_2.pdf*

EXPLANATION

- ❑ Crohn's disease (regional enteritis) chronic full thickness inflammatory process that can affect any part of the gastrointestinal tract from the lips to the anal margin more common in women than in men, and is most commonly diagnosed in young patients between the ages of 25 and 40 years
- ❑ Crohn's disease is a chronic (long-term) inflammatory disease of the bowel (intestines).

General information

Crohn's disease is one of the two major types of inflammatory bowel disease (IBD), the other being ulcerative colitis. The main difference between the two conditions is that, whereas Crohn's disease can affect any part of the digestive tract, ulcerative colitis affects only the large bowel and the rectum.

Risk factors

- ❑ Family history (genetics)
- ❑ Smoking

- Use of oral contraceptives
- Ethnicity
- Environment

Interaction between the predisposing genetic factors (making a person more inclined to develop the condition), environmental factors, host factors (e.g. a person's immune system function), and a triggering event (e.g. bacterial infection) may be responsible for the development of the disease.

Although diet may affect the symptoms in patients with Crohn's disease, it is unlikely that diet is responsible for the disease.

There is a clear genetic predisposition for Crohn's disease.

Environmental factors, especially cigarette smoking, are also clearly involved in this disease. Tobacco smoking doubles the risk of both initial and recurrent Crohn's disease.

Signs and symptoms

- Rectal bleeding
- Fever
- Weight loss, and loss of appetite
- Nausea, vomiting
- Malnutrition, and vitamin deficiencies
- Tiredness, lethargy
- Bone loss (osteoporosis)
- Depression, anxiety (associated with coping with the condition)
- Stunted growth in children (which may occur many years before digestive symptoms appear).

Diagnosis

Colonoscopy or sigmoidoscopy or mouth (gastroscopy).

Small samples (biopsies) of the lining of digestive tract can be taken for analysis. Endoscopic visualization and biopsy are essential in the diagnosis of Crohn's disease.

Barium radiographic studies of the small bowel reveal a number of characteristic findings, including a **cobblestone appearance of the mucosa** composed of linear ulcers, transverse sinuses, and clefts.

Colon is involved, sigmoidoscopy or colonoscopy may reveal characteristic **aphthous ulcers with granularity and a normal-appearing surrounding mucosa**.

The following are the most characteristic classically described histologic findings:

- Areas of chronic inflammation, comprising increased lamina propria plasma cells and lymphocytes, in association with chronic architectural distortion with patchy, mild to severe, neutrophilic inflammation, including neutrophilic cryptitis, crypt abscesses, or erosions/ulcers
- Skip lesions comprising focal, patchy erosions or ulcers, vertical fissures, and fistulas
- The hint of "skip lesions" – Mucosal fragments from the same level of the colon have variable microscopic findings.
- Transmural inflammation with multiple lymphoid aggregates
- Granulomas
- Submucosal fibrosis and neuromuscular hyperplasia of submucosa.

Indirect inspection involves the use of computerised tomography (CT) scan, which is a type of computerised X-ray, and barium X-ray studies, in which a chalky substance (barium) is swallowed or administered into the rectum and colon and X-rays taken. The barium, which can be seen on the X-rays, improves the contrast of the X-ray images.

Treatment

Medications

Four main categories of medication are used to treat inflammation in Crohn's disease:

Anti-inflammatory agents: Aminosalicylates, such as mesalazine (Pentasa) and sulphasalazine (Salazopyrin), are usually prescribed for mild-to-moderate Crohn's disease and are used to prevent flare-ups; corticosteroids, including budesonide (Entocort) and hydrocortisone acetate (Colifoam), are usually prescribed in short courses for active moderate-to-severe Crohn's disease. These medications act by reducing inflammation. The aminosalicylates and corticosteroids can be taken by mouth (orally) and into the rectum (as an enema or suppository).

Antibiotics: Such as ciprofloxacin (Cipflox), are used in the treatment of mild-to-moderate disease. It is thought that antibiotics work by altering the bacterial population of the intestine. They may also have an effect on the immune system.

Immunomodulators: Including methotrexate (Methoblastin) and azathioprine (Imuran) are sometimes used to treat moderate-to-severe Crohn's disease, disease that does not respond to corticosteroids, and to prevent flare-ups. These medications work by suppressing the immune system.

Disease-modifying agents: Such as infliximab (Remicade) and adalimumab (Humira) are used in the treatment of active moderate-to-severe Crohn's disease that has not responded to other medications. These medications act by disrupting the inflammatory process. Their use is somewhat restricted because they are expensive.

Other medications may be prescribed to address specific symptoms such as chronic diarrhea and abdominal cramps.

Surgery

Unlike ulcerative colitis, Crohn's disease does not have a surgical cure. Most people with Crohn's disease will, however, require surgery at some point in their lifetime either to control symptoms or to correct complications of the disease.

Major surgery, called resection, may be needed to remove severely inflamed or damaged portions of the small or large intestines. Abscesses or fistulae around the anus can be treated using local surgical drainage procedures.

People can be free of disease and symptoms for some time, often years, after a resection, and enjoy a marked improvement in their quality of life. In many people, however, Crohn's disease eventually returns, affecting previously healthy digestive tract. Half of patients can expect to have a recurrence of symptoms within four years of surgery. Certain drugs (e.g. mesalazine) can reduce the chance of the disease returning after surgery.

5. A 30-year-old male met an accident and he is unable to move his legs and pass urine since then. Trauma to cervical spine is suspected. Which of the following is best approach?

a. X-ray cervical spine lateral and anteroposterior view
b. Doctor accompany the patient and shift him to the X-ray table
c. Observe the patient for any neurological deficit.
d. Cervical collar immobilization and X-ray cervical spine

Ans. d. Cervical collar immobilization and X-ray cervical spine *Ref: Sabiston 20th/ed p495*

Explanation

In case of suspected cervical spine injury-immobilization of spine is the very first step advised.

Algorithm for cervical spine injury management

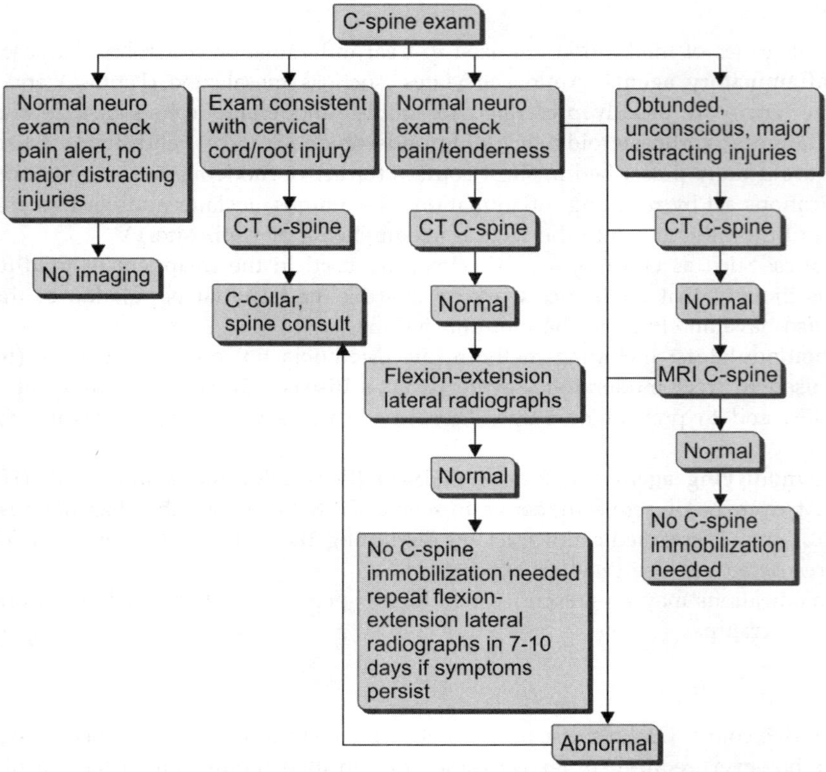

6. A 25-year-old male presented with breathing difficulty to emergency department after meeting an road traffic accident (RTA). On examination trachea was deviated to right side and respiratory sounds were diminished on left side with low blood pressure and thin pulse. Immediate modality of treatment is

a. Thoracocentesis
b. Thoracostomy
c. Tracheostomy
d. Needle thoracostomy

Ans d. Needle thoracostomy *Ref: Sabiston 20th/ed p415*

Explanation

This is a case of **tension pneumothorax**, in which immediate insertion of a wide bore needle in 2nd or 3rd intercostal space is life saving step.

Whenever **an RTA patient presents in emergency** with **dyspnea**, all of the following should be suspected:

- ❑ **Tension pneumothorax**
- ❑ **Massive hemothorax**
- ❑ **Flail chest with pulmonary contusion**

An immediate intervention is required in all of the above mentioned situation to prevent mortality, therefore a **clinical diagnosis is must.**

Tension pneumothorax: Deviation of the trachea in the sternal notch with unilaterally absent or diminished breath sounds and cardiopulmonary compromise.

Immediate chest decompression alarmed.

Massive hemothorax: Tube **thoracostomy** with evacuation of blood and reexpansion of lung.

Flail chest and pulmonary contusion: Mechanical ventilation

7. A 70-year-old patient who is chronic smoker and have chronic cough with sputum. He complains of recurrent hemoptysis for last 3 years. Which of the following is not done?

a. Pneumectomy
b. Embolization of bronchial vessels
c. Ligate bronchial artery
d. Ligate pulmonary artery

Ans. d. Ligate pulmonary artery *Ref: Harrison 19th/ed p246*

EXPLANATION

Hemoptysis

Bleeding in hemoptysis most commonly arises from the **small- to medium-sized airways**. Irritation and injury of the bronchial mucosa can lead to small-volume bleeding.

More significant hemoptysis can result from the **proximity of the bronchial artery** and vein to the airway, with these vessels and the bronchus running together in what is often referred to as the ***bronchovascular bundle***.

In the smaller airways, these blood vessels are close to the airspace, and lesser degrees of inflammation or injury can therefore result in their rupture into the airways.

Algorithm for hemoptysis management.

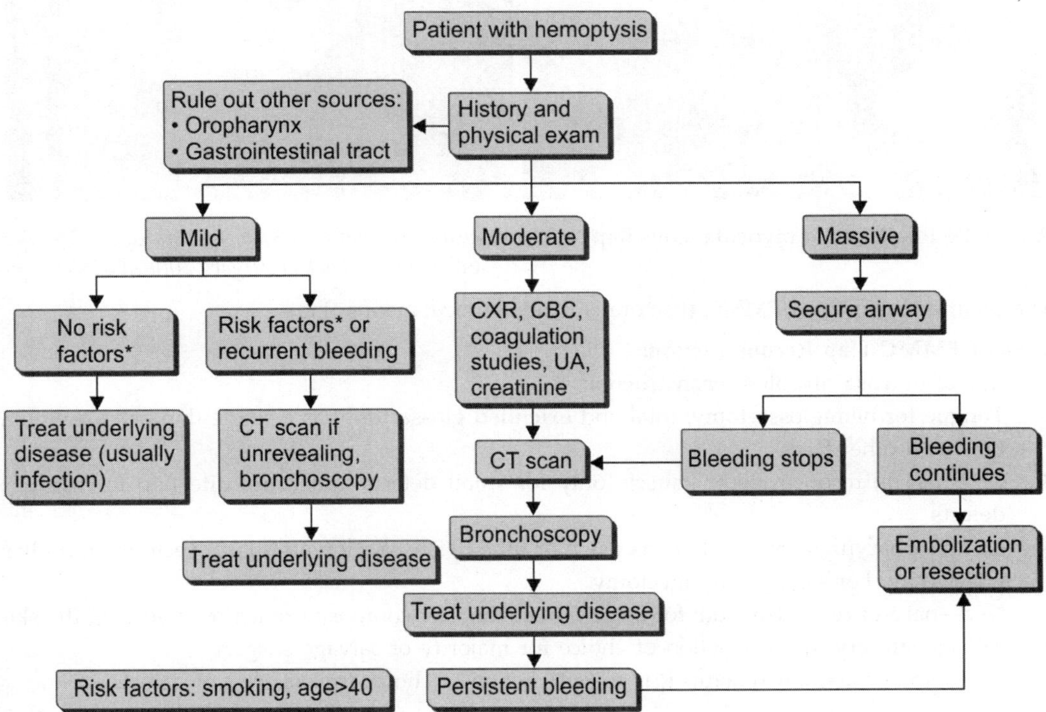

8. Percentage of metastatic axillary lymph nodes picked up by USG of axilla for clinically negative Lymph nodes?

a. 10 – 20%
b. 20 – 30%
c. 30 – 50%
d. 50 – 60%

Ans. d. 50–60% *Ref: Breast Imaging: The Requisites By Debra Ikeda, Kanae Kawai Miyake 3rd/ed p446*

EXPLANATION

PET can detect axillary lymph node involvement with higher sensitivity in patients with higher nodal stages: 41% in pN1, 67% in pN2, and 100% in pN3. USG is 41.2% sensitivity and 93% specificity for detecting metastatic axilla.

9. Which of the following is the flap shown in the picture?

a. Pectoralis major myocutaneous flap
b. TRAM flap
c. VRAM flap
d. Serratus anterior flap

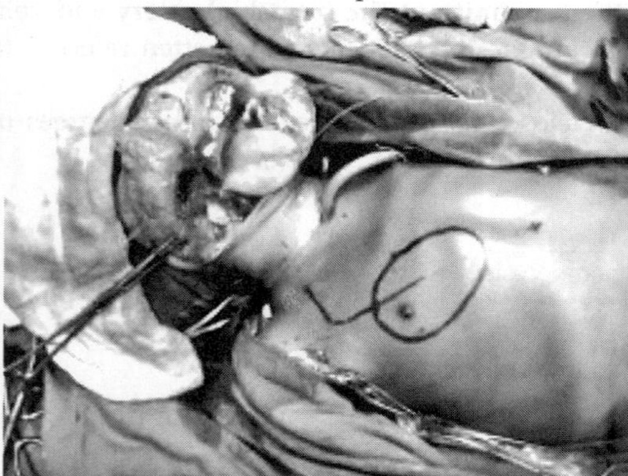
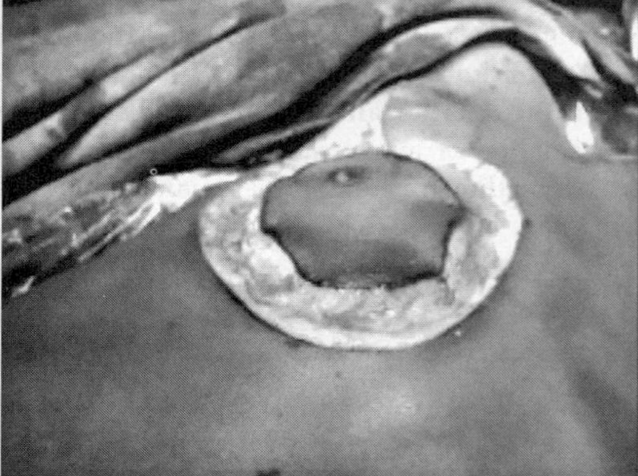

Ans. a. Pectoralis major myocutaneous flap *Ref: Schwartz Principles of Surgery 10th/ed p1872–1875, Sabiston Textbook of surgery 20th/ed p1953 -1954*

The picture shown is of PMMC (Pectoralis major Myocutaneous flap)

Uses of PMMC Flap Reconstruction:

1. Buccal mucosa–alveolus reconstruction
2. Tongue for hemiglossectomy, total and extended glossectomy as a single flap or in combination with other flaps
3. Oropharynx reconstruction: muscle only for small defects and composite flap for complex defects
4. Larynx–pharynx reconstruction: as patch or tube reconstruction after laryngectomy and pharyngectomy. For salvage laryngectomy
5. Neck–parotid reconstruction: for large skin cover after composite resection involving the skin
6. Salvage surgery: reconstruction of choice for majority of salvage surgery
7. In resource constrained setup it is reconstruction of choice for majority of defects

Limitations of PMMC flap

1. Reach not enough for maxilla and skull base defects
2. Difficult to cover defects above the zygoma
3. Flaps drags down in some cases due to its weight.

10. Hot water was spilled by mistake over a 5-year-old boy. He developed painful pink colored wound over medial aspect of forearm. Which of the following dressings will be done?

a. Silver sulfadiazine
b. Paraffin dressing
c. Normal dressing and leave it
d. Caspofungin

Ans. c. Normal dressing and leave it *Ref: Bailey and Love 26th/ed p392*

EXPLANATION

Since it is a **scald burn** it is generally **superficial burn** (deep burns dressed by nano-crystalline silver).

Also **pain** indicates superficial burn.

Since its because of hot water inside the house so chances of **contamination are low** (contaminated burns are dressed by silver sulfadiazine).

Therefore normal dressing is advised.

11. A 23-year-old lady with 20 weeks pregnancy was having a thyroid swelling. On fine needle aspiration cytology papillary carcinoma was diagnosed. Which of the following cannot be done to treat?

a. I-131 radioablation
b. Total thyroidectomy
c. Total thyroidectomy with lymph node dissection
d. Right lobectomy

Ans d. Right lobectomy *Ref: Love and Bailey 26th/ed p766*

EXPLANATION

Patients with large, locally aggressive or metastatic differentiated thyroid cancer (DTC) require **total thyroidectomy, with excision of adjacent involved structures if necessary, and appropriate nodal surgery followed by radioiodine ablation with long-term TSH suppression.**

Current guidelines advocate **routine total thyroidectomy**, often necessitating early reoperation and second lobectomy following a diagnostic first lobectomy with **routine central compartment node dissection for all tumors greater than 1 cm.**

Total thyroidectomy facilitates the use of radioiodine for postoperative scanning to detect and subsequently ablate metastases results in lower thyroglobulin levels.

Total thyroidectomy is recommended for tumors greater than 2 cm and those with nodal involvement or metastases and lobectomy for the remainder.

Also in papillary carcinoma multiple and bilateral lesions are commonly seen.

12. After laparoscopic cholecystectomy, drain was removed on 3rd day. Patient develops fever and tachycardia. USG shows 5 × 5 cm subhepatic collection. Next step will be:

a. Antibiotics and pigtail catheter under USG guidance
b. Re-exploration and t-tube insertion
c. USG guided aspiration of fluid
d. Reassure and discharge the patient

Ans. a. Antibiotics and pigtail catheter under USG guidance *Ref: Bailey and Love 26th/ed p1104*

Explanation

If a fluid collection is present in the subhepatic space drainage catheters may be required. These can be **inserted under radiological control** or if this expertise is not available then **open operation considered**.

PGI May 2017

1. All of the following syndromes are associated with brain tumors in children:

a. Neurofibromatosis
b. Turner's syndrome
c. Tuberous sclerosis
d. Peutz-jeghers syndrome
e. Li-Fraumeni syndrome

Ans. a. Neurofibromatosis and e. Li-Fraumeni syndrome

Ref: Sabiston; Table 28.3 Familial Cancer Syndrome 20th/ed p691

Syndrome	Genes	Locations	Cancer sites and associated traits
Breast/ovarian syndrome	BRCA1	17q21	Cancers of the breast, ovary, colon, prostate
	BRCA2	13q12.3	Cancers of the breast, ovary, colon prostate, gallbladder and biliary tree, pancreas, stomach; melanoma
Cowden disease	PTEN	10q23.3	Cancer of the breast, endometrium, and thyroid
Failial adenomatous polyposis	APC	5q21	Colorectal carcinoma, duodenal and gastric neoplasms, medulloblastomas, osteomas
Familial melanoma	P16; CDK4	9p21; 12q14	Melanoma, pancreatic cancer, dysplastic nevi, atypical moles
Hereditary diffuse gastric cancer	CDH1	16q22	Gastric cancer
Hereditary nonpolyposis colorectal	hMLH1; hMSH2;	3p21; 2p22-21	Colorectal cancer, endometrial cancer, transitional cell carcinoma of the ureter
Hereditary nonpolyposis colorectal cancer	hMLH1; hMSH2; hMSH6; hPMS1; hPMS2	3p21; 2p22-21; 2p16; 2q31.1; 7p22.2	Colorectal cancer; endometrial cancer; transitional cell carcinoma of the ureter and renal pelvis; and carcinomas of the stomach, small bowel, pancreas, and ovary
Hereditary papillary renal cell carcinoma	MET	7q31	Renal cell cancer

Contd....

Contd....

Syndrome	Genes	Locations	Cancer sites and associated traits
Hereditary paraganglioma and pheochromocytoma	SDHB; SDHC; SDHD	1p36.1p35; 1q21; 11q23	Paraganglioma, pheochromocytoma
Juvenile polyposis coli	BMPRIA SMAD4/ DPC4	10q21-q22 18q21.1	Juvenile polyps of the gastrointestinal tract, gastrointestinal malignant neoplasms
Li-Fraumeni	p53 hCHK2	17p13 22q12.1	Breast cancer, soft tissue sarcoma, osteosarcoma, brain tumors, adrenocortical carcinoma, Wilms tumor, phyllodes tumor (breast), pancreatic cancer, leukemia, neuroblastoma
Multiple endocrine neoplasia type 1	MEN1	11q13	Pancreatic islet cell tumors, parathyroid hyperplasia, pituitary adenomas
Multiple endocrine neoplasia type 2	RET	10q11.2	Medullary thyroid cancer, pheochromocytoma, parathyroid hyperplasia
MYH-associated adenomatous polyposis	MYH	1p34.3-p32.1	Cancer of the colon, rectum, breast, stomach
Neurofibromatosis type 1	NF1	17q11	Neurofibromas, neurofibrosarcoma, acute myelogenous leukemia, brain tumors
Neurofibromatosis type 2	NF2	22q12	Acoustic neuromas, meningiomas, gliomas, ependymomas
Nevoid basal cell carcinoma	PTC	9q22.3	Basal cell carcinoma
Peutz-Jeghers syndrome	STK11	19q13.3	Gastrointestinal carcinomas, breast cancer, testicular cancer, pancreatic cancer, benign pigmentation of the skin and mucosa
Retinoblastoma	RB	13q14	Retinoblastoma, sarcomas, melanoma, malignant neoplasms of the brain and meninges
Tuberous sclerosis	TSC1; TSC2	9q34; 16q13	Multiple hamartomas, renal cell carcinoma astrocytoma
von Hippel-Lindau syndrome	VHL	3p25	Renal cell carcinoma, hemangioblastomas of the retina and central nervous system, pheochromocytoma
Willms tumor	WT	11p13	Wilms tumor, aniridia, genitourinary abnormalities, mental retardiation

2. All is/are true for posterior mediastinal tumors:

a. Most common tumor is of neurogenic origin
b. Paragangliomas are rarely seen in posterior mediastinum

c. Thyroid and parathyroid tumors are also seen
d. Mostly malignant in adults
e. Mostly benign in children

Ans. a. Most common tumor is of neurogenic origin and c. Thyroid and parathyroid tumors are also seen *Ref: Sabiston 20th/ed p1609*

EXPLANATION

- Neurogenic tumors are usually the most common primary tumors of the mediastinum, and approximately 25% of these tumors are malignant. These tumors are located within the **paravertebral sulcus (posterior mediastinum)**.

Neurogenic tumors are usually located in the posterior mediastinum and originate from the **sympathetic ganglia** (ganglioma, ganglioneuroblastoma, and neuroblastoma), the **intercostal nerves** (neurofibroma, neurilemoma, and neurosarcoma), and the **paraganglia cells** (paraganglioma).

Although the peak incidence occurs in adults, neurogenic tumors make up a proportionally greater percentage of mediastinal masses in children.

Although most neurogenic tumors in **adults are benign**, a greater percentage of neurogenic tumors are **malignant in children**.

Mediastinal paragangliomas are **rare tumors**, representing less than 1% of all mediastinal tumors and less than 2% of all pheochromocytomas.

Amongst mediastinal ones, most are found in the paravertebral sulcus ***(option b)***

Option c:

- Although substernal extension of a cervical goiter is common, totally intrathoracic thyroid tumors are rare and make up only 1% of all mediastinal masses in collected series.
- These tumors arise from heterotopic thyroid tissue, which occurs most commonly in the anterosuperior mediastinum but may also occur in the middle mediastinum between the trachea and the esophagus as well as in the posterior mediastinum.

3. All of the following is/are premalignant conditions of esophagus:

a. Esophageal ring
b. Peterson Kelly
c. Achalasia
d. Barrett's esophagus

Ans. d. Barrett's esophagus *Ref: Sabiston 20th/ed p1023*

EXPLANATION

Barrett's esophagus is **most common precancerous** lesion of esophagus

Barrett's esophagus is a metaplastic change in the lining mucosa of the esophagus in response to **chronic gastroesophageal reflux.**

Intestinal metaplasia is an important risk factor for the development of adenocarcinoma.

Risk factors

Gastroesophageal reflux disease (GERD) increases risk for developing Barrett's esophagus. Chronic reflux can cause changes, or metaplasia, in the lining of the esophagus.

Barrett's esophagus can also occur in people who don't have symptoms of GERD. Most people with chronic GERD symptoms don't develop Barrett's esophagus.

The following **risk factors** can also increase chance of developing Barrett's esophagus:

- Obesity
- Smoking
- Alcohol

Symptoms

- ❑ Heartburn
- ❑ Acid reflux
- ❑ Indigestion
- ❑ Nausea and vomiting
- ❑ Difficulty swallowing
- ❑ Bringing up, or regurgitating, stomach acid

Diagnosis

Tests used to diagnose Barrett's esophagus include:

- ❑ Upper gastrointestinal (GI) endoscopy
- ❑ Biopsy

Endoscopic ultrasound (EUS) may be done if high-grade dysplasia is found with endoscopy and biopsy.

Treatments

Drug therapy with proton pump inhibitors and H2 blockers can be used to treat the reflux and control how much acid the stomach makes.

Endoscopic mucosal resection (EMR) may be used to treat high-grade dysplasia in the esophagus. The doctor uses an endoscope to do EMR. It removes the inner layer, or mucosa, of the esophagus that contains the abnormal areas.

Radiofrequency ablation (RFA)
Photodynamic therapy (PDT)
Electrocoagulation
Argon plasma coagulation
Fundoplication
Esophagectomy

Peterson Kelly is a risk factor for esophageal carcinoma, but not a premalignant lesion.

4. All are true about torsion of testis *except*:

a. Doppler used for diagnosis
b. Differentiated from epididymitis only by radionuclide scan
c. Intravaginal torsion is associated with bell clapper deformity
d. Most of the cases are seen in children below 5 years

Ans. a. Doppler used for diagnosis and b. Differentiated from epididymitis only by radionuclide scan

Ref: Sabiston 20th/ed p1887

Explanation

Testicular torsion

Torsion of the testis is the **most common genitourinary tract emergency** of childhood.

Doppler can be used to determine flow of blood to testis, but diagnosis is usually made on the basis of clinical findings and history.

Extravaginal torsion is more common in **neonates,** in whom there can be torsion of the spermatic cord along its course outside the tunica vaginalis.

Torsion of the testis occurs most frequently in **early adolescence** with a peak incidence at 14 years of age.

Pain is most common presenting symptom.

- ❑ On examination, the testis that has undergone torsion may be high-riding, edematous, and significantly tender. Urinary tract symptoms, such as frequency, urgency, dysuria, and fever, tend to occur more frequently with infectious or inflammatory conditions, such as epididymitis

- **Prehn's sign** (named after urologist Douglas T Prehn) is a medical diagnostic indicator that was once believed to help determine whether the presenting testicular pain is caused by acute epididymitis or from testicular torsion. Although elevation of the scrotum when differentiating epididymitis from testicular torsion is of clinical value, Prehn's sign has been shown to be inferior to Doppler ultrasound to rule out testicular torsion.

5. All are true about unilateral absent testis in scrotum:

a. Undescended testis are macroscopically normal in childhood
b. Most common site for ectopic testis is superficial inguinal pouch
c. Appropriate time for surgery is around puberty
d. Spontaneous decent does not occur

Ans. a. Undescended testis are macroscopically normal in childhood and b. Most common site for ectopic testis is superficial inguinal pouch *Ref: Sabiston 20th/ed p1886*

EXPLANATION

Above condition is known as **cryptorchidism.**

Cryptorchidism

- Incomplete descent of the testis occurs when the testis is arrested in some part of its normal path to the scrotum
- About **4%** of boys are born with one or both testes incompletely descended.
- About **two thirds** of these reach the scrotum during the first **three months** of life, but full descent after that is uncommon.
- The incidence of testicular maldescent at the age of **one year is around 1%.**
- Incompletely descended testes are often **macroscopically normal** in early childhood, but by **puberty** the testis is typically **smaller** compared with its intrascrotal counterpart.
- Microscopic changes are apparent from 1–2 years, including loss of Leydig cells, **degeneration of Sertoli cells and decreased spermatogenesis**.

The higher the testis, the greater the degree of histological change. An undescended testis has had its descent halted somewhere along the path of normal descent and is **most commonly located in the inguinal canal.**

Algorithm for management

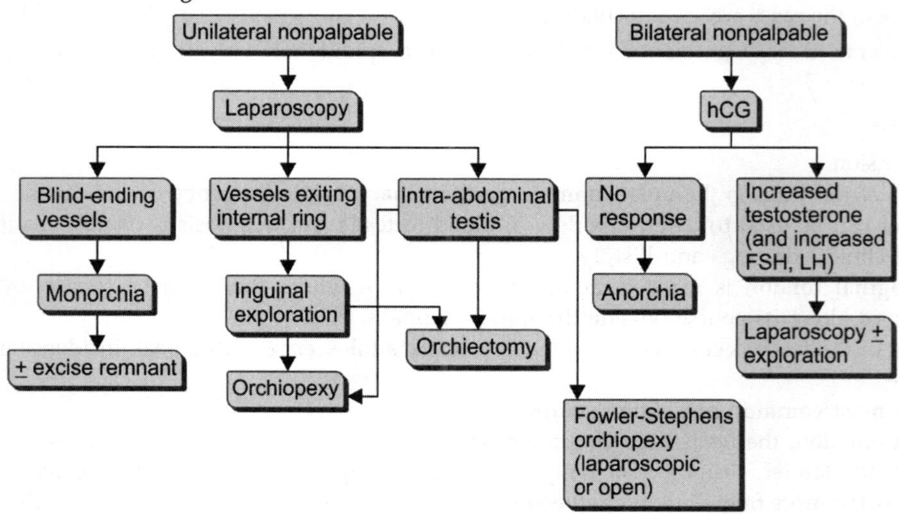

6. All are true about hernias *except*:

a. Strangulation is seen more commonly indirect than in direct inguinal hernias.
b. Inguinal hernia is more common than femoral hernia in females
c. Femoral hernia are ten times more common in women compared to men
d. Any hernia can strangulate

Ans. a. Strangulation is seen more commonly in indirect than direct inguinal hernias.

Ref: Bailey and Love 26th/ed p949

Explanation

Hernias

5% of the population will develop an abdominal wall hernia, but the prevalence may be even higher.

About **75%** of all hernias occur in **the inguinal** region.

Two thirds of these are **indirect** and the remainder are direct inguinal hernias.

Femoral hernias represent only **3%** of all groin hernias.

Men are 25 times more likely to have a groin hernia than women.

An indirect inguinal hernia is the most common hernia, regardless of gender.

In **men, indirect hernias** predominate over direct hernias at a ratio of 2:1. Indirect hernias are by far the **most common type of hernia in women**.

The female-to-male ratio for femoral and umbilical hernias, however, is about 10:1 and 2:1, respectively.

Although femoral hernias occur more frequently in women than in men, **inguinal** hernias remain the **most common hernia in women**. Femoral hernias are rare in men.

Indirect inguinal and femoral hernias occur more **commonly on the right** side. This is attributed to a **delay in atrophy of the processus vaginalis** after the normal slower descent of the right testis to the scrotum during fetal development.

The predominance of right-sided femoral hernias is thought to be caused by the **tamponading effect of the sigmoid colon on the left femoral canal.**

The prevalence of hernias **increases with age, particularly for inguinal, umbilical, and femoral hernias.**

The likelihood of **strangulation** and need for hospitalization also **increase** with aging.

Most strangulated hernias are indirect inguinal hernias.

Femoral hernias have the highest rate of strangulation (15% to 20%) of all hernias, and it is therefore recommended that all femoral hernias be repaired at the time of discovery.

7. Not included in surgical safety checklist:

a. Sign in
b. Sign out
c. Time in
d. Time out
e. Preanesthetic checkup

Ans. c. Time in and e. Preanesthetic checkup

Ref: http://apps.who.int/iris/bitstream/10665/44186/2/9789241598590_eng_Checklist.pdf

Explanation

WHO surgical safety checklist

Sign in →	Time out →	Sign out
Before induction of anesthesia	**Before skin incision**	**Before patient leaves operating room**
(with at least nurse and anesthetist)	(with nurse, anesthetist and surgeon)	(with nurse, anesthetist and surgeon)
Has the patient confirmed his/her identity, site, procedure, and consent? ☐ Yes	☐ **Confirm all team members have introduced themselves by name and role**	**Nurse verbally confirms:** ☐ The name of the procedure ☐ Completion of instrument, sponge and needle counts ☐ Specimen labeling (read specimen labels aloud, including patient name) ☐ Whether there are any equipment problems to be addressed
Is the site marked? ☐ Yes ☐ Not applicable	☐ **Confirm the patient's name, procedure, and where the incision will be made**	
Is the anesthesia machine and medication check complete? ☐ Yes	**Has antibotic prophylaxis been given withing the last 60 minutes?** ☐ Yes ☐ Not applicable	**To surgeon, anesthetist and nurse:** ☐ What are the key concerns fro recovery and management of this patient?
Is the pulse oximeter on the patient and functioning? ☐ Yes	**Anticipated Critical Events** **To surgeon:** ☐ What are the critical or non-routine steps? ☐ How long will the case take? ☐ What is the anticipated blood loss? **To anesthetist:** ☐ Are there any patient-specific concems? ☐ To Nursing team: ☐ Has sterility (including indicator results) been confirmed? ☐ Are there equipment issues or any concerns?	
Does the patient have a: **Known allergy?** ☐ No ☐ Yes **Difficult airway or aspiration risk?** ☐ No ☐ Yes, and equipment/assistance available **Risk of > 500 ml blood loss (7 ml/kg in children)?** ☐ No ☐ Yes, and two IVs/central access and fluids planned	**Is essential imaging displayed?** ☐ Yes ☐ Not applicable	

8. Cholecystectomy is considered completely safe in which of the following stages of gallbladder carcinoma?

a. 1a
b. 1b
c. 2
d. 3
e. 4

Ans. a. 1a *Ref: Bailey and Love 26th p1117; https://www.ncbi.nlm.nih.gov/pmc/articles/PMC4214932/;*

Explanation

Carcinoma gallbladder

Incidence

This is a **rare** disease, but extremely variable by geographical region and racial–ethnic groups.

The highest incidence is among Chileans, American Indians and residents in **parts of northern India**, where it accounts for as much as **9%** of all biliary tract disease.

Women appear to have a **higher incidence** across all geographic areas.

Pathology

The majority **(90%)** of cases are **adenocarcinoma.**

Squamous carcinomas also occur and are believed to arise from areas of mucosal squamous metaplasia.

Clinical features are similar to other gallbladder diseases.

Staging

T-groups for gallbladder cancer

TX: The primary tumor's extent cannot be assessed.

T0: There is no evidence of primary tumor.

Tis: Cancer cells are only found in the epithelium (the inner layer of the gallbladder) and have not grown into deeper layers of the gallbladder. This is also known as *carcinoma in situ*.

T1: The tumor has grown into the lamina propria or the muscle layer (muscularis).

- ❑ **T1a:** Tumor has grown into lamina propria.
- ❑ **T1b:** Tumor has grown into the muscularis.

T2: The tumor has grown into perimuscular fibrous tissue.

T3: The tumor has grown through the serosa (the outermost covering of the gallbladder) and/or it has grown from the gallbladder directly into the liver and/or a nearby structure such as the stomach, duodenum (first part of the small intestine), colon, pancreas, or bile ducts outside the liver.

T4: The tumor has grown into one of the main blood vessels leading into the liver (portal vein or hepatic artery) or it has grown into 2 or more structures outside of the liver.

N groups for gallbladder cancer.

NX: Nearby (regional) lymph nodes cannot be assessed.

N0: The cancer has not spread to nearby lymph nodes.

N1: The cancer has spread to lymph nodes near the gallbladder, such as those along the cystic duct, common bile duct, hepatic artery, and portal vein.

N2: The cancer has spread to lymph nodes in the abdomen that are farther away from the gallbladder, such as the lymph nodes along the aorta (periaortic), the vena cava (pericaval), the superior mesenteric artery, and the celiac artery.

M groups for gallbladder cancer

M0: The cancer has not spread to tissues or organs far away from the gallbladder.

M1: The cancer has spread to tissues or organs far away from the gallbladder.

Treatment

For **T1a** GB cancer, the optimal treatment modality is **simple cholecystectomy**, which can be carried out as either a laparotomy or a laparoscopic surgery.

For **T1b** GB cancer, either **simple or an extended cholecystectomy** is appropriate.

An extended cholecystectomy is generally recommended for patients with GB cancer at stage **T2 or above**. In extended cholecystectomy, a wedge resection of the GB bed or a segmentectomy IVb/V can be performed and the optimal extent of lymph node dissection should include the cystic duct lymph node, the common bile duct lymph node, the lymph nodes around the hepatoduodenal ligament (the hepatic artery and portal vein lymph nodes), and the posterior superior pancreaticoduodenal lymph node.

Gallbladder cancer for most patients is a **lethal disease** with a **grim prognosis**. The **median survival is less than six months** and a **five-year survival figure of 5% reported**.

9. Acute fluid collection after acute pancreatitis is:

a. Synonymous with pseudocyst
b. Mostly infectious
c. Ill defined wall
d. Mostly resolve spontaneously

Ans. c. Ill defined wall and d. Mostly resolve spontaneously *Ref: Bailey and Love 26th/ed p1131*

EXPLANATION

Acute fluid collection

- ❑ This occurs **early in the course** of acute pancreatitis and is located in or near the pancreas.
- ❑ The wall encompassing the collection **is ill defined.(option c)**
- ❑ The fluid is sterile and most such collections **resolve spontaneously.(option d)**
- ❑ **No intervention** is necessary unless a large collection causes symptoms or pressure effects.

If symptomatic

- ❑ Percutaneously aspirated under ultrasound or CT guidance.
- ❑ Transgastric drainage under EUS guidance is another option.

Complications

- ❑ Pseudocyst (**option a)**
- ❑ Abscess; if it becomes infected (**option b**)

10. All are true about Meckel's diverticulum;

a. A persistant remnant of vitellointestinal duct
b. Presents with gastrointestinal bleeding
c. Hematuria may be seen
d. Sometimes haemoptysis also observed

Ans. a. A persistant remnant of vitellointestinal duct and b. Presents with gastrointestinal bleeding. *Ref: Bailey and Love 26th/ed p1169*

EXPLANATION

Features of Meckel's diverticulum

- ❑ Remnant of **vitellointestinal duct (option a)**
- ❑ Occurs in 2% of patients, 2 inches (5 cm long), 2 feet (60 cm) from the ileocecal valve, 20% heterotopic epithelium
- ❑ **Should be looked for when a normal appendix is found at surgery for suspected appendicitis**
- ❑ If a Meckel's is found incidentally at surgery, it can be left provided it has a wide mouth and is not thickened
- ❑ Can be source of **gastrointestinal bleeding** if it contains ectopic gastric mucosa

11. Gastroesophageal reflux disease confirmed by:

a. Manometry
b. Upper gastrointestinal endoscopy
c. 24 hr pH monitoring
d. Barium meal

Ans c. 24 hr pH monitoring *Ref: Bailey and Love 26th/ed p996*

EXPLANATION

Investigation for gastroesophageal reflux disease (GERD)

Radiography

- ❑ Barium radiology is, however, inaccurate in the diagnosis of gastroesophageal reflux, unless reflux is gross.
- ❑ CT to differentiate from neoplasms

Endoscopy

- ❑ Upper gastrointestinal endoscopy is most appropriate examination if GERD is associated with dysphasia

Esophageal manometry

- ❑ Pressure of lower esophageal shincture is also required
- ❑ 24 hour pH and combined pH impedance monitoring
- ❑ Gold standard for diagnosis

12. All are true about lower GI bleed *except*:

a. Less common reason for hospitalization as compared to upper GI bleed
b. Aspirin is one of the commonest cause
c. Cured by angiography and treated
d. Colonic bleed is commoner than small intestinal bleed

Ans b. Aspirin is one of the commonest cause and c. Cured by angiography and treated

Ref: Sabiston 20th/ed p1151

EXPLANATION

Lower GI bleed

Compared with upper GI hemorrhage, lower GI bleeding is a **less frequent reason for hospitalization**

In more than **95% of patients** with lower GI bleeding, the source of hemorrhage is the **colon.**

Compared with endoscopy in upper GI bleeding, **no diagnostic modality is as sensitive or specific in making an accurate diagnosis in lower GI bleeding.**

Algorithm for diagnosis and management of lower GI bleed

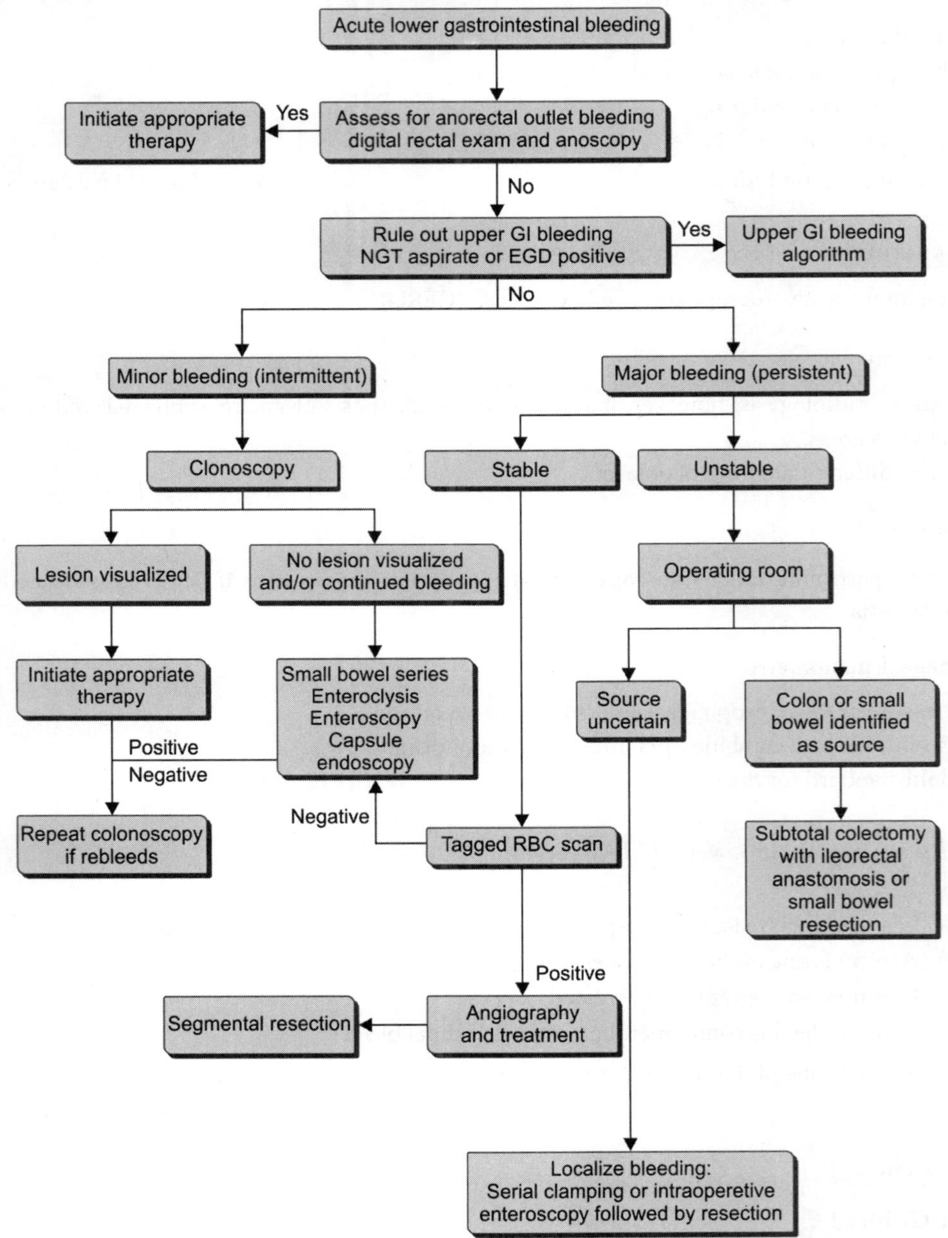

13. All are true about appendicitis *except*:

a. Pain on flexion and external rotation
b. Pain on flexion and internal rotation
c. Pain in right illiac fossa on deep palpation of left iliac fossa
d. Right illiac fossa tenderness

Ans a. Pain on flexion and external rotation *Ref: Question 1 Surgery AIIMS Paper*

14 All are radiological feature/s of Crohn's disease:

a. Hosepipe colon
b. Cracked appearance
c. Loss of haustrasion
d. Cobblestone appearance
e. String sign of kantor

Ans. e. String sign of kantor *Ref: Bailey and Love 26th/ed p1279*

EXPLANATION

Hosepipe colon and loss of haustration are radiological feature of **ulcerative colitis.**

Cobblestone appearance is seen in Crohn's disease but is seen on **endoscopy (Option d).**

The involved areas tend to be **narrowed, irregular** and, sometimes, when a length of terminal ileum is involved, there may be the **string sign of Kantor**.

CT scans with luminal contrast are widely used in the investigation of abdominal symptoms and can demonstrate fistulae, intra-abdominal abscesses and bowel thickening or dilatation.

15. Which of the following used for reducing intracranial pressure (ICP) in head injury patient?

a. Mannitol infusion
b. Barbiturates
c. Use of diuretics like furosemide
d. Hypotonic solution
e. Glucose based crystalloids

Ans. a. Mannitol infusion; b. Barbiturates and c. Use of diuretics like furosemide *Ref: Bailey and Love 26th/ed p319*

EXPLANATION

Hierarchy of raised ICP treatment

Initial
- ❑ Head up
- ❑ Loosen collar
- ❑ Optimize ventilation (pO_2>11, pCO_2−4.5 kPa)
- ❑ Optimize electrolyte balance (hypertonic fluids if necessary), treat hyperglycemia
- ❑ Sedation barbiturates, etc.
- ❑ Seizure control

Intermediate
- ❑ Mannitol, furosemide, hyperventilation as temporizing measures
- ❑ Heavy sedation
- ❑ Paralysis
- ❑ CSF drainage externally
- ❑ Cooling (controversial)

Final
- ❑ Induction of thiopentone coma
- ❑ Decompression craniotomy

16. All of the following conditions are associated with bilateral breast cancer *except*:

a. Lobular carcinoma of breast
b. Ductal carcinoma of breast

c. Pagets disease
d. DCIS

Ans. a. Lobular carcinoma of breast *Ref: Love and Bailey 26th/ed p809*

Explanation

Lobular carcinoma of breast

- Up to **15%** of cases
- Multiple foci and usually **bilateral**
- Classical type carries better prognosis than pleomorphic variety

Immunohistochemical analysis using **e-catherin** antibody is confirmatory in cases of mixed histology.

17. All are true about thyroid malignancies *except*:

a. Male to female sex ratio is 3:1
b. Dysphagia is an early symptom
c. Incidence in old age is associated with better prognosis.
d. Recurrent laryngeal nerve paralysis is a marker of locally advanced disease

Ans. a. Male to female sex ratio is 3:1; b. Dysphagia is an early symptom and c. Incidence in old age is associated with better prognosis.

Ref: Bailey and Love 26th/ed p764

Explanation

- Thyroid malignancies
- The annual incidence is about 3.7 per 100 000 of the population and the sex ratio is **three females to one male**.
- The overall mortality should be low because most patients are in a low-risk Category.
- **Older patients** have more aggressive disease with a **worse prognosis**.
- The most common presenting symptom is a thyroid swelling and a five-year history is far from uncommon in differentiated growths.
- Enlarged cervical lymph nodes may be the presentation of papillary carcinoma.
- **Recurrent laryngeal nerve paralysis** is very suggestive of **locally advanced** disease.

18. Chemoradiation therapy true is/are:

a. Chemotherapy is given with radiation dose
b. Less side effects as compared to chemotherapy and radiotherapy alone
c. Chemotherapy is better than radiotherapy in terms of side effects
d. Radiotherapy can reach to such sites where drugs cannot reach effectively

Ans. a. Chemotherapy is given with radiation dose and d. Radiotherapy can reach to such sites where drugs cannot reach effectively *Ref Love and Bailey 26th/ed p158*

Explanation

Reasons for combination therapy

- By the time of diagnosis, many tumors will contain cancer cells that, through **spontaneous mutation**, have **acquired resistance to cytotoxic drugs**.
- Unlike antibiotic resistance, there is no need for previous exposure to the drug.

- Spontaneous mutation rates are high enough to allow chance to permit the development, and subsequent expansion, of clones of cells resistant to drugs to which they have never been exposed.
- If drugs were used as **single agents**, then the further expansion of these *de novo* resistant **subclones would limit cure.**
- **In considering the combination of radiotherapy and chemotherapy, radiation could be considered as just another drug.**
- Chemotherapy is a systemic treatment; radiotherapy **is not, but it is able to reach sites, such as the central nervous system and testis,** which drugs may not reach effectively, e.g. cranial irradiation in leukemia.

19. Neoadjuvent chemotherapy states for:

a. Primary cytoreductive surgery followed by chemotherapy
b. Secondary cytoreductive surgery following chemotherapy
c. Chemotherapy followed by surgery
d. Primary cytoreductive surgery following chemotherapy

Ans. c. Chemotherapy followed by surgery and d. Primary cytoreductive surgery following chemotherapy *Ref: Bailey and Love 26th/ed p1011*

EXPLANATION

According to national cancer society:

Neoadjuvant therapy is defined as first step to shrink the tumor before the main treatment, which is usually surgery, is given. Examples of neoadjuvant therapy include radiation therapy, chemotherapy, and hormone therapy. It is a type of induction therapy.

20. Which of the following is/are inflammatory dental cyst:

a. Periapical
b. Dentigerous cyst
c. Follicular cyst
d. Residual cyst
e. Primordial cyst

Ans. a. Periapical and d. Residual cyst

Ref: http://www.mastereditora.com.br/periodico/20140716_144203.pdf

EXPLANATION

Odontogenic cysts are the most common osteolytic lesions (90% to 97% of reported cysts) in the oral region.

Most frequently seen **in jaw and mandible.**

Inflammatory dental cyst

The inflammatory cysts are lesions that originate from the **infection of root canals from caries or occurrence of a trauma that generated pulp changes.**

The appearance of these cysts occurs from the pre-existence of a periapical granuloma or by induction of epithelial rests of **Malassez.**

The inflammatory cysts can be classified as: inflammatory **periapical cyst** (apical radicular cyst and lateral periodontal cyst or apical), **residual cyst** and cyst **paradental.**

Dentigerous, primordial and follicular cyst belong to developmental cysts (*option b, c and d*).

JIPMER Pattern Based

1. In which of the following conditions operative repair is favored over conservative management?

a. Boerhaave's syndrome
b. Perforation of cervical Esophagus
c. Esophageal rupture confined to mediastinum
d. Flexible endoscopic perforation of esophagus

Ans. a. Boerhaave's syndrome *Ref. Bailey and Love 26th/ed p993*

Explanation

Question adopted as such from bailey and love table

The decision between operative and non-operative management depends on four factors. These are:

1. The site of the perforation (cervical versus thoracoabdominal esophagus);
2. The event causing the perforation (spontaneous versus instrumental);
3. Underlying pathology (benign or malignant);
4. The status of the esophagus before the perforation (fasted and empty versus obstructed with a stagnant residue).

Nonoperative management	Operative repair
Small septic load	Large septic load
Minimal cardiovascular upset	Septic shock
Perforation confined to mediastinum	Boerhaave's syndrome
Cervical esophagial perforation	Pleura breached
Perforation by flexible endoscope	Perforation of abdominal esophagus

Boerhaave's syndrome:

This occurs classically when a person vomits against a closed glottis. The pressure in the esophagus increases rapidly, and the esophagus bursts at its weakest point in the lower third, sending a stream of material into the mediastinum and often the pleural cavity as well. The condition was first reported by Boerhaave. A large volume of material is released into the mediastinum, which causes rapid chemical irritation in the mediastinum and pleura followed by infection if untreated.

2. A 40-year-old female presented with fresh bleeding per rectum and lower abdominal pain for 2 months. There was no history of tenesmus. All of the following can be considered as differential diagnosis *except*:

a. Ischemic colitis
b. Bleeding piles
c. Carcinoma rectum
d. Endometrioma

Ans. c. Carcinoma rectum *Ref: Bailey and Love 26th/ed p1216*

Explanation

Symptoms in the question are associated with all the pathologies mentioned above. However,

1. **Age** mentioned is not so commonly associated with carcinoma incidence.
2. **No history of tenesmus** is an important clue for the answer.

Tenesmus described by the patient as 'I feel I want to go, but nothing happens', this is normally an ominous symptom of rectal cancer, but can occur with any rectal pathology.

Main symptoms of rectal disease

- Bleeding per rectum
- Altered bowel habit
- Mucus discharge
- Tenesmus
- Prolapse

3. A 30-year-old woman with 15 weeks pregnancy was diagnosed with invasive ductal carcinoma with no axillary involvement. All of the following can be done *except*:

a. Use of technitium sulfur colloid for **sentinel** node detection
b. Breast conserving surgery followed **by** radiation
c. Full course chemotherapy
d. Axillary dissection is avoided

Ans. b. Breast conserving surgery followed by radiation *Ref: Sabiston 20th/ed p2058*

Explanation

The **mainstay** of therapy for pregnancy associated breast cancer is surgical resection, and resection can be offered during every trimester

- **Modified radical mastectomy** classically has been the **first choice** for local control of breast cancer because it eliminates the need for adjuvant radiation and its risk to the fetus, but it is not mandatory especially when performed later in pregnancy.
- **Axillary lymph node dissection** can be **avoided** in most pregnant women, especially after the first trimester, **as a sentinel lymph node biopsy using technetium sulfur colloid can be recommended (option a and d)**
- In patients in whom breast cancer is diagnosed during **the late second trimester or later,** immediate **breast-conserving lumpectomy and axillary dissection followed with radiation postpartum** is a treatment option. **(option b)**
- If the diagnosis of breast cancer is made in **the first or early second trimester of pregnancy, lumpectomy and axillary dissection can be followed by chemotherapy after the first trimester and radiation after delivery (option c)**
- **Chemotherapy** is indicated for node-positive cancers or node-negative tumors **greater than 1 cm**. Current chemotherapeutic regimens are **relatively safe after the first trimester, when the teratogenic risk is greatest (option c)**

4. A 35-year-old male met with an accident and was brought to emergency with severe pain and swelling in thigh. On examination fracture shaft of femur was suspected. Vitals were unstable with decreased urine output, on further investigation myoglobin in urine was detected. What is the further line of management?

a. Conservative management
b. Decompression in thigh region
c. Immediate intermedullary nail insertion
d. None of the above

Ans. b. Decompression in thigh region *Ref: Sabiston 20th/ed p2004*

Explanation

This is a typical case of **compartment syndrome**—pain and swelling in a closed space, circulatory failure and myoglobinuria (due to muscle death).

Compartment syndrome

Compartment syndrome results in symptoms and signs-caused **by increased pressure within a limited space that compromises circulation and function of the tissues in that space.**

Various injuries are known to cause compartment syndrome:

- **Decreased compartment volume** (e.g., from externally applied tight dressings or casts, lying on a limb in a comatose state)
- **Increased compartment content** (e.g., from bleeding or trauma with fractures or finger injuries; increased capillary permeability, such as reperfusion after ischemic injury; electrical burn injuries)
- **Other injuries** (e.g., snakebites, high-pressure injection injuries). The diagnosis of compartment syndrome is based primarily on **clinical evaluation.**

Muscle ischemia that lasts for more than 4 hours leads to muscle death and may also cause significant myoglobinuria. After 8 hours of total ischemia, irreversible nerve changes are complete. The hallmark of muscle and nerve ischemia **is pain**, which is progressive and persistent.

The pain is accentuated by **passive muscle stretching**.

Treatment is release of pressure by **surgically splitting** the covering fascia.

5. A 48-years-old male had a road traffic accident and was brought to emergency. All of the following are done as a part of primary survey *except*:

a. CT abdomen for bleeder identification
b. Airway checking
c. BP recording
d. Cervical spine stabilization

Ans. a. CT abdomen for bleeder identification *Ref: Sabiston 20th/ed p413*

Explanation

This initial assessment, also termed the *primary survey,* follows the mnemonic ABCDE:

- Airway and cervical spine protection
- Breathing
- Circulation
- Disability or neurologic condition
- Exposure and environmental control

Algorithm for management of a trauma victim:

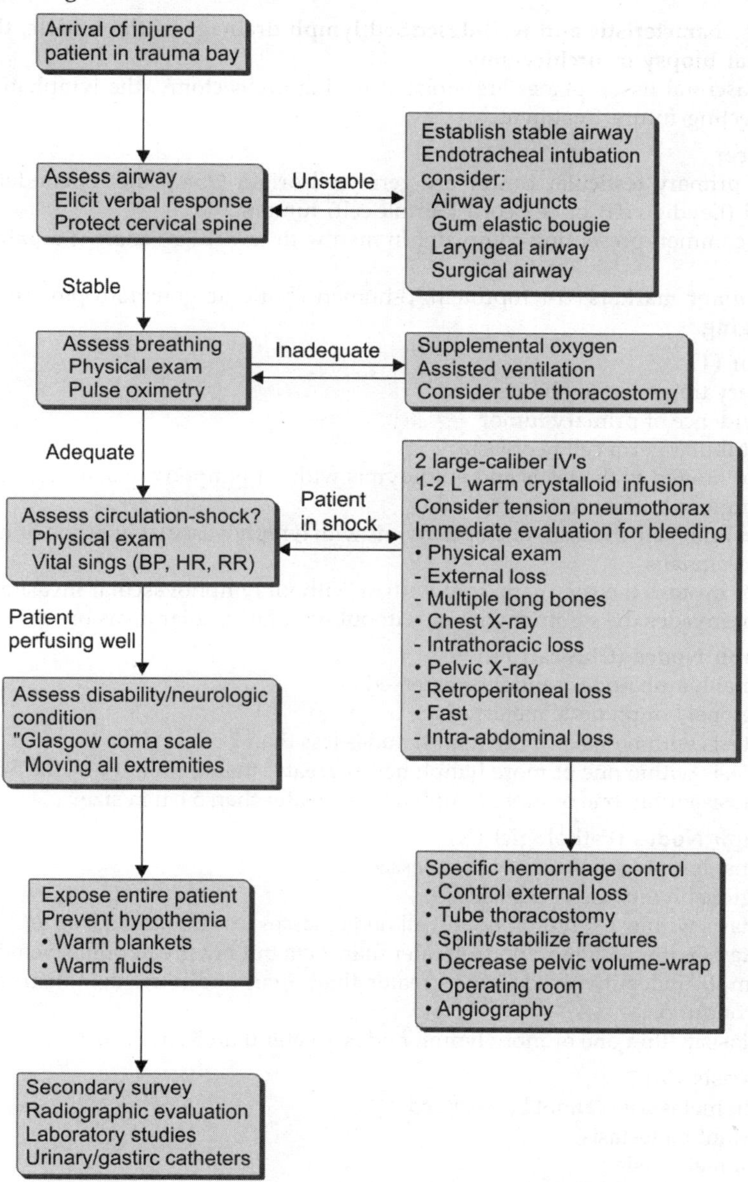

6. A 55-year-old male presented to surgery OPD with complaints of scrotal swelling. Patient also gives a history of anorexia and weight loss. On examination the swelling was hard. All of the following investigations are advised *except*:

a. Incisional biopsy
b. High frequency ultrasonography of scrotum
c. Serum human chorionic gonadotropin (hCG) levels
d. Serum lactate dehydrogenase (LDH) levels

Ans. a. Incisional biopsy *Ref: Sabiston 20th/ed p2102*

EXPLANATION

Because of the characteristic and well-described lymph drainage of the testicle, there is no role for trans-scrotal biopsy or orchiectomy.

If the intrascrotal tissue planes are violated during orchiectomy, the lymphatic drainage can be altered, affecting future treatment.

Testicular cancer

Most cases of primary testicular cancer are germ cell origin (95%); the remainder are predominantly stromal (Leydig cell) or sex cord (Sertoli cell) tumors.

The most common presenting complaint in men with testicular cancer is a **painless testicular mass.**

Specific tumor markers: α-fetoprotein, β-human chorionic gonadotropin, and lactate dehydrogenase **staging.**

Primary Tumor (T)

- pTX Primary tumor cannot be assessed
- pT0 No evidence of primary tumor
- pTis Intratubular germ cell neoplasia
- pT1 Tumor limited to the testis and epididymis without lymphovascular invasion, may invade tunica albuginea but not tunica vaginalis
- pT2 Tumor limited to the testis and epididymis with lymphovascular invasion or tumor involving the tunica vaginalis
- pT3 Tumor invades the spermatic cord with or without lymphovascular invasion
- pT4 Tumor invades the scrotum with or without lymphovascular invasion

Regional Lymph Nodes (Clinical) (N)

- NX Regional lymph nodes cannot be assessed
- N0 No regional lymph node metastasis
- N1 Metastasis within one or more lymph nodes less than 2 cm in size
- N2 Metastasis within one or more lymph nodes greater than 2 cm but less the 5 cm in size
- N3 Metastasis within one or more lymph nodes greater than 5 cm in size

Regional Lymph Nodes (Pathologic) (N)

- NX Regional lymph nodes cannot be assessed
- N0 No regional lymph node metastasis
- N1 Metastasis within 1–5 lymph nodes; all node masses less than 2 cm in size
- N2 Metastasis within a lymph node greater than 2 cm but not greater than 5 cm in size, or more than 5 lymph nodes involved, none greater than 5 cm and none demonstrating extranodal extension of tumor
- N3 Metastasis within one or more lymph nodes greater than 5 cm in size

Distant Metastasis (M)

- MX Distant metastasis cannot be assessed
- M0 No distant metastasis
- M1 Distant metastasis
- M1a Nonregional nodal or pulmonary metastasis
- M1b Distant metastasis at site other than nonregional lymph nodes or lung

Serum Tumor Markers (S)

- SX Tumor markers not available or performed
- S0 Tumor markers within normal limits
- S1 LDH <1.5× normal, hCG <5000 IU/L, alpha-fetoprotein (AFP) <1000 ng/mL
- S2 LDH 1.5-10× normal, hCG 5000–50,000 IU/L, alpha-fetoprotein (AFP) 1000–10,000 ng/mL
- S3 LDH >10× normal, hCG >50,000 IU/L, AFP >10,000 ng/mL
- Initial treatment of suspected testicular tumor is radical inguinal orchiectomy, which involves removal of the testicle and spermatic cord at the level of the inguinal ring.

Second-line treatment is directed by tumor histology and lymph node staging

- **For seminoma stage IA and IB disease**, treatment options include surveillance, radiotherapy to the regional lymph nodes (20 Gy), and one or two cycles of carboplatin-based chemotherapy.
- For seminoma stage IIA and IIB, radiotherapy of the retroperitoneal lymph nodes is standard therapy; for stage IIC or III, platinum-based chemotherapy is standard therapy.
- For non-seminomatous germ cell tumors (NSGCT) stage I disease, the options include surveillance, retroperitoneal lumph node dissection (RPLND), and cisplatin-based chemotherapy.
- **For NSGCT stage IIA**, either primary RPLND (in patients with normal levels of tumor markers) or three or four cycles of cisplatin-based chemotherapy is standard;
- **For NSGCT stage IIB**, three or four cycles of cisplatin-based chemotherapy is standard, followed by RPLND or surveillance.

7. A 40-year-old male presents to the hospital with severe abdominal pain. On investigation a fluid filled cyst with fibrous wall in pancreatic region and gas in retroperitoneal space was detected. Cystic fluid amylase was raised but CEA was normal. Patient is a known alcoholic and gives history of an episode of acute pancreatitis one month back. Management is:

a. Percutaneous drainage of the cyst under radiological guidance
b. Laparoscopic cystogastrostomy
c. Conservative management
d. Surgical intervention

Ans. d. Surgical intervention *Ref: Bailey and Love 26th/ed p1120*

Explanation

- This is a case of **complicated pseudocyst of pancreas**
- **Pancreatic pseudocyst** is a collection of amylase-rich fluid enclosed in a wall of fibrous or granulation tissue.
- **Pseudocysts** typically arise following an attack of acute pancreatitis, but can develop in chronic pancreatitis or after pancreatic trauma.
- Formation of a pseudocyst requires 4 weeks or more from the onset of acute pancreatitis. It may be **single or multiple in numbers**. Usually identified on **USG or CT scan.**
- Pseudocysts **will resolve spontaneously** in most instances, but complications can develop.
- Pseudocysts that are **thick-walled or large (over 6 cm in diameter), have lasted for a long time (over 12 weeks)** or have arisen in the context of chronic pancreatitis are less likely to resolve spontaneously, but these factors are not specific indications for intervention.
  Therapeutic interventions are advised only if the pseudocyst causes **symptoms, if complications** develop or a distinction has to be made between a pseudocyst and a tumor.

Three **possible approaches** to draining a pseudocyst:

- Percutaneous,
- Endoscopic and
- Surgical

Complications best managed surgically are:

- Abscess
- Systemic sepsis
- GI bleed
- Internal fistula
- Peritonitis
- Bowel obstruction
- Obstructive jaundice
- Hemorrhage into cyst
- Hemoperitoneum

8. A 65-year-old male is having a swelling on the back of lower thigh. On investigation it was found to be a high grade liposarcoma of 5 cm in size. Best management is:

a. Amputation of limb at mid thigh
b. Wide local excision
c. Chemotherapy
d. Radiotherapy

Ans. b. Wide local excision *Ref: Sabiston 20th/ed p762*

Explanation

Liposarcoma is one of the types of **soft tissue sarcoma (STS).** Liposarcoma is the **most frequent STS** subtype and represents **45% of all retroperitoneal sarcoma.** It is composed **of three histologic** varieties (listed in order of **decreasing frequency**):

i. Well-differentiated and dedifferentiated liposarcoma,
ii. Pleomorphic liposarcoma, and
iii. Myxoid/round cell liposarcoma.

Well differentiated and dedifferentiated liposarcomas more typically arise from the retroperitoneum versus the extremities, whereas the inverse is true for pleomorphic and myxoid/round cell liposarcoma.

Mainstay of treatment for STS is **surgery.**

Algorithm for STS management is as follows:

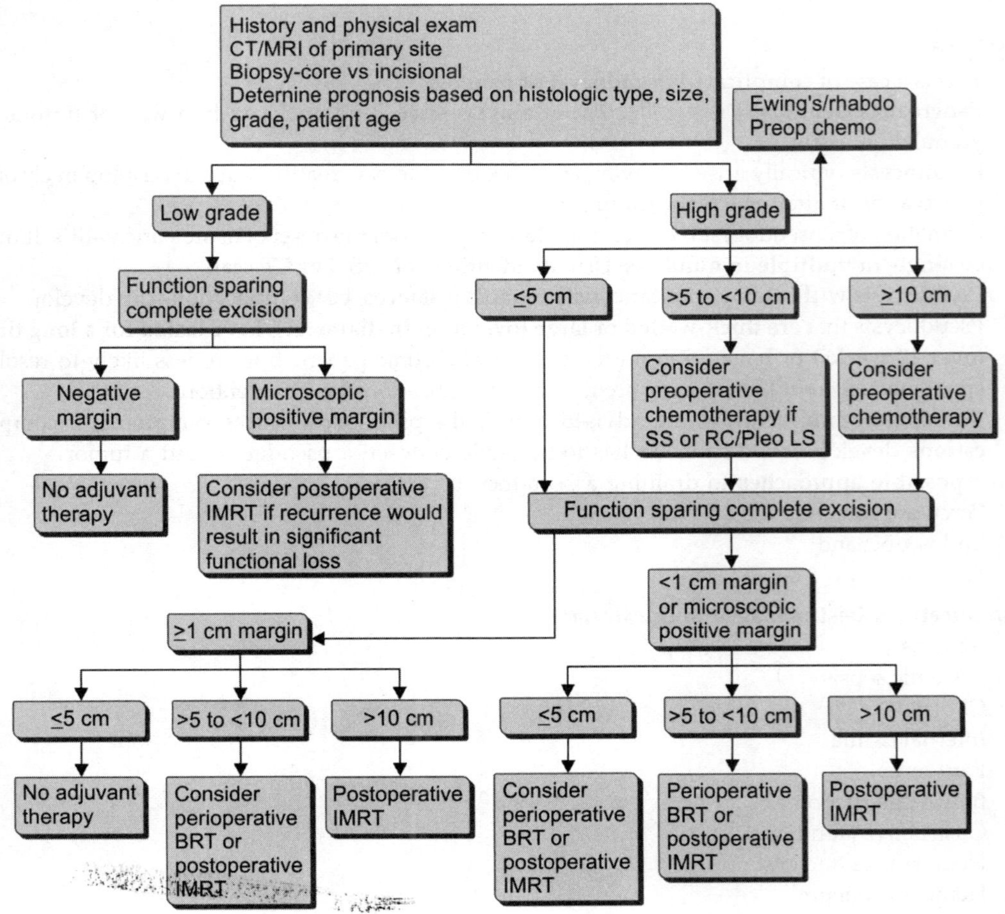

9. Head injury, worrisome and should require CT imaging is:

a. Antegrade amnesia for more than 30 minutes
b. Concussion and memory loss
c. One episode of Projectile vomiting
d. Option not recalled

Ans. a. Antegrade amnesia for more than 30 minutes *Ref Bailey and Love 26th/ed p314*

Explanation

- This question is directly adapted from a table in Love and Bailey, which mentions all indications of CT scan in case of head injury
- **National Institute for Health and Clinical Excellence (NICE) guidelines for computed tomography (CT) in head injury.**
  - GCS <13 at any point
  - GCS 13 or 14 at 2 hours
  - Focal neurological deficit
  - Suspected open, depressed or basal skull fracture
  - More than one episode of vomiting
  - Any patient with a mild head injury over the age of 65 years or with a coagulopathy, for instance warfarin use, should be scanned urgently
  - Dangerous mechanism or injury or antegrade amnesia >30 minutes warrants CT within 8 hours

10. All of the following are current surgical options for bariatric surgery, *except*:

a. Gastric fundoplication
b. Gastric bypass
c. Sleeve gastrectomy
d. Rouex-en-Y gastric bypass

Ans. a. Gastric fundoplication *Ref: Bailey and Love 26th/ed p1062*

Explanation

Bariatric surgery

Surgical management of obesity

- **Comorbidities** of obesity which can be alleviated by surgery
- Metabolic syndrome
  - Type II diabetes mellitus
  - High blood pressure
  - Dyslipidemia
- Obstructive sleep apnea
- Venous and lymphatic stasis
- Osteoarthritis
- Decreased mobility
- Chronic respiratory hypoventilation (Pickwickian syndrome)
- Hypertrophic cardiomyopathy
- Pseudotumor cerebri (idiopathic intracranial hypertension)
- Poor quality of life
- Urinary stress incontinence
- Gastroesophageal reflux disease

Not all patients of obesity are candidates for surgery

Criteria for surgery

- Body mass index (BMI) >40 kg/m^2 or BMI 35–39 kg/m^2 with serious comorbid disease treatable by weight loss
- Minimum of 5 years obesity
- Failure of conservative treatment
- No alcoholism or major untreated psychiatric illness
- Avoid if likely to get pregnant within 2 years
- Age limits 18–55 (relative)
- Acceptable operative risk on preoperative assessment

Types of bariatric surgery

Restrictive

Adjustable gastric banding
Sleeve gastrectomy

Bypass

Proximal gastric bypass/Roeux-en-Y gastric bypass
Biliopancreatic diversion (BPD) with or without duodenal switch

Outcome from bariatric surgery

	Restrictive	Gastric bypass	BPD
Weight loss (%)	48–68	62	72
Resolution of diabetes mellitus type 2 (DM2) (%)	48–72	84	98
Resolution of hypertension (HTN) (%)	28–73	75	81
Improvement in dyslipidemia (%)	71–81	94	100
Mortality due to surgery (%)	0.1	0.5	1.1

Fundoplication is a surgery for gastrointestinal reflux disease and hiatal hernia

11. A 20-year-old male presented with a midline soft tissue swelling in front of neck. On examination it is a cystic mass of 2 × 2 cm in size, which moves with deglutition and swallowing. No other significant finding observed. Which of the following is the definitive management for this condition:

a. Reassure the patient and regular follow-up
b. Surgical removal of cyst
c. Steroid injection into the cyst
d. Sistrunk's operation

Ans. d. Sistrunk's operation *Ref: Bailey and Love 26th/ed p677*

EXPLANATION

The thyroid gland descends early in fetal life from the **base of the tongue towards its position in the lower neck with the isthmus lying over the second and third tracheal rings.**

At the time of its descent, the hyoid bone has not been formed and the track of the descent of the thyroid gland is variable, **passing in front, through or behind the eventual position of the hyoid body**.

Thyroglossal duct cysts represent a persistence of this track and may therefore be found anywhere in or adjacent to the midline from the tongue base to the thyroid isthmus.

The cysts **almost always arise in the midline** but, when they are adjacent to the thyroid cartilage, they may lie slightly to one side of the midline. **Classically, the cyst moves upwards on swallowing and with tongue protrusion**.

Thyroglossal cysts may become infected and rupture onto the skin of the neck presenting as **a discharging sinus**.

Often occur in children, they may also present in adults, even as late as the sixth or seventh decade of life.

Treatment

Includes excision of the whole thyroglossal tract, which involves removal of the body of the hyoid bone and the suprahyoid tract through the tongue base to the vallecula at the site of the primitive foramen caecum, together with a core of tissue on either side (**Sistrunk's operation**).

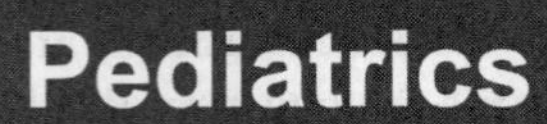

Pediatrics

Author: Jyotsana Priya, Co-author: Muhammad Awais

AIIMS May 2017

1. An 18-month-old child comes to subcenter with history of breathlessness, fever and cough. On examination weight was 11.5 kg, respiratory rate was 46/min, and there was no chest indrawing. Which is the most appropriate management?

a. IV antibiotics at PHC and observe
b. Give first dose of IV antibiotics and refer to higher center
c. Oral cotrimoxazole for 5 days and send home
d. Home remedies

Ans. c. Oral cotrimoxazole for 5 days and send home *Ref: Ghai Essential Pediatrics 8th/ed p759*

Explanation

Child is having fast breathing but no chest indrawing, stridor or any other general danger signs, so we will classify the disease as "pneumonia".

If the child is	Fast breathing is
2 months up to 12 months	50 breaths per minute or more
12 months up to 5 years	40 breaths per minute or more

Signs	Classify as	Identify treatment (Urgent pre-referral treatments are in bold print)
Any general danger sign, or • Chest indrawing, or • Stridor in calm child	Severe pneumonia or very severe disease	***Give first dose of injectable chloramphenicol, (If not possible give oral amoxicillin)*** **or** ***Refer URGENTLY to hospital***
Fast breathing	Pneumonia	Give Amoxicillin for 5 days • Soothe the throat and relieve the cough with a safe remedy if child is 6 months or older • Advise mother when to return immediately • Follow up in 2 days
No signs of pneumonia or very severe disease	No pneumonia: cough or cold	• If coughing more than 30 days, refer for assessment • Soothe the throat and relieve the cough with a safe • Home remedy if child is 6 months or older • Advise mother when to return immediately • Follow up in 5 days if not improving

2. Which of the following is true regarding congenital CMV infection?

a. Diagnosed only by persistent presence of IgM antibody after 6 months
b. It is the most common cause of non-syndromic sensorineural hearing loss

c. All babies born are symptomatic
d. Mothers of developing countries who transmit the virus are usually symptomatic

Ans. b. It is the most common cause of non-syndromic sensorineural hearing loss

Ref: Ghai Essential Pediatrics 8th/ed p273; Nelson Textbook of Pediatrics 20th/ed p3047

EXPLANATION

- ❑ *Option a:* Diagnosed only by persistent presence of IgM antibody after 6 months—**Incorrect**
  - A positive CMV IgM after the first 2 weeks of life can also occur due to postnatal transmission and is not an accurate method for diagnosis. (*Ghai Essential Pediatrics 8th/ed p273*).
- ❑ *Option b:* It is the most common cause of non-syndromic sensorineural hearing loss—**Correct**
  - The most common infectious cause of congenital SNHL is **cytomegalovirus** (*Nelson Textbook of Pediatrics 20th/ed p3047).*
- ❑ *Option c:* All babies born are symptomatic—**Incorrect**
  - The transmission risk with reactivation or reinfection is only 1% and only 5–10% of infected babies are symptomatic *(Ghai 8th/ed p273).*
- ❑ *Option d:* Mothers of developing countries who transmit the virus are usually symptomatic—**Incorrect**
  - CMV remains latent in the body and can reactivate any time; similarly reinfections can also occur (*Ghai 8th/ed p273*).

3. Which of the following is not seen in fetal alcohol syndrome?

a. Microcephaly
b. Macrocephaly
c. Holoprosencephaly
d. Thinning of corpus callosum

Ans b. Macrocephaly *Ref: Smith's Recognizable Patterns of Human Malformation; 7th/ed p728*

EXPLANATION

A specific pattern of malformation identified in fetus due to high levels of alcohol ingestion in mother known as *fetal alcohol syndrome.*

- ❑ **Growth:** Prenatal and postnatal onset of growth deficiency.
- ❑ **Performance:** Average IQ of 65 with a range of 20–120
  - Fine motor dysfunction manifested by weak grasp, poor eye-hand coordination, or tremulousness
  - Irritability in infancy, hyperactivity in childhood
  - Problems with executive function, working memory, and spatial processing
  - Poor impulse control, problems in social perception, deficits in higher level of receptive and expressive language.
- ❑ **Craniofacial:**
  - Mild-to-moderate microcephaly
  - Short palpebral fissures
  - Maxillary hypoplasia
  - Short nose, smooth philtrum with thin and smooth upper lip.
- ❑ **Skeletal:**
  - Joint anomalies, including abnormal position or function
  - Altered palmar crease patterns
  - Small distal phalanges
  - Small fifth fingernails.
- ❑ **Cardiac:**
  - Heart murmur, frequently disappearing by 1-year of age
  - Ventricular septal defect most common, followed by atrial septal defect.

4. A 5-year-old child comes to hospital with history of loose stools but no history of fever or blood in stools. Mother says he is irritable and drinks water if given. On examination eyes sunken and Skin pinch test—the skin retracted within two seconds but not immediately. What will be the appropriate management?

a. Administer the first dose of IV antibiotic and immediately refer to higher center
b. Give oral antibiotics and ORS and ask the mother to continue the same and visit again next day
c. Consider severe dehydration start IV fluids, IV antibiotics and refer to higher center
d. ORS with zinc for 14 days

Ans. d. ORS with zinc for 14 days *Ref: Ghai Essential Pediatrics 8th/ed p292-95*

Explanation

Child has no fever or blood in stool so there is no need to give oral or intravenous antibiotics (*options a and b—incorrect*)

Child is in moderate dehydration (option c incorrect) so we will give him ORS according to Plan B and zinc supplementation.

Look at Condition	Well alert	Restless, irritable	Lethargic or unconscious; floppy
Eyes	Normal	Sunken	Very sunken and dry
Tears	Present	Absent	Absent
Mouth and tongue	Moist	Dry	Very dry
Thirst	Drinks normally; not thirsty	Thirsty, drinks eagerly	'Drinks poorly' or is not able to drink
Feel Skin pinch	Goes back quickly	Goes back slowly	Goes back very slowly
Decide	The patient has no signs of dehydration	If the patient has ≤ 2 signs, there is some dehydration	If the patient has ≥ 2 signs, there is severe dehydration
Treat	Use treatment **Plan A (Oral)**	Weigh the patient, if possible, and use treatment **Plan B (Oral)**	Weigh the patient and use treatment **Plan C** urgently **(Intravenous Fluid)**

Plan A		
Age	**Amount of ORS to give after each loose stool**	**Amount of ORS to provide for use at home**
<24 month	50–100 mL	500 mL/day
2–10 year	100–200 mL	1000 mL/day
>10 year	Ad lib	2000 mL/day
Plan B		
75 mL/kg ORS over a period of 4 hours		

Plan C (100 mL/kg Intravenous fluid)		
Age	First give 30 mL/kg in:	Then give 70 mL/kg in:
< 12 months	1 hr	5 hr
> 12 months	30 min	2.5 hr

Zinc is recommended to be supplemented as *sulphate, acetate or gluconate*[Q] formulation, at a dose *of 20 mg*[Q] of elemental zinc per day for children >6 months for a period of *14 days.*[Q]

PGI May 2017

1. True for a 2-year-old boy:

a. Weight four times that of birth weight
b. Rides tricycle
c. Climbs up and down the stairs with alternating steps
d. Both upper and lower canines erupted
e. Ossification center for radius

Ans. a. Weight four times that of birth weight; c. Climbs up and down the stairs with alternating steps and d. Both upper and lower canines erupted *Ref: Ghai Essential Pediatrics 8th/ed p10-13*

Timing of dentition				
Primary dentition	Time of eruption, months		Time of fall, years	
	Upper	Lower	Upper	Lower
Central incisors	8–12	6–10	6–7	6–7
Lateral incisors	9–13	10–16	7–8	7–8
First molar	13–19	14–18	9–11	9–11
Canine	16–22	17–23	10–12	9–12
Second molar	25–33	23–31	10–12	10–12
Permanent teeth eruption				
First molar	6–7	First premolar		10–12
Central incisors	7–8	Second premolar		10–12
Lateral incisors	8–9	Second molar		12–13
Canine	10–12	Third molar		17–21

Approximate anthropometric values by age			
Age	Weight (kg)	Length or height (cm)	Head circumference (cm)
Birth	3	50	34
6 months	6 (2 times)	65	43
1 year	9 (3 times)	75	46
2 years	12 (4 times)	90	48
3 years	15 (5 times)	95	49
4 years	16	100	50

Age	Milestone
3 months	Neck holding
5 months	Rolls over
6 months	Sits in tripod fashion (sitting with own support)
8 months	Sitting without support
9 months	Stands holding on (with support)
12 months	Creeps well; walks but falls; stands without support
15 months	Walks alone; creeps upstairs
18 months	Runs; explores drawers
2 years	Walks up and downstairs (2 feet/step); jumps
3 years	Rides tricycle; alternate feet going upstairs
4 years	Hops on one foot; alternate feet going downstairs

Ossification center for radial head appears at 3–6 years.

2. A 2-year-old child presented with hepatomegaly. Cause may be:

a. Biliary atresia
b. Hepatoblastoma
c. Cirrhosis
d. Glycogen storage disease
e. Gauchers

Ans. All *Ref: Ghai Essential Pediatrics 8th/ed p310*

Chronic liver disease (cirrhosis or chronic hepatitis): Wilson disease, chronic hepatitis B and C, autoimmune liver disease, Budd-Chiari syndrome, cryptogenic	***Metabolic or storage disorders:*** Glycogen storage disease, Gaucher disease, Niemann-Pick disease, progressive familial intrahepatic cholestasis, nonalcoholic fatty liver disease
Infective: Viral hepatitis, liver abscess (pyogenic or amebic), tuberculosis, salmonella, malaria, kala-azar, hydatid disease	***Tumors:*** Lymphoma, leukemia, histiocytosis, neuroblastoma, benign hemangioendothelioma, mesenchymal hamartoma, hepatoblastoma, hepatocellular carcinoma
Biliary: Caroli disease, choledochal cyst, congenital hepatic fibrosis, cystic disease of liver; extrahepatic biliary obstruction	***Miscellaneous:*** Congestive heart failure, constrictive pericarditis, sarcoidosis

3. Eisenmenger complex is:

a. ASD with PDA
b. VSD with pulmonary hypertension
c. Pulmonary vascular obstructive disease with VSD
d. Pulmonary hypertension with ASD
e. Pulmonary stenosis with PDA

Ans. c. Pulmonary vascular obstructive disease with VSD

Ref: Ghai Essential Pediatrics 8th/ed p408; Nelson Textbook of Pediatrics 20th/ed p2242

Eisenmenger Complex denote the presence of ventricular septal defect with pulmonary vascular obstructive disease.

Nelson Textbook of Pediatrics 20th/ed p2242

- ❑ The term ***Eisenmenger syndrome*** refers to patients with a ventricular septal defect in which blood is shunted partially or totally from right to left as a result of the development of pulmonary vascular disease.
- ❑ **Eisenmenger physiology** is usually defined by an absolute elevation in pulmonary arterial resistance to greater than 12 Wood units (resistance units indexed to body surface area) or by a ratio of pulmonary to systemic vascular resistance of ≥ 1.0.

4. Wilms tumor true is/are:

a. In stage 2 tumor extend into inferior vena cava
b. Most common presentation is asymptomatic abdominal mass
c. Exploration of contralateral kidney while surgery
d. Patient with stage 1 requires radiation therapy after chemotherapy
e. Prognosis depends upon histology and staging

Ans. b. Most common presentation is asymptomatic abdominal mass; c. Exploration of contralateral kidney while surgery and e. Prognosis depends upon histology and staging

Ref: Nelson Textbook of Pediatrics 20th/ed, p2467

Wilms tumor (WT), also known as nephroblastoma, is the most common primary malignant renal tumor of childhood.

Staging of Wilms Tumor	
Stage I	Tumor *confined to the kidney* and completely resected. Renal capsule or sinus vessels not involved. Tumor not ruptured or biopsied. Regional lymph nodes examined and negative.
Stage II	Tumor extends *beyond the kidney* but is completely resected with negative margins and lymph nodes. At least 1 of the following has occurred: (a) penetration of renal capsule, (b) invasion of renal sinus vessels.
Stage III	*Residual tumor* present following surgery confined to the abdomen, including gross or microscopic tumor; spillage of tumor preoperatively or intraoperatively; biopsy prior to nephrectomy, regional lymph node metastases; tumor implants on the peritoneal surface; extension of tumor thrombus into the inferior vena cava including thoracic vena cava and heart.
Stage IV	*Hematogenous metastases* (lung, liver, bone, brain, etc.) or lymph node metastases outside the abdominopelvic region.
Stage V	*Bilateral* renal involvement by tumor

The Children's Oncology Group has specific drug dose and schedule recommendations for risk-adapted treatment of WT.

- ❑ Nephrectomy alone may be sufficient for patients younger than 2 year of age with stage I disease and a tumor weighing < 550 g.
- ❑ Patients with stages I and II disease receive chemotherapy with 2 drugs, vincristine and actinomycin D, every 1–3 weeks for a total of 18 weeks (regimen EE4A).
- ❑ Patients with stage III or IV disease receive chemotherapy with 3 drugs (vincristine, doxorubicin, and actinomycin D) every 1–3 week for a total of 24 weeks (regimen DD4A) and radiation therapy.

Overall, the survival of children with WT approaches 90%, with some prognostic factors (low stage, favorable histology, young age, low tumor weight) conferring even better outcomes.

5. Congenital adrenal hyperplasia with hypotension due to deficiency of enzymes:

a. Aromatase
b. 5 a reductase
c. 17 b hydroxylase
d. 21 hydroxylase
e. 11 hydroxylase

Ans. d. 21 hydroxylase and e. 11 hydroxylase *Ref: Nelson Textbook of Pediatrics, 20th/ed, p2057*

Explanation

Congenital adrenal hyperplasia (CAH) is a family of autosomal recessive disorders of cortisol biosynthesis. Enzymes involved are:

1. 21-Hydroxylase (P450c21) deficiency
2. 11β-Hydroxylase (P450c11) deficiency
3. 3β-Hydroxysteroid dehydrogenase defect
4. 11β-Hydroxylase (P450c11)
5. 17α-Hydroxylase (P450c17)

6. Benign neonatal seizures true is/are:

a. Common in late preterms
b. Followed by febrile seizures
c. Followed by infantile spasms
d. Prolonged seizures
e. Also called fifth day fits

Ans. a. Common in late preterm and e. Also called fifth day fits
Ref: Swaiman's Pediatric Neurology Principles and Practice 6th/ed p552

Explanation

Benign neonatal seizures

- This is a benign electroclinical syndrome that is seen in neonates. It is also referred to as the *fifth day fits* or *benign idiopathic neonatal convulsions.*
- These seizures occur in term and late preterm infants born after an uneventful pregnancy, labor, and delivery.
- The prevalence is estimated to be between 4% and 38% of neonatal seizures with males constituting about 62% of the cases.
- Seizures occur within the first week of life, and 90% of the seizures occur between days 4 and 6 of life.
- Often, there is no family history of epilepsy, and the neonates are otherwise asymptomatic with normal neurologic examinations between the seizures.
- The presentation is in the form of repetitive seizures lasting from 1 to 2 minutes, sometimes recurring in clonic status epilepticus that last hours. Seizures may recur during a period of 24 to 48 hours but often do not persist beyond that period.

7. H type TEF presents with:

a. Dysphagia
b. Aspiration
c. Hematemesis
d. Hemoptysis
e. Recurrent pneumonia

Ans. b. Aspiration and e. Recurrent pneumonia *Ref: Nelson Textbook of Pediatrics 20th/ed p1783*

- Esophageal atresia (EA) is the most common congenital anomaly of the esophagus, with a prevalence of 1.7 per 10,000 live births. Of these, >90% have an associated tracheoesophageal fistula (TEF).

- ❑ In the most common form of EA, the upper esophagus ends in a blind pouch and the TEF is connected to the distal esophagus (type C).
- ❑ Most often associated with the VATER or VACTERL (vertebral, anorectal, [cardiac], tracheal, esophageal, renal, radial, [limb]) syndrome.

Presentation: TEF typically presents with:

- ❑ Frothing and bubbling at the mouth and nose soon after birth.
- ❑ Coughing, cyanosis, and respiratory distress.
- ❑ Feeding exacerbates these symptoms.
- ❑ The infant with an isolated TEF in the absence of EA ("H-type" fistula) might come to medical attention later in life with chronic respiratory problems, including refractory bronchospasm and recurrent pneumonias.

Diagnosis

- ❑ Early-onset respiratory distress.
- ❑ Inability to pass a nasogastric/orogastric tube in the newborn.
- ❑ Absence of the infant stomach bubble on antenatal USG and maternal polyhydramnois might be indicative of esophageal atresia.
- ❑ A coiled feeding tube in the esophageal pouch and/or an air-distended stomach, indicating the presence of a coexisting TEF.
- ❑ In isolated TEF (H type), an esophagogram with contrast medium injected under pressure can demonstrate the defect.

Management

- ❑ Initially, maintaining a patent airway, prone positioning, preoperative proximal pouch decompression to prevent aspiration of secretions and use of antibiotics to prevent consequent pneumonia are paramount.
- ❑ Endotracheal intubation with mechanical ventilation is to be avoided.
- ❑ *Surgical ligation of the TEF and primary end-to-end anastomosis of the esophagus via right-sided thoracotomy* constitute the current standard surgical approach.
- ❑ In the premature or otherwise complicated infant, a primary closure may be delayed by *temporizing with fistula ligation and gastrostomy tube placement.*

If the gap between the atretic ends of the esophagus is >3–4 cm, primary repair cannot be done; options include using *gastric, jejunal, or colonic segments interposed as a neoesophagus.*

JIPMER Pattern Based

1. Most common location of congenital cyst in lung:

a. Right bronchus
b. Left bronchus
c. Pleural surface
d. Perihilar intrapulmonary

Ans. a. Right bronchus *Ref: Nelson Textbook of Pediatrics 20th/ed p2057*

Explanation

- ❑ Bronchogenic cysts arise from abnormal budding of the tracheal diverticulum of the foregut before the 16th week of gestation and are originally lined with ciliated epithelium.
- ❑ They are more commonly found on the right and near a midline structure (trachea, esophagus, carina), but peripheral lower lobe and perihilar intrapulmonary cysts are not infrequent. Cysts are rarely demonstrable at birth.

2. Right atrial isomerization syndrome is associated with all of the following *except*:

a. Spleen is absent
b. Always associated with dextrocardia
c. Cyanosis is present
d. Bilateral right atria are present

Ans. b. Always associated with dextrocardia *Ref: Nelson Textbook of Pediatrics 20th/ed p2235*

EXPLANATION

Determination of **viscera atrial situs** (position of atria in relation to abdominal viscera) can be made by radiography demonstration of the position of the abdominal organs and the tracheal bifurcation for recognition of the right and left bronchi and by echocardiography.

- **Situs solitus:** The viscera are in their normal positions (stomach and spleen on the left, liver on the right), the 3-lobed right lung is on the right, and the 2-lobed left lung on the left; the right atrium is on the right, and the left atrium is on the left.
- **Situs inversus:** The abdominal organs and lung lobation are reversed, the left atrium is on the right and the right atrium on the left.

If the viscera atrial situs cannot be readily determined, a condition known as **situs indeterminus** or **heterotaxia/isomerism.**

- **Right isomerism or bilateral right-sidedness (asplenia syndrome)** is associated with a centrally located liver, absent spleen, and 2 morphologic right lungs/right atria.
- **Left isomerism or bilateral left-sidedness (Polysplenia syndrome),** which is associated with multiple small spleens, absence of the intrahepatic portion of the inferior vena cava, and 2 morphologic left lungs/left atria.

3. Landau-Kleffner syndrome is characterized by all of following *except*:

a. Seizure
b. Loss of language skill
c. Normal EEG during sleep
d. Normal brain CT scan

Ans. c. Normal EEG during sleep *Ref: Nelson Textbook of Pediatrics 20th/ed p2837*

EXPLANATION

Landau-Kleffner syndrome is a condition of unknown cause characterized by:

- Loss of language skills attributed to auditory agnosia in a previously normal child
- Seizures (focal, generalized tonic–clonic, atypical absence, partial complex, and, occasionally, myoclonic seizures).
- High-amplitude spike-and-wave discharges ON EEG which are always more apparent during non–rapid eye movement sleep; thus, a child in whom Landau-Kleffner syndrome is suspected should have an EEG during sleep, particularly if the awake record is normal.
- CT and MRI studies typically yield normal results.

4. RBC life span in preterm:

a. 75–90 days
b. 40–60 days
c. 25–40 days
d. 15–25 days

Ans. b. 40–60 days *Ref: Nelson Textbook of Pediatrics 20th/ed p2319*

EXPLANATION

In premature infants, the physiologic Hb decline may be intensified by blood loss from repeated phlebotomies obtained to monitor ill neonates. Demands on erythropoiesis are further heightened by the premature infant's shortened RBC life span (40–60 days).

5. Investigations required for evaluation of 4 months old baby with first episode of urinary tract infection:

a. USG + MCU + DMSA Renal scan
b. USG + MCU
c. USG + DMSA Renal scan
d. Only USG

Ans. a USG + MCU + DMSA Renal scan *Ref: Ghai Essential Pediatrics 8th/ed p485*

Explanation

Evaluation following the first episode of urinary tract infection	
Age	**Evaluation**
Below 1 year	Ultrasound Micturating cystourethrogram (MCU) Dimercaptosuccinic acid (DMSA) renal scan
1–5 years	Ultrasound DMSA scan MCU, if ultrasound or DMSA scan is abnormal
Above 5 years	Ultrasound If ultrasound abnormal: MCU and DMSA scan

6. Baby presents with froth in mouth after 3 days of birth, coughing on feeding:

a. TE fistula
b. Choanal atresia
c. Cleft palate
d. Diaphragmatic hernia

Ans. a. TE fistula *Ref: Nelson Textbook of Pediatrics 20th/ed p1783*

Explanation

Condition	Presentation
TE fistula	Maternal polyhydramnois and single umbilical artery Excessive drooling soon after birth with frothing. Choking and cyanosis on feeding
Choanal atresia	Cyanosis which improves on crying
Cleft palate	Morphological defect present
Diaphragmatic hernia	Scaphoid abdomen, respiratory distress

7. Potts surgery:

a. Left pulmonary artery and descending aorta
b. Left pulmonary artery and ascending aorta
c. Main pulmonary artery and aorta
d. Left pulmonary artery and subclavian artery

Ans. a. Left pulmonary artery and descending aorta

Ref: Park's Pediatric Cardiology for Practitioners 6th/ed p129

Explanation

1. *Classic Blalock-Taussig (BT) shunt,* **anastomosed between the subclavian artery and the ipsilateral PA, is usually performed for infants older than 3 months because the shunt is often thrombozed in young infants.**

2. *Modified BT shunt,* a Gore-Tex interposition shunt is placed between the subclavian artery and the ipsilateral PA. This is the most popular procedure for any age. The surgical mortality rate is 1% or less.
3. *The Waterston shunt,* anastomosed between the ascending aorta and the right PA, is no longer performed because of a high incidence of surgical complications.
4. *The Potts operation,* anastomosed between the descending aorta and the left PA, is no longer performed.

8. A 6 months old female presented with tracheo-esophageal fistula, vaginal atresia and polydactyly, diagnosis is:

a. McKusick-Kaufman syndrome
b. Meckel-Gruber syndrome
c. McCune-Albright syndrome
d. Waardenburg syndrome

Ans. a. McKusick-Kaufman syndrome

Ref: Smith's Recognizable Patterns of Human Malformation; 7th/ed p765

Explanation

- **McKusick-Kaufman syndrome:** Vaginal atresia, cardiac defects, and postaxial polydactyly
- **Meckel-Gruber syndrome:** Occipital encephalomeningocele, microphthalmia; polydactyly (usually postaxial
- **McCune-Albright syndrome:** Polyostotic fibrous dysplasia, irregular skin pigmentation, sexual precocity
- **Waardenburg syndrome:** Lateral displacement of medial canthi, partial albinism, deafness.

McKusick-Kaufman syndrome, a disorder strikingly similar to Bardet-Biedl syndrome with overlapping features including vaginal atresia, cardiac defects, and postaxial polydactyly but lacking intellectual disability, obesity, retinal dystrophy, and deterioration of renal function.

Obstetrics and Gynecology

Author: Jyotsana Priya, Co-author: Sayeda Sarah

AIIMS May 2017

1. A 25-year-old female worked up for primary infertility. On hysterosalpingography there was bilateral cornual block. Which is the next step in management?

a. Hydrotubation
b. IVF
c. Tuboplasty
d. Hysteroscopy and laparoscopy guided surgery

Ans. d. Hysteroscopy and laparoscopy guided surgery

Ref: Telinde's 10th/ed p425,

Explanation

- **It must be noted that HSG has limitations:**
  i. Often does not indicate the exact nature of intrauterine lesions
  ii. It is associated with false-positive results with regard to cornual occlusion, and
  iii. It has a low positive predictive value in the diagnosis of periadnexal adhesions and endometriosis.
- For these reasons, laparoscopy and when necessary—hysteroscopy are undertaken to elucidate the diagnosis.
- HSG and laparoscopy are complementary, not competitive, procedures in the investigation of infertility associated with tubal and peritoneal factors.
- In many instances, HSG demonstrates the presence of severe tubal damage or conditions deemed inoperable. Severe intratubal adhesions and distal tubal occlusion in association with cornual lesions, such as salpingitis isthmica nodosa, are examples of contraindications of reconstructive surgery.
- In such instances, the couple may be advised of the significance of the findings, and IVF may be recommended as primary treatment, without recourse to laparoscopy.

2. A 59-year-old female with history of ovarian carcinoma in the mother achieved menopause with smooth transition. She is on hormone replacement therapy. She developed abdominal pain and right adnexal mass was palpable, non-tender. On routine examination she has a 3 × 3 cm smooth cyst in her ovary. What is the next step?

a. Do CA-125 levels, if normal advise regular check up
b. Confirm USG findings by ordering CT scan
c. Do an exploratory laparoscopy to visualize the nature of cyst
d. Reassure and do regular follow up once in 6 months

Ans. a. Do CA 125 levels, if normal advise regular check up

Ref: Telinde's 10th/ed, Chapter Ovarian Cancer p1312, Assessment of Risk of Malignancies in Ovarian Tumours.

Explanation

- ❑ When an ovarian tumor has been identified, it is important to establish its risk of malignancy to properly inform the patient and to **plan the most appropriate surgical approach.**
- ❑ Approximately **10–15%** of ovarian tumors in **pre**menopausal women, and **40%** of ovarian tumors in **post**menopausal women, are **malignant.**
- ❑ Tumor characteristics associated with malignancy include:
  - **Bilaterality,**
  - **Solid composition,**
  - **Fixation in the pelvis on bimanual examination, and**
  - **Increased size (>10 cm diameter).**
- ❑ Interestingly, extremely large ovarian tumors are often **benign mucinous or serous cystadenomas.**
- ❑ Other methods to predict the risk of malignancy are:
  - **Sonographically** determined tumor morphology,
  - **Serum markers**, and
  - **Color Doppler assessment** of tumor vasculature.
- ❑ A number of studies have concluded that sonographically generated tumor morphology can be used to differentiate benign from malignant ovarian tumors, particularly in postmenopausal women.
- ❑ Unilocular cystic tumors less than 5 cm in diameter have been shown to have an extremely low risk of malignancy, whereas complex ovarian tumors with solid or papillary projections from the cyst wall have a higher risk of malignancy.
- ❑ Serum biomarker levels have also been used both independently and in conjunction with sonographic findings. Morphology index used in evaluating sonographically confirmed ovarian tumors to differentiate benign from malignant ovarian tumors.
- ❑ An elevated serum CA-125 in a postmenopausal woman with a sonographically confirmed ovarian tumor had a PPV for malignancy of 80%.
- ❑ The sensitivity and specificity of an elevated serum CA-125 were highest in postmenopausal women.
- ❑ In patients with an elevated serum CA-125, the presence of abnormal ovarian morphology significantly increased the risk of ovarian malignancy.
- ❑ Logistic regression analysis revealed that sonographically determined ovarian morphology and serum CA-125 were the most significant predictors of malignancy in the ovarian tumors of postmenopausal women.

3. Ureteric injury is most commonly associated with which of the following?

a. Anterior colporrhaphy
b. Vaginal hysterectomy
c. Wertheim hysterectomy
d. Abdominal hysterectomy

Ans. d. Abdominal hysterectomy *Ref: Telinde's, 10th/ed, Chapter 38 p963*

Explanation

Ureteral injury associated with gynecologic surgery: "most common"

- ❑ **Most common site:** Pelvic brim near the infundibulopelvic ligament
- ❑ **Most common procedure:** Simple abdominal hysterectomy
- ❑ **Most common type of injury:** Obstruction
- ❑ **Most common "activity" leading to injury:** Attempts to obtain hemostasis

- **Most common time of diagnosis:** None: 50–50 split between intraoperative and postoperative
- **Most common long-term sequelae:** None.

Common sites of ureteral injuries

- Cardinal ligament where the ureter crosses under the uterine artery tunnel of Wertheim
- Intramural portion of the ureter dorsal to the infundibulopelvic ligament
- Near or at the pelvic brim
- Lateral pelvic sidewall above the uterosacral ligament.

General guidelines for management of ureteral injuries identified at time of surgery

- **Ureteral ligation:** Delegation, assessment of viability, stent placement
- **Partial transaction:** Primary repair over ureteral stent
- **Total transaction uncomplicated upper and middle-thirds:** Ureteroureterostomy over ureteral stent
- **Complicated**
  - **Upper and middle third:** Ureteroileal interposition
  - **Lower third:** Ureteroneocystostomy with psoas hitch over ureteral stent
- **Thermal injury:** Resection with management as per a transection.

4. Rh negative mother, ICT negative was given Anti-D during 28 week of pregnancy. Which of the following is the ideal one?

a. Give another dose of Anti-D 72 hour postpartum depending on the baby's blood group
b. Give another dose of Anti-D 72 hour postpartum irrespective of baby's blood group
c. No need of additional dose since she is ICT negative
d. None of the above

Ans. a. Give another dose of Anti-D 72 hour postpartum depending on the baby's blood group

Ref: https://www.acog.org/About-ACOG/ACOG-Departments/Deliveries-Before-39-Weeks/ACOG-Clinical-Guidelines

Explanation

- Anti-D immunoglobulin binds D antigen sites on fetal erythrocytes present in the maternal circulation.
- Presumably, blockade of these sites prevents immune recognition by B lymphocytes, and the transformation of activated B lymphocytes to IgG producing plasma cells never occurs.
- Anti-D immunoglobulin has a half-life of 24 days, and a standard 300-μg dose provides 12 weeks of protection against exposure to up to 30 mL of blood, or 15 mL of erythrocytes.
- Before the introduction of anti-D immunoglobulin, 10% of susceptible pregnancies developed hemolytic disease of the fetus and newborn. Approximately, 90% of these were due to fetomaternal hemorrhage at term. Administration of anti-D immunoglobulin within 72 hours of delivery reduces this incidence by 90%.
- The administration of an additional dose at 28 weeks produces a further decline in incidence from 2–0.1%.

ACOG Recommendations

Based on good and consistent scientific evidence (level A) Rh negative woman who is not Rh D-alloimmunized should receive anti–D immune globulin.

- At 28 weeks of gestation, unless father of the baby is known to be Rh D negative
- Within 72 hours after delivery of Rh D positive infant
- After a first trimester pregnancy loss

- ❑ After invasive procedures, (CVS, amniocentesis, FBS)
- ❑ Based on consensus and expert opinion (level C) anti-D immunoglobulin prophylaxis should be considered if patient experienced
- ❑ Threatened abortion
- ❑ Second or third trimester antenatal bleeding
- ❑ External cephalic version
- ❑ Abdominal trauma.

5. Endometriotic lesion is due to which hormone effect?

a. High estrogen
b. High progesterone
c. High cholesterol
d. High levels of prolactin

Ans. a. High estrogen *Ref: Robbin Basic Pathology 10th ed/p721, Shaw's Gynaec 15th ed/p466*

EXPLANATION

Whatever the initial genesis of endometriosis, its further development depends on the presence of hormones, mainly oestrogen.Various facts proving it are

- ❑ Pregnancy causes atrophy of endometriosis chiefly through high progesterone level.
- ❑ Regression follows oophorectomy and irradiation.
- ❑ Rarely seen before puberty and it regresses after menopause.
- ❑ Hormones with antioestrogenic activity also suppress endometriosis and are used therapeutically.

6. Drug of choice for strawberry vagina is:

a. Metronidazole
b. Tetracycline
c. Doxycycline
d. Fluconazole

Ans. a. Metronidazole *Ref: Novak's gynecology 15th ed/p560*

EXPLANATION

Drug of choice for *Trichomonas vaginalis* is Metronidazole or tinidazole, 2 g orally (single dose) or Metronidazole, 500 mg PO bid for 7 days.

7. A 32-year-old female came for routine PAP smear testing. The report came as carcinoma in situ. What is the next step?

a. Colposcopy and biopsy
b. Conization
c. Hysterectomy
d. HPV DNA testing

Ans. a. Colposcopy and biopsy *Ref: https://www.acog.org/About-ACOG/ACOG-Departments/Deliveries-Before-39-Weeks/ACOG-Clinical-Guidelines*

EXPLANATION

Question here is incomplete, may be, Pap smear should be reported as HSIL, since carcinoma in situ is a biopsy finding...

If its HSIL, then the answer would be a. **Colposcopy and biopsy.**

Algorithm for Pap smear:

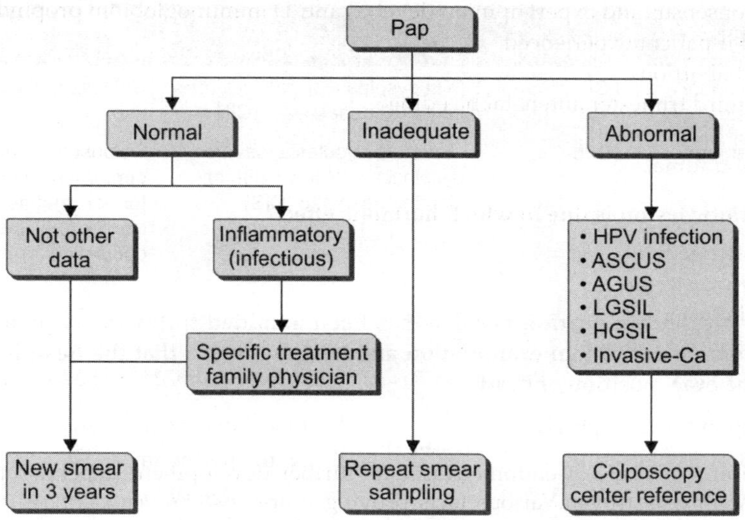

Fig. 1: Referral procedures for specific Pap smear results.

Pap smear guidelines	ACS 2012	USPSTF 2012	ACOG 2012
Age to start	Age 21	Age 21	Age 21
Women ages 21–29	Cytology every 3 years	Cytology every 3 years	Cytology every 3 years
Women ages 30–65	Cytology every 5 years (preferred or every 3 years with Pap alone)	Cytology every 5 years or every 3 years with Pap alone	Cytology every 5 years (preferred) or every 3 years with Pap alone
Women ages > 65	Discontinue after age 65 years (adequate screen)	Discontinue after age 65 years	Discontinue at age 65 years (adequate screen)
Total hysterectomy	Discontinue (if no history of CIN2+)	Discontinue (if no history of CIN2+)	Discontinue (if no history of CIN2+)
Screening among fully vaccinated	Same as for non-vaccinated	Not reviewed	Same as for non-vaccinated

Table 1: Pap test terms, follow-up, and testing strategies.

Pap test result	Abbreviation	Also known as	Test and treatments may include
Atypical squamous cells–undetermined significance	ASC-US		HPV testing repeat Pap test, colposcopy and biopsy, estrogen cream
Atypical squamous cells–cannot exclude HSIL	ASC-H		Colposcopy and biopsy
Atypical glandular cells	AGC		Colposcopy and biopsy and/or endocervical curettage
Endocervical adenocarcinoma in situ	AIS		Colposcopy and biopsy and/or endocervical curettage

Contd...

Contd...

Pap test result	Abbreviation	Also known as	Test and treatments may include
Low-grade squamous intraepithelial lesion	LSIL	Mild dysplasia or cervical intra-epithelial neoplasia–I (CIN I)	Colposcopy and biopsy
High-grade squamous	HSIL	Moderate dysplasia, severe dysplasia, CIN II, CIN III, or Carcinoma in situ (CIS)	Colposcopy and biopsy and/ or endocervical curettage, further treatment with LEEP, cryotherapy, laser therapy, conization, or hysterectomy

8. A 28-year-old female nearing her date has been admitted following regular contractions. The resident doctor did an examination and told the intern that the head is at +1 station. What is the exact position of head?

a. High up in the false pelvis
b. Just above ischial spine
c. Just below ischial spine
d. At the perineum

Ans. c. Just below ischial spine *Ref: Williams 24th/ed, p449, Chapter 22*

Explanation

- The level or **station** of the fetal presenting part in the birth canal is described in relationship to the **ischial spines**, which are half way between the pelvic inlet and the outlet.
- When the lowermost portion of the fetal presenting part is **at the level of spines**, it is designated **as 0** station.
- The classification of stations that divides the pelvis above and below the spines into fifths
- Each fifth represents **1 cm above and below the spines**, the designation is -5,-4,-3,-2,-1, then 0 station.
- **Below the spine** as the presenting part descends, it passes +1,+2,+3,+4 and +5 stations to delivery.
- **+5 station** corresponds to fetal head visible at the **introitus**.

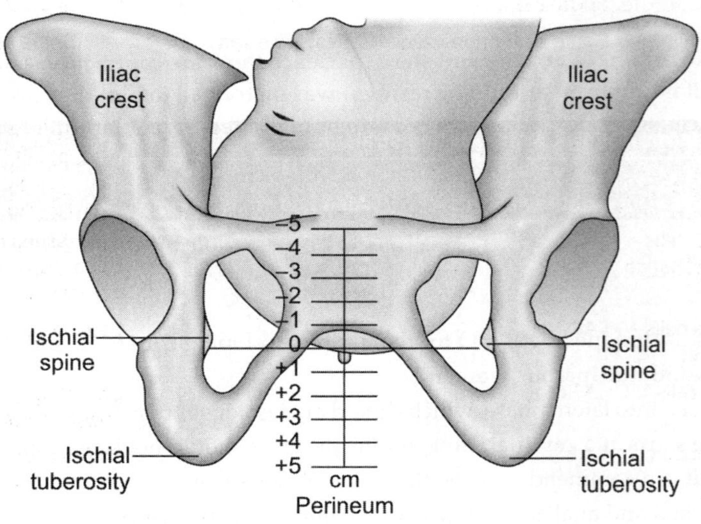

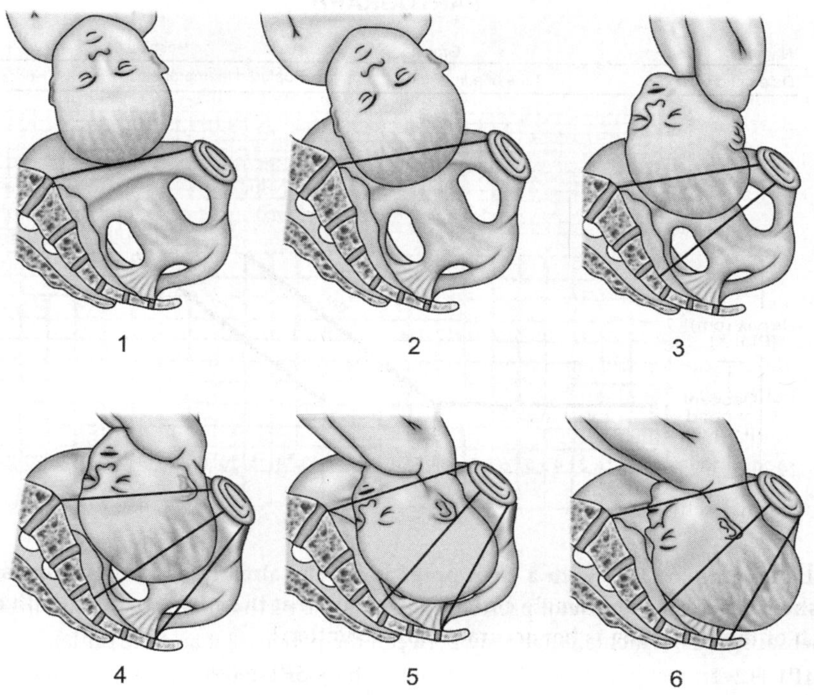

Fetal head station

- ❑ –2 (fixed to pelvic inlet)
- ❑ –1 (small segment of fetal head in pelvic inlet)
- ❑ 0 (large segment of fetal head in pelvic inlet)
- ❑ +1 (fetal head in plane of greatest dimension)
- ❑ +2 (fetal head in plane of least dimension)
- ❑ +3 (fetal head in the pelvic outlet)

9. A patient close to her due date and she experienced uterine contractions and was admitted in the hospital for observation. The resident was instructed to plot the partogram regularly. From what cm of cervical dilatation is partogram plotted in regular intervals?

a. 4 cm
b. 5 cm
c. 6 cm
d. 8 cm

Ans. a. 4 cm *Ref: Williams 24th/ed, p452, Chapter 22*

Explanation

- ❑ Partograph was designed by WHO for the use in developing countries, and it is **same for both multiparous and nulliparous women.**
- ❑ Labor is divided into latent phase, which should not last longer than 8 hours, and an active phase.
- ❑ **Active phase starts at 4 cm dilatation** and the progress should not be slower than 1 cm/hr.
- ❑ **A 4 hour wait** is recommended when the active phase is slow.
- ❑ Labor is graphed and analysis includes use of **alert and active lines.**

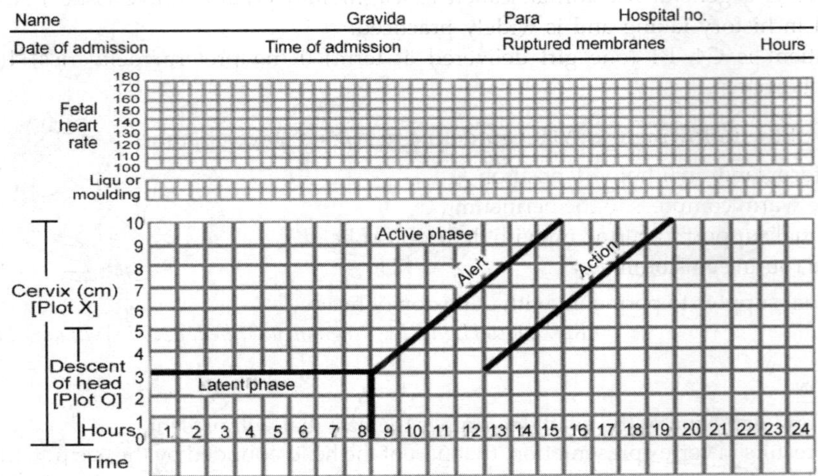

10. A patient came to OPD with a twin pregnancy. She already had 2 first trimester abortion and she has a 3-year-old female child who was born at the end of ninth month of gestation. Which of the following is her accurate representation?

a. G4P1 1+2+1
b. G5P1 2+0+1
c. G4P1 0+1+2
d. G5P0 1+0+2

Ans. c. G4P1 0+1+2 *Ref: Dutta's 7th/ed, p94-95, 131*

Explanation

- **Gravida:** Gravida denotes a pregnant state both present and past, irrespective of the period of gestation. A woman who delivers twins in first pregnancy is still a gravida one and para one.
- **Parity:** Parity denotes a state of previous pregnancy beyond the period of viability.
  Note: The 28th week is taken arbitrarily as the lower limit of fetal viability. (Dutta's obs 7th/ed, p131)
- Infants now considered to be at the threshold of viability are those born at 22, 23, 24, or 25 weeks (American College of Obstetricians and Gynecologists, 2012a,b). (Williams Obstetrics 24th/ed, p1712).
- For all purposes we will consider 28 weeks as the period of viability being a developing country.
  Past obstetric history is summarised by two methods
  Two digits (the first one relates with viable births and the second one relates with abortion) connected with a plus sign affixing the letter 'P'.
  Thus P2+1 denotes the patient had two viable births and one abortion.
  It is also expressed by four digits connected by dashes.
  PA–B–C–D, where
  A denotes number of term (37 to 42 weeks) pregnancies
  B – Number of preterm (28 to < 37 weeks) pregnancies
  C – Number of miscarriages (< 28 weeks)
  D – The number of children alive at present.
  The given patient is pregnant for the fourth time hence is G4, and P1-0-2-1.

But, this option is not given and considering that the given options are what were actually present, there is a general use format called as G(gravida) P(para) L(live issues) A (abortions) format used in history taking and is widely practiced.

Our patient is G4, P1 (one girl delivered at term) 0 (no preterm deliveries)+1(one living issue)+2 (2 abortions).

11. Which of the following is a WHO guideline in second stage of labor?

a. Perform labor in lithotomy position
b. Give warm compress to the perineum
c. Manual support to perineum with deflexion of head
d. Do a routine episiotomy

Ans. c. Manual support to perineum with deflexion of head

Ref: James High Risk Pregnancy, 3rd/ed, p2077, Williams 24th/ed, p538

EXPLANATION

- Flexion and deflexion of the head determines the part that will present.
- Flexion results in vertex presentation, that part of the head bounded by the occiput, the posterior part of the anterior fontanelle and the biparietal eminences.
- This results in the smallest dimensions of the head presenting themselves to the birth canal (9.5 cm × 9.5 cm).
- Flexion is promoted by efficient powers—uterine contractions in the first stage and the addition of maternal pushing in the second.
- Alternatively, if the expulsive efforts are inadequate, modified **Ritgen's Maneuver** can be employed.
- With this the gloved finger beneath a draped towel exert forward pressure on the fetal chin through the perineum just in front of the coccyx. Concurrently, the other hand presses superiorly over the occiput.
- It favors neck extension so that the head passes through the introitus with its smallest diameters.

PGI May 2017

1. Which of the following is most viable aneuploidy:

a. Klinefelter's syndrome
b. Down's syndrome
c. Edward syndrome
d. Turner syndrome
e. Patau syndrome

Ans. b. Down's syndrome

Ref: Williams 24th/ed, Chapter 13, p261

EXPLANATION

- Down's syndrome is the **most common non-lethal trisomy (Only viable trisomy).**
- Prevalence: 1:500 recognized pregnancy, abortuses, stillbirths and liveborn infants.
- ***Option c***: Trisomy 18-Edwards syndrome- prevalence- 1:2000, high rate of in utero lethality, 85% of them are lost between 10 weeks and term.
- ***Option e***: Trisomy 13-Patau syndrome-1:12000 live births, it is again highly lethal and is lost between 10 weeks and term.
- Turner's syndrome is monosomy ***(option d)***
- Klinefelter's is triploidy ***(option a)***

Other important points:

Table 2: Chromosomal findings in First-trimester Abortuses.

Chromosomal studies	Incidence range (%)
Embryonic	~50
Euploid	
46,XY and 46,XX	45–55
Aneuploid	
Autosomal trisomy	22–32
Monosomy X (45,X)	5–20
Triploidy	6–8
Tetraploidy	2–4
Structural anomaly	2
Anembryonic (blighted ovum)	~50

Data from Eiben, 1990; Kajii, 1980; Simpson, 1980, 2007.

2. Regarding Turner's syndrome true is/are :

a. Clinical features include long stature, narrow chest, high hairline
b. Most common cause of first trimester abortions for aneuploidy
c. 20% of all first trimester abortions
d. Incidence 1 in 50000
e. Prevalence 1 in 5000

Ans. c. 20% of all first trimester abortions and e. Prevalence 1 in 5000

Ref: *Williams 24th/ed, Chapter 13, 264.*

EXPLANATION

Turner's syndrome

- Only MONOSOMY compatible with life.
- The most common aneuploidy in abortuses and **accounts for 20% of first trimester losses**.
- **Prevalence: 1:5000 live births.**
- The missing X chromosome is paternally derived in 80% of the cases.
- Anomalies associated are,
  - Cardiac malformations—coarctation of aorta and bicuspid valve 30–50%
  - Horseshoes kidney
  - Hypothyroidism
  - **Short stature, broad chest** and widely spaced nipples, congenital lymphedema, webbed posterior neck and minor bone and cartilage abnormality.

3. Detection of aneuploidy in 1st trimester:

a. hCG and PAPP–A
b. hCG and AFP
c. hCG, PAPP–A and AFP
d. AFP and estriol

Ans. a. hCG and PAPP-A

Ref: William's 24th/ed, p289

Table 2: Selected Down syndrome screening strategies and their detection rate

Strategy	Analytes	Detection Rate[a] (%)
First-trimester screen	NT, PAPP-A, and hCG or free β-hCG	79-87
NT	NT alone	64-70
Triple test	MSAFP hCG OR free β-hCG, uE3	61-70
Quadruple (Quad) test	MSAFP, hCG or free β-hCG, uE3, inh	74-81
Integrated screen	First-trimester screen and Quad test; results withheld until Quad test completed	94-96
Stepwise sequential	First-trimester screen and Quad test 1% offered diagnostic test after first-trimester screen 99% proceed to Quad test, results withheld until Quad test completed	90-95
Contingent sequential screen	First-trimester screen and Quad test 1% offered diagnostic test after first-trimester screen 15% proceed to Quad test; results withheld until Quad test completed 84% have no additional test after first trimester screen	88-94
Cell-free fetal DNA testing (high-risk pregnancies)	No analytes—massively parallel genomic sequencing	98

[a]Based on a 5% positive screen rate.
Free β-hCG = free β-subunit hCG; hCG = human chorionic gonadotropin, inh = dimeric inhibin a; MSAFP = maternal serum alpha-fetoprotein; NT = nuchal translucency; PAPP-A = pregnancy-associated plasma protein-A; uE3 = unconjugated estriol.

4. Absolute contraindications to medical abortion:

a. Rheumatic heart disease
b. Ectopic pregnancy
c. Hypersensitivity to prostaglandins
d. Previous cesarean section
e. Myomectomy in last 1 year

Ans. b. Ectopic pregnancy and c. Hypersensitivity to prostaglandins

Ref: Williams 24th/ed, Chapter 18, p368

Explanation

Relative contraindications to medical abortions are:

- In situ intrauterine devices
- Severe anemia
- Coagulopathy
- Anticoagulants use
- Medical conditions—active liver disease, cardiovascular diseases, uncontrolled seizure disorder.

5. All are true about diabetes in pregnancy, *except*:

a. Macrosomia detected by amniocentesis
b. No poor fetal outcome
c. Risk of congenital malformations increases 10 folds with each pregnancy

d. Preeclampsia is commoner
e. Congenital anomalies more commoner

Ans. a. Macrosomia detected by amniocentesis and c. Risk of congenital malformations increases 10 folds with each pregnancy *Ref: James High Risk Pregnancy, 3rd/ed, Chapter 45, p1454*

EXPLANATION

'Maternal hyperglycemia leads to fetal hyperglycemia, and this in turn leads to hyperplasia of fetal pancreatic beta cells and increased fetal insulin concentrations.'

Diabetes in pregnancy:

- Insulin can be detected in increased amounts in the cord blood and amniotic fluid of diabetic women from **20 weeks** gestation onward.
- Many centers around the world continue to report that **approximately 3–8%** of infants of diabetic mothers suffer from **major congenital abnormalities.** Congenital anomalies account for between 20 and 50% of the perinatal deaths to diabetic women.
- The increased risk of **congenital anomaly** is found in type 1 and type 2 diabetics who had hyperglycemia during early pregnancy while women with gestational diabetes diagnosed later in pregnancy do not seem to be at risk.
- **Neural tube defects and cardiac malformations** are more common than in the nondiabetic population.
- **Caudal regression** (or sacral agenesis) is reported to be 200 to 400 times more common in infants of women with diabetes.
- The development of **proteinuric hypertension** is reported to complicate 12–40% of diabetic pregnancies.

6. Conditions worsened during pregnancy:

a. Diabetes mellitus
b. Hypertension
c. Rheumatoid arthritis
d. Anemia
e. Thyroid

Ans. a. Diabetes mellitus; b. Hypertension; d. Anemia and e. Thyroid
Ref: James High Risk Pregnancy, 3rd/ed

EXPLANATION

- Pregnancy is associated with a physiologic worsening of tissue insulin resistance and with renal and cardiovascular adaptations that might be expected to accelerate the progression of diabetic complications such as retinopathy and nephropathy.
- Diabetic women are more prone to developing hypertension in pregnancy, and the increased susceptibility to infection means that diabetic women are more likely to suffer from pyelonephritis and perhaps from other infection-mediated adverse obstetric events.
- Pregnancy is a state of relative iodine deficiency because of **increased renal loss** (increased glomerular filtration rate in the early first trimester) and **transfer of iodine to the developing fetus.**
  - To compensate, the **thyroid gland increases its uptake of iodine from the blood. If the supply is insufficient, cellular hyperplasia and goiter result.**
- Anemia may also worsen because of physiological dilution due to blood volume expansion starting from 2nd trimester.
- Literature suggests a **protective effect of pregnancy in development of rheumatoid arthritis.**

7. All are true about anti-phospholipid antibody syndrome (APLA) *except*:

a. Recurrent 2nd trimester abortion
b. In untreated patients only 10% chance of continuation of pregnancy
c. Fetal deaths are more common than early pregnancy losses
d. Option not recalled

Ans. a. Recurrent 2nd trimester abortion and b. In untreated patients only 10% chance of continuation of pregnancy *Ref: Williams 24th/ed, p1175*

Explanation

APLA

- **Incidence:** General population—5%, population with recurrent early pregnancy losses—20%
- **Fetal deaths are more common than 1st trimester losses.**
- Due to fetal growth abnormalities and stillbirths, serial sonographic assessment of fetal growth and antepartum testing is recommended by ACOG.
- Even with treatment the fetal loss rate remains at 20–30%.
- **Diagnosis of APLA—at least 2 clinical criteria:**
  - Unexplained fetal death (10 weeks)
  - Preterm birth for severe preeclampsia or placental insufficiency
  - Recurrent pre-embryonic and embryonic losses
- **And 2 lab criteria:**
  - Positive lupus anticoagulant or anti-cardiolipin antibodies
  - IgG or IgM in medium and high titers, should be positive on 2 occasions 6 weeks apart.

8. All of the following is/are risk factors of placental abruption, *except*:

a. Anxiety
b. Hypertension
c. Preeclampsia
d. Decreased coagulability of blood
e. H/o myomectomy 1 year back

Ans. a. Anxiety and e. H/o myomectomy 1 year back *Ref: Williams Obstetrics, 24th ed/ p1004*

Explanation

Risk factors for placental abruption are as follows:

- Prolonged deceleration
- Late deceleration
- PROM
- Fetoscopic laser ablation
- Intrauterine fetal surgeries
- Cigarate smoking
- Opoids narcotics
- Schizophrenia
- Hypothyroidism
- **Clotting factor deficiencies**
- **Thrombocytopenia**
- Sickle cell disease
- Hepatic adenoma
- **Hypertension**
- Eclampsia
- **Preeclampsia**

9. Magnesium sulfate use in eclampsia and severe eclampsia is/are:

a. Levels 4–7 are sufficient to control eclampsia
b. Used in eclampsia to control hypertension
c. Can be given as continuous IV infusion or IM intermittently
d. Toxicity can be treated by calcium gluconate

Ans. a. Levels 4–7 are sufficient to control eclampsia; c. Can be given as continuous IV infusion or IM intermittently and d. Toxicity can be treated by calcium gluconate

Ref: James High Risk Pregnancy, 3rd/ed, p1153, Williams 24th/ed, p759

Explanation

Blood level symptoms and signs

- **4–8 mg/dL:** Therapeutic
- **9–12 mg/dL:** Nausea, warmth, flushing, somnolence, double vision, slurred speech, weakness, loss of patellar reflexes
- **15–17 mg/dL:** Muscular paralysis and respiratory arrest
- **30–35 mg/dL:** Cardiac arrest

Parameters to be assessed:

- Respiratory rate
- Blood pressure
- Pulse rate
- Urine output
- Patellar reflexes

Note:

- Currently there is no recommendation of routine $MgSO_4$ level measurement.
- Disappearance of patellar reflexes- 10 mEq/L because of curariform action.
- It's a sign of impending $MgSO_4$ toxicity.
- Treatment: Withhold $MgSO_4$, **calcium gluconate 1g IV slowly reverses respiratory depression.**

Neuroprotective action:

- Reduces presynaptic release of glutamate
- Blockade of NMDA receptors
- Improved calcium buffering by the mitochondria
- Blockade of calcium channels.

Inhibition of uterine contractility 8–10 mEq/L

10. Features observed in HELLP syndrome:

a. Raised conjugated bilirubin
b. Increased transaminases
c. Low platelet count
d. Increased anti-thrombin level
e. Low LDH level

Ans. a. Raised conjugated bilirubin; b. Increased transaminases and c. Low platelet count

Ref: James High Risk Pregnancy, 3rd/ed, p1156

Explanation

HELLP syndrome

- HELLP syndrome is considered a complication of severe preeclampsia and eclampsia.
- HELLP syndrome occurred in approximately **20% of women with severe preeclampsia.**
- The diagnosis of HELLP syndrome is based on laboratory findings and includes the following:
  - Hemolysis. Microangiopathic hemolytic anemia is characterized by burr cells, schistocytes, and polychromasia on the peripheral smear.

- **An increased bilirubin level**, most of it **indirect (>1.2 mg/dL)**, and an **increased LDH level (>600 IU/L)** confirm the diagnosis.
- **Elevated liver enzyme levels.** Levels of SGOT, SGPT, and LDH are increased.
- **Right upper quadrant pain** may be associated with hepatic cell damage, which also causes an elevation in liver enzymes.
- The hepatic lesion **is parenchymal necrosis**, in which deposits of **fibrin-like material are seen in the sinusoids**. In severe parenchymal necrosis, bleeding can extend to the subcapsular region, leading to a **hematoma that stretches Glisson's capsule** and eventually may rupture.

❑ Diagnostic features:
- Low platelet count. The platelet count is less than 100,000/mm^3
- Right upper quadrant or epigastric pain (86–90%)
- Nausea or vomiting (45–84%)
- Headache (50%)
- Right upper quadrant tenderness on palpation (86%)
- Diastolic blood pressure greater than 110 mm Hg (67%)
- Proteinuria greater than 2+ on dipstick (85–96%)
- Edema (55–67%).

11. All are true about ventouse, *except*:

a. It can be applied at the cervical dilatation of 5 cm
b. Pressure is 0.6 to 0.8 kg/m^2
c. Applied 1.5 cm anterior to posterior fontanelle
d. Option not recalled

Ans. a. It can be applied at the cervical dilatation of 5 cm and b. Pressure is 0.6 to 0.8 kg/m^2

Ref: Williams 24th/ed, Chapter 29, p583

EXPLANATION

Ventouse

Flexion point-found along the sagittal suture, **3 cm in front the posterior fontanelle**, and 6 cm from the anterior fontanelle.

Flexion point

❑ Maximizes traction
❑ Minimizes cup detachment
❑ Flexes the head but also averts twisting of the head
❑ Delivers head though the smallest diameters.

Advantages

❑ Improves the overall success rate
❑ Lowers fetal scalp injury rates
❑ Lessens perineal trauma rate.

Gradual suction at an increment of 0.2 kg/m^2 till max of 0.8 kg/m^2

Contraindications of Ventouse

❑ CPD
❑ Preterm labor
❑ Present membranes
❑ Contracted pelvis

12. Bivalent HPV vaccine effective against:

a. HPV 45 and 52
b. HPV 35 and 58
c. HPV 31 and 33
d. HPV 6 and 11
e. HPV 16 and 18

Ans. c. HPV 31 and 33 and e. HPV 16 and 18 *Ref: DC Dutta, Gynaecology*

- HPV **vaccines** has been developed from the capsid coat of the virus.
- It has high immunogenicity.
- Bivalent vaccines (cervarix) against HPV types 16, 18 and quadrivalent (Gardasil) against HPV types 16, 18, 6, 11 are effective in prevention of about 90% cervical cancer.
- Both the vaccines have some cross protection against HPV types 31, 33 and 45.
- Vaccines are given to girls aged 12–18 years, in three doses IM over the deltoid muscle.
- The impact of vaccines is greatest when it is given to females who have not been already infected. This is the reason it is recommended to adolescent girls.
- Vaccines are safe and well tolerated.
- Vaccine induced neutralizing antibodies (IgG, IgA) works locally (cervix) by preventing the attachment of the virus to the cervical epithelium.
- Immune defense is type specific and is effective only when given prophylactically.
- **Vaccines are effective for at least 7.5 years.** However, screening with Pap test should be continued as the vaccines are type specific and do not protect against the other types of HPV.

13. All of the following are causes of vaginal prolapse after hysterectomy, *except*?

a. Level 1 support
b. Level 2 support
c. Level 3 support
d. Urogenital diaphragm
e. Inability to identify supports

Ans. a. Level 1 support *Ref: Telindes 10th/ed, Chapter 36, p861*

EXPLANATION

Level 1 defects lead to uterine prolapse not vaginal prolapse. *See below:*
Delancey's three levels of pelvic support:

- *Level 1:* The cardinal-uterosacral ligament complex provides apical attachment of the uterus and vaginal vault to the bony sacrum. Uterine prolapse occurs when the cardinal-uterosacral ligament complex breaks or is attenuated.
- *Level 2:* The arcus tendineous fascia pelvis and the fascia overlying the levator ani muscles provide support to the middle part of the vagina.
- *Level 3:* The urogenital diaphragm and the perineal body provide support to the lower part of the vagina.

14. HSIL on pap smear next step in management is:

a. Hysterectomy
b. Conization and biopsy
c. Repeat pap smear
d. HPV testing
e. Colposcopy and biopsy

Ans. e. Colposcopy and biopsy

EXPLANATION

Kindly Refer to Question 9 of AIIMS paper

15. About atrophic vaginitis, true is/are:

a. Estrogen gives temporary relief
b. Acidic vaginal pH
c. Estrogen cream is treatment of choice
d. No pain only spotting after intercourse
e. Regular intercourse prevents it

Ans. a. Estrogen gives temporary relief and c. Estrogen cream is treatment of choice

Ref: Dutta's Gynecology 6th/ed p181

Explanation

Senile vaginitis/atrophic vaginitis

- **Vaginitis in postmenopausal women is called atrophic vaginitis.**
- The term is preferable to senile vaginitis.
- There is atrophy of the vulvovaginal structures due to estrogen deficiency. The vaginal defense is lost.
- Vaginal mucosa is thin and is more susceptible to infection and trauma.
- There may be desquamation of the vaginal epithelium which may lead to formation of adhesions and bands between the walls.
- **Clinical features**
  - Yellowish or blood stained vaginal discharge.
  - Discomfort, dryness, soreness in the vulva.
  - Dyspareunia.
- **On examination**
  - Evidences of pruritus vulvae.
  - Vaginal examination is often painful and the walls are found inflamed.
- Improvement of general health and treatment of infection if present should be done.
- **Systemic estrogen therapy** may be considered if there is no contraindication. This **improves the vaginal epithelium, raises glycogen content**, and **lowers vaginal pH**. Intravaginal application of estrogen cream by an applicator is also effective.
- About one-third of the vaginal estrogen is systemically absorbed.

16. Chronic use of oral contraceptive pills prevent all of the following, *except*:

a. Dysmenorrhea
b. Menorrhagia
c. Break through bleeding
d. Migraine
e. Mood changes

Ans. c. Break through bleeding and d. Migraine *Ref: DC Dutta Gynecology, p486*

Explanation

Oral contraceptive pills (OCP)

Non-contraceptive benefits: *Improvement of menstrual abnormalities:*

- Regulation of menstrual cycle
- Reduction of **dysmenorrhea** (40%)
- Reduction of **menorrhagia** (50%)
- Reduction of premenstrual tension syndrome
- Reduction of Mittelschmerzs syndrome
- Protection against iron-deficiency anemia.

Protection against health disorders:

- ❑ Pelvic inflammatory disease (thick cervical mucus)
- ❑ Ectopic pregnancy
- ❑ Endometriosis
- ❑ Fibroid uterus
- ❑ Hirsutism and acne
- ❑ Functional ovarian cysts
- ❑ Benign breast disease
- ❑ Osteopenia and postmenopausal osteoporotic fractures
- ❑ Autoimmune disorders of thyroid
- ❑ Rheumatoid arthritis.

Prevention of malignancies:

- ❑ Endometrial cancer (50%)
- ❑ Epithelial ovarian cancer (50%)
- ❑ Colorectal cancer (40%).

About option c: Breakthrough bleeding (BTB)

- ❑ Commonly due to **subthreshold blood level of hormones**
- ❑ **Other causes of breakthrough bleeding** in pill takers are
  - Disturbance of drug absorption — diarrhea, vomiting
  - Use of enzyme inducing drugs, missing pills, use of low dose pills
  - Pregnancy complications (miscarriage)
  - Diseases—cervical ectopy or carcinoma.
- ❑ Usually, it settles after 3–4 cycles when there is no other specific cause for BTB.
- ❑ Exogenous estrogen (conjugated estrogen 1.25 mg or estradiol 2 mg) given daily for 7 days can control the bleeding.

Nausea, vomiting, headache and leg cramps: These are transient and often subside following continuous use for 2–3 cycles.

17. Contraindications to intrauterine devices contraceptive:

a. Rheumatic heart disease
b. Actinomycetes pelvic infection
c. Infected abortion in last 1 year
d. Undiagnosed genital bleeding
e. H/O Cervicitis and vaginitis

Ans. b. Actinomycetes pelvic infection and d. Undiagnosed genital bleeding

Ref: Dutta's Gynecology 6th/ed p495

- ❑ **Contraindications for Insertion of IUCD:**
  - **Presence of pelvic infection current or within 3 months**
  - **Undiagnosed genital tract bleeding**
  - Suspected pregnancy
  - Distortion of the shape of the uterine cavity as in fibroid or congenital uterine-malformation
  - Severe dysmenorrhea
  - Past history of ectopic pregnancy
  - Within 6 weeks following cesarean section
  - STIs—Current or within 3 months
  - Trophoblastic disease
  - Significant immunosuppression.
- ❑ Additionally for
  - **Copper-T** are:

- Wilson disease and
- Copper allergy.
- **LNG-IUS** are:
  - Hepatic tumor or hepatocellular disease (active)
  - Current breast cancer and
  - Severe arterial disease.

18. True about ovarian cyst:

a. Dermoid is derived from germ cells
b. Theca luteal cyst after clomiphene administration
c. Follicular cyst in adolescent
d. Corpus luteum cysts seen in reproductive age group
e. Theca lutein cyst in hydatidiform mole

Ans. a. Dermoid is derived from germ cells; b. Theca luteal cyst after clomiphene admininistration; d. Corpus luteum cysts seen in reproductive age group and e. Theca lutein cyst in hydatidiform mole

Ref: DC Dutta Gygecology 6e/p289

EXPLANATION

Follicular cyst

- Usually multiple and small as seen in cases of cystic glandular hyperplasia of the endometrium or in association of fibroid.
- **Hyperestrogenism is implicated as its cause:** However, an isolated cyst may be formed in unruptured Graafian follicle, which may be enlarged but usually not exceeding 5 cm.
- The cyst is lined by typical granulosa cells without lutein cells or the cells may be flattened due to pressure.
- In majority of cases, the detection is made accidentally on bimanual examination, sonography, laparoscopy or laparotomy.
- The cyst may remain asymptomatic or may produce vague pain.
- **Management:**
  - A follicular cyst < 3 cm requires no further investigations.
  - A simple cyst, < 8 cm unilocular, echo free without solid areas or papillary projections, with normal serum CA 125 should be followed up with repeat ultrasound in 3 to 6 months time.
  - Whenever a cyst persists or grow, it should be removed by laparoscopy/laparotomy.

Corpus luteum cysts

- Corpus luteum cyst usually occurs due to over activity of corpus luteum. There is excessive bleeding inside the corpus luteum.
- In spite of the blood filled cyst, the progesterone and estrogen secretion continues.
- As a result, the menstrual cycle may be normal or there may be amenorrhea or delayed cycle. It is usually followed by heavy and/or continued bleeding. It is then confused with a case of **threatened abortion**.
- If the intracystic bleeding is much, it may rupture producing features of acute intraperitoneal hemorrhage with clinical picture simulating disturbed **tubal ectopic pregnancy**.
- It may often be associated with pregnancy and persists for about 12 weeks.
- Spontaneous regression is expected.
- If features of acute abdomen appears, laparotomy with enucleation of the cyst is to be done along with resuscitative measures as in disturbed tubal pregnancy.

These two types of cysts are rather uncommon in women taking oral contraceptive pills. As such, if the cyst persists after three months of pill therapy, it is more likely to be a neoplastic cyst.

Lutein cysts

- Lutein cysts are usually bilateral and caused by excessive chorionic gonadotropin secreted in cases of gestational trophoblastic tumors.
- These may also be formed with administration of gonadotropins or even clomiphene to induce ovulation.
- These are usually lined either by theca lutein cells, called theca lutein cyst or by granulosa lutein cells, called granulosa lutein cyst.
- Spontaneous regression is expected within few weeks following effective therapy of the tumors with the gonadotropin level returning back to normal.

19. True about primary dysmenorrhea:

a. Due to myometrial contraction and ischemia
b GNRH analogues is treatment of choice
c. Psychological effect in some women
d. Starts 3 days before menses till day 1 of menstruation

Ans. a. Due to myometrial contraction and ischemia and c. Psychological effect in some women

Ref: DC Dutta, p178

Explanation

- The primary dysmenorrhea is one where there is no identifiable pelvic pathology.
- *Incidence:* The incidence of primary dysmenorrheal of sufficient magnitude with incapacitation is about 15–20%.
- With the advent of oral contraceptives and non-steroidal anti-inflammatory drugs, there is marked relief of the symptom.
- **Pain appears few hours before menstruation and usually persists for hours (rarely > 48 hours)**
- Causes of pain
  - Mostly confined to adolescents.
  - Almost always confined to ovulatory cycles.
  - The pain is usually cured following pregnancy and vaginal delivery.
  - The **pain is related to dysrhythmic uterine contractions and uterine hypoxia.**
- Drugs:
  - Prostaglandin synthetase inhibitors
  - Oral contraceptives (combined estrogen) and
  - Progestogen

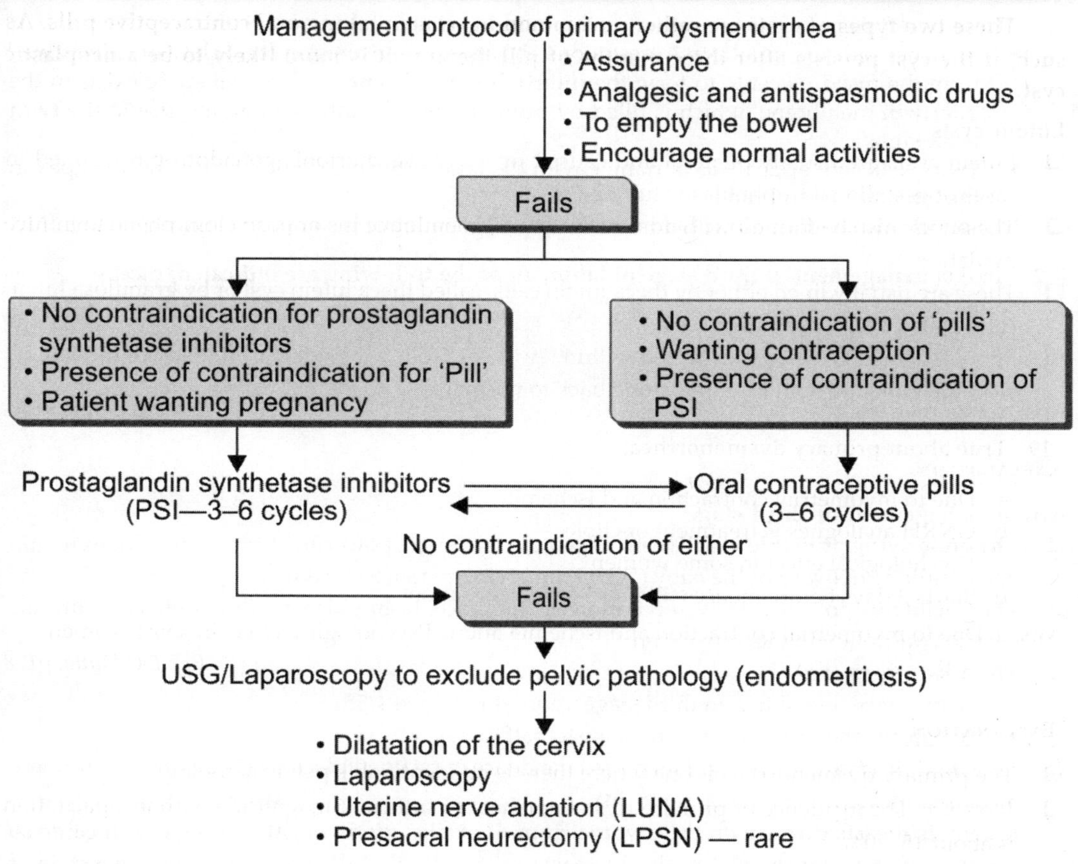

JIPMER Pattern Based

1. Twin peak sign seen in:

a. Monochorionic-diamniotic
b. Conjoined twins
c. Dichorionic diamniotic
d. Monochorionic monoamniotic

Ans. c. Dichorionic diamniotic *Ref: DC Dutta Obstetrics 7th/ed p203*

- **Dizygotic twins:**
  - There are two placentae, either completely separated or more commonly fused at the margin appearing to be one (9 out of 10).
  - There is no anastomosis between the two fetal vessels.
  - Each fetus is surrounded by a separate amnion and chorion.
  - **The intervening membranes consist of 4 layers**—amnion, chorion, chorion and amnion.
  - In fact in early pregnancy the **decidua capsularis of each sac** may be identified under the microscope in between the chorionic layers.

- **"Twin peak"** sign
  - In dichorionic diamniotic twin gestations, the chorion and amnion for each twin reflect away from the fused placenta to form the **intertwine membrane**. A potential space exists in the intertwin membrane, which is filled by proliferating placental villi giving rise to the **twin peak sign**.
  - Twin peak sign appears as a triangle with the base at the chorionic surface and the apex in the inter twin membrane.
- **In monochorionic-diamniotic twins,** the intertwine membrane is composed of two amnions only.

2. Active management of third stage of labor, all of the following are indicated, *except*:

a. Ergometrine
b. Oxytocin
c. Uterine massage
d. Controlled cord traction
e. Methergine

Ans. a. Ergometrine *Ref: DC Dutta, p141*

EXPLANATION

Active management of third stage:

- **The underlying principle in active management** is to excite powerful uterine contractions within one minute of delivery of the baby (WHO) by giving parenteral oxytocic.
- This facilitates not only early separation of the placenta but also produces effective uterine contractions following its separation.
- **The advantages are:**
  - To minimize blood loss in third stage approximately to 1/5th
  - To shorten the duration of third stage to half.
- **The only disadvantage** is slight increased incidence of retained placenta (1–2%) and consequent increased incidence of manual removal.
- **Ergometrine acts directly on the myometrium. It excites uterine contractions which come so frequently one after the other with increasing intensity that the uterus passes into a state of spasm without any relaxation in between. It should not be used in the induction of abortion or labor.**

3. A 30-year-female presented with milky white discharge with fishy odor and minimal itching. Causative organism is/are:

a. Gardnerella
b. Bacterial vaginosis
c. Trichomonas vaginitis
d. Candidiasis
e. Gonorrhea

Ans. b. Bacterial vaginosis *Ref: DC Dutta Textbook of Gynaecology, p152*

EXPLANATION

- **Bacterial vaginosis (BV)**
  - Is characterized by **malodorous vaginal discharge**.
  - The term vaginosis is preferred as there is no vaginal inflammation.
  - The discharge is homogeneous, grayish-white and adherent to the vaginal wall.
  - Clinical implications of BV, in pregnancy are:
    - Preterm rupture of membranes
    - Preterm labor
    - Chorioamnionitis

- **Amsel's four diagnostic criteria are:**
  - Homogeneous vaginal discharge.
  - Vaginal pH >4.5 (litmus paper test).
  - Positive **whiff tests.**
  - Presence of **clue cells** (> 20% of cells).
  - Gram stained vaginal smear (Hay/Ison).
  - Presence of more *Gardnerella* or mobiluncus morphotypes with few or absent lactobacilli.
- **Whiff test: Fishy (amine) odor** when a drop of discharge is mixed with 10% potassium hydroxide solution.
- **Clue cells:** A smear of vaginal discharge is prepared **with drops of normal saline on a glass slide** and is seen under a **microscope**. Vaginal epithelial cells are seen covered with these **coccobacilli** and the cells appear as **stippled or granular**. At times, the cells are so heavily stippled that the cell borders are obscured. **These stippled epithelial cells are called "clue cells"**.

4. Least common cause of ambiguous genitalia in female genotype:

a. 21 hydroxylase deficiency
b. 11 hydroxylase deficiency
c. Fetal steroid sulphatase deficiency
d. WT1 gene

Ans. c. Fetal steroid sulphatase deficiency *Ref: Speroff, 9th/ed, p119*

EXPLANATION

Placental sulfatase deficiency

- There is an X-linked metabolic disease characterized by a placental sulfatase deficiency in the syncytiotrophoblast, and postnatally, ichthyosis, occurring in about 1 in 2000–3000 newborn males.
- Patients with the placental sulphatase disorder are unable to hydrolyze DHAS or 16a-hydroxy-DHAS, and, therefore, the placenta cannot form normal amounts of estrogen.
- A deficiency in placental sulphatase is usually discovered when patients go beyond term and are found to have extremely low estriol levels and no evidence of fetal distress.
- All newborn children, with a few exceptions, have been male.
- The steroid sulfatase X-linked recessive ichthyosis locus (the steroid sulphatase gene) has been mapped to the distal short arm portion of the X chromosome.
- Family history of scaling in males (as well as repeated **postdate pregnancies**) should prompt a consideration for prenatal diagnosis.

WT1 gene

- The *WT1* gene is named after the Wilms' tumor nephroblastoma because it is one of the genes on chromosome 11 deleted in patients with this tumor. Mutant mice lacking *WT1* fail to develop kidneys and gonads.
- ***WT1* mutations**, however, could not be detected in 25 patients with a congenital absence of the uterus and vagina, indicating that ***WT1* may be necessary for normal renal and gonadal development, but not for early Müllerian duct development**.

5. A 25-year-old, 3 months pregnant lady presented with a growing vulval wart, all of the following can be a modality of management *except*:

a. Trichloroacetic acid application
b. Cryotherapy
c. Podophyllin application
d. Wide excision

Ans. c. Podophyllin application *Ref: William's Obstetrics 24th ed page 1294*

EXPLANATION

- There may be an incomplete response to treatment during pregnancy, but lesions commonly improve or regress rapidly following delivery.
- Wart eradication during pregnancy is usually not necessary.
- Therapy is directed toward minimizing treatment toxicity to the mother and fetus and debulking symptomatic genital warts.
- There is no definitive evidence that any one of the subsequently discussed treatments is superior to another.
- ***Trichloroacetic or bichloracetic acid,*** 80- to 90% solution, applied topically once a week, is an effective regimen for external warts.
- ***Cryotherapy***
- ***Laser ablation***, or
- *Surgical excision*
- **Agents not recommended in pregnancy:**
  - Podophyllin resin,
  - Podofilox 0.5% solution or gel,
  - Imiquimod 5% cream,
  - Interferon therapy, and
  - Sinecatechins

6. Maximum fetal skull diameter is:

a. Biparietal diameter
b. Mentovertical
c. Occipitobregmatic
d. Occipitofrontal

Ans. b. Mentovertical *Ref: DC Dutta. Chapter fetal skull and maternal pelvis, p85*

EXPLANATION

All diameters are as follows:

A. Suboccipito-bregmatic 9.5 cm
B. Suboccipito-frontal 10 cm
C. Occipitofrontal 11.5 cm
D. Mentovertical 14 cm
E. Submentovertical 11.5 cm
F. Submentobregmatic 9.5 cm

7. 25 years old died just after child birth. On autopsy, hair, fat and epithelial cells were found in pulmonary vessel. Probable cause of death is:

a. Amniotic fluid embolism
b. Fat embolism
c. DIC
d. Pulmonary thromboembolism

Ans. a. Amniotic fluid embolism *Ref: James High Risk Pregnancy, 3rd/ed p2317*

EXPLANATION

Amniotic fluid embolism

- Occurs during labor, during cesarean section, or within a short time after delivery.

- ❑ This condition may lead to maternal death as a result of severe pulmonary hypertension following embolization of the pulmonary vessels by fetal squames.
- ❑ If the mother survives this acute event, there may be an **anaphylactoid reaction** to the presence of the fetal tissues in the maternal circulation associated with **cardiovascular collapse, pulmonary edema, seizure activity,** and the development of an intractable bleeding diathesis due to severe DIC.
- ❑ The **diagnosis** is suggested by the detection of fetal squames within the maternal lungs at the time of **postmortem**.
- ❑ The incidence of successfully treated cases is difficult to determine as the diagnosis is only suggestive and cannot be proved.
- ❑ In most cases, the **maternal death is unpredictable and unavoidable**, and as obstetric care improves, amniotic fluid embolism has been responsible for an increasing proportion of maternal deaths.

8. Which is not a sling operation for prolapse:

a. Manchester
b. Shirodkar
c. Khanna
d. Abdomino cervicopexy

Ans. a. Manchester *Ref: DC Dutta, p232*

Explanation

Manchester operation

- ❑ Also known as **Fothergill's repair.**
- ❑ The **indications** are:
  - Preservation of reproductive function.
  - When the symptoms are due to vaginal prolapsed
- ❑ Associated with **elongation of the (supravaginal) cervix**
- ❑ **Steps** of this procedure include:
  - Preliminary D + C
  - Amputation of cervix
  - Plication of Mackenrodt's ligaments in front of cervix
  - Anterior colporrhaphy
  - Colpoperineorrhaphy

9. A case of cervical CA. Investigation all to be done *except*:

a. CT abdomen
b. Chest X-ray
c. Cystoscopy
d. IVP
e. CT pelvis

Ans. a. CT abdomen and e. CT pelvis *Ref: DC Dutta gyneology 6th/ed p357*

Staging of cervical cancer is based principally on clinical examination.

Staging procedures allowed by FIGO are:

- ❑ Inspection of cervix and vagina
- ❑ Pelvic examination (vaginal, rectovaginal) under anesthesia

- ❑ Lymph node palpation
- ❑ Colposcopy
- ❑ Hysteroscopy
- ❑ Cystoscopy
- ❑ Biopsy
- ❑ Endocervical curettage
- ❑ Conization
- ❑ Chest X-ray
- ❑ Skeletal X-ray
- ❑ Intravenous urogram
- ❑ USG
- ❑ Barium enema
- ❑ Proctoscopy

Final staging cannot be changed once therapy has begun.

If any doubt exists as to which stage should be assigned, the lower stage should be chosen.

10. Most common site of endometriosis:

a. Uterosacral ligament
b. Broad ligament
c. Ovary
d. Pouch of Douglas

Ans. c. Ovary *Ref: Telindes 10th/ed p439*

EXPLANATION

Incidence of endometriosis in different organs

- ❑ Ovary: 44%
- ❑ Uterus: 11%
- ❑ Broad ligament: 25%
- ❑ Pouch of Douglas: 34%
- ❑ Uterosacral ligaments: 15%

11. A women presented with complaints of menorrhagia. An endometrial biopsy was done and it showed tubular glands and cells with subnuclear vacuoles. This biopsy finding is suggestive of which phase of cycle?

a. Proliferative phase
b. Anovulatory cycle
c. Hyperplasia with atypia
d. Early secretory phase
e. Secretory phase

Ans. d. Early secretory phase *Ref: Dutta's Gynecology 6th/ed p88-95*

Secretory phase

- ❑ The changes of the components are due to the combined effects of estrogen and progesterone liberated from the corpus luteum after ovulation.
- ❑ The endometrium contains receptors for progesterone which are induced by estrogen.
- ❑ **Thus, the progesterone can only act on the endometrium previously primed by estrogen.**
- ❑ It begins on day 15 and ceases 5–6 days prior to menstruation.

- **The surface epithelium** becomes more columnar and ciliated at places. The glands show predominant changes.
- **The glands** increase in size. The lining epithelium become taller. There is appearance of vacuoles due to secretion of glycogen between the nuclei and the basement membrane.
- This is called **sub-nuclear vacuolation**, which is the **earliest (36–48 hours) evidence of progesterone effect (ovulation)**.
- **The subnuclear vacuolation persists until about 21st day of cycle**. The intracellular secretion then enters the gland lumina on the way to the uterine cavity pushing the nuclei back towards the basement membrane.
- The effect is a saw-toothed glandular epithelium. The fluid has got nutritive value for any fertilized ovum reaching the uterus during that time.
- **The glands become corkscrew-shaped. The blood vessels undergo marked spiraling.**

12. A women with history of obesity and hypertension presented with post- menopausal and was diagnosed with Ca Endometrium. On biopsy, invasion of more than 50% of myometrium with extension to vagina but no involvement of paraaortic or inguinal lymph nodes, Stage of the disease is

a. Stage 3A
b. Stage 3B
c. Stage 3C1
d. Stage 3C2

Ans. b. Stage 3B *Ref: DC Dutta's Gynecology 6th/ed p357*

Explanation

Table 1: FIGO surgical staging of endometrial carcinoma (2009)

Stage	Description
Stage I*	Tumor confined to the corpus uteri
IA*	No or less than half myometrial invasion
IB*	Invasion equal to or more than half of the myometrium
Stage II*	Tumor invades cervical stroma, but does not extend beyond the uterus**
Stage III*	Local and/or regional spread of the tumor
IIIA*	Tumor invades the serosa of the corpus uteri and/or adnexae*
IIIB*	Vaginal and/or parametrial involvement*
IIIC*	Metastases to pelvic and/or paraortic lymph nodes*
IIIC1*	Positive pelvic nodes
IIIC2*	Positive paraaortic lymph nodes with or without positive pelvic lymph nodes
Stage IV*	Tumor involves bladder and/or bowel mucosa, and/or distant
IVA*	Tumor invasion of bladder and/or bowel mucosa
IVB*	Distant metastases, including intra abdominal metastases and/or inguinal lymph nodes

* Either G1, G2 or G3. Depending upon the percentage of solid nonsquamous component, G1 has ≤5% G2 has 6-50% and G3 has > 50% of solid component.

** Endocervical glandular involvement only is considered as Stage I and no longer as Stage II

* Positive cytology has to be reported separately without changing the stage.

13. Best diagnosed with USG at first trimester

a. Anencephaly
b. NT defects
c. Meningocele
d. Option not recalled

Ans. a. Anencephaly *Ref: DC Dutta's obstetric p408*

EXPLANATION

In the first half of pregnancy, the diagnosis of anencephaly is made by elevated alpha-fetoprotein in amniotic fluid and confirmed by sonography.

Question not recalled properly: Imerslund-Gräsbeck syndrome, its cause was asked.

EXPLANATION

Caused by low levels of vitamin B12 (also known as cobalamin).
The characteristic features are

- Megaloblastic anemia.
- Proteinuria (~50% cases)
- Normal kidney function.

Typically begins in infancy or early childhood.
Symptoms include:

- An inability to grow and gain weight at the expected rate (failure to thrive),
- Pale skin (pallor),
- Excessive tiredness (fatigue), and
- Recurring gastrointestinal or respiratory infections.
- Other features include mild neurological problems, such as weak muscle tone (hypotonia), numbness or tingling in the hands or feet, movement problems, delayed development, or confusion.

Mutations in the *AMN* or *CUBN* gene. The AMN gene provides instructions for making a protein called amnionless, and the CUBN gene provides instructions for making a protein called cubilin which are in turn responsible for uptake of Vit b12 in body.

Management is symptomatic.

Dermatology

Author: Jyotsana Priya

AIIMS May 2017

1. A 12-year-old child presents with 4 hypopigmented lesions of on back and on front of left arm with loss of sensation. What should be the treatment of this child?

a. Rifampicin 600 mg once a month + dapsone 100 mg daily + clofazamine 300 mg once a month and 50 mg daily
b. Rifampicin 600 mg once a month + dapsone 100 mg daily
c. Rifampicin 450 mg once a month + dapsone 50 mg daily + clofazamine 150 once a month + 50 mg alternate days
d. Rifampicin 450 mg once a month + dapsone 50 mg daily + clofazamine 150 mg once a month + 50 mg daily

Ans. c. Rifampicin 450 mg once a month + dapsone 50 mg daily + clofazamine 150 once a month + 50 mg alternate days *Ref: http://apps.who.int/medicinedocs/en/d/Jh2988e/5.html*

Explanation

This is a case of multibacillary leprosy since more than 5 hypopigmented (4 + 4) lesions are present. A different regimen is followed in children below 14 years.

	Paucibacillary	Multibacillary
Definition	5 or less lesions	More than 5 lesions
Duration of therapy	6 months to be completed in 9 months	12 months to be completed in 18 months
Drug for adults		
Supervised (monthly)	Rifampicin, 600 mg	Rifampicin, 600 mg + Clofazimine, 300 mg
Not supervised (daily)	Dapsone, 100 mg	Dapsone, 100 mg + Clofazimine, 50 mg

WHO Recommended treatment regimens

Six-month regimen for paucibacillary (PB) Leprosy

	Dapsone	Rifampicin
Adult 50–70 kg	100 mg Given daily	600 mg Given once a month under supervision
Child 10–14 years[a]	50 mg Given daily	450 mg Given once a month under supervision

[a]Adjust dose appropriately for child less than 10 years. For example, dapsone 25 mg daily and rifampicin 300 mg given once a month under supervision.

Twelve-month regimen for multibacillary (MB) leprosy

	Dapsone	Rifampicin	Clofazimine		
Adult 50–70 kg	100 mg Given daily	600 mg Given once a month under supervision	50 mg Given daily	and	300 mg Given once a month under supervision
Child 10–14 years[b]	50 mg Given daily	450 mg Given once a month under supervision	50 mg Given every other day	and	150 mg Given once a month under supervision

[b]Adjust dose appropriately for child less than 10 years. For example, dapsone 25 mg daily, rifampicin 300 mg given once a month under supervision, clofazimine, 50 mg given twice a week, and clofazimine 100 mg given once a month under supervision.

Single lesion paucibacillary (SLPB) leprosy (one time dose of 3 medications taken together)

	Rifampicin	Ofloxacin	Minocycline
Adult 50–70 kg	600 mg	400 mg	100 mg
Child 5–14 years[c]	300 mg	200 mg	50 mg

[c]Not recommended for pregnant women or children less than 5 years.

2. A 30-year-old lady comes with a 2-month history of non-scarring patchy alopecia on the left side. There was no scaling or erythema. Most likely diagnosis is:

a. Alopecia areata
b. Trichotillomania
c. Telogen effluvium
d. Androgenic alopecia

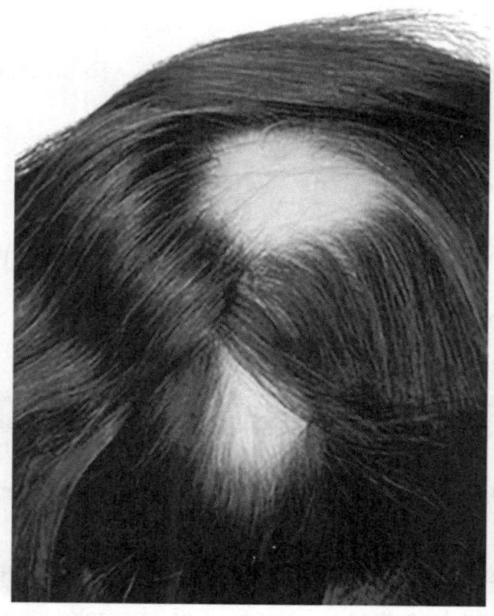

Ans. b. Trichotillomania *Ref: Fitzpatrick Clinical Dermatology p762*

Explanation

All the options are responsible for non-scarring alopecia. Since patchy hair loss is seen in the picture, so, alopecia areata and telogen effluvium can be ruled out.

Regarding androgenic alopecia, it is a type of pattern hair loss in which male have frontal and occipital hair loss, while females have increased thinning of hair in midline partition is seen. And the pattern in the picture is temporal loss.

Cause of hair loss non-scarring

Global hair loss (non-scarring)	Patchy hair loss
Failure of follicle production	Non-scarring
Hair shaft abnormality	• Production decline
Abnormality of cycling	Triangular alopecia
• Telogen effluvium **(option c)**	Androgenic alopecia
• Anagen effluvium	• Hair breakage
• Loose anagen syndrome	Trichotillomania
• Alopecia areata **(option a)**	Traction alopecia
	Tinea capitis
	Primary or acquired hair shaft abnormality
	• Unruly hair
	• Abnormality of cycling
	Alopecia areata
	Syphilis

3. A 3-year-old child, presented with itching and erythema over the patchy hair loss as shown in the picture. Which of the following will aid in the diagnosis?

a. KOH mount
b. Slit skin smear
c. Tzank smear
d. Gram stain

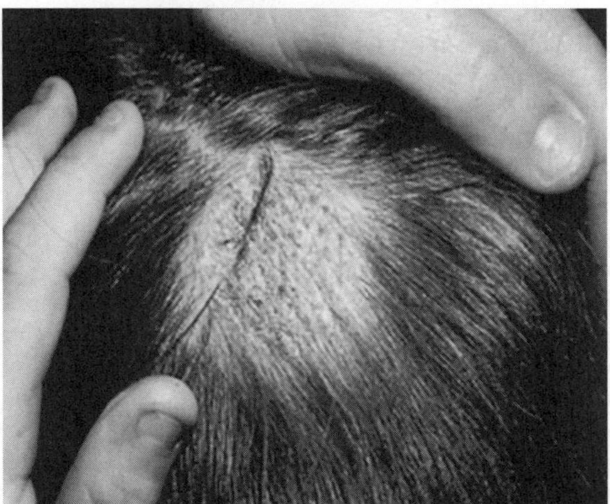

Ans. a. KOH mount *Ref: Dermatology by Neena Khanna p280*

Explanation

Characteristic tinea capitis lesion: A large, **round, hyperkeratotic plaque** of alopecia due to breaking off of hair shafts close to the surface.

Remaining hair shafts and scales exhibit a green fluorescence when examined with Wood's lamp.

DERMATOPHYTE INFECTIONS (RING WORM)

Etiology: Three genera of dermatophytes: *Trichophyton, Epidermophyton,* and *Microsporum.*
Morphology: *Prototype lesion:* Is an itchy, annular/arcuate polycyclic lesion with clear center and an active margin with papulovesicles and scaling. *Scalp lesions* manifest as discoid areas of non-cicatricial alopecia with easily pluckable hair.
Sites: Lesions modified by site and named variously as ***Tinea capitis* (scalp), *T. faciei* (face), *T. corporis* (trunk), *T. cruris* (groin), *T. pedis* (feet), *T. manuum* (hand), and *T. unguium* (nails).**
Diagnosis: Typical clinical morphology as well as demonstration of fungal elements, using **potassium hydroxide preparation**.
Treatment: Topical therapy with **imidazoles or allylamines** for localized infection while nail infection, scalp infection, and extensive skin infection need to be treated with oral **terbinafine or griseofulvin or itraconazole**.

Genera of dermatophyte and its relation with site of infection

Genera	Site of infection		
	Skin	Hair	Nails
Trichophyton	+	+	+
Microporum	+	+	–
Epidermophyton	+	–	+

Tinea capitis

Age

Invariably a **child** (as in question)

Morphology

- ❑ Discoid patch of partial alopecia from which the hair can easily and painlessly be plucked.
- ❑ Degree of inflammation varies, depending on the strain of fungus

Patterns

Three patterns are recognized:

- ❑ ***Noninflammatory tinea capitis:***
  - Caused by anthropophilic organisms (*e.g., T. verrucosum*), so less inflammation.
  - Human to human spread occurs, so may occur in **epidemics.**
  - Appear as **partially bald areas with scaling** most marked **at the periphery**. Hair present in the patch are lusterless, may break 3–4 mm from the scalp and can easily be plucked. The broken hair may appear as gray/black dots.
  - There is very little inflammation (**erythema**, papules, and pustules) (**given in question).**
- ❑ ***Inflammatory tinea capitis (kerion)***
  - Caused by zoophilic dermatophytes (*e.g., M. canis*), which elicit intense inflammation.
  - Presents as a **boggy swelling with pustulation**. Often, the pus discharges from multiple orifices. **Hair** from such a swelling is easily and **painlessly pluckable.**
  - Lymphadenopathy (especially occipital) invariable.

- **Favus:**
  - Caused by *T. schoenleinii.*
  - Characterized by presence of **foul-smelling, yellowish** cup-shaped **crusts entangling many scalp hair**.
  - Often results in **cicatricial alopecia.**

4. What is the diagnosis of the below histopathology picture?

a. Pemphigus vulgaris
b. Leishmaniasis
c. Mycosis fungoides
d. Psoriasis

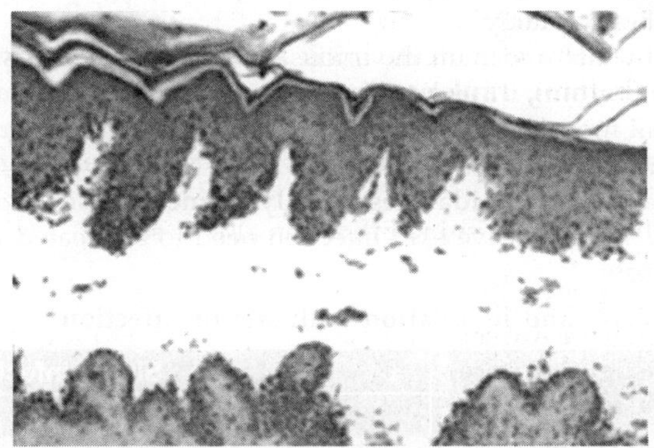

Ans. a. Pemphigus vulgaris *Ref. Lever's Histopathology of the Skin 3rd/ed p190, Rook's 8th/ed p40.2*

EXPLANATION

To be discussed in detail in question 6 of AIIMS dermatology

5. A child had hyperpigmented patch with hair on cheek since birth. Most likely diagnosis is:

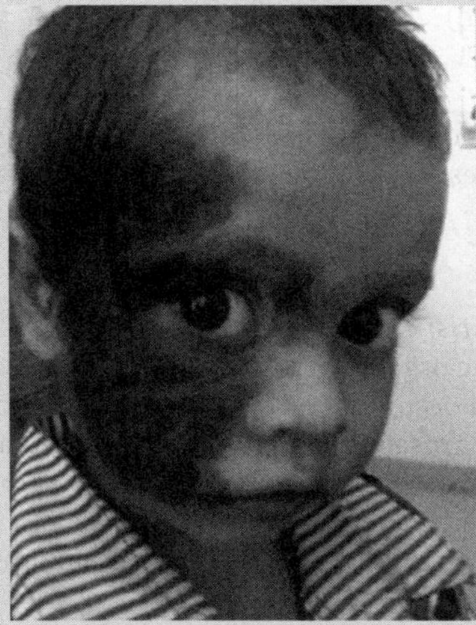

a. Congenital melanocytic nevus b. Hematoma
c. Verrucous epidermal nevus d. Melanoacanthoma

Ans. a. Congenital melanocytic nevi *Ref: Dermatology by Neena Khanna p353*

EXPLANATION

Congenital melanocytic nevi

- *Etiogenesis:* Derived from epidermal melanocytes and nevus cells have a predilection for deeper penetration.
- *Onset:* Present at birth.
- **Morphology:**
  - May be **single**, but are often **multiple**.
  - Color varies from **brown to black** and the lesions darken and enlarge as the child grows.
  - With age, the lesions also become raised and develop rugosities (**cerebriform appearance**).
  - **Coarse hair develops in 90% of lesions** and may have a vortex distribution.
  - Larger lesions may have satellite papules at the periphery.
  - Can occur anywhere on body.
  - Giant lesions are usually seen on the trunk and because they may cover large areas of the trunk, are called **"bathing trunk nevi"**.
- **Complications:**
  - The potential for **malignant transformation** is definitely more in giant congenital melanocytic nevi
  - **Meningeal involvement** and **spina bifida** can also be seen.
- **Treatment**
  - Most lesions can be left alone
  - Some lesions need to be excised
  - If cosmetically disfiguring (face)
  - In a trauma-prone area
  - If malignancy suspected

Verrucous epidermal nevus (option c)

- Multiple **brown papules** arranged **linearly**.
- Lesions either localized or generalized.

6. A patient presents with skin and oral lesions. Immunofluorescence picture is shown below. All are true *except*:

a. Dsg 3 antibodies
b. Dsg 1 antibodies
c. Antibody against hemidesmosome
d. IgG type is the most common

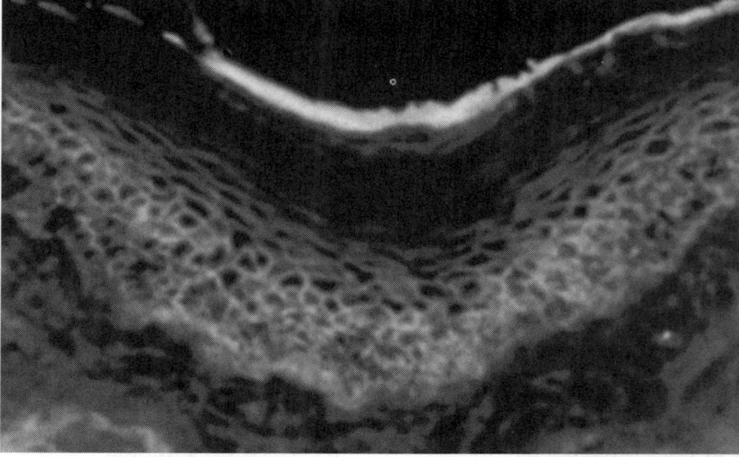

Ans. c. Antibody against hemidesmosome *Ref: Dermatology by Neena Khanna p72*

Explanation

- ❑ **Etiology:**
  - Autoimmune disease, characterized by acantholysis, **induced by deposition of IgG autoantibodies in an intercellular area of epidermis.**
  - IgG autoantibodies against **desmogleins (Dsg)** (present in desmosomes).
- ❑ ***Clinical features:*** Several variants
  - ***Pemphigus vulgaris:***
    Flaccid bullae that rapidly rupture to form painful erosions that heal slowly. Oral erosions universally present.
  - ***P. foliaceus:***
    Bullae superficial, rupture rapidly, so only scale crust seen; in seborrheic distribution. No oral lesions.
  - ***Others:*** *P. erythematosus, P. vegetans.*
- ❑ Investigations:
  - Diagnosis based on **Tzanck smear** (acantholytic cells),
  - **Histopathology (intraepidermal bulla with acantholytic cells),**
  - Immunopathology **(intercellular fishnet pattern IgG** deposit in epidermis on **DIF (Direct immunofluorescence); circulating IgG antibodies on IIF (Indirect immunofluorescence).**
- ❑ ***Treatment:*** Aggressive treatment. Supportive care is very important.
  - Steroids systemically (daily doses or as monthly bolus)
  - Immunosuppressive adjuvants (azathioprine, methotrexate, or cyclophosphamide).

7. A 12-year-old girl comes with red, itchy exudative lesions in cubital fossa, popliteal fossa and neck. What is most likely diagnosis?

a. Dermatitis herpetiformis
b. Pemphigus vulgaris
c. Psoriasis
d. Atopic dermatitis

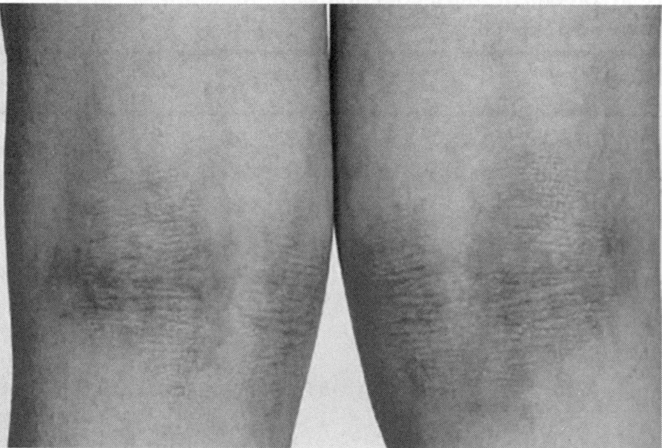

Ans. d. Atopic dermatitis *Ref: Fitzpatcrick's Dermatology in General Medicine 8th/ed p165*

Explanation

Atopic dermatitis

- ❑ ***Etiology:***
  - A strong genetic predisposition. Raised IgE level is most consistent immunological finding.

- ❑ ***Clinical features:***
  - Picture varies with age of patient.
  - *Infantile phase:* Begins at about 3 months, severely itchy, exudative lesions on face and other parts, sparing diaper area. Clears in 40%, by age of 18 months.
  - *Childhood phase:* Itchy, leathery flexural lesions.
  - *Adult phase:* Lichenified flexural lesions; sometimes a discoid pattern.
- ❑ ***Associated features:*** Ichthyosis vulgaris, lick cheilitis, nipple eczema, hand dermatitis, and asthma.
- ❑ ***Complications:*** Bacterial and viral infections.
- ❑ ***Treatment:*** Multipronged approach.
  - Avoid triggers like woollens and excessive degreasing. Rehydration followed by topical moisturizers forms the mainstay of therapy.
  - Topical therapy like **steroids (with oral antihistamines) during flares.**
  - **Tacrolimus and pimecrolimus to prevent flares.**
  - *Extensive lesions*:
    - Oral steroids, cyclosporine and azathioprine.
  - Antihistamines regularly used, though role debated.

Dermatitis herpetiformis (option a)
- ❑ Distribution is on extensor surface of extremities
- ❑ Intense itching seen

Pemphigus vulgaris
- ❑ Bullous disorder
- ❑ Distribution scalp, face, mucosa, flexures, trunk
- ❑ Painful erosions seen

Psoriasis (option c)
- ❑ Silvery scales present
- ❑ Extensor surface involvement (most commonly).

PGI May 2017

1. All of the following is/are sub-epidermal blisters:

a. Pemphigus vulgaris
b. Bullous pemphigoid
c. Bullous pemphigoid SLE
d. Pemphigus vegetans
e. Dermatitis herpetiformis

Ans. b. Bullous pemphigoid *Ref: Fitzpatrick's Dermatology in General Medicine, 8th/ed p106*

Explanation

Subepidermal lesions seen in:
- ❑ Pemphigus vulgaris **(blister)**
- ❑ Bullous pemphigoid **(blister)**
- ❑ Epidermolysis bullosa **(blister)**
- ❑ Dermatitis herpetiformis **(vesicles)**
- ❑ Linear IgA dermatosis **(vesicles)**

2. All are true about Basal cell carcinoma, *except*:

a. Rarely metastasizes
b. UV radiation is one of the important factor
c. Individual with light skin are less prone as compared to dark skinned.
d. Lymphadenopathy is common

Ans. c. Individual with light skin are less prone as compared to dark skinned and d. Lymphadenopathy is common *Ref Dermatology by Neena Khanna p362*

EXPLANATION

- *Etiology:*
  - Ultraviolet rays *(Option b)*, chemicals
  - Genetic predisposition (**more in light colored skin) (option c)**
- *Morphology:*
  - Translucent nodule with telangiectasia.
  - May ulcerate. Has a pearly, beaded edge, which is diagnostic.
  - Many variants (classical or noduloulcerative BCC, superficial BCC, morphoeic BCC and any of these may be pigmented).
  - Locally invasive, does not metastasize *(Option a)*.
  - **No lymphadenopathy** (**option d)**
- *Sites:* Face. Superficial variant on trunk.
- *Diagnosis:* Based on characteristic edge; histopathology diagnostic.
- *Treatment:*
  - Surgical excision mainstay of treatment. Use Moh's micrographic surgery in recurrent lesions
  - Radiotherapy in elderly.

LIST OF QUESTIONS THAT WERE NOT RECALLED PROPERLY

Question: On hypertrophic Scar

EXPLANATION

- A hypertrophic scar is a thickened, wide, often raised scar that develops where skin is injured. Scars are common during the wound healing process, but a hypertrophic scar is a result of an abnormal response to a trauma or injury.
- Myofibroblasts produce too much collagen during healing. This can happen simply as a result of a person's skin type and healing tendencies.
- The scars are a frequent complication of burn injuries, but can also form after piercings, cuts, or even acne. Hypertrophic scars are similar to keloid scars but tend to be milder and don't grow beyond the boundaries of the original skin injury.
- The scars aren't dangerous or life-threatening.

Medical Treatments

- *Corticosteroid treatments:* Corticosteroid injections are considered a first-line treatment for hypertrophic scars. Injecting a steroid into the scar every six weeks may help flatten and soften the scar. There's a limit to the number of times this can be performed, however, as the steroids may also weaken normal tissue around the scar.

- *Laser therapy:* Laser therapy is more effective in newly formed scars than in older scars. The lasers work by burning and flattening elevated scars. They also target the red and pink pigments in the scars to lighten them.
- *Bleomycin:* Bleomycin is a metabolite of a strain of soil bacteria. It is shown promising results when injected directly into a hypertrophic scar. It may help improve the scars appearance and relieve itching and pain. More clinical trials are needed to confirm its efficacy.
- *Cryotherapy:* In cryotherapy, a doctor or dermatologist freezes the scar tissue with liquid nitrogen to help flatten it. Cryotherapy has been shown to be successful, safe, nontoxic, and well-tolerated in a number of small studies.
- *Surgery:* After waiting at least a year, a hypertrophic scar can be excised, or cut out, and closed again with stitches. This treatment tries to re-heal the injury while eliminating the issues that may have caused the scar in the first place, such as infection, inflammation, or tension.

Hypertrophic Scars vs. Keloid Scars

- Before treating a hypertrophic scar, it is important to differentiate it from a similar type of scar called a keloid. Keloid scars are smooth, hard, benign growths that also form when scar tissue grows excessively. Even your doctor may have difficulty telling the difference between a hypertrophic scar and a keloid, but it is important to distinguish them because the treatment may be different.

  In general, Hypertrophic scars:
- Are raised, but rarely more than 4 millimeters above the skin
- Are red or pink in color
- Can develop anywhere on the body

  On the other hand, keloids usually:
- Are raised more than 4 millimeters from the skin
- Grow beyond the boundaries of the original incision or wound
- Are pink to purple in color
- Evolve and grow over time
- Form on the earlobes, shoulders, cheeks, and chest above the sternum.

Both scars tend to occur more commonly in darker skin types. Hypertrophic scars tend to be easier to treat than keloids, which have a high recurrence rate despite treatment.

Preventing hypertrophic scars

In you experience an injury, especially a burn injury, or if you have surgery, there are ways to help prevent hypertrophic scarring. These include:

- Cleaning and caring for the wound properly, such as by applying wound dressings to prevent infection
- Using silicone sheeting after a surgery
- Injecting a corticosteroid after a surgery.

Question: Premalignant condition of tongue was asked and options were like lichen planus, erythroplakia, Behcet's disease, Bowen's disease

Ref: *http://oralcancerfoundation.org/cdc/premalignant-lesions/*

EXPLANATION:

Leukoplakia:

- Most cases of leukoplakia are a hyperkeratotic response to an irritant and are asymptomatic, 20% of leukoplakic lesions show evidence of dysplasia or carcinoma at first clinical recognition

- Some anatomic sites (floor of mouth and ventral tongue) have rates of dysplasia or carcinoma as high as 45%.
- In one large study, lesions with an erythroplakic component had a 23.4% malignant transformation rate, compared with a 6.5% rate for lesions that were homogeneous.
- The term erythroleukoplakia has been used to describe leukoplakias with a red component.

Erythroplakia:

- An erythroplakia is a red lesion.
- Far less common than leukoplakia, erythroplakia has a much greater probability (91%) of showing signs of dysplasia or malignancy at the time of diagnosis.
- Such lesions have a flat, macular, velvety appearance and may be speckled with white spots representing foci of keratosis.

Lichen planus:

- The premalignant or malignant potential of lichen planus is in dispute.
- Some believe that the occasional epithelial dysplasia or carcinoma found in patients with this relatively common lesion may be either coincidental or evidence that the initial diagnosis of lichen planus was erroneous.
- It is frequently difficult to differentiate lichen planus from epithelial dysplasia
- One study found that 24% of oral lichen planus cases had 5 of the 12 World Health Organization (WHO) diagnostic criteria for epithelial dysplasia, and only 6% had no histologic features suggestive of that disorder.
- It is prudent practice to biopsy the lesion at the initial visit to confirm the diagnosis and to monitor it thereafter for clinical changes suggesting a premalignant or malignant change.

Other premalignant lesions include:

- Linea alba,
- Leukoedema, and
- Frictional keratosis.

Question: Urticaria was asked and options were related to its mediators, cause and treatment.

Ref: http://emedicine.medscape.com/article/137362-treatment

EXPLANATION:

- Urticaria (hives) is a vascular reaction of the skin marked by the transient appearance of smooth, slightly elevated papules or plaques (wheals) that are erythematous and that are often attended by severe pruritus. Individual lesions resolve without scarring in several hours.
- Most cases of urticaria are self-limited and of short duration; the eruption rarely lasts more than several days, it but may be recurrent over weeks.
- Chronic urticaria is defined as urticaria with recurrent episodes lasting longer than 6 weeks).

Pathophysiology

- It results from the release of histamine, bradykinin, leukotriene C4, prostaglandin D2, and other vasoactive substances from mast cells and basophils in the dermis.
- These substances cause extravasation of plasma into the dermis, leading to the urticarial lesion.
- The intense pruritus of urticaria is a result of histamine released into the dermis.

Medical Causes

- Viral infections like acute viral syndromes, hepatitis (A, B, and C), Epstein-Barr virus, and herpes simplex virus
- Streptococcal infection
- Chronic parasitic infections
- Cutaneous fungal infection
- Leukemia
- Cryoglobulinemias (e.g. associated with hepatitis C, chronic lymphocytic leukemia)
- Serum sickness
- Other immune complex–mediated inflammation
- Systemic lupus erythematosus, rheumatoid arthritis, juvenile rheumatoid arthritis, or other rheumatologic diseases (rare causes of urticaria)
- Hypothyroidism and hyperthyroidism, although euthyroid patients with antithyroid antibodies (i.e. vide infra) can be affected
- Lymphoreticular malignancies (e.g. chronic lymphocytic leukemia)
- Pregnancy (i.e. pruritic urticarial papules and plaques of pregnancy [PUPPP]).

Physical causes (physical urticaria):

- Cold
- Pressure
- Vibration
- Cholinergic (triggered by heat, exercise, or emotional stress)
- Sunlight
- Water
- Dermographism (can occur as an isolated condition)
- Exercise.

Treatment:

- H1 antagonist(both 1st and 2nd generation)
- Corticosteroids
- Sympathomimetic agents
- Immunomodulatory and anti-inflammatory therapy
- Tricyclic antidepressant.

JIPMER Pattern Based

1. A 1-year-boy presented with dry, scaly, eczematous, red vesicobullous crusted lesion. Lesions started in perioral and perigenital areas, later on scalp, flexural surfaces also get involved. On examination pallor seen. What is the probable diagnosis?

a. Acrodermatitis enteropathica
b. Psoriasis
c. Pemphigiod
d. Pemphigus vulgaris

Ans. a. Acrodermatitis enteropathica *Ref: Fitzpatrick's Dermatology in General Medicine 8th/ed p397*

Explanation

Acrodematitis enteropathica

- Acrodermatitis enteropathica is a **genetic disorder of zinc absorption.**
- **Autosomal recessive** trait.
- It occurs in **infants, bottle-fed with bovine milk, days to few weeks or in breastfed infants, soon after weaning.**
- *Skin Findings*:
  - Patches and plaques of dry**, scaly, sharply marginated** and brightly **red, eczematous dermatitis** evolving into **vesiculobullous, pustular**, erosive, and **crusted lesions.**
  - **Initially** occur in the **perioral** and **anogenital areas.**
  - **Later**, scalp, hands and feet, flexural regions, trunk. Fingertips glistening, erythematous, with fissures and **secondary paronychia**. Perlèche.
  - Lesions become secondarily infected with *Candida albicans, S. aureus*. Impaired wound healing.
  - **Diffuse alopecia, graying of hair. Paronychia, nail ridging, and loss of nails.**
  - **Red, glossy tongue; superficial aphthous-like erosions; secondary oral candidiasis**.
  - Photophobia; irritable, depressed mood.
  - Children with Acrodermatitis Enteropathica whine and cry constantly
  - **Failure of growth.**
  - **Anemia,** low serum/plasma zinc levels; reduced urinary zinc excretion.
  - **After zinc replacement, severely infected and erosive skin lesions heal within 1–2 weeks diarrhea ceases, and irritability and depression of mood improve within 24 hour.**
- *Management*:
  - Dietary or IV supplementation with **zinc salts in two to three times the required daily amount** restores normal zinc status in days to weeks.

Rest all options are explained in detail in questions discussed above.

2. Which of the following is the causative organism for kerion?

a. Tinea capitis
b. Malassezia furfur
c. Tinea versicolor
d. Staphylococcus aureus

Ans. a. Tinea capitis

Explanation

Refer to Question Number 3 in AIIMS Question

3. A 10-year-old child presented with erythematous lesion over flexural surface of arms and legs. Parents also gives history of episodes of respiratory illness. What is the most probable diagnosis?

a. Pemphigus vulgaris
b. Dermatitis herpetiformis
c. Bullous pemphigoid
d. Atopic dermatitis

Ans. d. Atopic dermatitis

Explanation

Refer to Question 7 from AIIMS Paper

4. A 9-month-old child presented with yellow greasy scales in head, itching and crusting in flexures of arm. Diagnosis is:

a. Seborrheic dermatitis
b. Atopic dermatitis
c. Allergic dermatitis
d. Contact dermatitis

Ans. a. Seborrheic dermatitis *Ref: Dermatology by Neena Khanna, p99*

EXPLANATION

Seborrheic dermatitis

- *Etiology:*
  - Overgrowth of yeast, *Malassezia furfur* may play an important role.
- *Age:*
  - Adults; infrequently seen in **infants**, but not in children.
- *Morphology:*
  - Follicular papules with **yellow greasy scales.**
  - Several other variants—eczematous, petaloid, flexural pattern.
- *Sites:*
  - Scalp, eyebrows/eyelashes (squamous blepharitis).
  - Nasolabial folds, retroauricular region, presternal and interscapular regions and flexures.
  - Sites involved in isolation or in combination.
- *Treatment:*
  - Topical and systemic antifungal agents along with topical antibiotics/corticosteroids.

Allergic contact dermatitis

- *Etiology:*
  - Common allergens are plants (parthenium), metals (nickel), cosmetics (hair dyes and fragrances), medicines and rubber.
- *Clinical features:*
  - Could manifest either as acute or chronic dermatitis. Distribution characteristic, depending on the antigen.
- *Investigations:*
  - Patch test confirmatory.
- *Treatment:*
  - Removal of antigen essential to prevent recurrences.
  - *Localized disease:* Treat symptomatically with topical steroids.
  - *Widespread disease:* Systemic steroids; other immunosuppressive drugs.

Irritant contact dermatitis

- *Etiology:*
  - Occupational/recreational exposure.
- *Morphology:*
  - Acute (with strong irritants) or
  - Chronic (with weak irritants) dermatitis.
- *Sites:*
  - Hands/forearms
- *Treatment:*
  - Absolute or relative withdrawal of exposure to irritant.
  - Topical corticosteroids for acute stage.
  - To prevent and minimize exposure.

5. A 4-month-old child presented with slightly raised brown papules on the back and scalp. whealing was seen on rubbing. Child is suffering from:

a. Atopic dermatitis
b. Contact dermatitis
c. Pemphigus vulgaris
d. Urticaria pigmentosa

Ans. d. Urticaria pigmentosa *Ref Fitzpatcrick's Dermatology in General Medicine 8th/ed p397*

EXPLANATION

Urticaria pigmentosa

- A type of generalized cutaneous mastocytosis
- **Morphology**
  - Tan macules to slightly raised tan to brown papules.
  - Disseminated, few or >100 with widespread symmetric distribution.
  - Darier sign (whealing) after rubbing; in infants, may become bullous.
  - Bright red diffuse flushing occurring spontaneously, after rubbing of skin, or after ingestion of alcohol or mast cell–degranulating agents.
- **Management**
  - Avoidance of precipitating factors
  - Antihistaminics and mast cell stabilizer. A detailed note on urticaria is at the end of PGI

6. Groove sign seen in:

a. Lymphogranuloma venereum (LGV)
b. Chanchroid
c. Donovanosis
d. Herpes

Ans. a. Lymphogranuloma venereum (LGV) *Ref: Dermatology by Neena Khanna p311*

EXPLANATION

Lymphogranuloma venereum

- *Etiology:*
  - *Chlamydia trachomatis* serovars L1, L2, and L3.
- *Clinical features:*
  - Genital lesion not noticed
  - Presenting feature is enlargement of inguinal, femoral, and sometimes external iliac group of lymph nodes
  - **Sign of groove characteristic**
- *Complications:*
  - Esthiomene
- *Treatment:*
  - Doxycycline (200 mg) or erythromycin base (2 g) daily for 21 days
  - Aspiration of buboes

Donovanosis

- *Etiology:*
  - *Klebsiella granulomatis*
- *Morphology:*
  - Single or few, asymptomatic ulcers with an elevated, serpiginous edge, and beefy red floor.
  - Subcutaneous nodules (pseudobuboes) in inguinal region may ulcerate
  - No lymphadenopathy

- ❑ *Sites:*
  - Genital and perianal areas
- ❑ *Complications:*
  - Large deforming lesions; malignant transformation
- ❑ *Investigations:*
  - Tissue smear and histopathology show organisms as **bipolar intracellular inclusions**
- ❑ *Treatment:*
  - Doxycycline (200 mg daily) or azithromycin (1 g once a week) for 3 weeks

Herpes genitalis

- ❑ *Etiology:*
  - *Herpes simplex virus* type II (less frequently HSV type I). Recurrent lesions
- ❑ *Classification:*
  - First episode and recurrent
- ❑ *Clinical features:*
  - Primary or first episode infection more severe, lasts longer. Lesions consist of grouped vesicular lesions on an erythematous base. Rupture to form polycyclic erosions
- ❑ *Investigations:*
  - Multinucleated giant cells **on Tzanck smear**
  - **Culture** confirmatory
- ❑ *Treatment:*
  - Symptomatic. Long-term suppressive acyclovir, given if six or more episodes/year

Difference between chanchroid and LGV

Chanchroid	LGV
Genital ulcer present	Transient or absent
Usually single lymph node group enlargement	Multiple group lymph node enlargement
Chanchroid ulcer	Ulcer with undermined edges
Occasional constitutional symptom	Frequent constitutional symptom

7. A 40-year-old man presented with white lacey pattern in cheeks, with severe burning sensation on food intake. What is the diagnosis?

a. Lichen planus
b. Candida
c. Oral hairy leucoplakia
d. Aphthous ulcer

Ans. a. Lichen planus *Ref: Dermatology by Neena Khanna p56*

Lichen Planus

- ❑ *Etiology:*
  - Common dermatosis of unknown etiology.
- ❑ *Morphology:*
  - **Pruritic, Polygonal, Purple** (but violaceous is the term to use!), **Plane** (flat topped), **Papules** (five Ps) with **Wickham's striae on surface**.
- ❑ *Sites:*
  - Wrists, legs.

- ❑ ***Associations:***
  - Always look in the **mouth (lacey pattern**) and examine the **scalp (follicular lesions and scarring alopecia**) and the **nails (thinning of nails, pterygium)**.
- ❑ ***Variants:***
  - Number of variants. Common ones being follicular, hypertrophic and linear.
- ❑ ***Treatment:***
  - Depending on extent and site.
  - *Localized lesions:* Topical steroids and antihistamines.
  - *Extensive lesions:* Dapsone, PUVA, acitretin and systemic steroids.
  - *Erosive oral LP:* Acitretin.

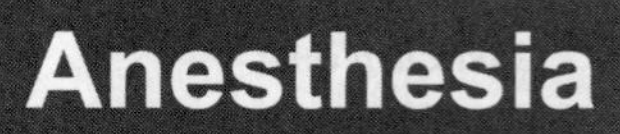

Author: Bahram Gor, Co-author: Abhijit

AIIMS May 2017

1. All of the following are true regarding the procedure performed with the instrument shown below *except*:

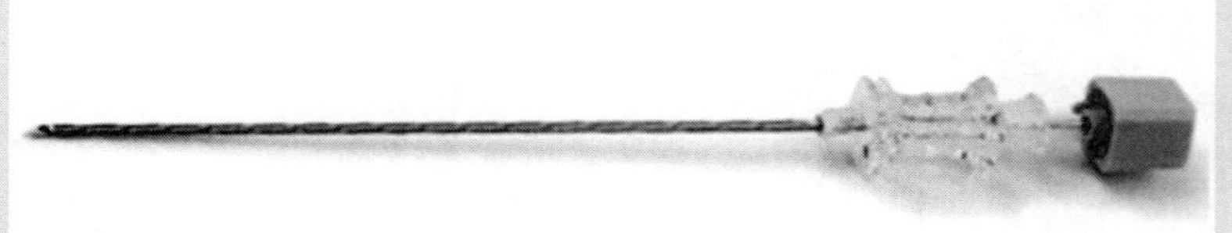

a. Absolutely contraindicated in coagulation disorder
b. Done in lateral recumbent position
c. Bevel of needle faces upwards
d. Breath holding not required

Ans. a. Absolutely contraindicated in coagulation disorder *Ref: Miller's 8th/ed p1691*

Explanation

- There are few absolute contraindications to neuraxial blockade
  1. Patient refusal
  2. Localized infection
  3. An allergy to any of the drugs
  4. Patient's inability to maintain stillness during needle puncture, which can expose the neural structures to traumatic injury.
  5. Raised intracranial pressure, which may theoretically predisposes to brainstem herniation.
- ***Option c:*** It is not necessary to keep the bevel side of the needle upwards. But as a standard practice, bevel side is introduced laterally to lessen PDPH and bevel side is kept up while injecting the drug.

PGI May 2017

1. Agents used for induction:

a. Thiopentone
b. Ketamine
c. Propofol
d. Diazepam
e. Midazolam

Ans. a. Thiopentone; b. Ketamine; c. Propofol; d. Diazepam and e. Midazolam

Ref: Miller's 8th/ed p832,841,849

EXPLANATION

All the drugs mentioned can be used for induction.

- Drugs that can be used for IV induction of anesthesia:
  1. Thiopentone
  2. Propofol
  3. Etomidate
  4. Droperidol
  5. Ketamine
  6. Midazolam
  7. Diazepam
  8. Lorazepam
  9. Dexmedetomidine

2. Adrenaline used for:

a. CPR (Cardiopulmonary resuscitation)
b. Pain
c. Bronchial asthma
d. Anaphylaxis
e. As adjuvant for local anesthetic

Ans. a. CPR (Cardiopulmonary resuscitation); c. Bronchial asthma; d. Anaphylaxis and e. As adjuvant for local anesthetic *Ref: Stoelting's 4th/ed p297*

EXPLANATION

Not used for pain, though it has some analgesic property through alpha 2 receptors ***(Option b)***

- Clinical uses of epinephrine are:
  1. Addition to local anesthetic solutions to decrease systemic absorption and prolong the duration of action of the anesthetic ***(Option e)***
  2. Treatment of life-threatening anaphylactic reactions ***(Option d)***
  3. Administration during cardiopulmonary resuscitation as the single most important therapeutic drug ***(Option a)***
  4. Continuous infusion to increase myocardial contractility. The administration of supraphysiologic doses (100 μg/kg) of epinephrine during cardiopulmonary resuscitation has not been shown to be more effective than standard doses (10 μg/kg) of this.
- ***(Option c)*** Adrenaline is not extensively used in bronchial asthma but there are studies on adrenaline being used in severe acute asthma. The results were not very promising so not recommended these days.

3. Bupivacaine toxicity treatment:

a. Intralipid
b. $CaCl_2$
c. Esmolol
d. Bretylium
e. Adrenaline

Ans. a. Intralipid; d. Bretylium and e. Adrenaline *Ref: Stoelting's 4th p193*

EXPLANATION

Important medications for treatment of Bupivacaine toxicity are intralipid for binding of the bupivacaine, Bretylium for induced dysrrhythmia and adrenaline as per ACLS protocol.

About ***Option b,*** though some references mentioned Calcium channel blockers enhance features of Bupivacaine toxicity, there are evidences that support Calcium chloride prolongs duration of action of Bupivacaine as well as other local anesthetics.

Bupivacaine Toxicity Review

- Most potent cardiotoxic LA with maximum safe dose 2.5–3 mg/kg.
- **CNS toxicity**:
  - Feelings of light headedness and dizziness.
  - Visual and auditory disturbances such as difficulty focusing and tinnitus.
  - Disorientation and drowsiness.
  - Shivering and muscular twitching and tremors initially involving muscles of the face and distal parts of the extremities.
  - Generalized convulsions of a tonic-clonic nature occur.
  - If a sufficiently large dose or rapid intravenous injection of a bupivacaine accidentally is administered, the initial signs of CNS excitation are rapidly set in followed by a state of generalized CNS depression.
- It has lower CV to CNS toxic ratio unlike lignocaine.
- **Cardiotoxicity**:
  - Depresses the rapid phase of depolarization in Purkinje fibers and ventricular muscle more than lidocaine does.
  - Increase in the PR interval and duration of the QRS complex. VPCs and variable AV blocks may be seen.
  - Extremely high concentrations depress spontaneous pacemaker activity in the sinus node, thereby resulting in sinus bradycardia and sinus arrest refractory to CPR.
- **Treatment**:
  - Prompt and effective airway management is crucial to preventing hypoxia and acidosis, which are known to potentiate toxicity.
  - If seizures occur, they should be rapidly halted with benzodiazepines. If benzodiazepines are not readily available, small doses of propofol or thiopental are acceptable. Future data may support the early use of lipid emulsion for treating seizures.
  - If cardiac arrest occurs, standard ACLS protocol should be followed with the following modifications:
    - If epinephrine is used, small initial doses (10–100 mcg boluses in the adult) should be given.
    - If ventricular arrhythmias develop, amiodarone is preferred.
    - Bretylium, 20 mg/kg IV, reverses bupivacaine induced cardiac depression and increases the threshold for ventricular tachycardia.
  - Vasopressin and CCBs are not recommended.
  - Lipid emulsion therapy:
    - Consider administering at the first signs of CNS features, after airway management.
    - Dosing:
    - 1.5 mL/kg 20% lipid emulsion bolus followed by 0.25 mL/kg per minute of infusion, continued for at least 10 minutes after circulatory stability is attained.
    - If circulatory stability is not attained, consider re-bolus and increasing infusion to 0.5 mL/kg per minute.

- Approximately 10 mL/kg lipid emulsion for 30 minutes is recommended as the upper limit for initial dosing
- Propofol is not a substitute for lipid emulsion.

4. Drug that can cause malignant hyperthermia:

a. Succinyl choline
b. Halothane
c. Rocuronium
d. Fentanyl
e. Propofol

Ans. a. Succinyl choline and b. Halothane *Ref: Miller's 8th p1294*

EXPLANATION

- Drugs causing malignant hyperthermia in order
  - Succinyl choline > Halothane > Methoxyflurane > Enflurane > Isoflurane > Desflurane > Sevoflurane > Ether > Cyclopropane > Lidocaine > TCA > MAOI > Phenothiazine
- Malignant hyperthermia syndrome (MHS)
  - Triggered by above agents in susceptible individuals
  - Cause unknown
  - Not necessary to occur on every exposure
  - Majority of mutations that confer MHS reside in the *RyR (Ryanodine 1 receptor)* gene, recently three mutations in the *CACNA1S* gene encoding for the CaV1.1 (Voltage sensitive calcium channel) subunit of skeletal muscle have been linked to MHS.

5. Malignant hyperthermia is suspected by:

a. Hypotonia
b. Seizure
c. Masseter stiffness
d. Rhabdomyolysis
e. Hypokalemia

Ans. c. Masseter stiffness and d. Rhabdomyolysis *Ref: Miller's 8th p1297*

EXPLANATION

In MHS Masseter stiffness (hypertonia not hypotonia), Rhabdomyolysis (leading to hyperkalemia not hypokalemia) occurs. Literature does not support development of seizure solely because of MHS, but may happen secondary to hypoxemia.

Early signs of MHS (Malignant Hyperthermia Syndrome)

1. Unexplained elevation of end-tidal carbon dioxide ($ETCO_2$)
2. Unexplained hypoxemia
3. Increase in body temperature above 38.8°C with no obvious cause
4. Tachypnea and/or tachycardia
5. Masseter spasm (along with pterygoids), if succinylcholine has been used (Jaw muscle rigidity with limb muscle flaccidity)
6. Generalized muscle rigidity
7. Mixed metabolic and respiratory acidosis
8. Profuse sweating
9. Mottling of skin

10. Cardiac arrhythmias
11. Unstable blood pressure.

Late signs of MHS

1. Hyperkalemia
2. Rapid increase of core body temperature
3. Elevated creatine phosphokinase levels
4. Gross myoglobinemia and myoglobinuria
5. Cardiac arrest
6. Disseminated intravascular coagulation.

6. Spinal versus epidural anesthesia, true is/are:

a. Needle used in epidural is of small size
b. Drug used are of same concentration
c. Onset of action faster in epidural anesthesia
d. More volume of drug required in epidural anesthesia
e. Density of motor blockade is more in epidural anesthesia

Ans. d. More volume of drug required in epidural anesthesia

Ref: Ward's Anaesthetic Equipment 6th/ed 316-317; Miller's 8th/ed 1704

EXPLANATION

- ❑ ***Option a:*** Needles used for spinal anesthesia are of 25 to 27 G but for epidural anesthesia needles used are of 16–18 G.
- ❑ ***Option b:*** For spinal anesthesia we use mostly fixed concentrations (0.5% Bupivacaine, 5% lignocaine) but for epidural one we can use different concentrations as per need. (0.5% Bupivacaine for complete motor, till 0.25% for sensory and autonomic blockade).
- ❑ ***Options c and e:*** As drug has to cross the fatty tissue and dural sheath in epidural space to block nerve roots, so effective concentration becomes less. That is why in epidural anesthesia motor blockade is less dense.
- ❑ ***Option d***: For epidural anesthesia, the amount of drug required is 1.5–2 mL per segment to be blocked and there are barriers (dura matter and fatty tissues) to act on nerves. But as in spinal anesthesia drug is mixed with CSF, the amount of drug required is less.

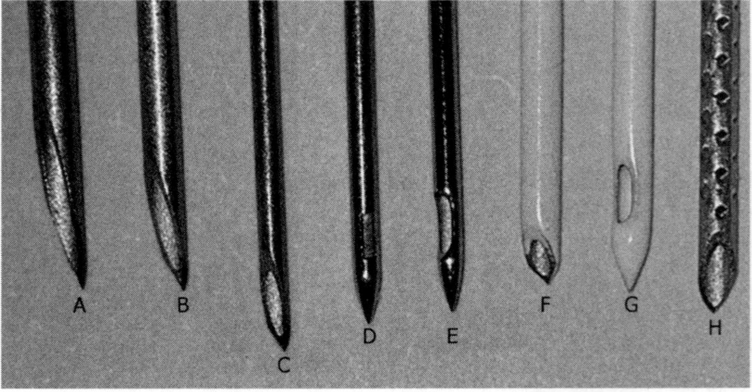

Needle tips for comparison: **A.** 21 G Hypodermic needle. Spinal needles: **B.** 22 G Quincke, **C.** 25 G Quincke, **D.** 25 G Whitacre, **E.** 25 G Sprotte. Peripheral nerve block needles: **F.** 21 G Locoplex (*Vygon, France*), Teflon coated, **G.** 22 G Pencil point Polymedic (*te me na SAS, France*), Teflon coated, **H.** 22 G SonoPlex (*Pajunk, Germany*), proprietary NanoLine coating over embossed pattern.

Diagram below is of different epidural needles

- 4, 16G Tuohy needle;
- 5, 17G Barkers spinal needle;
- 6, Large gauge spinal needle;
- 7, 18G Crawford needle

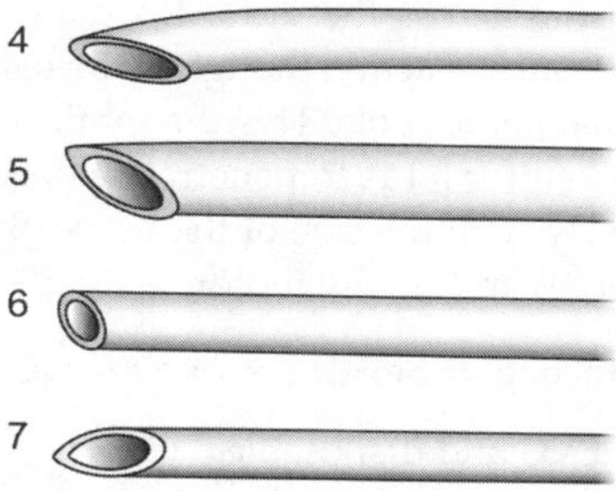

4

5

6

7

Table 1 below shows analgesics administered epidurally with their concentration, onset and duration in a fixed 20 mL volume.

Table 1: Comparative onset times and analgesic durations of local anesthetics administered epidurally in 20- to 30-mL volumes

Drug	Concentration (%)	Onset (min)	Duration (min)	
			Plain	1:200,000 Epinephrine
2-Chloroprocaine	3	10–15	45–60	60–90
Lidocaine	2	15	80–120	120–180
Mepivacaine	2	15	90–140	140–200
Bupivacaine	0.5–0.75	20	165–225	180–240
Etidocaine	1	15	120–200	150–225
Ropivacaine	0.75–1.0	15–20	140–180	150–200
Levobupivacaine	0.5–0.75	15–20	150–225	150–240

Table 2 below shows dose, block height, onset times and duration of spinal anesthetics:

Table 2: Dose, block height, onset times, and duration of commonly used spinal anesthetics

Local anesthetic mixture	Dose (mg)		Duration (min)		Onset (min)
	Till T10	Till T4	Plain	Epinephrine (0.2 mg)	
Lidocaine 5% (with/without dextrose)	40–75	75–100	60–150	20–50%	3–5
Mepivacaine 1.5% (no dextrose)	30–45	60–80	120–180	—	2–4
Chloroprocaine 3% (with/without dextrose)	30–40	40–60	40–90	N/R	2–4
Bupivacine 0.5–0.75% (no dextrose)	10–15	12–20	130–230	20–50%	4–8
Levobupivacaine 0.5% (no dextrose) (ref B)	10–15	12–20	140–230	—	4–8
Ropivacaine 0.5–1% (with/without dextrose)	12–18	18–25	80–210	—	3–8

From above mentioned tables, it is evident that both spinal and epidural anesthesia does not require same concentration.

- ❑ Mechanism of action of epidural anesthesia produced by LA is thought to be the result of a combination of three potential mechanisms.
  1. LA may diffuse into the paravertebral areas through the intervertebral foramina and block nerves distal to their dural sheaths, resulting in multiple paravertebral blocks.

2. Diffusion of LA across the dura into the subarachnoid space → acts on nerve roots.
3. After diffusion across the dura, LA may act directly on the spinal cord.

- The primary sites of action thought to be responsible for epidural anesthesia produced by LA are the spinal nerve roots. This theory fits the observed gravity effect on the block.
- The time taken for a LA to penetrate a nerve trunk and the concentration of drug achieved vary inversely with the size of the nerve. Sympathetic nerves are affected first, followed by sensory nerves and finally motor.

7. About endotracheal tube, all are true *except*:

a. Is made of PVC and disposable
b. Can be introduced through oral or nasal route
c. High volume low pressure preferred
d. Rubber tubes used in children
e. Un-cuffed tubes preferred in children and made up from red rubber
f. More tendency to go to right bronchus thereby decreasing left lung ventilation

Ans. d. Rubber tubes used in children and e. Un-cuffed tubes preferred in children and made up from red rubber *Ref: Ward's Anaesthetic Equipment 6th/ed p160*

Explanation

- ***Option a: is true.*** Preferred materials for Endotracheal tubes (ETT) Silicone > Polyurethane > PVC > Red rubber > Natural latex.
- ***Option b: is true.***
- ***Option c: is true.*** Preferred cuffs for ETT- High volume (total of 20 cc) low pressure (HVLP) > Low volume high pressure (LVHP).
  - Other types of cuffs are: Foam cuffs, Laser flex double contoured cuffs.
  - According to shape of Cuffs: Cylindrical > Conical > Globular.
- ***Options d and e: are false.*** *Tubes are made of PVC not red rubber;* Previously un-cuffed tubes were preferred in children in fear of tracheal mucosal ischemia but nowadays it has been seen that cuffed tubes with HVLP cuffs produce lesser tracheal mucosal ischemia. But total outer diameter of the tube increases because of the cuff. So, still now un-cuffed tubes are being used these days.
- ***Option f: is true.*** As right bronchus is in 20–30° from midline in relation to left one which is 40–50°, ETT tends to go into right bronchus. If it enters right bronchus it will only ventilate the right lung decreasing the left lung ventilation.
- These days mostly PVC tubes are being used.
- Previously red rubber tubes were being used but not preferred these days because it is opaque, inadequate cleaning and foreign bodies within the lumen of the tube might be overlooked. Repeated sterilization causes degradation, with the potential for weakening leading to kinking or rupture. The materials themselves are potentially allergenic and irritant when used for long periods, being implicated in the development of laryngeal granulomata.
- Currently, plastics (PVC and more recently polyurethane) and to a lesser extent, silicone rubber, have replaced red rubber and natural latex as primary materials for the following reasons:
  - They are non-irritant and are now inexpensive enough to allow single-patient use and hence sterilization at manufacture.
  - As the material is usually clear, foreign bodies and blockages may be seen more easily.
  - Manufacturing tolerances are much better with plastics, so that there is much less variation in the size of the lumen (most important in neonatal tracheal tubes).

- ❑ Cuffs of rubber tubes are usually thick and require high intra-cuff pressures to inflate them; inadvertent over-distension of the cuff may result in this pressure being transmitted to the tracheal mucosa with a risk of mucosal ischemia or necrosis during prolonged use.
- ❑ As a standard practice high volume low pressure cuff tubes are being used to prevent tracheal mucosal ischemia and low volume high pressure cuff tubes are abandoned.

8. Ventilator setting depends on:

a. Age b. Gender
c. Weight d. Height
e. Clinical condition of the patient

Ans. a. Age; c. Weight; d. Height and e. Clinical condition of the patient

Ref: The ICU Book by Paul L Marino 4th/ed p498

EXPLANATION

Ventilator settings does not vary as per gender of the patient.

For ventilator settings, the basic parameters to be considered are:

- ❑ **Mode:** Depends on
  - Clinical condition and
  - Age
- ❑ **Tidal volume/target airway pressure:** Depends on
  - Clinical condition
  - Weight [Ideal body weight (IBW) can be calculated from height]
- ❑ **Respiratory rate:** Depends on
  - Clinical condition and
  - Age
- ❑ **PEEP** (Positive end expiratory pressure): Depends on
  - Clinical condition
- ❑ **Pressure support above PEEP:** Depends on
  - Mode and
  - Clinical condition

Just have a note on ideal body weight calculation:

IBW (kg) males:
50 + 2.3 (height in inches – 60)
or 50 + 0.91 (height in cm – 152.4)
IBW (kg) females:
45.5 + 2.3 (height in inches – 60)
or 45.5 + 0.91 (height in cm – 152.4)

JIPMER Pattern Based

1. Inhalational anesthetic that can be used for induction:

a. Sevoflurane b. Desflurane
c. Enflurane d. Nitrous oxide

Ans. a. Sevoflurane

Ref: Miller's 8th p640; Goodman and Gilman's the Pharmacological Basis of Therapeutics, 12th/ed p530

EXPLANATION

Option a: Sevoflurane with a comparative higher MAC and sweet smell. Ideal for inhalational induction. Halothane also has similar property, so it can also be used as induction agent.

Option d: As MAC of Nitrous is 104, even if we use 100% nitrous patient can not be induced.

Options b and c: Desflurane and enflurane are pungent smelling and not used during induction. These may result in choking and breath holding while induction.

Agent	MAC[a] (vol %)	MAC_{AWAKE}[b] (Vol %)	Vapor pressure (mm Hg, 20°C)	Partition coefficient at 37°C			% Recovered as metabolities
				Blood / Gas	Brain / Blood	Fat / Blood	
Halothane	0.75	0.41	243	2.3	2.9	51	20
Isoflurane	1.2	0.4	250	1.4	2.6	45	0.2
Enflurane	1.6	0.4	175	1.8	1.4	36	2.4
Sevoflurane	2	0.6	160	0.65	1.7	48	3
Desflurane	6	2.4	664	0.45	1.3	27	0.02
N_2O[c]	105	60.0	Gas	0.47	1.1	2.3	0.004
Xe	71	32.6	Gas	0.12	—	—	0

[a]MAC (minimum alveolar concentration) values are expressed as vol% the percentage of the atmosphere that is anesthetic. A value of MAC > 100% means that hyperbaric conditions would be required.
[b]MAC_{AWAKE} is the concentration at which appropriate responses to commands are lost.
[c]EC_{50} for memory supression (vol %): isoflurane, 0.24; N_2O, 52.5; values not available for other agents.

2. Postpartum lady after 48 hours of cesarean section, suffering from headache and signs of meningism. Headache gets relieved on lying down. Immediate treatment would be:

a. Epidural blood patch
b. Do lumbar puncture
c. Foot end elevation
d. Sumatriptan

Ans. a. Epidural blood patch *Ref: Morgan 5th/ed p969*

EXPLANATION

As patient has signs of meningism, the treatment would be epidural blood patch.

The Lybecker classification of severity for PDPH:

1. Mild PDPH (Score 1)
   - Postural headache with slight restriction of daily activities.
   - Not bedridden.
   - No associated symptoms.
   - Responds well to non-opiate analgesics (Paracetamol, NSAID, Caffeine).
2. Moderate PDPH (Score 2)
   - Postural headache with significant restriction of daily activities.
   - Bedridden part of the day associated symptoms may or may not present.
   - Requires the addition of opiate derivatives.
3. Severe PDPH (Score 3)

- Postural headache with complete restriction of daily activities.
- Bedridden all day associated symptoms present (photophobia, diplopia, tinnitus, nausea, vomiting).
- Not responsive to the above conservative management.

If the question was like this:

A lady after delivering by c section develops headache which increases on sitting and decreases on lying down. What needs to be done?

a. Lumbar puncture
b. Foot end elevation
c. Epidural blood patch
d. NSAIDs

Ans. d. NSAIDs

3. Eight hours after spinal anesthesia, 28-year-old lady complaining of backache and progressive weakness of both lower limbs. Suspected cause:

a. ASA syndrome
b. Intraprocedural neurologic injury
c. Neuraxial hematoma formation
d. Epidural abcess

Ans. c. Neuraxial hematoma formation *Ref: Morgan 5th/ed, p970*

Explanation

Early development of backache and weakness of lower limbs suggests development of Epidural hematoma.

- ❑ *Options a and b:* ASA syndrome and intraprocedural neurologic injury develops suddenly within 6 hours.
- ❑ Epidural hematoma develops after 6 hours and needs surgical decompression within 8 to 12 hours.
- ❑ *Option d:* Epidural abscess develops after a median time of 5 days.

4. Minimum alveolar concentration (MAC) denotes:

a. Efficacy
b. Potency
c. Solubility
d. Diffusibility

Ans. b. Potency *Ref: Miller's 8th p640*

Explanation

MAC is an indicator of gas potency. The blood:gas partition coefficient is an indicator of solubility, which affects the rate of induction and emergence; it is NOT related to MAC.

MAC: Alveolar concentration of a gas at which 50% of subjects do not respond to surgical incision.

MAC of Inhaled Anesthetics

Gas	Blood: Gas partition coefficient	MAC*
Halothane	2.4	0.75%
Enflurane	1.9	1.7%
Isoflurane	1.4	1.2%
Sevoflurane	0.65	2.0%
N_2O	0.47	104%
Desiflurane	0.42	6.0%

*MAC values for adults 36–49 years old.

Important points:

- ❑ Remarkably consistent across species.
- ❑ MAC is a population average; not a true predictor of an individual's response.
- ❑ MAC is an ED50 concentration. The ED95 is ± 25%, so at 1.3 MAC, 95% of patients will not respond to incision.
- ❑ MAC values are additive (e.g. 0.5 MAC isoflurane + 0.5 MAC N_2O = 1 MAC)
  - ▪ MAC-Awake (a.k.a. MAC-Aware): The MAC necessary to prevent response to verbal/tactile stimulation. – Volatiles: ~0.4 MAC; N_2O: ~0.6 MAC
  - ▪ MAC-BAR: The MAC necessary to "blunt the autonomic response" to a noxious stimulus – ~1.6 MAC
  - ▪ MAC-intubation: The MAC necessary to prevent laryngeal response to "endotracheal intubation" – ~1.3 MAC

5. All true *except*:

a. Patient on warfarin is contraindicated to LP
b. LMWH should be stopped 24 hours prior to LP
c. IV Heparin should be stopped 6 hours before LP
d. Aspirin is not a contraindication to lumbar puncture

Ans. c. IV Heparin should be stopped 6 hours before LP *Ref: Miller's 8th p1693*

Explanation

Low dose aspirin < 150 mg per day aspirin is not a contraindication to LP.

Drug	Time to stop before LP	Time after LP to start anticoagulation
Heparin	2–4 hours	2 hours
LMWH	24 hours (Therapeutic)	4 hours
Fondaparinux	72 hours	12 hours
Rivaroxaban	72 hours	6 hours
Dabigatran	120 hours	6 hours
Apixaban	72 hours	6 hours
Prasugrel	7–10 days	6 hours
Ticagrelor	5–7 days	6 hours
Clopidogrel	7 days	2 hours

Radiodiagnosis and Radiotherapy

Author: Jyotsana Priya, Co-author: Anjuna R

AIIMS May 2017

1. A young female came with complaints of bone pain and abdominal cramps. Her family members suggested that she is behaving abnormally over few days. Attending physician made a provisional diagnosis. Next best investigation to arrive at a definitive diagnosis will be:

a. USG
b. ^{99m}Tc SestaMIBI
c. FDG PET
d. CT

Ans. b. ^{99m}Tc SestaMIBI *Ref: Textbook of Radiology and Imaging by David Sutton 7th/ed p1507,1510,1514*

Explanation

- The condition described above is hyperparathyroidism, which presents clinically with "stones, bones, groans, moans", i.e. renal stones, bone and joint pain, abdominal pain and psychosis.
- In 80% cases, primary hyperparathyroidism results from a single adenoma.
- Imaging is used to localize parathyroid adenomas, hyperplastic glands or ectopic sources of excessive parathyroid hormone secretion.
- **The preferred radiopharmaceutical for parathyroid imaging is** ^{99m}Tc- **m**ethoxy**i**so**b**utyl**i**sonitrile (MIBI).
- *(Option a)* USG: Normal parathyroid glands have lower reflectivity than normal thyroid and the echogenic capsule will separate one from the other. Calcification is rare in parathyroid adenomas but may be seen in hyperplastic parathyroid glands and in parathyroid carcinomas. Cystic changes may be seen. 90% of adenomas are hypervascular.
- *(Option d)* CT can identify ectopic parathyroid adenomas in the neck or upper mediastinum.

2. A 55-year-old man came for an ultrasound to renew his medical insurance. On ultrasound examination, a complex cyst was found in right kidney. On contrast enhanced CT (CECT) examination, the cyst is solid, exophytic and encroaching on the adjacent structure. Most likely diagnosis is:

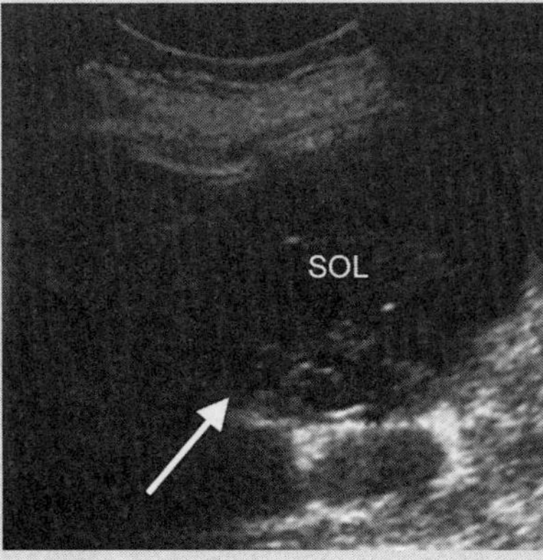

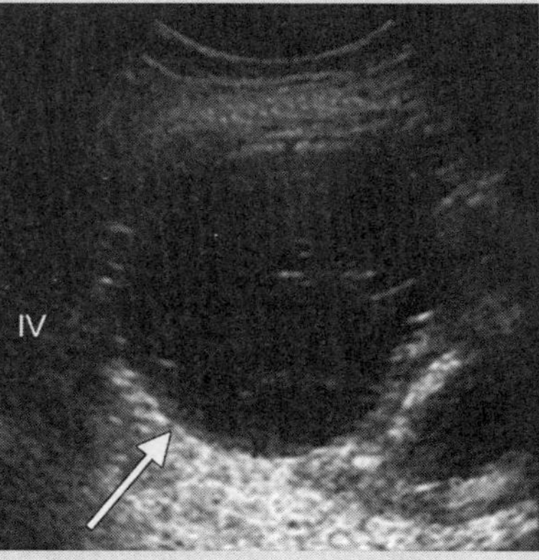

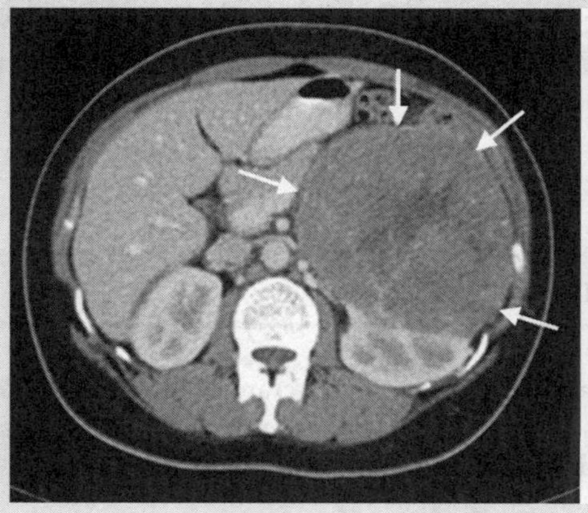

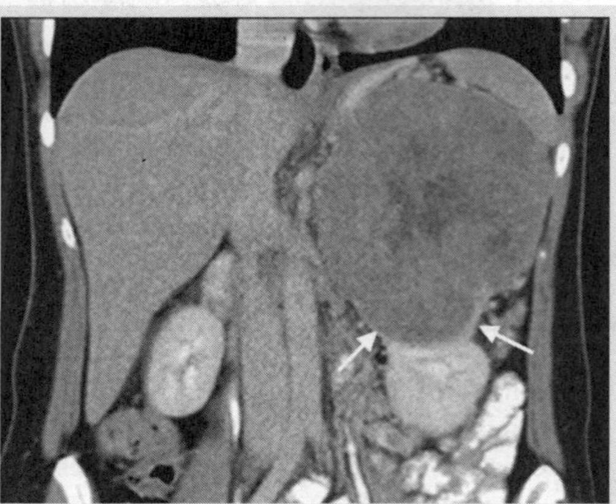

a. Angiomyolipoma
b. Parapelvic cyst
c. Renal cell carcinoma
d. Simple renal cyst

Ans. c. Renal cell carcinoma *Ref: CT and MRI of the Whole Body by John R. Haaga, p1875,1912*

EXPLANATION

The Bosniak classification system for renal cysts is as follows:

Category	Description
I	Simple cyst (0–20 HU attenuation on CECT) without septa, calcification or solid components. No further evaluation needed.
II	Cyst with few thin hairline septa/fine calcification in wall or septa. High density cyst <3 cm size which do not enhance are also included in this group: No further evaluation needed.
IIF	Cyst with multiple hairline septa or minimal smooth thickening of wall or septa, with thick, nodular calcification but without measurable enhancement. Non-enhancing high density cysts >3 cm are also included in this category. Require follow up studies.
III	Cysts with thickened irregular or smooth walls or septa with measurable enhancement. Require surgical removal
IV	Complex cysts with enhancing soft tissue component. Require surgical removal.

- In the case described above, the lesion is an exophytic complex cystic lesion on ultrasound with enhancing solid components on contrast enhanced CT, suggesting Bosniak grade IV cyst. This is highly in favor of malignancy. Hence, ***option c*** (renal cell carcinoma) is the right option here.

Arrows in the above figures indicate pseudocapsule of Renal Cell Carcinoma

- ***(Options b and d)*** are suggestive of simple benign renal cysts (Bosniak grade I) and hence are excluded.

- (*Option a*) (Angiomyolipoma) is predominantly solid lesion and contains fat, blood vessels and smooth muscle. It is seen in association with tuberous sclerosis. The diagnosis is made on CT by detection of intralesional fatty tissue (attenuation of -10 HU or lower). On ultrasound the fatty areas appear hyperechoic.
- Also the clinical findings given in question like, male sex, 55-year-old and incidental finding on routine investigation also favor RCC.

3. Below is radioactive testing scan for thyroid pathology. Which of the following is the most probable diagnosis?

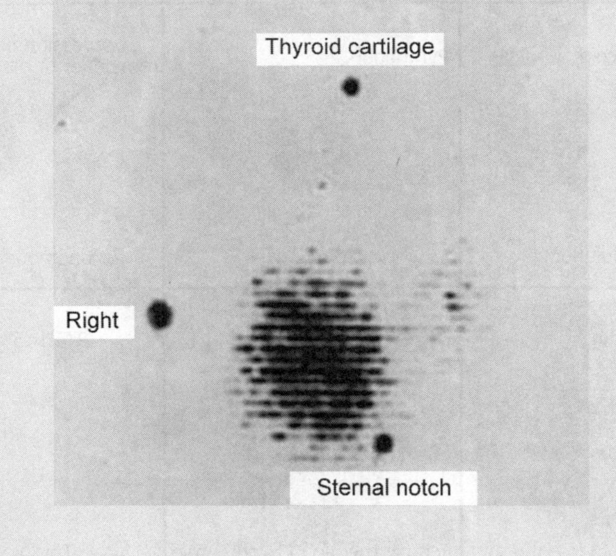

a. Lateral aberrant thyroid
b. Hypersecretory adenoma
c. Grave's disease
d. Papillary carcinoma of thyroid

Ans. b. Hypersecretory adenoma *Ref: Grainger & Allison's Diagnostic Radiology 5th/ed ch7, Essentials of Nuclear Medicine imaging. Fred A Milter. p605*

EXPLANATION

In the given scan right lobe uptakes the isotope tracer while left lobe does not, there is no ectopic thyroid tissue hence Lateral aberrant thyroid and retrosternal extension can be ruled out. There is one single hot nodule suppressing the uptake of the remaining gland, hence Toxic nodule/ Hypersecretory adenoma.

Option d: In malignancy there is cold nodule.

- Tc 99m (Technetium) is the isotope of choice for diagnosis of thyroid disorders as it is cheap, involves less radiation, less time 20 minutes, and 99mTc half life is 6 hours.

Note: Only absolute indication in modern days is Autonomous toxic nodule in toxic thyroid showing hot nodule

The image on next page shows radioactive scans in various thyroid pathologies.

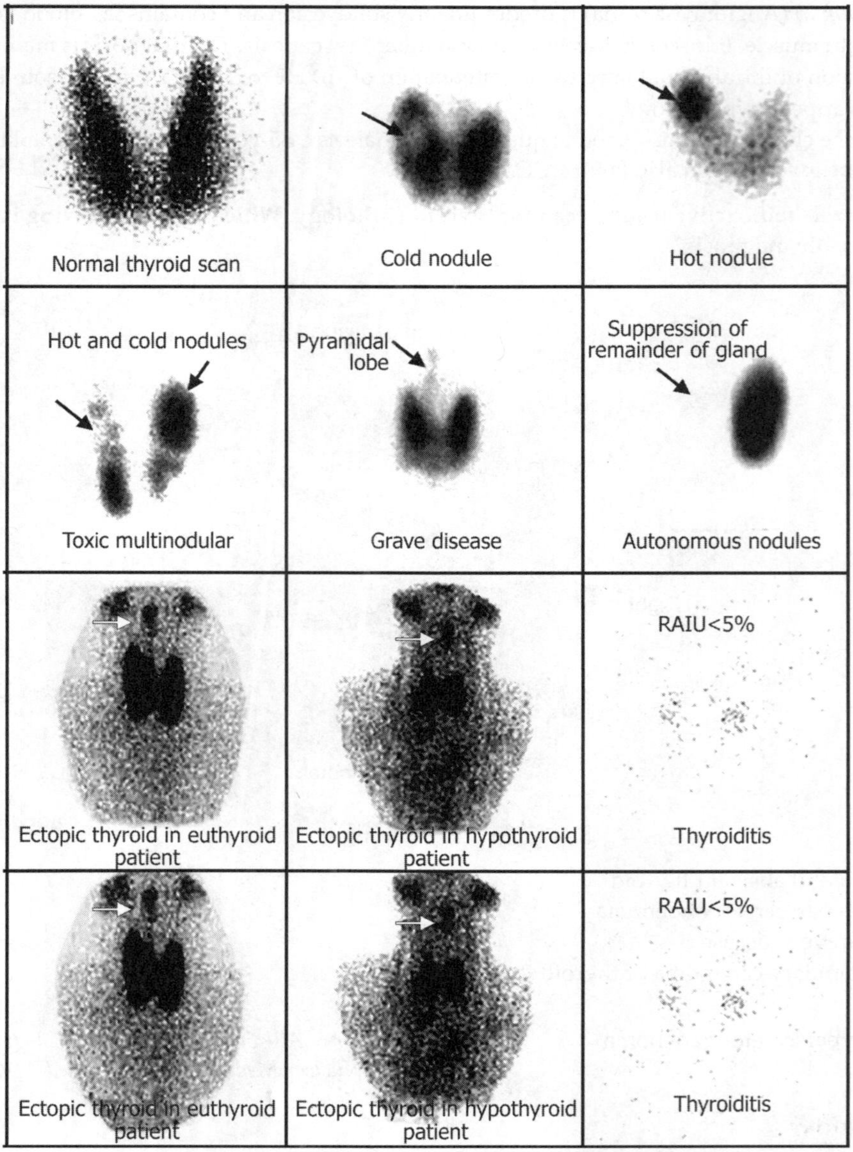

Normal thyroid scan	Cold nodule	Hot nodule
Hot and cold nodules Toxic multinodular	Pyramidal lobe Grave disease	Suppression of remainder of gland Autonomous nodules
Ectopic thyroid in euthyroid patient	Ectopic thyroid in hypothyroid patient	RAIU<5% Thyroiditis
Ectopic thyroid in euthyroid patient	Ectopic thyroid in hypothyroid patient	RAIU<5% Thyroiditis

4. Which of the following is not seen in the following chest X-ray?

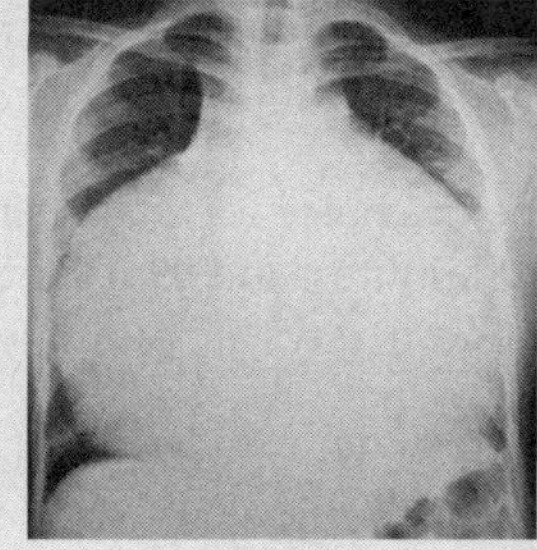

a. Decreased cardiac output
b. Narrow vascular pedicle
c. Decrease pulmonary blood flow
d. Pulmonary venous hypertension

Ans. d. Pulmonary venous hypertension

Ref: Textbook of Radiology and Imaging by David Sutton 7th/ed p332,333

EXPLANATION

- The above figure shows gross cardiomegaly with water bottle appearance, suggestive of (s/o) gross pericardial effusion.
- **Pericardial effusion** is suspected when there is diffuse cardiac silhouette enlargement without specific chamber enlargement, along with a narrow vascular pedicle ***(option b)***.
- Filling of the retrosternal space, enlargement of normal cardiac borders, development of "flask" configuration seen in larger effusions.
- In the lateral projection, *'epicardial fat pad' sign* or *'oreo-cookie sign'* is diagnostic of pericardial disease. This is positive when the anterior pericardial stripe, bordered by the epicardial fat and mediastinal fat on either side, is seen to be thicker than 2 mm.
- When intrapericardial pressure exceeds intracardiac pressure, diastolic filling of both ventricles decreases, leading to decreased pulmonary blood flow ***(option c)*** and cardiac output ***(option a)***.
- Impaired right heart filling leads to congestion of SVC, IVC and azygos vein. However, in gross pericardial effusion, pulmonary venous hypertension is not described and lung fields are usually oligemic ***(option d)***.
- Pulmonary venous hypertension is typically seen in cardiogenic pulmonary edema and features include cephalization of pulmonary veins, interstitial edema in the form of Kerley lines and alveolar edema.

5. A patient presented with mucopurulent sputum and fever. His WBC count was 28000. The chest X-ray was as follows. The microorganism causing pneumonia is:

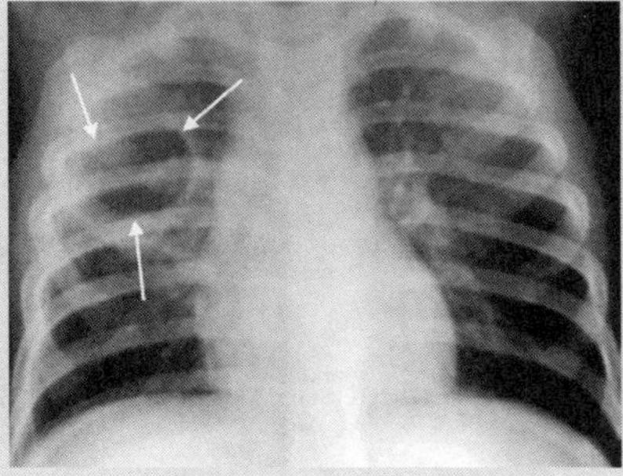

a. *Staphylococcus aureus*
b. *Streptococcus pneumoniae*
c. *Chlamydia*
d. *Aspergillus fumigatus*

Ans. a. *Staphylococcus aureus*

Ref: Thoracic Imaging by W. Richard Webb, p384

EXPLANATION

- In the above chest radiograph (frontal view), there is a cystic lesion located in the upper and mid zones of right lung, with thin walls, arrows indicate wall of pneumatocele. This is the classic appearance of pneumatocele.
- ***(Option a)*** *S. aureus* is the **most common organism causing pneumatoceles.**
  - It usually causes a bronchopneumonia, with homogeneous or patchy consolidation, which may often be multifocal.

- It causes pneumatoceles, especially in children.
- Pneumatoceles, unlike abscesses, appear as thin-walled cystic structures that may contain air-fluid levels. The inner wall of a pneumatocele is usually thin and regular, unlike that of a pulmonary abscess.
- Pneumatoceles tend to resolve spontaneously in weeks or a few months following infection. The **next most common organism causing pneumatocele is** *Klebsiella*.

- ❑ ***(Option b)*** *Streptococcus pneumonia* is the **most common cause of pneumonia associated with Gram-positive cocci**. It usually causes lobar pneumonia with *air bronchogram*. *Strep. pneumonia* is a very rare cause of pneumatocele.
- ❑ ***(Option c)*** *Chlamydia* causes atypical pneumonia/ interstitial pneumonia seen as *reticular opacities on chest radiograph*.
- ❑ ***(Option d)*** *Aspergillus fumigatus* causes aspergilloma which is seen as a *fungal ball in a pre-existing cavity*, with crescent of air above **('air crescent sign')**.

6. Patient admitted with complaints of abdominal pain. Plain X-ray abdomen erect showed the following findings. What is your diagnosis?

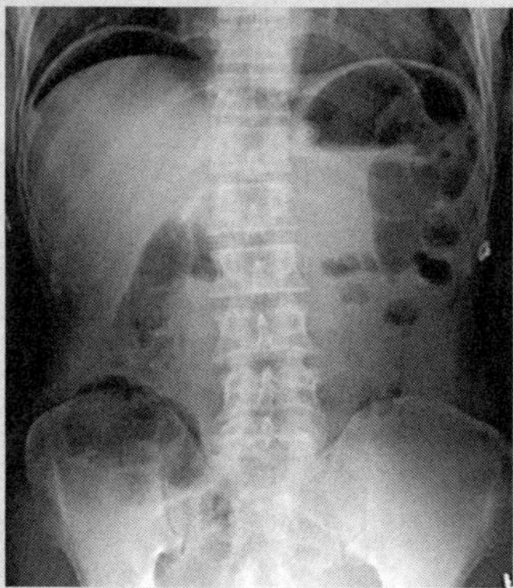

a. Pneumoperitoneum
b. Pneumothorax
c. Intestinal obstruction
d. Subdiaphragmatic abscess

Ans. a. Pneumoperitoneum *Ref: Textbook of Radiology and Imaging by David Sutton 7th/ed p666*

EXPLANATION

- ❑ This is an erect X-ray abdomen of a patient showing **free air under the right hemidiaphragm**, s/o pneumoperitoneum.
- ❑ Erect chest radiograph is superior to the erect abdominal film for the demonstration of pneumoperitoneum. In patients who are unfit to sit or stand for an erect film, left lateral decubitus is the projection of choice to show a small pneumoperitoneum. Patient should be in position for 10 min before the film is taken in erect or decubitus position, for it takes this time for free gas to rise to the highest point in the abdomen.
- ❑ Only in 75–80% of perforations is free gas under diaphragm demonstrable in erect film. 56% of patients with a pneumoperitoneum may have free gas detectable on a supine radiograph.
- ❑ CT is the **most sensitive method for the detection of peritoneal free gas**.
- ❑ Findings of pneumoperitoneum on supine radiograph:
  - Collection in the right upper quadrant adjacent to the liver and lying mainly in the subhepatic space and the hepatorenal fossa (Morison's pouch), and visible as an oval or linear collection of gas.

- Visualization of the outer as well as the inner wall of a loop of bowel (**Rigler's sign**) is a valuable indication of pneumoperitoneum.
- Small triangular collections of gas between loops of bowel.
- Relatively large amounts of gas may accumulate beneath the diaphragm (the **'cupola' sign**) or in the center of the abdomen over a fluid collection (the **'football' sign**).
- Falciform ligament, medial and lateral umbilical ligaments and the urachus can occasionally be identified when relatively large amounts of gas are present. Free gas may also be identified in the fissure for the ligamentum teres.

7. A patient presented with fever and pain abdomen. He has history of diarrhea for several months. Abdominal X-ray is shown below. What is the most probable diagnosis?

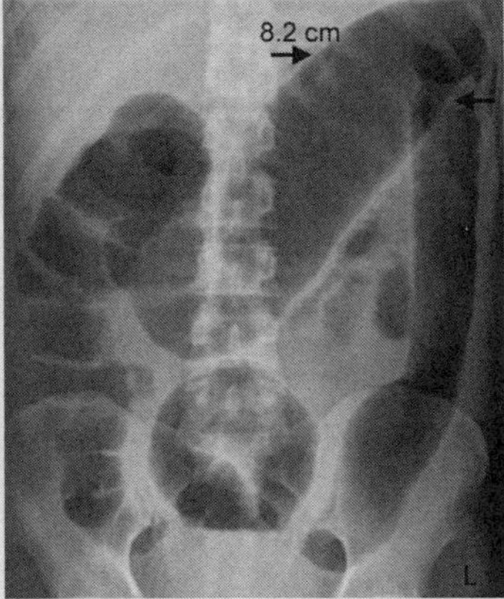

a. Pneumatosis intestinalis
b. Toxic megacolon
c. Volvulus
d. Intestinal perforation

Ans. b. Toxic megacolon

Ref: Textbook of Radiology and Imaging by David Sutton 7th/ed p646,647,653,664

EXPLANATION

- This is the X-ray abdomen of patient showing dilated colon, with maximum diameter of 8.2 cm at level of distal transverse colon (as per marking). Also there is lack of haustra in transverse, descending and sigmoid colon. This is characteristic of toxic megacolon, an acute complication in ulcerative colitis.
- Ulcerative colitis is characterized by relapsing and remitting proctitis. The rectum is always affected but proximal spread occurs in a continuous fashion in approximately two-thirds of patients, half of whom will have total colitis at the time of presentation.
- Attacks are characterized by bloody diarrhea with or without constitutional symptoms.
- Plain abdominal radiography is used to detect acute toxic dilatation/megacolon (diagnosed when transverse colonic diameter exceeds 5.5 cm).
- Transverse colon is the **segment most often dilated on plain films**, due to the patient's supine position. The haustra will be effaced or blunted, indicating that ulceration is transmural, causing neuromuscular degeneration. There will be no or little residue. The mucosal line is irregular, producing so-called '**mucosal islands**' because of adjacent mucosal ulceration and sloughing. The colon has a consistency akin to wet blotting paper, so patients are at risk of perforation and ultimately death.

- *(Option c)* An inverted 'U' without haustra or **coffee bean sign** suggests **sigmoid volvulus** and its apex frequently overlaps the transverse colon, with inferior converging margins towards left. There may be considerable proximal colonic gas and possibly small bowel gas but there is no rectal gas.
- The cecum is often ectopic in **cecal volvulus** (e.g. in the left upper quadrant), with inferior converging margins towards right and well preserved haustra. Distal colonic gas not visualized.
- *(Option a)* **Pneumatosis coli** (pneumatosis cystoides intestinalis) is defined by multiple gas-filled cysts that lie submucosally or subserosally; overlying mucosa is normal. The idiopathic condition is rare but may be confused with life-threatening colonic disease. The small bowel is also affected. Pneumatosis may be secondary to bowel necrosis, for example, necrotising enterocolitis or mesenteric thrombosis. It can also follow endoscopy or chronic obstructive pulmonary disease. Cysts are seen on plain films and are commonest in sigmoid and descending colon.
- *(Option d)* ***Intestinal perforation***: refer to question above.

PGI May 2017

1. Diffuse axonal injury detected by:

a. MRI with diffusion weighted imaging
b. DSA
c. Doppler
d. CT
e. MR elastography

Ans. a. MRI with diffusion weighted imaging and d. CT

Ref: Osborn's Brain: Imaging, Pathology and Anatomy p37,38

Explanation

- MR findings of diffuse axonal injury.
  - As most DAIs are nonhemorrhagic, **T1 scans** are often normal, especially in the early stages.
  - **T2WI** may show hyperintense foci in the subcortical white matter and corpus callosum. Multiple lesions are the rule, and a combination of DAI and contusions or hematomas is very common. T2* scans (T2* = a special sequence in MRI called gradient echo sequence, which detects calcification and bleed specifically) are very sensitive to the microbleeds of DAI and typically show multifocal ovoid and linear hypointensities.
  - **DWI** (Diffusion weighted MRI) may show restricted diffusion, particularly within the corpus callosum.
  - **DTI** tractography (Diffusion tensor MRI) may be useful in depicting white matter disruption.
  - **MR** elastography ***(option e)*** has been speculated to have a role in pathogenesis of DAI. However, no established role in diagnosis of DAI is described in literature.
- *(Option d)* Initial NECT is often normal or minimally abnormal. Mild diffuse brain swelling with sulcal effacement may be present. A few small round or ovoid subcortical hemorrhages may be visible.

JIPMER Pattern Based

1. Scalloping of edge of sigmoid colon on barium enema is seen in:

a. Pseudomembranous colitis
b. Intussusception
c. Ulcerative colitis
d. Ischemic colitis

Ans. c. Ulcerative colitis

Ref: Textbook of Gastrointestinal Radiology, Gore and Levine 2nd/ed p1114-1116

EXPLANATION

Features of ulcerative colitis on barium enema are as follows:

Acute ulcerative colitis	Chronic ulcerative colitis
• Fine mucosal granularity (due to edema) • Scalloping of edges of colon, especially sigmoid colon • Collar button ulcers • Pseudopolyps • Toxic megacolon	• Lead pipe colon due to loss of haustrations • Shortened and narrowed colon • Backwash ileitis • Thickened rectal valve • Widened presacral space (>1.5 cm at S4 vertebral level) • Benign stricture • Colorectal carcinoma

- Sign seen on barium enema in other options given in question is as follows:
  - *(Option a)* Pseudomembranous colitis → '**Accordion sign**'.
  - *(Option b)* Intussusception → '**Pincer sign**'.
  - *(Option d)* Ischemic colitis → '**Thumb printing sign**'.
- **Scalloping of edge of sigmoid colon can also be seen in** cases of large pelvic masses or pseudomyxoma peritonei causing extrinsic compression on sigmoid colon.

2. Which is the best modality to assess cardiac viability?

a. SPECT
b. Dobutamine stress echocardiography
c. PET scan
d. Cardiac MRI

Ans. d. Cardiac MRI

Ref: Ahmed Talib, Caroline Cheese, Iqbal Elfigih et al Assessment of Myocardial Viability: A Review of Current Non-invasive Imaging Techniques. ICF Journal 2014. Vol 3; 113-117

EXPLANATION

- The options given above are all modalities to assess myocardial viability. However, the **most widely accepted imaging technique** now is cardiac MRI with a sensitivity of 95%, followed by PET scan with a sensitivity of 92%.
- *(Option c)* For the assessment of viability, N-13 Ammonia or Rubidium-82 is used as perfusion agent and F-18 fluoro-2- deoxy-D-glucose (F-18 FDG) as metabolic tracer in PET scan.
- *(Option a)* Single-photon emission computed tomography (SPECT) involves the administration of a radioactive tracer such as thallium-201 or Technetium Tc-99m, with ^{99m}Tc Sestamibi being the **most widely used in clinical practice**.
- *(Option b)* Dobutamine stress echocardiography is the **initial imaging modality to assess myocardial viability** routinely.

3. Best imaging modality in detection of patients with renal hypertension is:

a. Renal Doppler
b. MR angiography
c. CT angiography
d. Digital subtraction angiography (DSA)

Ans. d. Digital subtraction angiography (DSA)

Ref: Kjell Tullus, Derek J. Roebuck, Clare A. McLaren, Stephen D. Marks. Imaging in the Evaluation of Renovascular Disease. Pediatr Nephrol. 2010 Jun; 25(6):1049–1056.

- DSA provides images of the lumens of the renal arteries and their branches with the best spatial and temporal resolution and is the platform for endovascular intervention. Hence DSA is considered **gold standard in evaluation of renovascular hypertension**.
- ***(Option a)*** Ultrasound doppler is well tolerated, safe and easy to perform. However, sensitivity of abnormality detection has been found to be less in most studies.
- ***(Option b)*** MR Angiography performed using gadolinium-based contrast agents has inadequate spatial resolution, problems related to movement artefacts and gadolinium toxicity.
- ***(Option c)*** CTA offers better spatial resolution than does MRA, but at the price of the patient's exposure to ionizing radiation.

4. New emerging technology in detection of metastases:

a. SPECT
b. PET/CT
c. Bone scan
d. MRI

Ans. b. PET/CT

Ref: GJ Mallarajapatna, Rajul Rastogi, Fusion Imaging: The Current Trends. JIMSA 2013 Vol. 26;73-5.

Explanation

- Latest trend in oncological imaging is towards fusion or hybrid imaging using combination of two modalities (like PET and MRI), the most widely used techniques being PET/CT and PET/MRI. This has led to **better detection of metastases using any of the techniques alone**.
- F18-FDG used for detection of osseous metastases is more sensitive than MDP bone scans ***(option c)***. It gives an extra-advantage of detecting occult primary and associated visceral and unsuspected metastases in addition to osseous metastases.
- PET-MRI has applications mainly in head and neck imaging especially CNS tumors.
- Other emerging hybrid modalities are SPECT/CT and SPECT/MRI.
- **SPECT:** **S**ingle-**ph**oton **e**mission **c**omputed **t**omography is a nuclear medicine tomographic imaging technique using gamma rays.

5. Saw-tooth appearance on barium enema is seen in:

a. Carcinoma colon
b. Ulcerative colitis
c. Crohn's disease
d. Diverticular disease

Ans. d. Diverticular disease

Ref: Textbook of Radiology and Imaging by David Sutton 7th/ed p645,646.

Explanation

- **Diverticulosis** describes the mucosal herniations through vascular entry sites into pericolic fat, often between the mesenteric and antimesenteric taeniae. **Diverticulitis** implies superimposed inflammation, whereas the term **diverticular disease** encompasses both concepts.
- Diverticula themselves appear as flask-like or rounded outpouchings on barium enema. When seen enface they produce ring shadows. Differentiation from a polyp is a common problem but the definitive signs are projection beyond bowel wall and presence of fluid level within it. Muscular changes result in **concertina/serrated/saw tooth appearance *(answer)***.
- **Hinchey classification** is used in grading of diverticular disease.
- Note the saw-tooth appearance in diverticulosis in below image of barium enema:

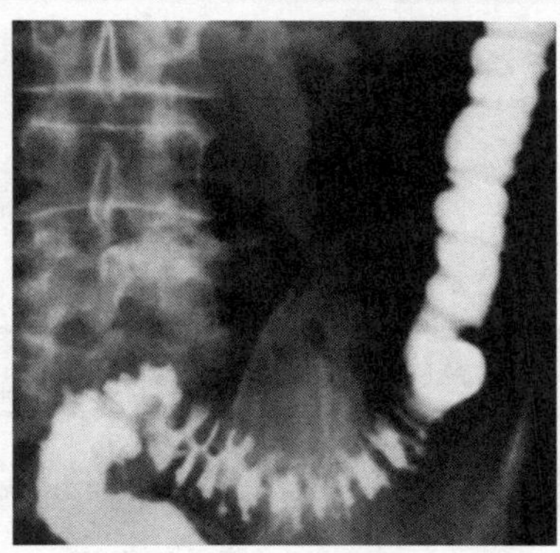

- *(Option a)* In annular carcinoma colon, the sign seen on barium enema is **'Napkin ring sign'**.
- *(Option b)* In ulcerative colitis, the appearance on barium enema is **Pipe stem colon** due to lack of haustrations in colon.
- *(Option c)* In Crohn's disease, the sign seen on barium enema is **'String sign of Cantor'** due to thin column of barium in strictured segment.

6. Kidney cortical scars not seen by:

a. DMSA
b. DTPA
c. Ultrasound
d. CT

Ans. b. DTPA *Ref: Textbook of Radiology and Imaging by David Sutton 7th/ed p947*

EXPLANATION

- Ultrasound, CT and radionuclide imaging (DMSA) will all demonstrate the areas of renal scarring.
- 99Tc- DMSA (static/anatomical imaging) is **best for evaluation of scars in reflux nephropathy**.
- *(Option b)* 99Tc- DTPA (dynamic or functional imaging) is useful for **evaluating** perfusion **or function of kidneys**.

7. Not done for bone metastasis detection:

a. MRI
b. CT
c. Radionuclide scan
d. Ultrasound

Ans. d. Ultrasound *Ref: Textbook of Radiology and Imaging by David Sutton 7th/ed p1251*

EXPLANATION

Imaging in Bone Metastases

- Plain radiographs are often done as the first line investigation in patients with bone pain. However, radiography is considered insensitive to screen for asymptomatic metastases. The radiographic presence of such lesions very often lags behind their detectability by scintigraphy, CT or MRI.
- Plain radiographs are recommended to assess abnormal radionuclide uptake or the risk of pathological fracture.
- *(Option a)* **MRI** is the imaging modality of choice for assessing metastatic spread in the **marrow cavity** due to its excellent soft tissue resolution.
- *(Option b)* **CT** has excellent resolution of **cortical and trabecular bone** and is the imaging modality of choice for evaluating the ribs which have a high cortex to marrow ratio.
- *(Option c)* Radionuclide scan/bone scintigraphy is the **imaging modality of choice in general for evaluation of bone metastases**. Main agent used is metastable technetium 99 labeled diphosphonates, most commonly methylene diphosphonate (^{99m}Tc-MDP).
- *(Option d)* Ultrasound is not the imaging modality of choice in assessment of bony pathologies due to dense acoustic shadowing from bony surface.

Psychiatry

Author: Bahram Gor, Co-author: Pawan Vilas Khot

AIIMS May 2017

1. Mutism and akinesis in a person, who appears awake and even alert, is best described as:

a. Oneiroid state
b. Stupor
c. Twilight state
c. Delirium

Ans. b. Stupor *Ref: Ahuja Textbook of Psychiatry 10th/ed, p59*

Explanation

Akinesis (no movement) with mutism but with evidence of relative preservation of conscious awareness is called stupor. It is one of the features of retarded catatonia. The term akinetic mutism originated with Cairns and colleagues. They described a young woman who, although appearing wakeful, became mute and rigidly motionless when a craniopharyngiomatous cyst expanded to compress the walls of third ventricle and frontal lobe.

Option (a) Oneiroid state: Oneiroid Schizophrenia: Described first by Mayer-Gross, this is a subtype of schizophrenia with an acute onset, clouding of consciousness, disorientation, dream-like states (oneiroid means 'dream'), and perceptual disturbances with rapid shifting.

Option (b) Stupor is an imprecise term for 1. State of decreased reactivity to stimuli, 2. Unresponsiveness with immobility. 3. Mutism but retention of consciousness and often with open eyes that follows external objects.

Option (c) Twilight state: Describes disturbed consciousness with hallucinations. Appears as waking dreams that portray desires, wishes or fears in a direct or symbolic way. A transitory disturbance of consciousness during which many acts, sometimes very complicated may be performed without the subjects conscious volition and without any remembrance of them.

Option (d) Delirium: According to ICD 10, diagnosis of delirium must include impairment of consciousness and attention (on a continuum from clouding to coma; reduced ability to direct, focus, sustain, and shift attention), global disturbance of cognition, psychomotor disturbances, disturbance of sleep-wake cycle, and emotional disturbances.

2. Which of the following mood stabilizers has anti-suicide properties?

a. Lithium
b. Carbamazepine
c. Valproate
d. Lamotrigine

Ans. a. Lithium

Explanation

"Clinical studies have shown that lithium reduces the incidence of suicide in patients with bipolar I disorder sixfold or sevenfold."................. *Kaplan's 10th/ed p492*

"Initial treatment of BPD includes lithium or valproic acid or SSRI such as bupropion, sertraline, citalopram and escitalopram. One advantage of lithium salt is that it also possesses an anti-suicidal effect" ....*Trends in Neurochemistry Research By Robert Milton Coleman-Page 169.*

3. A 20-year-old female has thoughts of cutting her fingers, she plans and imagines doing it but never actually does it. She says she is not having any guilt of having such thought. And also says the thoughts are distressing her and she is unable to control them. The thoughts vanish either by ending with a seizure or automatically subsides on its own. Which of the following is the cause?

a. Obsession
b. Thought insertion
c. Forced thinking
d. Crowding of thoughts

Ans. c. Forced thinking *Ref: Lishman's Organic Psychiatry p321,335*

Explanation

Note: Crowding of thoughts is a component of Forced thinking but not vice versa. Provided the symptoms ends with epilepsy, Forced thinking is best suited.

- One of the clues to diagnosis is by the thoughts vanishing in seizure.
- Forced thinking (FT) is a rare epileptic phenomenon which is usually seen in patients with temporal as well as frontal lobe epilepsy. It is a comparatively often found type of psychic seizure. ***This type of psychic aura is called 'forced thinking,' characterized by recurrent intrusive thoughts, ideas, or crowding of thoughts.***
- It is an autonomous appearance of a fixed thought induced by seizure activities.
- Patients may experience distortion of thoughts such as forced thinking, which describes a feeling of being compelled to think about a specific topic or word; or crowding of thoughts, which describes a feeling of racing, disorganized thoughts.
- Subtle but disturbing changes in the quality of perception are reported, including derealization and depersonalization, distortions in the perception of time and changes in the significance of objects.
- These latter are often impossible for patients to describe but may involve a sense that a specific object in their environment seems changed and has a heightened but mysterious personal relevance.
- The seizures of prefrontal origin are characterized by forced actions, forced thinking and motor automatism followed by brief duration of seizure activity less than 1 minute or some time less than few seconds after that thoughts subside by its own.

Option (a) Obsession: There is no guilt, no compulsion no attempt to stop these thoughts

Option (b) Thought insertion: Seen in Schizophrenia. There is no description that thoughts were inserted by some external agency. Also thoughts were subsided by episode of seizures

Option (c) Crowding of thoughts were also seen in Schizophrenia, as no history of delusion, hallucinations, etc. mentioned plus patient experience the thoughts were too fast, excessive in amount, unexplainable (patient is not able to explain the type/kind of thought) patient can anatomically locate the location of thoughts—being crowded in back of my head and being controlled by some outside agency.

PGI May 2017

1. How many items are there in Mini mental state examination (MMSE)?

a. 10
b. 15
c. 20
d. 30

Ans. d. 30 *Ref: Lishman's Organic Psychiatry, A Textbook of Neuropsychiatry 4th/ed, p110*

EXPLANATION

MMSE or Folstein test is a simplified form of routine cognitive status examination. It is routinely used to track improvement and deterioration. It includes following points:

a. Orientation to time-5
b. Orientation to place-5
c. Registration-3
d. Attention and calculation-5
e. Recall-3
f. Language-2
g. Repetition-1
h. Complex commands-6

Total score-30, score less than 24 indicates cognitive impairment.

2a. Essential criteria for major depression are all *except*:

a. Bodyache and pain
b. Absence of pleasure
c. Insomnia
d. Hypersomnia
e. Guilt or self loathing for being ill

Ans: b. Absence of pleasure

Ref: Kaplan & Sadock's Comprehensive Textbook of Psychiatry 10th/ed p4194

EXPLANATION

Five (or more) of the following symptoms should be present during the same 2-week period:

a. Sadness of mood (S)
b. Loss of interest (I)
c. Guilt (G)
d. Loss of energy (E)
e. Decreased concentration (C)
f. Appetite increased or decreased (A)
g. Psychomotor agitation or retardation (P)
h. Sleep increased or decreased (S)
i. Recurrent suicidal ideation (S)

Mnemonic for MDD (Major depressive disorder): SIGECAPS

2b. Criteria for major depressive episode:

a. Insomnia
b. Anorexia
c. H/o past trauma
d. Long duration
e. Benzodiazepines are drug of choice

Ans. a. Insomnia and b. Anorexia

EXPLANATION

See above explanation

3. Naltrexone is used for:

a. Cocaine
b. Alcohol dependence
c. Anorexia
d. Cannabis toxicity
e. Bulimia

Ans. b. Alcohol dependence *Ref: Kaplan & Sadock's Synopsis of Psychiatry 10th/ed p1075*

EXPLANATION

- ❑ Naltrexone is a opioid receptor antagonist used to reduce or eliminate the subjective high associated with consumption of opioid and alcohol.
- ❑ It is approved by US FDA for alcohol dependence and for blockade of effects of exogenously administered opioids.

4. Nicotine withdrawal feature/s seen is/are:

a. Irritability
b. Anorexia
c. Decreased concentration
d. Weight gain
e. Hypersomnia

Ans. a. Irritability and c. Decreased concentration
Ref: Kaplan & Sadock's Comprehensive Textbook of Psychiatry 10th/ed p3468

EXPLANATION

- ❑ Tobacco withdrawal follows use for at least many weeks and either cessation or reduction in use resulting in:
  a. Anxiety, depressed mood;
  b. Irritability, frustration, or anger;
  c. Insomnia, difficulty concentrating;
  d. Restlessness, and
  e. Increased appetite.
- ❑ To meet withdrawal criteria at least four of the seven signs or symptoms listed above must apply within 24 hours of abrupt cessation or volume reduction.
- ❑ Contrary to DSM-IV classification of withdrawal, DSM-5 omitted reduced heart rate or weight gain symptoms.

5. True about generalized anxiety disorder is/are:

a. Insomnia
b. Hypersomnia
c. Episode lasts for several days
d. Free floating anxiety
e. Benzodiazepine is treatment of choice
f. Autonomic symptoms

Ans. a. Insomnia; c. Episode lasts for several days and d. Free floating anxiety
Ref: Kaplan & Sadock's Comprehensive Textbook of Psychiatry 10th/ed p,4425-26,4570-71

EXPLANATION

Generalized anxiety disorder is associated with excessive anxiety and worry (apprehensive expectation), occurring more days than not for at least 6 months, about a number of events or activities. The anxiety and worry are associated with three (or more) of the following six symptoms (with at least some symptoms having been present for more days than not for the past 6 months):

1. Restlessness or feeling keyed up or on edge
2. Being easily fatigued
3. Difficulty concentrating or mind going blank

4. Irritability
5. Muscle tension
6. Sleep disturbance (difficulty falling or staying asleep, or restless, unsatisfying sleep).

❑ **Treatment:** SSRI and SNRI are drugs of choice in GAD.

6. Lithium causes:

a. Acne
b. Rash
c. Psoriasis
d. Pemphigus
e. Blisters
f. Angioneurotic edema
g. Photosensitivity

Ans. a. Acne; b. Rash and c. Psoriasis

Ref: Kaplan & Sadock's Comprehensive Textbook of Psychiatry 10th/ed, p7908

EXPLANATION

A. Uses of lithium:

a. Lithium is an established, first line, FDA approved antimanic drug but it is not approved by the FDA for the acute treatment of bipolar depressive episodes.
b. Lithium appears to have antiaggressive effects independent of its mood stabilizing action.

B. Onset: Its onset of action is relatively slow, with clinical improvement usually occurring over the first 1 to 3 weeks of treatment.

C. Dosage: Lithium is typically started at 900 mg/day and serum levels measured after 5 days of consecutive therapy, 12 hours after the last dose. Serum levels between 0.8 and 1.2 mEq/L are likely required to treat acute mania effectively, although lower levels may be appropriate in elderly.

D. Toxicity: Lithium levels of ≥1.5 mEq/L can lead to symptoms of lithium toxicity and this should be treated as a medical emergency. Patients should be educated and clinically monitored for signs of lithium toxicity that may include gastrointestinal (vomiting and diarrhea), neurological (coarse tremor, agitation, dysarthria, drowsiness, lethargy, ataxia) renal (polyuria and polydipsia), and cardiovascular (syncope, dizziness, arrhythmias) symptoms.

E. Adverse effects:

Neurological: Generally benign

- **Nontoxic:** Dysphoria, lack of spontaneity, slowed reaction time, memory difficulties
- **Tremor:** Postural, occasional extrapyramidal
- **Toxic:** Course tremor, dysarthria, ataxia, neuromuscular irritability, seizures, coma, death
- **Miscellaneous:** Peripheral neuropathy, benign intracranial hypertension, myasthenia gravis-like syndrome, reduced creativity, lowered seizure threshold.

Endocrine

Thyroid: Goiter, hypothyroidism, exophthalmos, hyperthyroidism (rare).

Parathyroid: Hyperparathyroidism, adenoma.

Cardiovascular

Benign T-wave changes, sinus node dysfunction.

Renal

Concentrating defect, morphological changes, polyuria (nephrogenic diabetes insipidus), reduced glomerular filtration rate, nephrotic syndrome, renal tubular acidosis.

Dermatological

Acne, hair loss, psoriasis, rash.

Gastrointestinal

Appetite loss, nausea, vomiting, diarrhea.

Miscellaneous

Altered carbohydrate metabolism, weight gain, fluid retention.

JIPMER Pattern Based

1. Gilles de la Tourette's syndrome treatment, all true *except*:

a. Clonidine
b. Carbamazepine
c. Verapamil
d. Haloperidol

Ans. c. Verapamil *Ref: Kaplan & Sadock's Comprehensive Textbook of Psychiatry, 10th/ed, p9279-91*

EXPLANATION

Tourette syndrome (named for Georges Gilles de la Tourette, who first described this disorder in 1885) is a condition that causes a person to make repeated, quick movements or sounds that they cannot control. Treatment of Gilles de la Tourette syndrome is as follows:

A. **Medical management:**
1. **Alpha adrenergic agonist:** Clonidine, guanfacine are used for treatment of tics.
2. **Neuroleptics:** Haloperidol and pimozide are Food and Drug Administration (FDA) approved but other like risperidone, ziprasidone, aripiprazole, olanzapine are also used for treatment of tics.
3. **Selective serotonin reuptake inhibitors:** Fluoxetine, fluvoxamine, sertraline and paroxetine are commonly used to treat obsessions and compulsions associated with Tics.
4. **Tricyclic antidepressants:** Clomipramine, desipramine are also used.
5. **Benzodiazepines** like clonazepam are used to treat comorbid anxiety symptoms
6. Comorbid attention-deficit hyperactivity disorder (ADHD) can be treated with Methylphenidate and atomoxetine.

B. **Surgical management:**
1. Bilateral capsulotomy
2. Deep brain stimulation for intractable Tics.
3. Transcranial magnetic stimulation.

2. Not useful in ADHD is:

a. Verapamil
b. Clonidine
c. Atomoxetine
d. Tricyclic antidepressants

Ans. a. Verapamil *Ref: Kaplan & Sadock's Comprehensive Textbook of Psychiatry, 10th/ed p9154-66.*

EXPLANATION

A. **Stimulants:**
a. Methylphenidate
b. Dexmethylphenidate
c. Dextroamphetamine

B. **Non-stimulant:**
a. Atomoxetine
b. Long acting Alpha Adrenergic agents like clonidine and guanfacine.
c. Tricyclic antidepressants like imipramine, desipramine and nortryptiline.
d. Bupropion
e. Other drugs like lithium, carbamazepine.

C. **Psychosocial treatment:**
   a. Parental training
   b. Intensive behavior modification
   c. Social skills training
   d. Academic organization skills

3. Drug not effctive in treating pediatric acute mania is:

a. Lithium
b. Divalproex
c. Oxcarbazepine
d. Carbamazepine

Ans. c. Oxcarbazepine *Ref: Kaplan & Sadock's Comprehensive Textbook of Psychiatry, 11th/ed p379 and p1300*

Explanation

Use of mood-stabilizing agents in pediatric patients (page 1300)
- Classic mania in children and adolescents is treated as it is treated in adults.
- Use of **lithium** in treating adolescent mania has been supported in many open trials. ***(Option a)***
- **Divalproex** is used frequently to treat bipolar disorder in children and adolescents. ***(Option b)***
- **Quetiapine** is at least as effective as divalproex in treating acute manic symptoms. Reduction of symptoms occurred more quickly with quetiapine compared with divalproex.
- **Propranolol** (Inderal) has been chosen as an agent to control aggression in open trials, although no evidence supports its use in children and adolescents.
- **Carbamazepine** (Tegretol) has not been shown to be effective in controlling aggression in child and adolescent conduct disorders. ***(Option d)***

About carbamazepine and oxcarbazepine (page 379)
- Carbamazepine has been used worldwide for decades as a first-line treatment for acute mania but has only gained approval in the United States in 2004.
- Typical doses of carbamazepine to treat acute mania range between 600 and 1,800 mg/day associated with blood levels of between 4 and 12 μg/mL.
- Oxcarbazepine (keto congener of carbamazepine), possess similar antimanic properties as carbamazepine. Higher doses than those of carbamazepine are required because 1,500 mg of oxcarbazepine approximates 1,000 mg of carbamazepine.

Thus based on above discussion oxcarbazepine seems to be possible answer

4. Which is not a DSM-5 criteria for ADHD?

a. Children under 7 years
b. Children under 12 years
c. Symptoms in 2 or more settings
d. Option not recalled

Ans. a. Children under 7 years

Ref: Kaplan & Sadock's Comprehensive Textbook of Psychiatry, 10th/ed p9142-43

Explanation

DSM-5 criteria for ADHD include:

A. Onset before 12 years of age
B. Duration greater than 6 months

C. Children must have at least 6 symptoms from the inattention and/or impulsive/hyperactive symptom list
D. Several symptoms must be present in 2 or more settings and interfere with functioning.
E. Symptoms do not occur along with other psychotic disorder or mental disorder.

5. Which of the following is true regarding treatment of tremors?

a. Diazepam is helpful in reducing
b. Haloperidol is used to reduce tremors in parkinsonism
c. Phenytoin induced tremors are cured after withdrawal
d. Commonly seen with beta blockers

Ans. a. Diazepam is helpful in reducing

Ref: Kaplan & Sadock's Comprehensive Textbook of Psychiatry, 10th/ed, p1449-56,4567

EXPLANATION

A. **Diazepam is used to treat alcohol withdrawal tremors.**
B. **In Parkinsonism slow resting tremors 3–6 Hz are seen. Treatment of parkinsonism is with:**
   a. Anticholinergic drugs like trihexiphenidyl, Benztropine, amantadine and selegiline
   b. Dopamine agonist like Pramipexole, Ropinirole, Pergolide
   c. Levodopa
C. **Beta blockers are used for treatment of tremors in performance anxiety.**

6. Least suicidal tendency is seen with which drug?

a. Carbamazepine
b. Lithium
c. Valproate
d. Option not recalled

Ans. b. Lithium *Ref: Kaplan & Sadock's Comprehensive Textbook of Psychiatry, 10th/ed p7894*

EXPLANATION

A. A meta-analysis of 31 studies of major affective disorders found a fivefold reduction in suicides and attempted suicides during lithium treatment compared to those not taking the drug.
B. In a retrospective study, patients at high risk of suicidal behavior were grouped into excellent, moderate, and poor lithium responders. No further suicide attempts occurred in 93.3%, 82.7%, and 48.8%, respectively, suggesting that the antisuicidal effect of lithium extends beyond its mood stabilizing property.
   Initial treatment of BPD includes lithium or valproic acid or SSRI such as bupropion, sertraline, citalopram and escitalopram. One advantage of lithium salt is that it also possesses an anti-suicidal effect" .... Trends in Neurochemistry Research By Robert Milton Coleman- Page 169.